PATHOPHARMACOLOGY

Bruce J. Colbert, MS, RRT
Kurtis Pierce, MBA, RRT

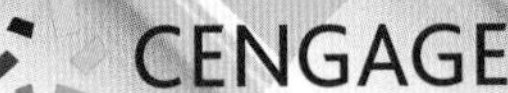
CENGAGE

Australia • Brazil • Mexico • Singapore • United Kingdom • United States

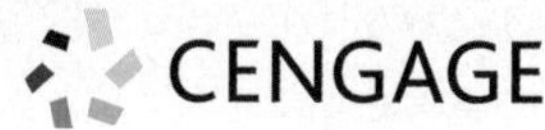

Pathopharmacology

Authors: Bruce J. Colbert, MS, RRT
Kurtis Pierce, MBA, RRT

SVP, GM Skills & Global Product Management: Jonathan Lau

Product Director: Matthew Seeley

Senior Product Manager: Laura Stewart

Product Assistant: Nicholas Scaglione

Executive Director, Content Design: Mara Bellegarde

Learning Design Director: Juliet Steiner

Senior Learning Designer: Deb Myette-Flis

Vice President, Strategic Marketing Services: Jennifer Ann Baker

Marketing Manager: Jonathan Sheehan

Director, Content Delivery: Wendy Troeger

Senior Content Manager: Kenneth McGrath

Digital Delivery Lead: Lisa Christopher

Senior Art Director: Jack Pendleton

Production Service: SPi Global

Cover image(s): © Shutterstock.com/ponsulak
© iStock.com/Eraxion

Library of Congress Control Number: 2018946349

ISBN: 978-0-3571-0798-0

Cengage

20 Channel Center Street
Boston, MA 02210
USA

Cengage is a leading provider of customized learning solutions with employees residing in nearly 40 different countries and sales in more than 125 countries around the world. Find your local representative at **www.cengage.com.**

Cengage products are represented in Canada by Nelson Education, Ltd.

To learn more about Cengage platforms and services, register or access your online learning solution, or purchase materials for your course, visit **www.cengage.com**.

Printed in the United States of America
Print Number: 01 Print Year: 2018

Contents

MODULE 4

Drug Administration and Dosage Forms 105

MODULE 5

Cancer and Antineoplastic Pharmacology 138

MODULE 6
Pathopharmacology of the Musculoskeletal System 163

MODULE 7
Pathopharmacology of the Integumentary System 207

MODULE 8
Gastrointestinal Diseases and Medications 241

MODULE 9
Pathopharmacology of the Endocrine System 287

MODULE 10
Pathopharmacology of the Urinary System 312

Module 1

Core Concepts of Disease

Module Introduction

You probably have heard the term **disease** or **pathology** used before to describe an illness, but what exactly is the meaning of these terms? Literally, the word disease means "not at ease." A disease is the deviation from the body's normal or away from the homeostatic state of the body. In other words, the body attempts to maintain a constant balance of all bodily functions; however, a disease alters the ability of the body to function properly.

LEARNING OBJECTIVE 1.1 Interpret disease medical terminology.

KEY TERMS

Acute disease Disease that has a rapid onset.

Chief complaint (CC) Main reason the individual sought medical attention.

Chronic disease A long-term disease.

Death rate A statistical measurement of deaths caused by a disease of a certain population over a specific time period.

Diagnosis Identifying the disease.

Etiology Cause or origin of the disease.

Exacerbation Acute disease flare up or attack from a chronic condition.

Idiopathic Disease occurring spontaneously with an unknown cause.

Metastasize Spread of disease.

Morbidity rate Statistical measurement of how often a disease occurs in a certain time-frame within a population.

Mortality rate Statistical measurement of deaths caused by a disease of a certain population over a specific time period; also known as death rate.

Pathogen Any organism causing disease to its host.

Pathogenic Used to describe organisms that produce disease.

Pathologist Individual who studies disease.

Prognosis Expected outcome or the prediction of an ailment.

Relapse Reappearance of the disease or condition.

Remission Period where disease is treated successfully and the patient is free of symptoms.

Survival rate Length of time a patient's lives after being diagnosed with a disease.

Terminal Condition or disease resulting in imminent death.

1-1 TERMS ASSOCIATED WITH DISEASE

Let's build a little on the term pathology. The individual who studies disease is a **pathologist**. The pathologist will examine samples taken from the patient to identify the pathogens involved. A **pathogen** is any organism causing disease to its host. For example, microorganisms that can potentially cause disease are bacteria, fungi, helminths (worms), and protozoans, which will be further covered in Module 4. Some microorganisms may not be harmful within the body, but when they become harmful, the term **pathogenic** is used to describe those organisms that produce disease. For example, *Escherichia coli*, more commonly known as *E. coli*, is a bacterium normally found in the intestines, which assists in maintaining a healthy intestinal tract. However, if this bacterium reaches another location in the body where it should not be an infection will develop.

CLINICAL CONNECTION 1.1

It should also be noted that any disease occurring spontaneously with an unknown cause is termed **idiopathic**. A politically incorrect way to help remember this term is to think: "don't ever feel like an idiot if you can't determine the cause of a disease because some are just idiopathic in nature." Besides, no one should ever feel like an idiot in the first place.

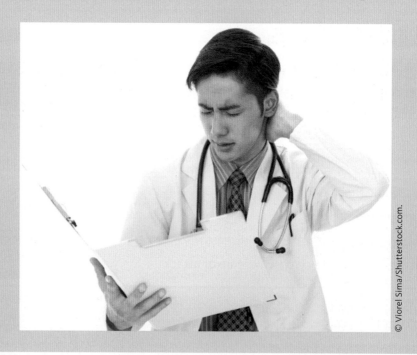

© Viorel Sima/Shutterstock.com.

1-1a Diagnosis

So what are some of the medical terms related to identifying and treating diseases? We have all heard the terms diagnosis and prognosis, but what is the difference and how do they relate to disease?

To understand more about a disease, it is important to determine the **etiology**. The etiology is the fancy term for the cause or origin of the disease. For example, the etiology of the common cold is the rhinovirus. Makes you wonder what they call a rhino with a cold?

When presenting to a medical facility, the patient will complain of a specific ailment or issue that is being experienced. This is called the **chief complaint (CC)**, or the main reason the individual sought medical attention. The chief complaint along with signs, symptoms, and diagnostic testing assists with identifying the disease or reaching a **diagnosis**.

1-1b Prognosis

Once a patient is diagnosed with a disease, the individual's future is at question. The expected outcome or the prediction of an ailment is known as the **prognosis**. For example, multiple sclerosis (MS) is not a fatal disease or one that will significantly shorten the life span of those affected. However, the prognosis of MS is that the patient will likely become progressively disabled. Now, let's continue to lay our foundation and build our vocabulary with more terms associated with a patient's disease.

A disease can come on very suddenly or it can always be with you. If the disease is short-term and has a rapid onset, it is known as an **acute disease**. A disease that affects the patient long-term is a **chronic disease**. Let's see how these two terms are used in an actual patient scenario.

Consider a patient with Chronic Obstructive Pulmonary Disease (COPD). COPD is a combination of chronic diseases, meaning the disease state is not cured and is everlasting. Because COPD is incurable, it can only be maintained with proper medications and care. Even though the patient has a long-term disease, sudden uncontrolled attacks can occur. When a patient has an acute flare-up or attack from a chronic disease, it is known as an **exacerbation**, or a sudden worsening of a condition.

Besides having acute flare-ups or exacerbations of their underlying chronic disease, acute diseases can also occur. For example, someone with COPD can acutely develop pneumonia. While the acute condition of pneumonia can be cured, the chronic underlying obstructive pulmonary disease will always be there.

CLINICAL CONNECTION 1.2

At this point, we have an understanding of some of the terms associated with disease. Now, let's put this vocabulary to use in a real world setting with the following case.

A patient presents (shows up) at the Emergency Department (ED) at 4 am with a shortness of breath (SOB). Dr. Jay DeWayne interviews, assesses the patient, Alex Sherry, and finds the following:

Alex is a 74-year-old Caucasian male in respiratory distress. He has difficulty breathing and speaking without interrupting to catch his breath. Alex manages to say he has been diagnosed with Chronic Obstructive Pulmonary Disease 4 years ago, but has been having difficulty over the past week. The doctor does a sputum culture and finds he has bacterial pneumonia. The doctor prescribes antibiotics and tells him he should feel better in a day or two.

1-2 MORE DISEASE TERMINOLOGY

Once a disease is established, several terms can be used to describe the progression or current status. Disease status can worsen when "complications" arise such as an unexpected fever or coughing up blood. Sometimes the worsening of the disease may indicate it is spreading. For example, if a patient has prostate cancer, there is potential for it to **metastasize**, or spread, to other regions of the body such as the bones, further complicating the patient's disease process.

Diseases can have several different outcomes. If the disease prognosis is that it will result in imminent death, it is deemed **terminal**. However, if the disease is treated successfully and the patient is free of symptoms, the patient is in **remission**. While the patient may have thought they were cured, there is potential for a **relapse** in which the disease reappears. Once a patient has been diagnosed with a disease, the length of time a patient's lives afterward is the **survival rate**.

Other rates associated with disease are morbidity rate and mortality rate. **Morbidity rate** is a statistical measurement showing how often a disease occurs in a certain time-frame within a population. Let's take a look at an example to better understand this concept. Imagine there is a classroom of 10 people being observed over the course of 1 year and 7 of those people develop asthma. The morbidity rate of asthma for those 10 people in the classroom is 70%. The key point to keep in mind is those seven people are living with, and have not died from, the disease.

The **mortality rate**, sometimes called **death rate**, is a statistical measurement of deaths caused by a disease of a certain population over a specific time period. This is expressed in a ratio of 1,000 per year. For example, the number of deaths in the United States caused by pancreatic cancer was 40,000 in 2015. See Figure 1-1.

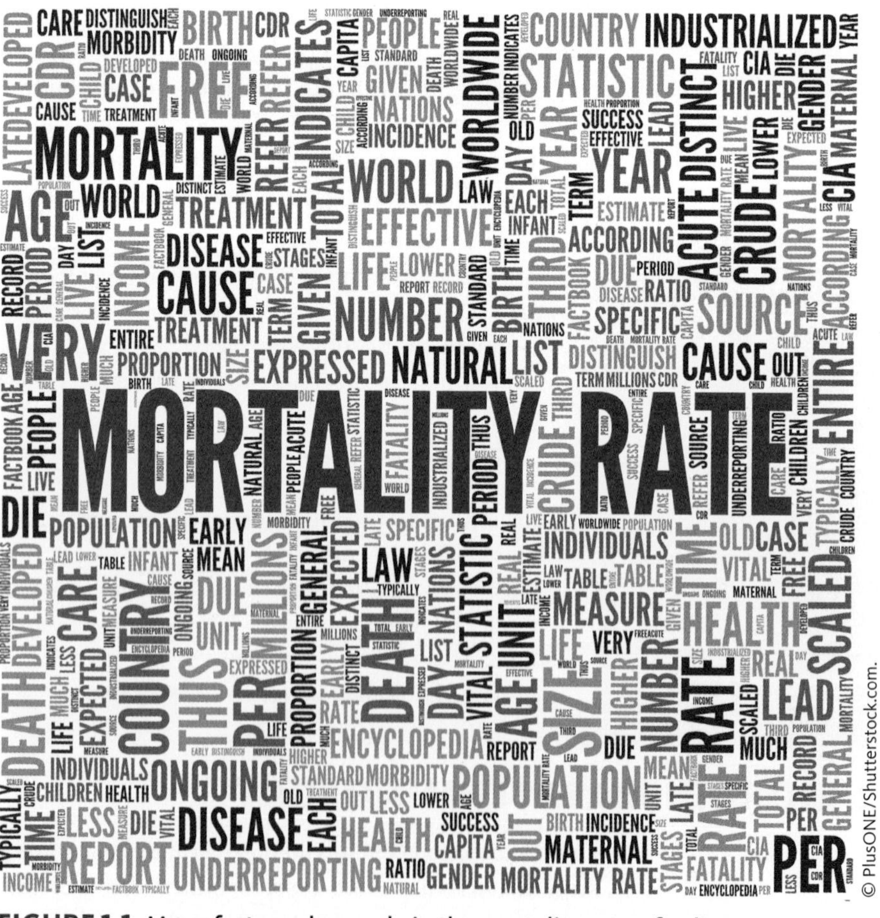

FIGURE 1-1 Many factors play a role in the mortality rate of a disease.

LEARNING OBJECTIVE 1.2 Describe how disease is transferred.

KEY TERMS

Airborne transmission Pathogenic transmission by way of coughing, sneezing, talking, and laughing.

Biological vector Animal or insect that spreads pathogen to other hosts by a bite or injection.

Centers for Disease Control and Prevention (CDC) Agency responsible for recording and tracking diseases not only domestically but also abroad.

Common vehicle Any medium such as food or blood that acts as a vehicle to transport pathogens.

Communicable Contagious and spread from one source to another whether it is person–person, animal–person or even an object–person via bacterial or viral microorganisms.

Contagious Potential to cause infection and spread rapidly.

Direct contact Making physical contact with another person or body fluids that spreads infection.

Endemic Disease found in a certain region or specific population.

Epidemic Sudden spread of illness to large amount of people.

Epidemiology Study of disease transmission, occurrence, distribution, and control for a population.

Healthcare-associated infection (HAI) Infection caused by medical intervention.

Host The susceptible individual who can harbor pathogen.

Iatrogenic Disease caused by medical intervention.

Incubation period Period of pathogen reproduction causing symptoms to occur within the host.

Indirect contact Host coming into contact with a contaminated surface.

Infectious The ability to cause disease.

Inoculation period Period of pathogen introduction without symptoms.

Mechanical vector Pathogen transmitted by an animal or insect simply by coming into contact with a microorganism and then physically transporting it to the host.

Mode of transmission The way a pathogen is transported from the source of infection to the host.

Pandemic Disease affecting the population of a vast geographic area such as a country or possibly worldwide.

Pathogenesis Creation or progression of disease development.

Portal of entry Pathogen point of entry to host such as by way of mouth, eyes, and nose or other mucous membrane.

Portal of exit A point where pathogen leaves the body.

The chain of infection Chain-like illustration made up of a series of steps or links that demonstrate how pathogens infect others.

1-3 TRANSMISSION OF DISEASE

This section will further explain the different methods by which disease can be transferred.

Many terms are used to describe the characteristics of disease. Before understanding how diseases are transmitted, let's discuss the meaning of the terms communicable, contagious, and infectious diseases.

1-3a Communicable and Contagious

Communicable diseases are contagious and spread from one source to another whether it is person–person, animal–person, or even an object–person via bacterial or viral microorganisms. For example, the virus Hepatitis C can be spread from one person to another via the exchange of bodily fluids or from an object such as a shared needle. A **contagious** disease is also communicable; however, it is differentiated by "rapidly" spreading from person to person by direct or indirect contact. For example, a fungal infection such as athlete's foot is certainly communicable but not highly infectious. On the other hand, the flu, or influenza, is highly contagious and spreads rapidly through the population.

1-3b Infectious

Infectious disease has the ability to be communicable, but that is not always the case. It can also be spread from a food source to a person or animal. Botulism is caused by an infectious bacterium called botulinum. This bacterium enters the body from ingesting spoiled food products, and the results are better known as food poisoning. Therefore, an individual may become ill from the infected food, but will not pass the infection to another. We will discuss more about routes of transmission later in this module.

1-3c Healthcare-Associated Infection

A very important type of infection that everyone working in health care should be aware of is a **healthcare-associated infection (HAI)**. The older term for this was nosocomial infection, which meant a hospital-acquired infection. HAI is a much more inclusive term because patients are treated in other facilities besides a hospital. This type of infection may also be called **iatrogenic**, meaning the infection was caused by medical intervention. A HAI can occur in the healthcare setting but might not show symptoms until long after the patient is discharged. Figure 1-2 shows all the hiding places microorganisms lurk in plain sight.

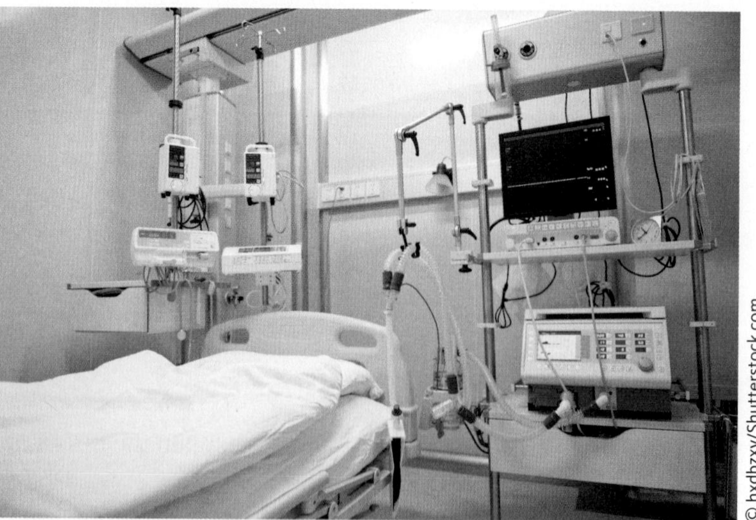

FIGURE 1-2 The healthcare environment has a lot of potential for causing an infection due to improperly cleaned equipment, poor hand hygiene, and poor infection control.

According to the Centers for Disease Control and Prevention (CDC), in the United States, approximately 1 in 25 patients has at least one infection contracted during the course of their hospital care, adding up to about 722,000 infections in 2011. Figure 1-3 is an informative poster from the CDC on HAI.

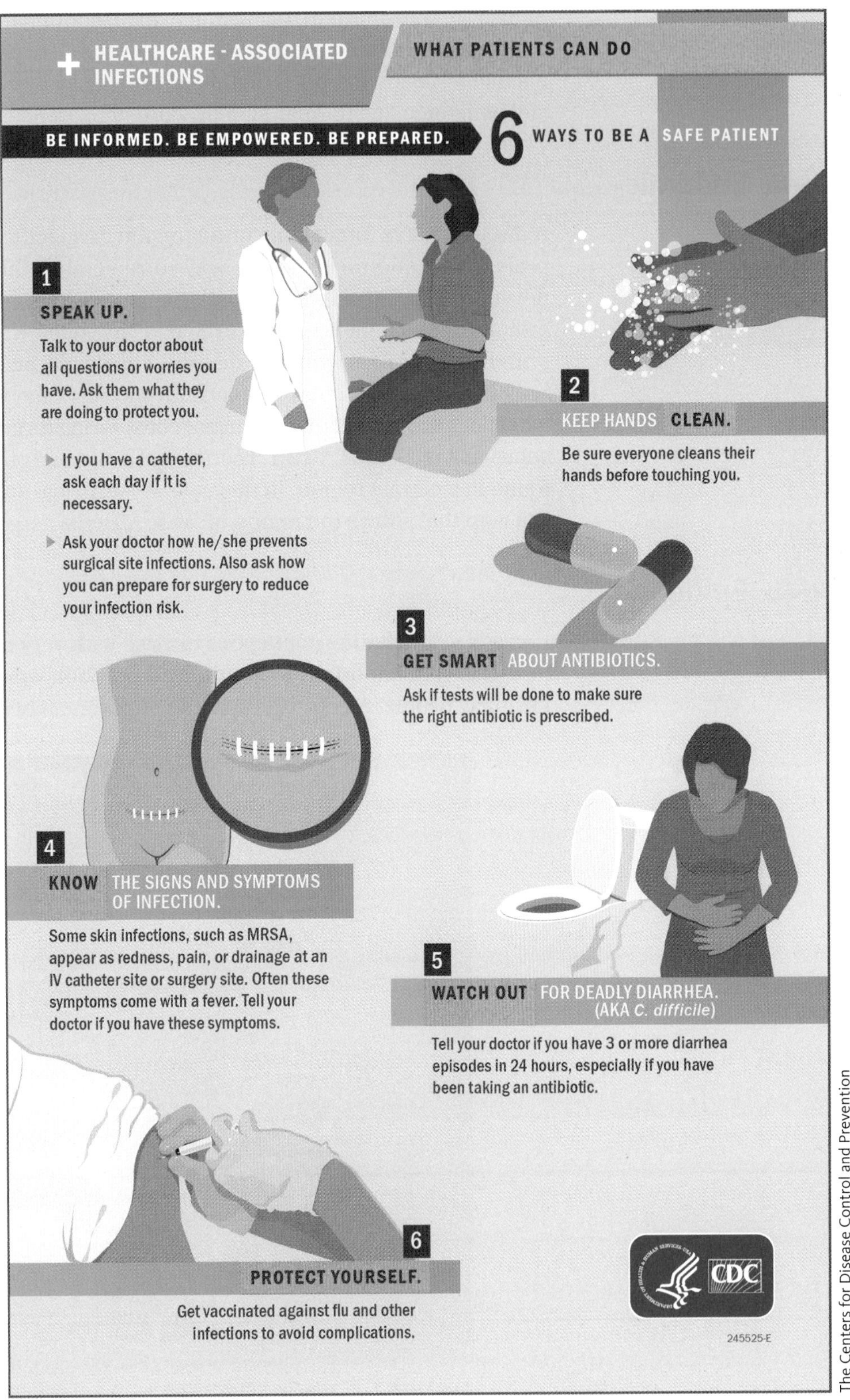

The Centers for Disease Control and Prevention

FIGURE 1-3 Steps to prevent HAIs.

1-4 EPIDEMIOLOGY

The Centers for Disease Control and Prevention (CDC) records and tracks diseases not only domestically but also abroad in an effort to monitor possible threats. One aspect monitored by the CDC is epidemiology, which is the study of disease transmission, occurrence, distribution, and control for a population of people. You often hear in the news how the CDC is monitoring an epidemic or pandemic. Just what does that mean? It is easy to confuse endemic, epidemic, and pandemic due to their similar word appearances.

1-4a Endemic

A disease that is found in a certain region or specific population on a continual basis is an endemic. Another way to remember this word is to think of it as never "ending." It will continually be in a certain location affecting a certain group of people, hence the word "end" in endemic. Ebola in West Africa is a prime example of an endemic disease. The deadly and highly contagious disease has been confined to Guinea, Sierra Leone, and Liberia for over a year and fortunately has not spread out of control considering its great potential. It has spread somewhat to Central Africa. Therefore, Ebola is an endemic disease because it is found in a certain region, in this case West Africa, and nowhere else. Figure 1-4 is a map that shows the region of West Africa where Ebola cases are found.

1-4b Epidemic

Ebola is a devastating contagious disease with very high mortality rates. Therefore, it is very important to monitor for an Ebola epidemic that can spread and kill many people. An epidemic is a sudden spread of illness to a large number of

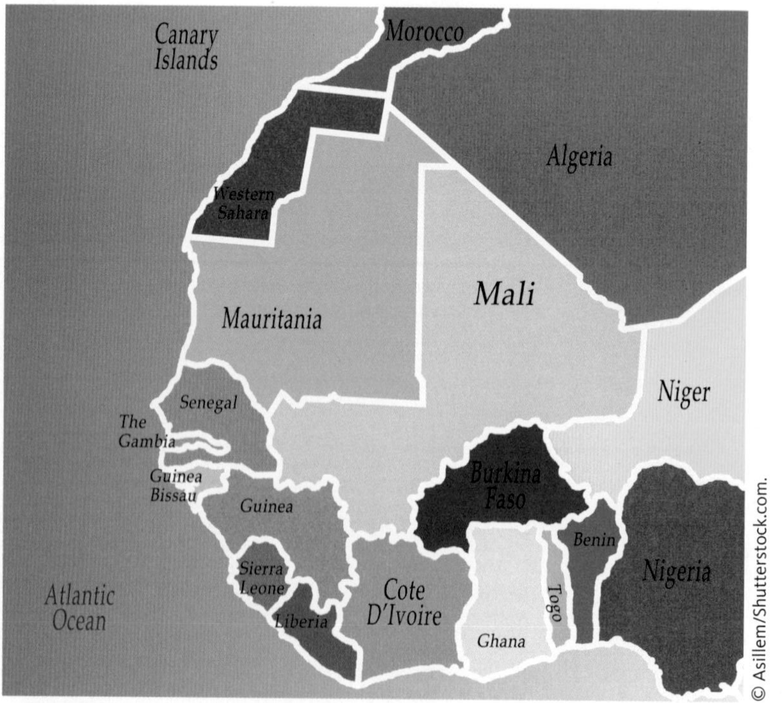

FIGURE 1-4 A map of West Africa, where Ebola is found.

people. This occurred in West Africa when the endemic Ebola virus re-emerged in, and spread throughout, the population, killing thousands.

A learning strategy to assist in recalling the meaning of epidemic is to think of an EpiPen. Epidemic and EpiPen both have "epi" in the word. Even though the meanings of the two words are totally different, it will assist you in remembering the meaning of epidemic. When someone has a sudden allergic reaction an EpiPen is used for immediate relief of sudden symptoms. The key words both have in common is sudden.

In early 2016, the Zika virus was declared an epidemic and global emergency. A sudden occurrence of microcephaly, a small head and mental retardation was found in many newborns. At that time, it was thought to be caused by the mother being exposed to the Zika virus while pregnant. It was also thought the virus is transmitted to humans via mosquitos and can then be transmitted to other humans via contaminated body fluids. To further the alarm, the virus has become a pandemic moving throughout the Americas. A lot is yet to be discovered in regards to this virus. See Figure 1-5.

1-4c Pandemic

A disease affecting the population of a vast geographic area such as a country or possibly the globe is known as a **pandemic**. A way to remember the meaning

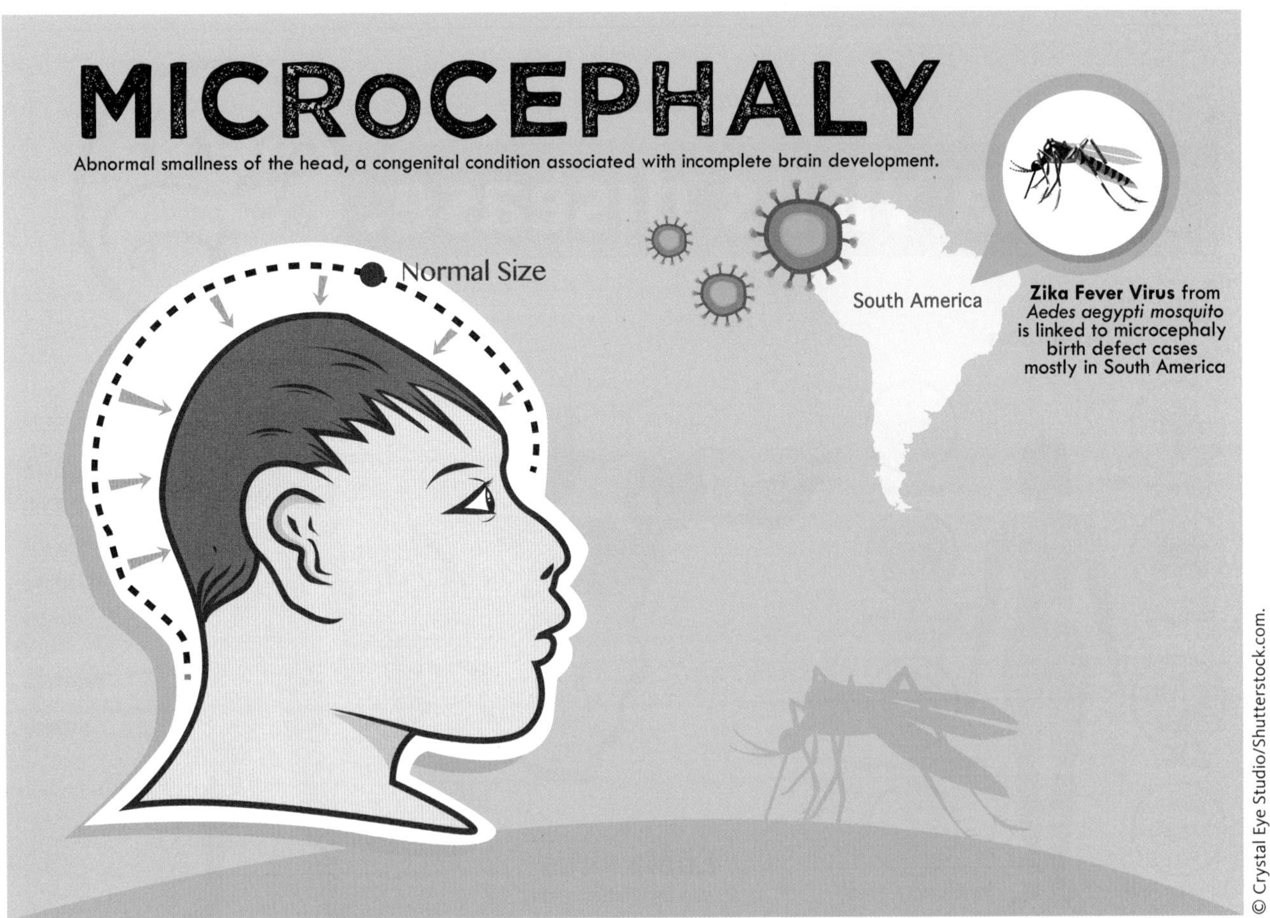

FIGURE 1-5 Microcephaly is a congenital defect as a result of the Zika virus.

of this word is by associating it with a word you may be more familiar with—panoramic. A panoramic photograph is the widest picture one can take with a camera. A panoramic picture is used to photograph a very large area or a huge group of people.

There was much fear that the Ebola virus (shown in Figure 1-6) might become a pandemic if not contained within West Africa. More about Ebola can be found in Figure 1-7.

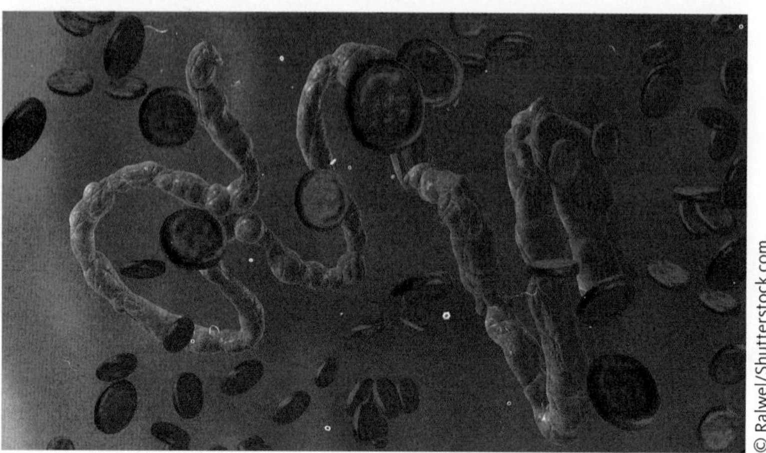

FIGURE 1-6 Ebola virus in the bloodstream.

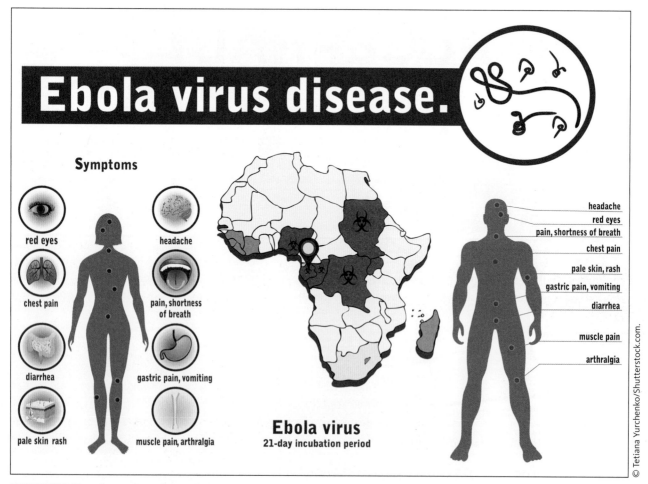

FIGURE 1-7 Infographic of the Ebola virus.

There's a lot of information for this learning objective, so let's stop and test your knowledge on some of the terms discussed thus far.

1-5 CONTACT TRANSMISSION

There are many different routes a disease can take to enter your body. Some are fairly "straightforward" and some more "indirect."

1-5a Direct Contact

Pathogens are spread by two common routes of transmission, or simply by direct and indirect contact. **Direct contact** is when a person carrying a pathogenic microorganism comes into physical contact with another person or when body fluids make contact with an open sore or mucous membrane. Infectious disease is most commonly spread through direct contact. For example, if an individual fails to wear gloves when dealing with contaminated body fluids and the fluid breaches the skin through a cut on a finger, the pathogen now can gain entry into the body. Kissing would be another form of potential direct contact transmission.

1-5b Indirect Contact

Indirect contact occurs when a person comes into contact with a contaminated surface, such as a doorknob, and then touches a mucous membrane or wound. This is why it is so important to use new or sterilized medical instruments and equipment. It should also be noted that droplets can transmit disease via the indirect route. If a contaminated person sneezes in a doorway and particles land on a door knob and moments later another person opens the door, that person has come into indirect contact with a pathogen.

Another method of indirect contact is by puncturing oneself with a dirty needle. A hollow needle has greater risk for transmitting disease than solid needles, due to the possibility of body fluids remaining inside the needle and releasing upon contact.

1-5c Airborne Transmission

There are other routes by which disease can be transmitted to a susceptible host. One of these routes is **airborne transmission**, which occurs when a pathogen is released into the air by way of coughing, sneezing, talking, and laughing. As seen in Figure 1-8, if an infected individual is in close proximity to a potential host, the pathogen is transferred through droplets in the air.

1-6 COMMON VEHICLE

We have discussed a lot of routes that pathogens can take to enter your body; however, there is yet another route. This route is called **common vehicle**. Just like a vehicle can transport passengers, a common vehicle can be used to transport pathogens. For example, any consumable item, such as food, can serve as a common vehicle for infection. You've probably heard on the news of food poisoning outbreaks that have occurred as a result of the spread of *Salmonella* or *E. coli* from contaminated food or water sources.

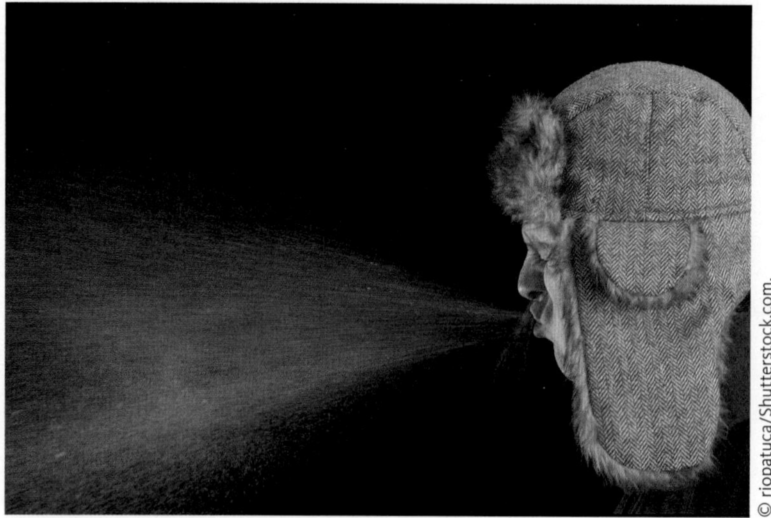

FIGURE 1-8 Droplets traveling through the air from a sneeze.

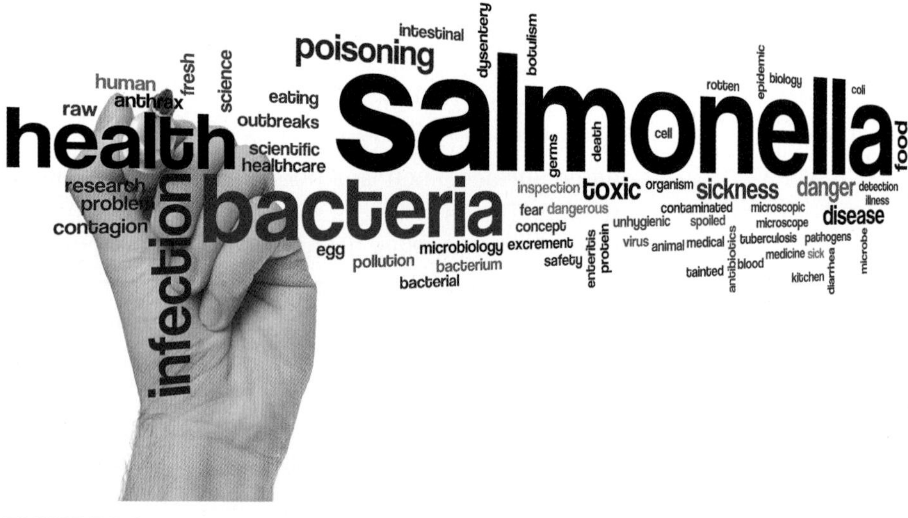

FIGURE 1-9 Common vehicle word cloud.

Common vehicles are not limited to food or water. Medical products such as blood, injectable medications, and IV solutions can cause a sudden spread of the same disease to many patients. Common vehicles do not happen only in health care, but from a consumer standpoint, such as consuming contaminated food products. See Figure 1-9.

1-7 CARRIERS OF DISEASE

Now that we have discussed the various routes a pathogen can take, we need to take a closer look at the actual carriers that can assist the pathogen in entering the body.

The carriers that assist pathogens are termed vectors. A vector is any living organism (person, plant, or animal) that carries and transmits disease to another living organism. A vector-borne exposure can occur in two ways, mechanical and biological. A **mechanical vector** is involved when a pathogen is transmitted by an animal or insect simply by coming into contact with a microorganism and then physically transporting it to the host, as shown in Figure 1-10. Imagine a fly landing on feces or a deceased animal that contains pathogens, then landing on an open sore. The carrier does not develop the disease but rather acts as the mechanical vector and transports the microorganisms from one location to another.

A pathogen can actually live inside a host such as an animal or insect. The host can then harbor the disease. The pathogen can then spread to other hosts by a bite or injection, as shown in Figure 1-11. A prime example is a tick infected with Lyme disease. The tick bites the victim to feed on the host's blood and in the process transmits Lyme disease through its saliva, symptoms illustrated in Figure 1-12. The tick in this example is the **biological vector**.

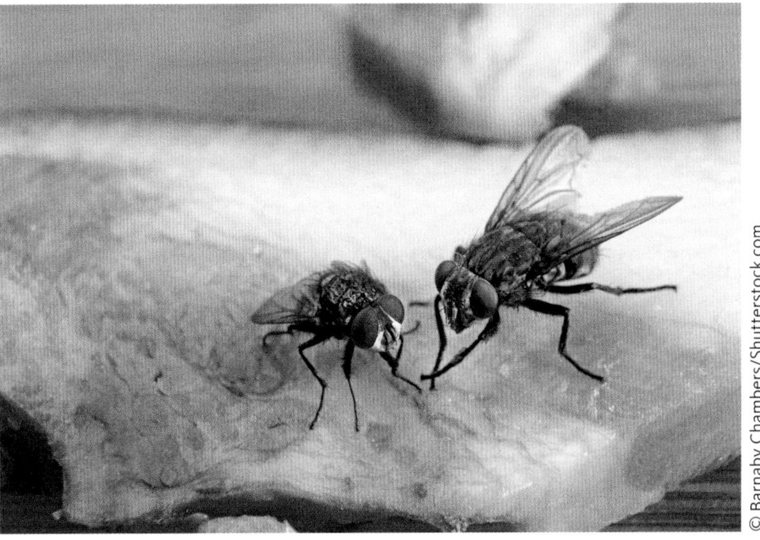

FIGURE 1-10 Flies touching a piece of meat.

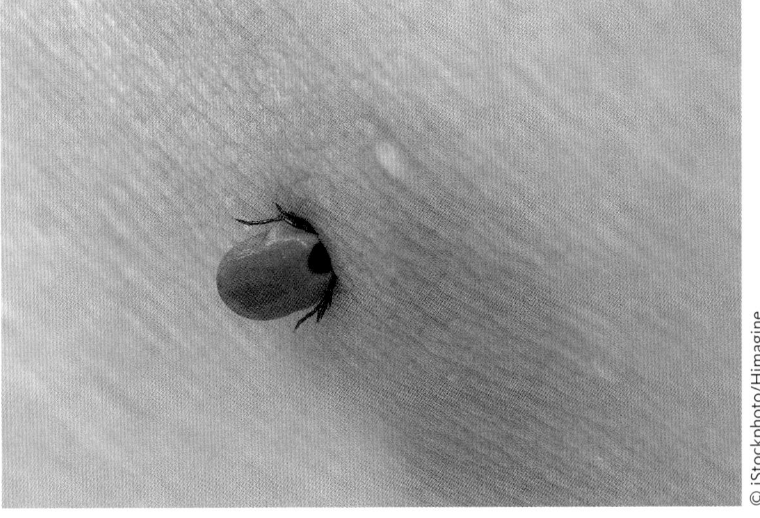

FIGURE 1-11 A tick feeding off a host.

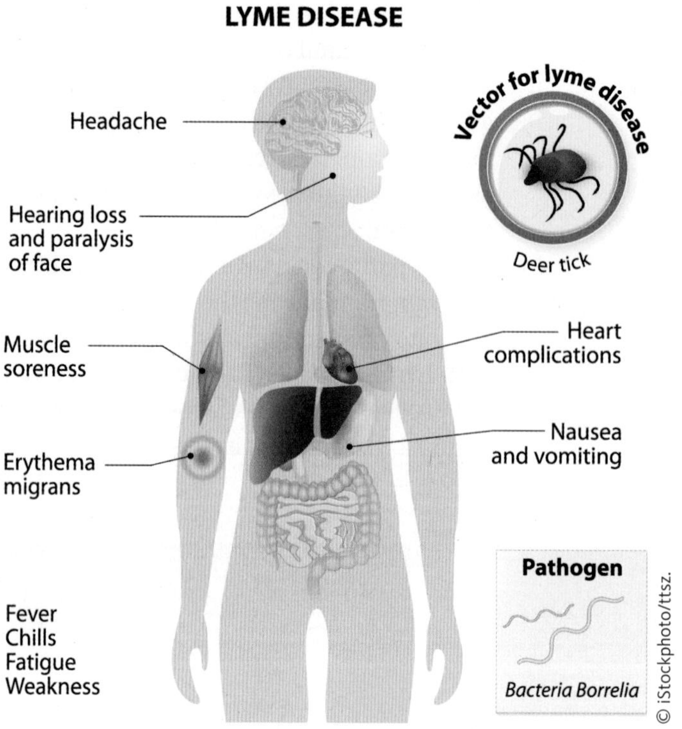

FIGURE 1-12 List of symptoms caused by Lyme disease.

1-8 CHAIN OF INFECTION

So, how do many of these concepts all "link" together? A model called the "chain of infection" demonstrates the linkages in the disease process. The chain is a great analogy because it not only shows the interconnectedness but also shows how a chain becomes useless when a link is broken. You will soon learn that there are many ways to break the chain of infection and prevent the spread of disease, Figure 1-13.

The chain of infection is made up of a series of steps or links. In Figure 1-13, the first link at 12 o'clock is the causative agent or pathogen. Moving clockwise, to survive the pathogen it needs to find the second link, a reservoir or environment such as an animal, human, soil, or water in which to thrive. The pathogen then finds a **portal of exit** or the third link, in other words, a way out of the body or reservoir where they are growing. The pathogen is now seeking to spread. The fourth link is the **mode of transmission** that can either be directly or indirectly transmitted from the source of infection to the host by way of the fifth link, the **portal of entry**. The pathogen can enter the new host by way of mouth, eyes, and nose to name just a few portals. Now, the microorganism has made it to the sixth and final link, the susceptible **host**.

This creation or progression of disease development is cumulatively known as **pathogenesis**. Now that the pathogen has made it to the new host the **inoculation period** begins. At this stage, the pathogen has just been introduced into the body. There are no signs or symptoms at this time. The inoculation period is followed by the **incubation period**. During incubation, the pathogen multiplies to pathogenic levels causing symptoms to occur within the host.

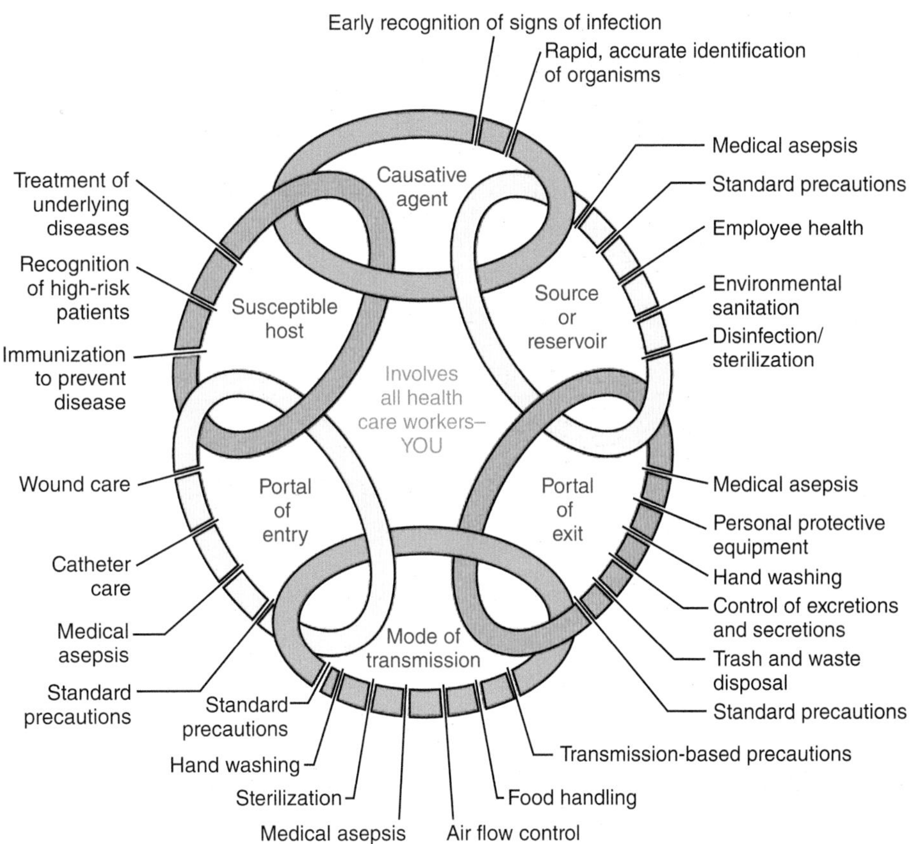

FIGURE 1-13 Illustration of the chain of infection with ways it can be broken.

1-8a Breaking the Chain of Infection

Now that you understand the links of the chain of infection, let's focus on ways to break the chain. It is important to remember that any break in the chain will prevent the spread of infection.

The chain of infection shown in Figure 1-13 has subsections that break each link into smaller pieces. Each piece gives an example of how each link can be broken, stopping the pathogen before it has an opportunity to further grow and spread. For instance, following standard precautions will protect a clinician from a source of disease, such as an infected patient. Hand washing also breaks the chain of infection at the portal of exit and the mode of transmission links, preventing the pathogen from spreading to others.

CLINICAL CONNECTION 1.3

Before moving on, let's take a look at a case study to put the material we covered into real-world perspective.

James, a 33-year-old outdoorsman went camping with his girlfriend, Lauren, in late July. The morning was very humid and sunny without a cloud in the sky. The couple decided to leave their campsite around 10 am to go hiking and picnic in the mountains. A few miles into the hike, Lauren noticed a black spot on the back of James' knee.

CLINICAL CONNECTION 1.3 (*Continued*)

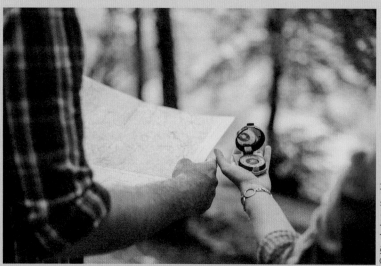

The two stopped for a closer look and it was a tick embedded in James' skin. James removed the tick and the couple decided to picnic in a clearing. As they unpacked their food, Lauren noticed that the ice packs were no longer cold. Lauren told James that it was probably not a good idea to eat the potato salad because it was warm. James did not take the warning seriously and ate the potato salad anyway. The couple finished their meal and headed back to camp. Later in the evening, James did not feel well. Thinking he had food poisoning, the couple ended their camping trip early and went home.

The next day, James was very nauseated and was experiencing abdominal cramps and pain. James vomited throughout the day and decided to go to the hospital. The physician confirmed that James did have food poisoning and was dehydrated from vomiting and not eating or drinking most of the day. The physician ordered a nurse to give James fluids via an intravenous (IV) route. The nurse, not using proper techniques, placed the needle into James' arm. At first there were no signs of infection, but later the injection site became very sore, swollen, and red, the results of a staph infection.

LEARNING OBJECTIVE 1.3 State risk factors associated with disease.

KEY TERMS

Environment Surrounding in which one lives.

Hereditary Diseases are passed down from parents to their offspring.

Lifestyle The way in which an individual lives his or her life.

1-9 RISK FACTORS

Risk factors, or predisposing factors, increase the risk of an individual becoming affected by an illness. Predisposing factors can be grouped into different categories. Let's discuss each in more depth.

1-9a Age

The risk of disease is not only for the elderly. Upon entering the world, newborn infants are at greater risk of infection. The newborn has not fully developed an immune system that will deter illness. On-the-other-hand, as the body ages it becomes more susceptible to heart disease, coronary artery disease, pneumonia, and, as the brain ages, decreasing cognitive ability. In fact, even though we may not feel any different from year to year our bodies are aging. Some people dread their birthdays and maybe for good reason. Did you know we lose 1% of our body function at age 30? So, Happy 30th Birthday!

1-9b Environment

The **environment** in which one lives can play a major role in whether or not an individual is at a greater risk of encountering a particular disease. From the way we live at home to where we work, the environment can play a major role in our overall health. At home, we may be exposed to mold, pollen, or dust from a local cement plant. Exposures at work can also increase the odds of developing a disease as a result of prolonged exposure. Imagine the dust breathed into the lungs of a coal miner. Before knowing the disastrous effects, miners would work in the mines with no masks, resulting in black lung disease. Coal dust can be seen on the miner's face in Figure 1-14.

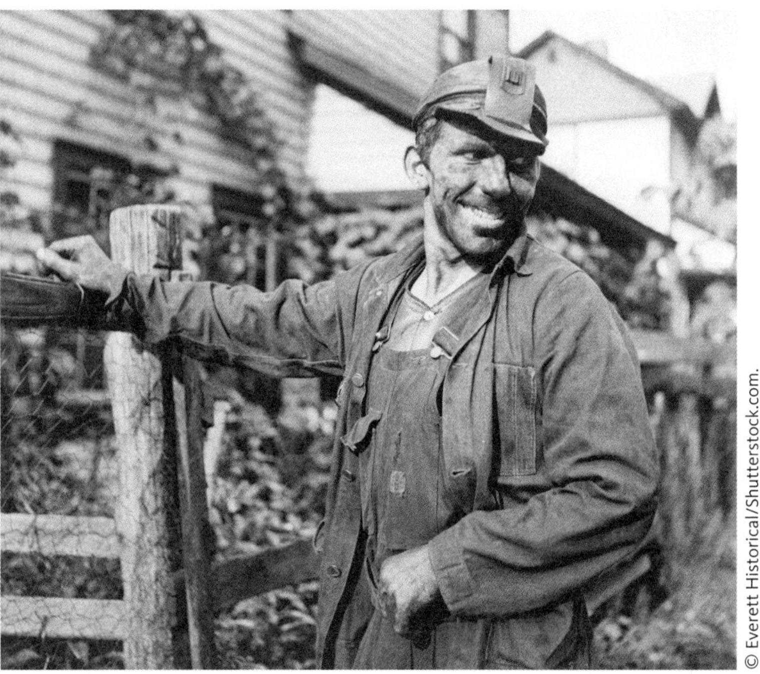

FIGURE 1-14 Smiling Polish-American miner, in work clothes and covered with coal dust, arriving home from work in Capels, West Virginia. 1938 photo by Marion Post Wolcott.

1-9c Lifestyle

The way in which an individual lives his or her life is their **lifestyle**. A person has control over how he or she chooses to live. Poor decision-making can have an everlasting impact on an individual's lifespan. Poor nutrition can lead to deficiencies of the vitamins and minerals that the body needs to function correctly. If a poor diet and lack of portion control is present, the person will gain excess weight, causing strain on the body's systems. Obesity is a major problem in our society and can be avoided with proper eating habits and routine exercise. Smoking is another poor choice one can avoid. Smoking has been known to significantly increase the risk of cancers and is the number one cause of chronic obstructive pulmonary disease. Stress is also known to wreak havoc on the body. Although easier said than done, it is important to set aside time to relax and rest. Increased stress levels can cause one to burn out, suffer increased memory loss, and become more susceptible to illnesses. Figure 1-15 illustrates healthy choices that you can control.

1-9d Heredity

Unlike lifestyle, what is inherited cannot be avoided by healthy choices. **Hereditary** diseases are passed down from our parents. We are all born with certain traits and characteristics; however, some of these can increase the odds of getting a disease. Cystic fibrosis is passed on to a child and will be present at

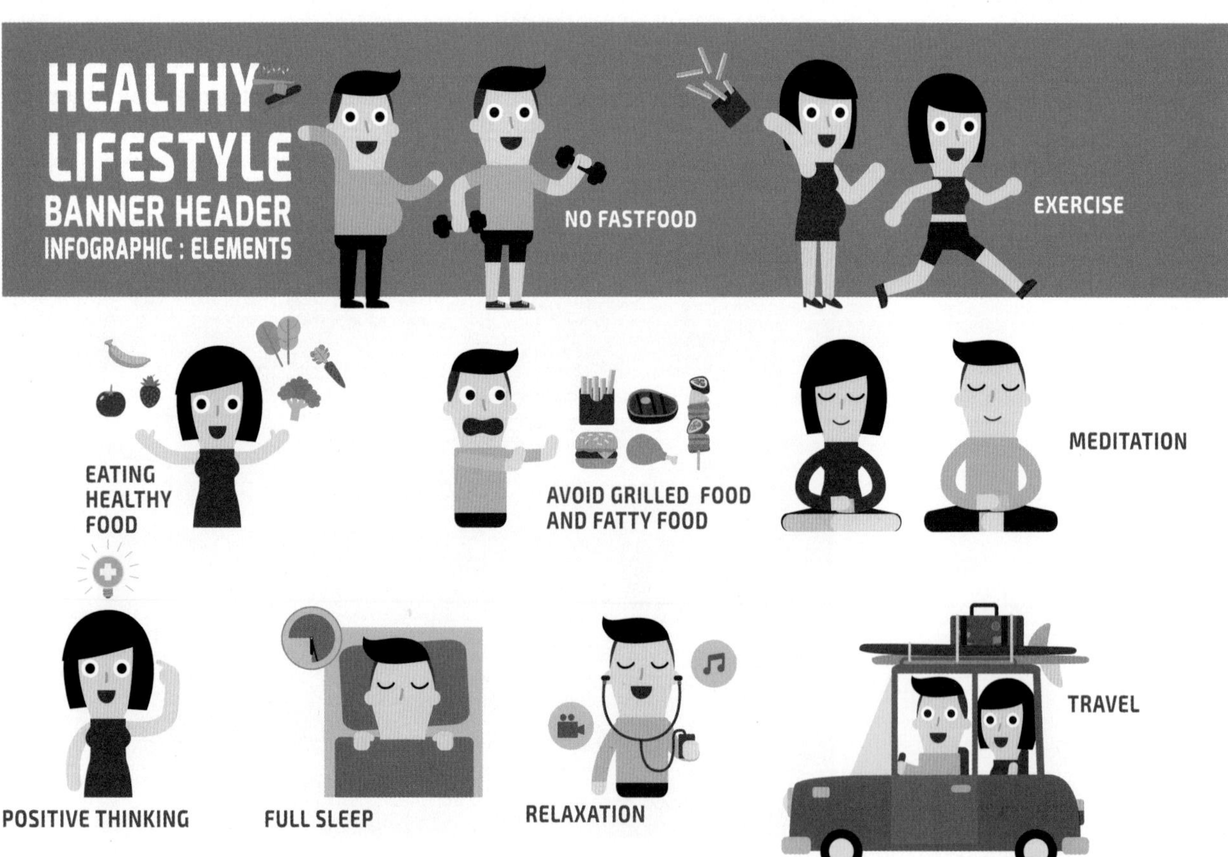

FIGURE 1-15 Examples of healthy choices.

birth, drastically shortening the life-expectancy to 37.5 years of age. The BRCA or breast cancer gene is passed down the generations to children as well. Those with the BRCA gene are more susceptible to breast cancer. A blood test can be taken to examine DNA and determine if you are a carrier.

Do you ever wonder why doctors ask you about your family history? Maybe you thought they were just nosey. However, physicians ask patients questions about their family history to identify if your relatives have been diagnosed with certain diseases that may have a tendency to run in the family. This gives the physician an idea of what disease you will be most likely to encounter, so it can be better prevented. For instance, heart disease is known to be inherited and if the patient's predecessors have heart disease they are at a greater risk of developing the disease themselves.

1-9e Gender

Discrimination readily exists with disease, meaning some diseases affect more men than women, while other diseases affect women more than men. In women, multiple sclerosis, osteoporosis, and rheumatoid arthritis are more prevalent. Men have an increased risk of heart disease and Parkinson's disease. The reason for this may derive from hormones or genetics. Researchers are exploring potential causes of this phenomenon to gain a better understanding.

LEARNING OBJECTIVE 1.4 Describe the importance of patient history.

KEY TERMS

Auscultation Listening with a stethoscope to examine breath, and heart and bowel sounds to determine if any abnormalities are present.

Direct or closed questioning Asking questions that require a yes or no answer.

Disorder Describes disruption from the normal functioning of the mind or body. Typically used when a disease is not an appropriate term to describe condition.

Family history Interview to identify diseases the patient is susceptible to according to heredity.

History of present illness (HPI) History of the current condition or disease.

Inspection Visually looking for anything out of the norm.

Medication history Listing of all current prescriptions, over-the-counter (OTC) drugs, and herbal supplements and any adverse drug reactions.

NKA Abbreviation for no known allergies.

Occupational history Listing of what the patient does or did for a living.

Open-ended questioning Asking the patient simple, broad questions that require more than a yes or no to answer.

Palpation Process of touching a patient in an effort to evaluate abnormalities.

Past medical history (PMH) Listing of previous medical illnesses and procedures.

Patient interview Process where clinician gathers patient information.

Percussion Tapping with fingers in areas on the body such as the chest, to check body cavities for excess fluid or air.

Physical examination Process of physically examining a patient in a systematic manner.

Signs Objective measurements of body functions.

Social history Information obtained on the type of lifestyle the patient lives such as marital status, social or frequent drinking history, smoking history, or illicit drug use.

Symptoms Observable subjective states or behaviors that rely on the patient to state how they feel.

Syndrome A particular set of signs and symptoms that when grouped together is indicative or characteristic of a certain disease or disorder.

Vital signs Measured signs that are vital for life; heart rate, respiration rate, blood pressure, and body temperature.

1-10 THE IMPORTANCE OF INFORMATION GATHERING

Have you ever heard of the computer phrase, "garbage in, garbage out?" The same can be said for information gathering. If the information you collect is useless or inaccurate, the ability to properly diagnose and treat the patient will be compromised. The patient's information should be in chronological order, clear, correct, complete, and concise. We will start by discussing basic patient interview techniques because what better source to learn about the patient than the patient?

1-11 THE PATIENT INTERVIEW

How can we get the patient to open up and explain how they are feeling in detail? During the **patient interview** process the clinician has the opportunity to make the patient feel comfortable and build a relationship. The clinician should maintain an open body posture by not crossing their arms or avoiding eye contact. It is also recommended to avoid standing in or near the door. It makes it appear as though the clinician is ready for the quickest possible exit. Another pointer is to avoid using medical jargon; the complicated, foreign sounding words will alienate the patient and only cause confusion. A patient is more likely to open up to questioning and elaborate on current and past history if she or he feels comfortable. We will further explore open and closed questioning.

1-12 PATIENT QUESTIONING

When interviewing a patient, the clinician may want the patient to elaborate on the condition being discussed. In this case, it is best to ask open-ended questions. **Open-ended questioning** is conducted by asking the patient simple, broad questions that require more than a yes or no to answer. For example, "So, what made you decide to visit us today?" and "Tell me about your knee pain." are simple and effective ways to get the patient to open up about their condition. However, if you are looking for less patient engagement and a direct answer, then closed questioning is used.

Direct or closed questioning is used when it is not necessary for the patient to elaborate and only a short answer such as yes or no is desired to obtain specific facts. If the clinician is looking for certain details that may not have been answered during the interview or wants to regain control of the conversation, closed questioning is acceptable. During the interview it is also important to take the patient's body language into account. The patient may be indicating that they are in pain, which you can then direct your questions toward. See Figure 1-16.

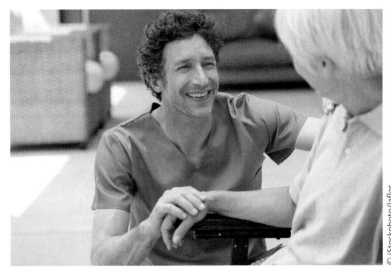

FIGURE 1-16 Friendly communication with a patient.

1-13 HISTORY OF PRESENT ILLNESS

A clinician is like a detective. To uncover the **history of present illness (HPI)**, the clinician must use a line of questioning to help aid in determining the patient's diagnosis. It is important for the clinician to not only question the patient to gather information but also listen to the patient and not solely rely on tests to diagnose. The data listed in this section should only pertain to what recently happened in regards to the chief complaint, such as asking the patient when the issue first occurred and whether any other symptoms arose since then. Other details include, how long has this symptom been occurring? Has it been getting progressively worse or remaining constant? Has the condition improved at all since its first onset? Does anything alleviate or make the symptom(s) worse?

For example, let's say a middle-aged woman named Jessica comes into the physician's office with complaints of shortness of breath (SOB). The doctor asks when she has trouble breathing. Jessica states that she has her breathing under control most of the time. However, the physician discovers that she has many cats in her apartment and she has trouble breathing when she vacuums the carpet. Then Jessica further explains she only has difficulty for about an hour or so and then her breathing returns to normal after she stops vacuuming. The doctor asks how often has this been happening and finds it has started over that last few months. Based on this information the doctor has found probable cause for her SOB. Now further testing can be done to determine if the patient has an allergic asthma and if it is from the vacuum releasing cat dander, dust, or other irritants into the air (Figure 1-17).

1-14 PAST MEDICAL HISTORY

The patient's **past medical history (PMH)** is a list of previous medical illnesses and procedures from the past. It is listed from the most relevant to the chief complaint to the least.

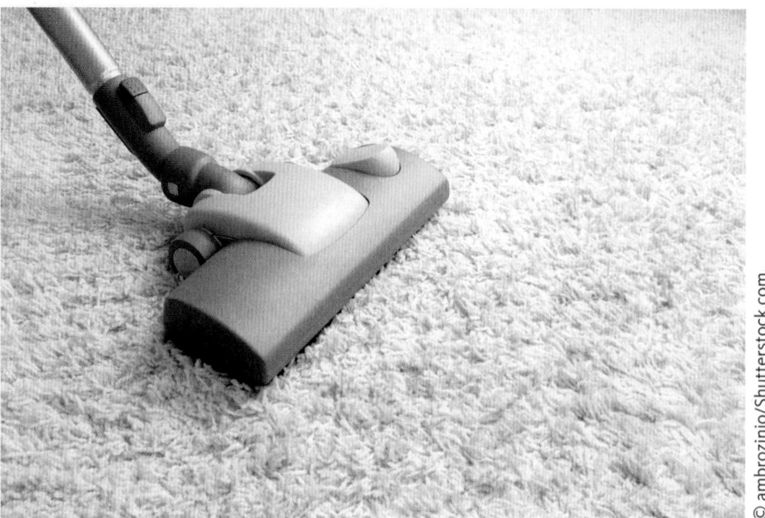

© ambrozinio/Shutterstock.com.

FIGURE 1-17 Vacuuming can cause allergens to become airborne.

1-15 FAMILY MEDICAL HISTORY

Why does a physician ask about your family history? A **family history** can help identify diseases the patient is susceptible to and likely to develop over his or her lifetime. As parents pass their physical traits on to their children, other characteristics are also inherited such as the predisposition to diseases. Heart disease and stroke are known to be hereditary. It is important to determine what illnesses a patient's parents or close relatives have or that caused their death. A family history of heart disease would make it more likely that a patient might develop heart disease. If a female patient's mother or grandmother had, or passed away from, ovarian or breast cancer, the odds of the patient encountering the disease is greatly increased. If this information is known, preventive measures can be taken to catch the disease in its earliest stage to increase the rate of survivability. For men, a cancer such as prostate cancer tends to run in the family. Therefore, men should be examined regularly when there is an increased chance of developing the disease.

1-16 SOCIAL HISTORY

The **social history** gives the caretaker an insight into the patient's lifestyle. Marital status, social or frequent drinking history, smoking history, or illicit drug use are important data findings. The social history obtained may aid in providing clues as to why the patient presents as is and can determine potential diseases the patient is at risk of developing. The patient may be living a risky lifestyle and may be more prone to certain ailments. For instance, if a patient states he smokes, the clinician can infer lung disease.

Other factors included under this category are sexual and travel history as well as education level. Have you ever been asked if you recently traveled to Africa? Why do you think that happens? There are many diseases that can be acquired abroad, so it is best practice to know if the patient may have been exposed to those potential pathogens. For example, Africa is known for the Ebola virus, while South and Central America is known for the Zika virus.

1-17 OCCUPATIONAL HISTORY

It is important to know what the patient does or did for a living. The patient's **occupational history** may aid in the understanding of what caused the patient to present to the emergency department or physician's office. A patient's work environment can have a significant impact on their overall health. A worker exposed to inorganic or organic dust can develop many possible diseases causing permanent destruction to the lungs and possibly lead to cancer. Individuals exposed to chemicals and radiation over periods of time can also develop long-term effects resulting in possible disability or death. This history, like others, can be found within the forms given to the patient to fill out prior to being seen by the attending physician. See Figure 1-18.

1-18 MEDICATIONS

Obtaining a proper **medication history** is a very important component of the information and history gathering process. A proper medication history should include all current medications, including over-the-counter (OTC) drugs, and herbal supplements. Also, questioning the patient whether he or she takes all his or her medicines as prescribed or if any adverse drug reactions (side-effects) have ever occurred is critical. Gathering a list of medications will prevent the risk of medicine errors. The odds of an error occurring is increased in elderly patients prescribed different medications for the same ailment. Patients may self-medicate and take a variety of supplements to further treat a condition for which their doctor has already prescribed medication. The patient does not realize or consider the potential dangers that can occur from mixing over-the-counter drugs with prescribed medications. Elderly patients with multiple prescriptions can easily get their medications confused. Not only is this dangerous, but it can be frustrating for the patient, Figure 1-19.

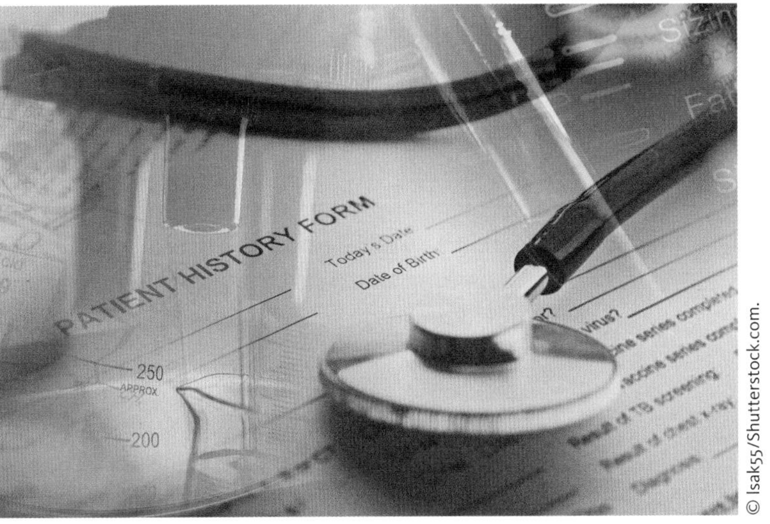

FIGURE 1-18 An example of a patient history form.

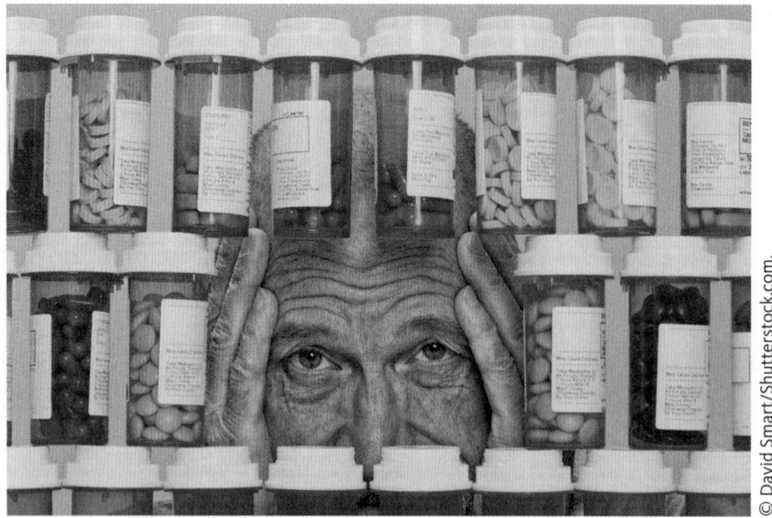

FIGURE 1-19 Elderly patient confused by all of his medication.

1-19 ALLERGIES

It is important to ask and make note of any patient allergies. Common patient allergies seen in the hospital are latex, dyes, and medications, all of which can cause a wide array of adverse effects. If the patient has no known allergies the abbreviation used in the chart is NKA. When a patient is first exposed to an allergen a mild reaction may present. Allergic reactions can occur within seconds, or hours after the initial exposure. An anaphylactic reaction results in a loss of blood pressure, making it the most serious and potentially life-threatening allergic reaction, requiring immediate medical intervention.

1-20 PHYSICAL EXAMINATION

After the clinician reviews the patient's medical history, the next step is examining the patient. Now, we will discuss the **physical examination** process in more depth.

Commonly performed by the clinician at the beginning of a physical exam is the HEENT, which stands for Head, Eyes, Ears, Nose, and Throat. The physician will visually inspect the head for any abnormalities such as facial symmetry and palpate, or feel using their fingers, to search for any irregularities. The examination will proceed downwards to the neck to assess lymph nodes and thyroid. The eyes are checked to note the patient's ability to track a moving object to determine the movement ability, pupil dilation, contraction in response to light as well as equal and overall condition of the eyes. The ears are examined for hearing acuteness, redness, and inflammation with the use of an otoscope. An examination of the lungs and chest use four general principles, inspection, auscultation, palpation, and percussion.

The **inspection** is done by visually looking for anything out of the norm. A few examples are accessory muscle use while breathing that is an indicator of respiratory distress, any scars that may be a result of a previous trauma or surgery, distention of veins and edema (swelling) in the extremities.

Auscultation is listening with a stethoscope to examine breath, and heart and bowel sounds to determine if any abnormalities are present, Figure 1-20.

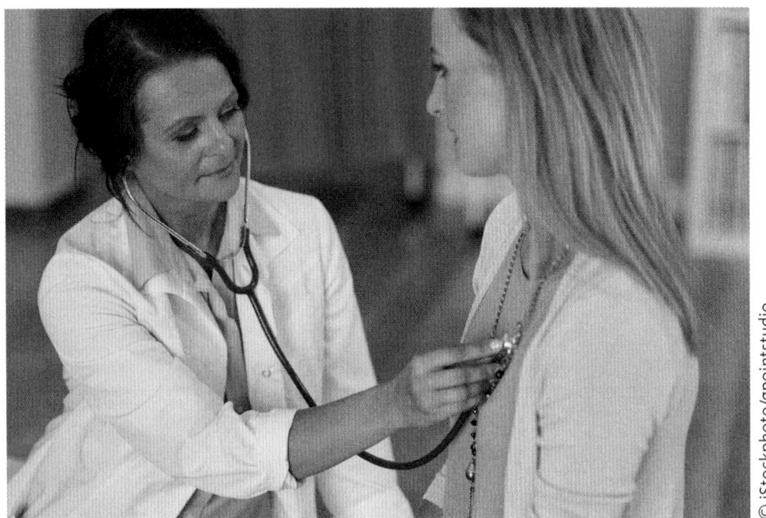

FIGURE 1-20 Physician auscultating patient.

Palpation is the process of touching a patient in an effort to evaluate chest abnormalities, tenderness, and tone of respiratory muscles.

Percussion involves tapping areas on the body such as the chest, to check body cavities for excess fluid or air.

During the exam, the patient's general appearance is noted as well as age and sex that are taken into account during the exam. Differences will vary by gender and whether the patient is a neonate, pediatric, adult, or geriatric patient. Vitals taken during the exam are temperature, blood pressure, heart rate, respiratory rate. We will discuss the normal ranges a little later in this section but first, let's determine what exactly are vital signs.

1-21 DIFFERENTIATING BETWEEN SIGNS AND SYMPTOMS

Signs are objective measurements such as height and weight that can be consistently obtained by different clinicians without bias and personal judgement. **Vital signs** are all vital to life in the form of heart rate, respiration rate, blood pressure, and body temperature. Vital signs (listed in Table 1-1) vary according to patient age, sex, weight, and overall fitness level. To differentiate signs from

Table 1-1 Normal values for adult vital signs

VITAL SIGNS	NORMAL RANGES (ADULT)
Blood pressure	120/80 mm/Hg
Breathing	12 to 20 breaths per minute
Pulse	60 to 100 beats per minute
Temperature	97.8°F to 99.1°F (36.5°C to 37.3°C) average 98.6°F (37°C)

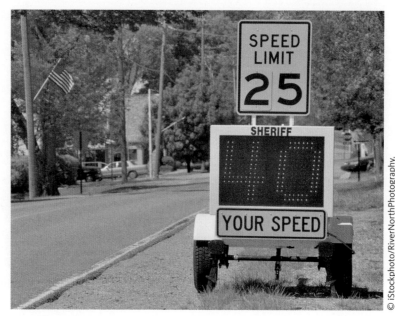

© iStockphoto/RiverNorthPhotography.

FIGURE 1-21 Example of signs and how they give clinicians a measurement.

symptoms, think of a road sign, more specifically a speed limit sign. A speed limit sign displays numbers showing how fast motorists can travel (Figure 1-21), and in health care a sign is measured numerically on a monitor or counted.

Symptoms are observable states or behaviors that are subjective. The diagnosis relies on the patient stating how she or he feels, and how the clinician interprets the patient. This is more difficult to measure, hence it is not a definitive measurement and is rather an estimation that is compared with other patients' answers to the same questions. For instance, when a patient is asked how nauseated or dizzy they feel, or how much pain is being experienced, there is no clear way to know, as a clinician, what the patient is actually experiencing. Everyone has different perceptions and tolerance levels.

1-22 SYNDROME

Now, how are signs and symptoms related to a syndrome? A **syndrome** refers to a particular set of signs and symptoms that when grouped together is indicative or characteristic of a certain disease or disorder. Down syndrome results when an individual has an extra partial or extra whole chromosome 21. Symptoms seen in affected individuals include mental impairment, flat face, slanted eyes, a short neck, low set ears, flaccid muscles, and obesity to list a few similar qualities, Figure 1-22.

1-23 DISORDER

Although disease and disorder is frequently used interchangeably, a **disorder** is a term used to describe a disruption from the normal functioning ability of the mind or body. Typically, disorder is used when a disease is not an appropriate term to describe a condition. For example, posttraumatic distress disorder

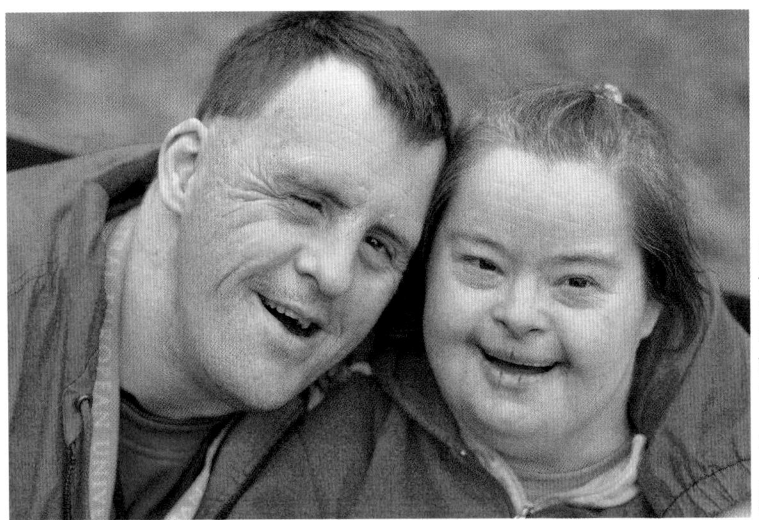

FIGURE 1-22 Similar characteristics of two individuals with Down Syndrome.

(PTSD) is not classified as a disease. The individual's bodily functions are not deviated from functioning properly as in disease states. PTSD has symptoms such as anxiety, which is caused from witnessing or experiencing a traumatic event. Sadly, society has a stigma against mental health disorders and many veterans see PTSD as a label and choose to not seek help with the disorder.

LEARNING OBJECTIVE 1.5 Describe common methods used to treat and diagnose diseases.

KEY TERMS

Blood glucose Sugar found in the bloodstream used for energy.

Chest X-ray (CXR) Imaging used to examine the thoracic cavity.

Complete Blood Count (CBC) Blood sample analyzing types and numbers of cells within the bloodstream.

Computerized tomography (CT or CAT) scan Imaging utilizing x-rays and a computer to produce cross-sectional slices of the body.

Culture and sensitivity (C&S) Laboratory sample from a patient that grows and identifies the pathogen and tests what drug will kill it.

Electrocardiogram (ECG or EKG) Recorded display of electrical impulses produced by the heart.

Electrocardiograph Instrument used to record heart rhythms.

Electrolytes Minerals dissolved in blood needed by the body to function properly, (calcium, potassium, sodium, phosphate, magnesium, and chloride).

Hematocrit (HCT) Ratio of total cellular volume to total volume of blood.

Hemoglobin (Hgb) Protein in the red blood cell that carries oxygen.

Holistic medicine A care plan that not only focuses on the disease, but the patient as a whole, including body, mind spirit and emotions, in a quest for optimal health and wellness.

Magnetic resonance imaging (MRI) Imaging uses magnets and radio waves to produce high resolution images of organs and soft tissue with no radiation exposure to patient.

Patient care plan Set of steps used to explain patient's care regarding possible treatments and expected outcomes.

Patient education Instructing patients in various aspects of their care such as how to properly perform treatments.

Platelets (PLT) Cellular fragments that clots blood.

Red blood cells (RBC) Cells within blood that transport oxygen.

Urine analysis (UA) Testing a urine sample for abnormalities.

Urine color Observing urine color to help identify a disease or dehydration.

Urine concentration Measurement to determine if kidney failure is present.

Urine odor Determining the smell of the urine to help determine presence of illness.

White blood cells (WBC) Cells within bloodstream that fights infection.

X-ray Imaging technique utilized to determine any bone breaks and defects in the body.

1-24 THE IMPORTANCE OF DIAGNOSTIC ACCURACY

Technology today, allows clinicians to take a multifaceted approach to ensure an accurate diagnosis. If an incorrect diagnosis is made, it will delay proper treatment and increase the odds of an adverse outcome, not to mention the possible legal action taken by the patient if he or she is wrongfully diagnosed. Could you imagine being diagnosed with cancer only to find out it was a mistake? It would take an emotional toll on the patient and their family members. Therefore, diagnostic labs and tests are performed to ensure accuracy at all times.

1-24a X-ray

Let's begin by taking a look at X-rays. A **chest X-ray (CXR)** is used to examine the thoracic cavity. An X-ray is also utilized to determine any bone breaks and defects elsewhere in the body. An **X-ray** has four main body densities, gas/air (black), water/blood (gray), tissue/fat (gray), and metal/calcium (white). The X-ray machine projects into the body a ray of electrons which are either scattered or deflected by body tissue. Some rays pass directly through the patient and reach the film, while others are absorbed by body tissues. A film is placed behind the targeted area and that film reflects the different contrasts of shades and shadows producing the image in Figure 1-23.

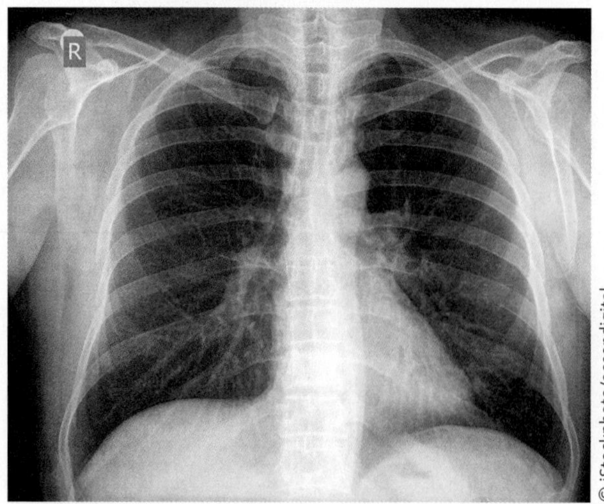

FIGURE 1-23 Chest X-ray.

1-24b Computerized Tomography

Another important tool is a CT scan. A **computerized tomography (CT or CAT) scan** has the ability to take a more detailed image of the patient than an X-ray. A CT produces cross-sectional slices of the body at various angles. It is capable of imaging bone, vessels, and organs such as the lungs. It is widely used to examine the extent of trauma such as a cranial hemorrhage. The scan uses a combination of an X-ray and computer making it more precise than a traditional X-ray and it is much faster and cheaper than an MRI, but not as detailed, Figure 1-24.

1-24c Magnetic Resonance Imaging

Magnetic Resonance Imaging (MRI) uses magnets and radio waves to produce high-resolution images of organs and soft tissue; therefore, the patient is not exposed to any radiation. However, metal objects are contraindicated due to the magnetic field produced, this also includes pacemakers. Although not utilizing X-rays to produce images, MRIs have the capability to develop 3D images of the body at any desired plane. MRIs are widely used for making detailed images of ligaments, tendons, and other soft tissues such as the brain. However, an MRI can take up to two hours to complete, Figure 1-25.

1-24d Electrocardiogram

How can we monitor the activity of the heart? An **electrocardiogram (ECG or EKG)** is a quick, noninvasive, and painless technique used to record electrical impulses produced by special cells in the heart. These electrical impulses can be detected on the surface of the body as the impulse travels through the

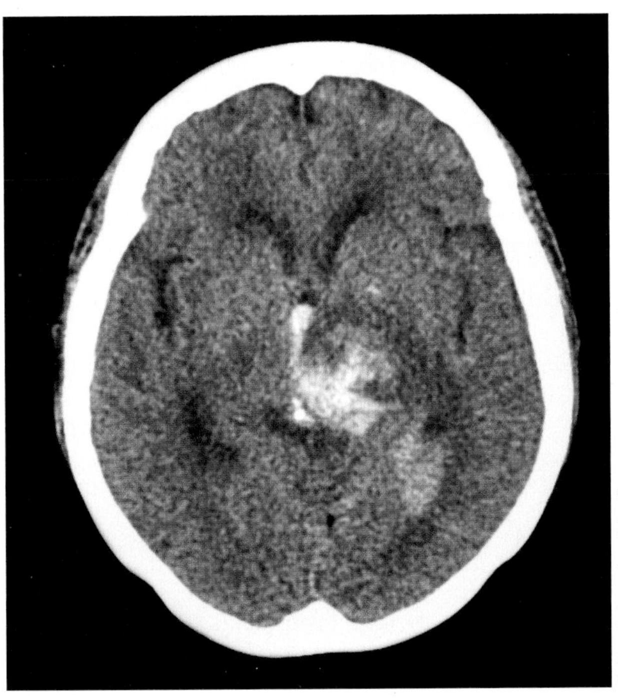

FIGURE 1-24 CT scan of stroke.

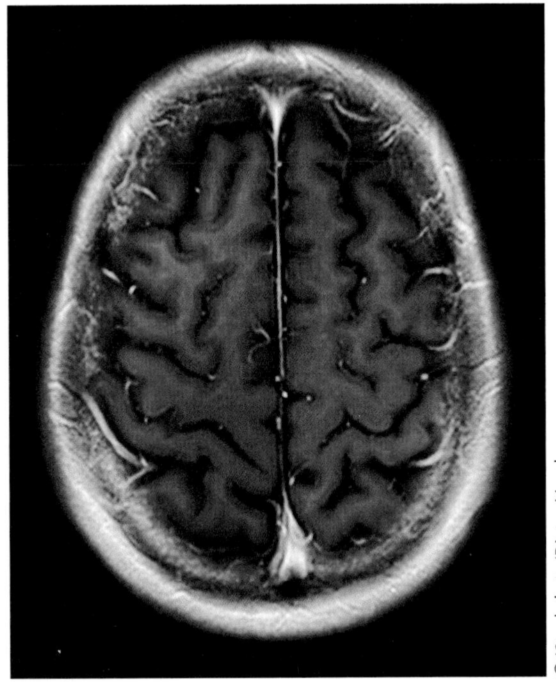

FIGURE 1-25 MRI of Brain.

heart. The heart rhythms are recorded using an **electrocardiograph**, while the actual display of the rhythms recorded is an electrocardiogram. If a patient has an arrhythmia, an irregular heartbeat, it can be identified and treated.

1-24e Culture and Sensitivity

If a patient has an infection, it is important to determine if it is viral or bacterial. In order to identify the bug, a **culture and sensitivity (C&S)** needs to be completed. A C&S uses body secretion samples from a patient. The sample is placed in a sterile container designated for laboratory samples. Care must be taken to prevent contamination of the inside of the container and bottom of the lid, as this may cause an erroneous result. Once the sample is collected and properly labeled with the patient's information, it is promptly sent to the lab. The sample is grown (cultured) to determine the type of bacteria present and which antibiotics will destroy the microorganism. If the results show that it is viral microorganism, the patient can be treated with anti-viral medications.

1-24f Complete Blood Count

Blood is a very valuable tool to assess the overall condition of the body. A **Complete Blood Count (CBC)** is a blood sample analyzed to determine if any anomalies are present. An increase or decrease from the normal cell ranges assists in the identification, monitoring, and examination of a disease. A CBC also displays the effectiveness of the treatment and overall system analysis of all blood components. Table 1-2 illustrates the cell types and normal values.

Table 1-2 Types of blood cells and normal ranges

CELL TYPE	DESCRIPTION	NORMAL RANGE
Red blood cells (RBC)	Transport oxygen	**Men:** 4.32–5.72 trillion cells/L or (4.32–5.72 million cells/mcL) **Women:** 3.90–5.03 trillion cells/L or (3.90–5.03 million cells/mcL)
Hemoglobin (Hgb)	Protein in the red blood cell that carries oxygen	**Men:** 13.5–17.5 grams/dL or (135–175 grams/L) **Women:** 12.0–15.5 grams/dL or (120–155 grams/L)
Hematocrit (HCT)	Ratio of volume of red blood cells to total volume of blood	**Men:** 38.8–50.0 percent **Women:** 34.9–44.5 percent
Platelets (PLT)	Clot blood	50–450 billion/L (150,000 to 450,000/mcL)
White blood cells (WBC)	Fight infection	.5–10.5 billion cells/L (3,500 to 10,500 cells/mcL)

1-24g Electrolytes

Another important component measured from a blood sample is **electrolytes**. Electrolytes are highly important minerals (calcium, potassium, sodium, phosphate, magnesium, and chloride) that must to be maintained at a proper concentration level to enable the body to function efficiently. Each electrolyte plays a significant role in the way the body functions. When an imbalance occurs a disorder will present. Electrolyte imbalances may result from too much or not enough fluid in the body. Dehydration, vomiting, diarrhea, sweating, and burns cause decreases in electrolytes. Electrolyte increases may result from excess fluid intake from an intravenous (IV) solution. The severity of symptoms can vary greatly from nonlife threatening (muscle cramps) to a medical emergency (heart arrhythmias and organ failure).

1-24h Blood Glucose

Blood glucose (blood sugar) is sugar found in the bloodstream. Glucose is transported throughout the body to provide energy to cells. Blood sugar levels are maintained by the body to sustain normal function. Glucose levels can be monitored with a glucose meter, which requires a very small blood sample. A lancet or small needle sticks the patient to draw a drop of blood. The blood sample is collected with a test strip, which is then placed into the meter where the sample is read. Another method used to measure blood sugar levels is with urine.

1-24i Urine Analysis

A **Urine Analysis (UA)** may also be indicated to further explain a medical condition. Urine is a waste product of the body's metabolism. Assuming an individual takes in normal amounts of fluid, about 2 liters of urine is produced a day. The kidneys act as a filter and remove dissolved waste in the bloodstream. Urine is secreted from the body to maintain homeostasis. A lot of information can be learned from a urine specimen. Color, consistency, and odor can indicate certain body dysfunctions.

A **urine odor** may be benign or a possible cause for alarm. Normal urine does not have a putrid acidic smell. Certain foods such as beets and asparagus can cause an odd odor and may catch you off guard, but it is not a problem. An ammonia scent indicates dehydration, while urinary infections and cancer can produce an offensive odor. A sweet smelling urine is indicative of glucose or sugar in the urine as a result of diabetes.

Urine concentration is measured to determine if renal (kidney) failure is present. The more concentrated a sample the more dissolved particles will be present. Think of it this way, the strength of a cup of tea depends on how long it sits. As time passes, the tea bags have more time to release particles from the tea bag to further increase the concentration or strength of the tea. In regards to a urine concentration test, fluid is withheld from the patient for several hours prior to collecting a specimen to determine the kidney's ability to concentrate urine with decreased hydration. A clean catch technique is used to prevent any contamination with the sample.

A lot can be learned by looking at the color of urine. Normal **urine color** is typically a pale straw or light or dark yellow color. If clear, it is an indicator that too much hydration is being had, while darker amber to brown coloration indicates a lack of fluid intake. Brown and orange may indicate liver disease, while orange can also be caused by medication used for urinary tract infections. Pink and red colored urine can be associated with certain foods, cancer, blood, infection, or medications. Blue and green colors can be derived from medication, certain bacterial infections, and certain food dyes. A milky, cloudy color is indicative of excess protein in the urine.

1-25 RECOGNIZING DIFFERENT TYPES OF TREATMENT

A **Patient Care Plan** is derived by the physician once the diagnosis is determined. This plan is used to explain the next steps in the patient's care regarding possible treatments and expected outcomes. When the care plan not only focuses on the disease but the patient as a whole, it is known as **holistic medicine**. The idea behind holistic medicine is that the patient should be treated like a person and not just a disease. Components of holistic medicine are physical, social, emotional, and spiritual, and include lifestyle changes. Many departments must work together in the common interest of the patient. Therefore, instead of fixing the ailment with only pharmaceuticals, a holistic approach will facilitate treatment by alternative methods to cure the disease and not mask the symptoms.

1-25a Patient Education

Patient education in all aspects of their care is highly important. A patient should always understand the importance of each treatment and procedure. Instructing how to properly perform each treatment and explaining the purpose will greatly increase the chances of the patient continuing therapy on her or his own. It should be mentioned that including the patient's family members in patient education helps to reinforce proper technique, as well as ensure the likelihood of the patient continuing therapy once discharged.

LEARNING OBJECTIVE 1.6 **Describe the use of standard precautions and personal protection equipment.**

KEY TERMS

Gloves Latex, vinyl, or nitrile; worn to protect hands from coming into contact with any type of patient fluid or mucous membrane secretions.

Gowns Protective garment used to protect clothing and skin from infectious exposures.

Masks Facial covering to protect a clinicians face, nose and mouth from body fluids and secretions.

Personal Protective Equipment (PPE) Clothing and equipment used to prevent bodily fluid contact.

Respirator Specialized mask used for droplet airway infections.

Standard precautions Set of steps and procedures that protects not only the clinician, but the patient from exposure to infectious microorganisms.

1-26 STANDARD PRECAUTIONS

To ensure total protection for both patient and clinician, it is assumed that every patient has an infectious disease. **Standard precautions** are a basic form of protection that protects not only the clinician, but the patient from exposure to infectious microorganisms. These precautions are used whether or not a patient has a confirmed or suspected disease, Figure 1-26.

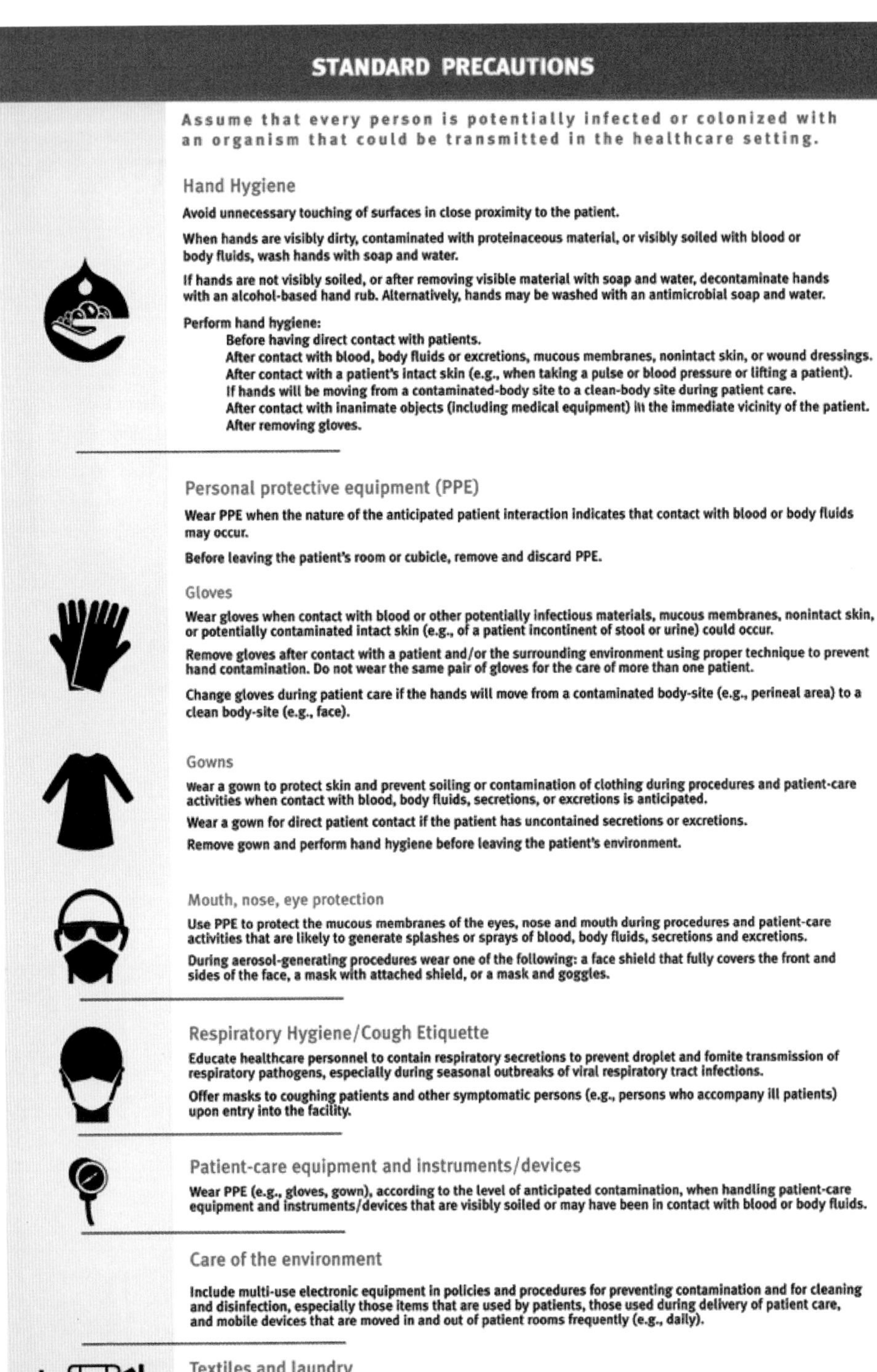

STANDARD PRECAUTIONS

Assume that every person is potentially infected or colonized with an organism that could be transmitted in the healthcare setting.

Hand Hygiene

Avoid unnecessary touching of surfaces in close proximity to the patient.

When hands are visibly dirty, contaminated with proteinaceous material, or visibly soiled with blood or body fluids, wash hands with soap and water.

If hands are not visibly soiled, or after removing visible material with soap and water, decontaminate hands with an alcohol-based hand rub. Alternatively, hands may be washed with an antimicrobial soap and water.

Perform hand hygiene:
- Before having direct contact with patients.
- After contact with blood, body fluids or excretions, mucous membranes, nonintact skin, or wound dressings.
- After contact with a patient's intact skin (e.g., when taking a pulse or blood pressure or lifting a patient).
- If hands will be moving from a contaminated-body site to a clean-body site during patient care.
- After contact with inanimate objects (including medical equipment) in the immediate vicinity of the patient.
- After removing gloves.

Personal protective equipment (PPE)

Wear PPE when the nature of the anticipated patient interaction indicates that contact with blood or body fluids may occur.

Before leaving the patient's room or cubicle, remove and discard PPE.

Gloves

Wear gloves when contact with blood or other potentially infectious materials, mucous membranes, nonintact skin, or potentially contaminated intact skin (e.g., of a patient incontinent of stool or urine) could occur.

Remove gloves after contact with a patient and/or the surrounding environment using proper technique to prevent hand contamination. Do not wear the same pair of gloves for the care of more than one patient.

Change gloves during patient care if the hands will move from a contaminated body-site (e.g., perineal area) to a clean body-site (e.g., face).

Gowns

Wear a gown to protect skin and prevent soiling or contamination of clothing during procedures and patient-care activities when contact with blood, body fluids, secretions, or excretions is anticipated.

Wear a gown for direct patient contact if the patient has uncontained secretions or excretions.

Remove gown and perform hand hygiene before leaving the patient's environment.

Mouth, nose, eye protection

Use PPE to protect the mucous membranes of the eyes, nose and mouth during procedures and patient-care activities that are likely to generate splashes or sprays of blood, body fluids, secretions and excretions.

During aerosol-generating procedures wear one of the following: a face shield that fully covers the front and sides of the face, a mask with attached shield, or a mask and goggles.

Respiratory Hygiene/Cough Etiquette

Educate healthcare personnel to contain respiratory secretions to prevent droplet and fomite transmission of respiratory pathogens, especially during seasonal outbreaks of viral respiratory tract infections.

Offer masks to coughing patients and other symptomatic persons (e.g., persons who accompany ill patients) upon entry into the facility.

Patient-care equipment and instruments/devices

Wear PPE (e.g., gloves, gown), according to the level of anticipated contamination, when handling patient-care equipment and instruments/devices that are visibly soiled or may have been in contact with blood or body fluids.

Care of the environment

Include multi-use electronic equipment in policies and procedures for preventing contamination and for cleaning and disinfection, especially those items that are used by patients, those used during delivery of patient care, and mobile devices that are moved in and out of patient rooms frequently (e.g., daily).

Textiles and laundry

Handle used textiles and fabrics with minimum agitation to avoid contamination of air, surfaces and persons.

SPR

©2007 Brevis Corporation www.brevis.com

FIGURE 1-26 Standard precautions chart.

Hand hygiene is a simple, yet highly effective way to prevent the spread of infectious diseases. Even if gloves were worn, hand washing is done before and after patient contact. Another way to cleanse hands is by using an alcohol hand rub. Hand sanitizer is a temporary method of cleaning hands before and after coming in contact with a patient. That being said, it is important to remember that hand sanitizer does not replace proper hand washing with soap and water. In addition, there are situations when hand washing is not enough and personal protective equipment should be donned. It is also important to keep in mind that proper hand washing techniques should be done before and after putting on personal protective equipment.

1-27 PERSONAL PROTECTIVE EQUIPMENT

Personal Protective Equipment (PPE) is worn during specific procedures that greatly increase the odds of the provider coming into contact with body fluids. PPE consists of gloves, gowns, eye protection (goggles or face shields), and masks, or respirators, Figure 1-27.

Let's begin by protecting our hands. **Gloves** come in latex, vinyl, or nitrile versions; because patients can have latex allergies, it may be less likely to find latex gloves in the field. Gloves must be worn when coming into contact with any type of patient fluid or mucous membrane secretions. Gloves are single use only and are not to be reused and should be properly disposed of after each use.

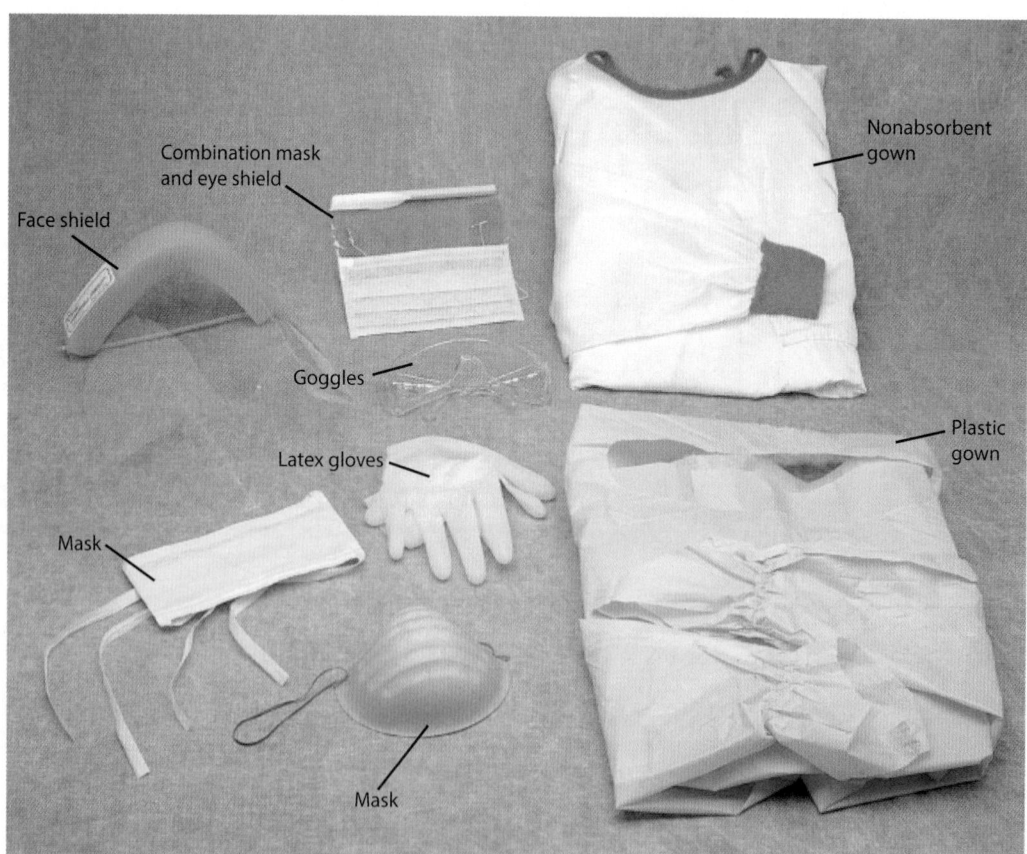

FIGURE 1-27 Examples of personal protective equipment.

In addition, not all types of gloves can be used for sterile procedures. For example, the boxes of gloves located in a patient's room are clean, but not sterile. Sterile gloves come in special packaging and kits.

Occasionally, blood and other body fluids may potentially splash or spray. In these situations, **gowns** are used to protect clothing and skin from exposures. Gowns are worn like a backwards robe and should be tied to remain secure and prevent falling during a procedure. Gowns should only be used once and should be discarded after the procedure.

So, what do we use to protect our face? **Masks** should be worn to protect a clinicians face, nose, and mouth from body fluids and secretions generated from the patient care procedures. Masks also protect the patient from the clinician during invasive procedures. Some masks have shields attached to protect the eyes, which is a convenient form of eye protection. Always keep in mind that eye glasses are not a substitute for a face shield or googles.

To protect our lungs, we can wear a respirator. A **respirator** is utilized when dealing with droplet airway infections and a regular mask will not be enough. Tuberculosis is an example of a time when this type of device is needed.

Module 2

Mechanism of Disease

Module Introduction

In Module 1, we discussed the basic principles of disease. Now, let's build on those concepts by identifying the mechanisms of disease. As you can imagine, diseases have many sources, which can make the topic quite overwhelming. To help make it easier to understand, we will break up the sources into several distinct categories.

LEARNING OBJECTIVE 2.1 Explain the various sources of disease.

KEY TERMS

Benign Noncancerous tumor.

Cachexia Describes thin and wasting away appearance.

Cancer Malignant cell growth.

Chromosomal disorders Abnormality of a whole or partial chromosome.

Congenital disease An inherited disease at birth that may not be experienced until later in life or fetal damage due to maternal trauma.

Enteral route Administering substances through the GI tract, including oral, feeding tubes, and rectal routes.

Hyperplasia An overgrowth of tissue in response to a stimulus.

Malignant Cancerous cell growth.

Malnutrition Poor nutrition.

Multifactorial disorders Caused by the abnormality of many genes.

Nasogastric tube (NG) A tube that is passed through the nasal passage and into the stomach for a short-term feeding solution.

Neoplasm A new growth called a tumor.

Parenteral route Substance given by an injection.

Percutaneous endoscopic gastrostomy procedure The procedure for inserting a feeding tube through the abdomen and into the stomach.

Percutaneous endoscopic gastrostomy (PEG) tube The actual tube used to administer fluids, medications, and nutrition.

Single gene Likely to be a recessive or an inherited disorder.

Tissue degeneration Tissues cannot replace the cells as efficiently with old age.

Total parenteral nutrition (TPN) All nutrition is received through a vein.

Trauma Physical injury or a disturbing experience.

2-1 CONGENITAL DISEASE

Many diseases can occur during one's life, and many of them can be avoided by making healthy decisions. However, sometimes diseases can still occur regardless of the choices made, especially if someone is born with a certain genetic predisposition or inherited characteristic. An individual's genetic or hereditary traits can greatly increase the risk of certain diseases. Some people might be affected by an inherited disease at birth or they might not experience the disease until later in their lifetime, either way, it is known as a **congenital disease**. It is important to realize that the disease being passed onto the fetus from the parents' DNA is only one cause of congenital disease. A congenital disease can also occur during pregnancy in different ways, such as if the mother is in an accident that injures the fetus or if she ingests drugs or alcohol during her pregnancy. An example of this type of congenital disease is fetal alcohol syndrome.

Hereditary disorders are classified into three different categories:

- Chromosomal
- Single gene
- Multifactorial.

Chromosomal disorders arise from an abnormality of a whole or partial chromosome. An example is Turner syndrome, which occurs when a female does not inherit an X chromosome from either the mother or father, resulting in one less X chromosome than normal. A **single-gene** abnormality is more likely to be a recessive or an inherited disorder. If both parents have abnormal genes, it is possible the child will have an abnormality. An example is cystic fibrosis, in which the individual will have pancreatic dysfunction resulting in the inability to properly absorb nutrients as well as pulmonary involvement causing excessive mucus production in the airways. **Multifactorial disorders** derive from the abnormality of many abnormal genes, resulting in brain and heart diseases (see Figure 2-1).

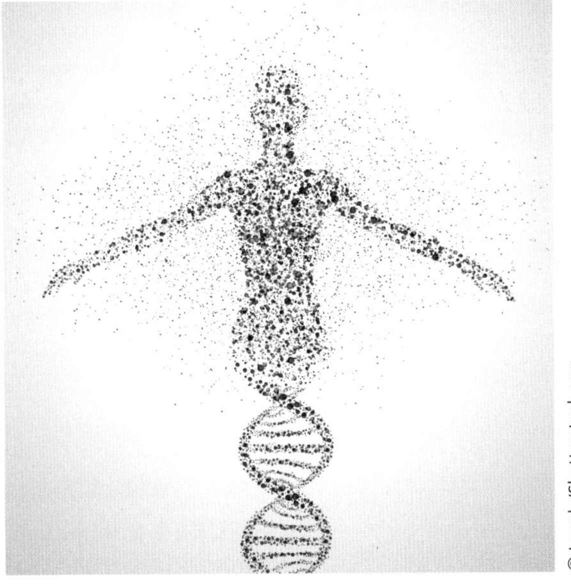

© Lonely/Shutterstock.com.

FIGURE 2-1 Our genes make up who we are.

2-2 AGE

Another factor that can be a source of disease is age because as we get older our body has more difficulty maintaining homeostasis. As a person ages, **tissue degeneration** that occurs makes it difficult to fight infection and repair itself as efficiently. Bone density peaks around age 35; after that, it decreases in both men and women. More precisely, 1% of bone density is lost every year from ages 55 to 75. Also occurring as we age is a decrease in lean body mass. Our body fat increases, particularly accumulating in the abdominal region between 25 and 45 years of age, peaking at age 40. Even though this sounds terrible, there is still a light at the end of the tunnel. On a much lighter note, in spite of the accumulation of fat and slowing of reflexes that accompanies aging, people are living longer lives now than any time in history. Thanks to advances in research and technology, we have a growing older population.

2-3 NUTRITION IMBALANCES AND DISEASE

Proper nutrition is vital to maintain a healthy body. Nutrition follows the concepts of, "good in, good out" and "garbage in, garbage out." If you put diesel fuel in a car that uses unleaded gasoline, its function will be greatly impaired. In a person, poor nutrition or **malnutrition** will result in poor body development and decreased cognitive ability and, in severe cases, death can occur (see Figure 2-2).

It is important to recognize that malnutrition can happen in different ways. A disease can impair the body's ability to break down and absorb nutrients. Also, what people consume can have a direct effect on their body's nutrition. Those most likely to be affected by poor nutrition are children and senior citizens.

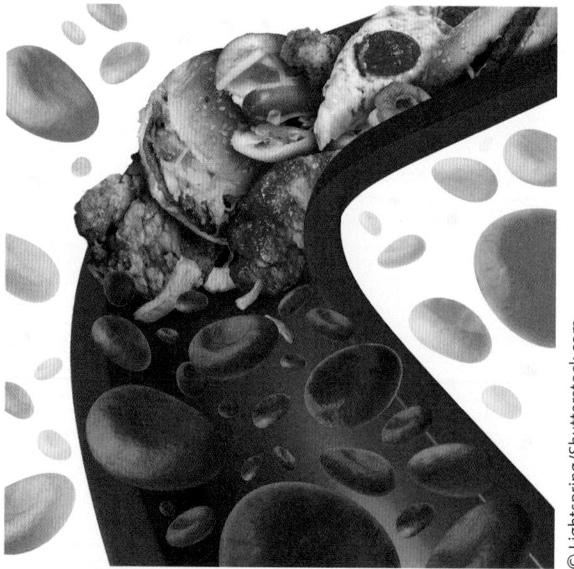

FIGURE 2-2 Although this picture is an exaggeration, it shows that what we consume does make it to our bloodstream.

2-4 MALNUTRITION

Diseases such as cancer can cause malnutrition. For instance, cancer cells grow quickly and out of control, and this rapid growth takes a lot of energy, causing the patient to burn through calories that would otherwise be used for the body's nutrition. Nutritional supplements can be given to the patient to help combat a poor nutritional state. If patients are too weak to eat or drink, they will be provided nutrition via the **parenteral route**, which is given by an injection. When a patient receives all nutrition through a vein, it is known as **total parenteral nutrition (TPN)**.

Another method to provide nutrition is by way of the **enteral route** meaning via the gastrointestinal or GI system. If patients cannot orally consume their food, a **percutaneous endoscopic gastrostomy procedure** is done to insert a feeding tube or **percutaneous endoscopic gastrostomy (PEG) tube**. As shown in Figure 2-3, a PEG tube is used to administer medications, fluids, and nutrition from a small, flexible, plastic tube that is inserted into the abdomen and through the stomach wall. A PEG tube is used as a long-term solution.

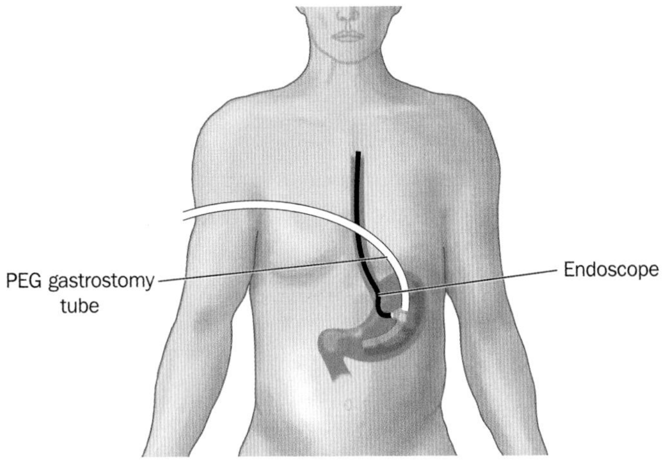

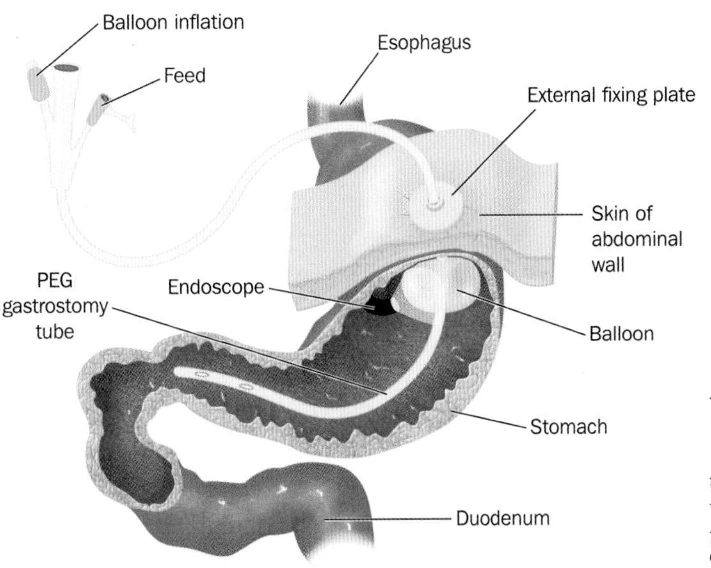

FIGURE 2-3 Illustration of a PEG tube inside the stomach.

Now, what if the patient requires only a short-term solution? If this is the case, a **nasogastric tube (NG)** would be used instead. The feeding tube is passed through the patient's nasal passage and then into the stomach. Once the patient can resume normal feedings, the tube is removed.

CLINICAL CONNECTION 2.1

MEDICATION ADMINISTRATION WITH A PEG TUBE

We discussed what a PEG tube is used for, but did you know medications can be given via this route? Here are a few clinical pearls to keep in mind. When administering drugs through a PEG tube, the drugs must be either in liquid form or crushed and mixed with water. Remember that it is important to make sure the medications can be delivered in this manner. Also, since fluid is given with the drugs, the patient's fluid intake must be carefully monitored, which includes the fluid used to flush the PEG tube itself after each dose.

2-5 VITAMIN/MINERAL EXCESS AND DEFICIENCY

Another aspect to consider is whether an individual gets the proper amount of minerals and vitamins their body needs to function efficiently. Therefore, too much or too little of a good thing can have undesired consequences. If an individual does not get the necessary amounts of minerals and vitamins, it might result in fatigue and a weakened immune system. For example, if a patient lacks calcium (hypocalcemia) needed for bone growth, he or she will be more likely to have weak bones and be likely to suffer from osteoporosis. However, if a person has too much calcium (hypercalcemia), instead of going to the bones, the excess mineral will go to the arteries, causing plaque that can clog the arteries and increase the risk of a heart attack or stroke.

Caution must be taken when using supplements. As with all the other drugs that will be discussed in this text, adverse side effects can occur if not taken properly. Supplements can also affect other medications the patient is taking. Therefore, it is extremely important to notify your physician of any OTC supplements you are using (see Figure 2-4).

2-6 OBESITY

Looking at Figure 2-5, it should be no surprise that obesity puts more stress on the body, especially the heart. The obesity epidemic is also a main contributor to disease, such as heart disease, cancer, diabetes, and problems with joints. Obesity costs the United States $150 billion per year, which is nearly 10% of the nation's healthcare budget. Unhealthy foods replace nutritious choices and are readily consumed with little regard to portion sizes. Lack of exercise also can contribute to obesity. Ultimately, these poor choices shorten the life expectancy of the individual and prevent the body from getting the nutrition needed to thrive. If we consider the risk factors for disease studied in Module 1, obesity would fall under lifestyle choices, because almost all cases are preventable.

For example, type II diabetes occurs when a person consumes more calories, sugars, and fats than his or her body can burn and properly maintain. Type II diabetes is predominately seen in middle-aged and older Americans; however, cases are increasing among school children because of poor diets. In an effort to

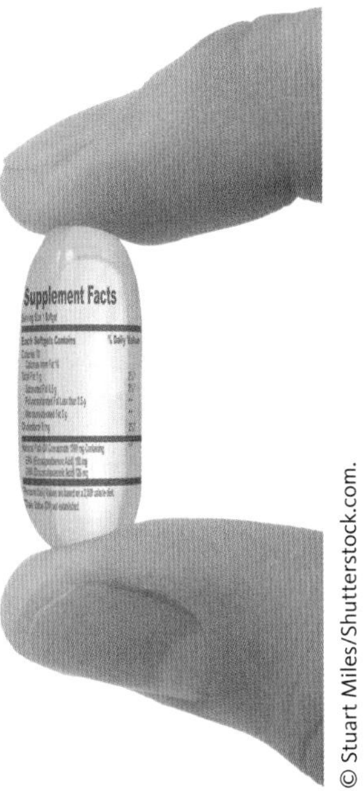

FIGURE 2-4 OTC supplements can interact with prescribed medications. Consult with your physician before taking.

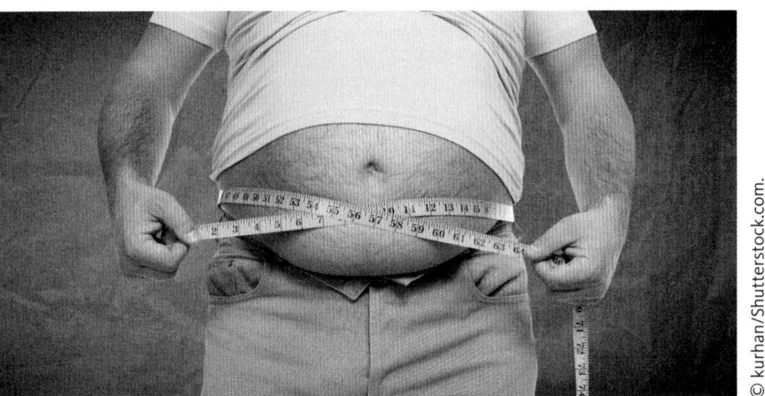

FIGURE 2-5 Overweight male.

help prevent students from becoming overweight or diabetic, school administrators have been pulling vending machines from cafeterias. Some people view this as a positive change, while others claim it is unfair and overreaching. However, when one in three adults and one in six children are obese, it is evident that changes need to be made somewhere.

2-7 NEW AND EXCESSIVE GROWTHS

New and excessive growths can occur in any body tissue and therefore anywhere in the body. As expected, it is very frightening for a patient when a new growth is discovered. A new growth can be either a **hyperplasia** or **neoplasm**. A hyperplasia is an overgrowth of the *same* tissue in response to some sort of a stimulus. Neoplasms, or tumors in layman's terms, are *new growths* made up of different cells or tissues. The word "neoplasm" literally means "new growth," and this new growth can be either benign (noncancerous) or malignant (cancerous).

Cancer cells grow out of control, depleting the body of the nutrition it would use as fuel for more cell growth. This causes malnutrition in the patient, making them thin and weak. The term used to describe this wasting away from an ailment is cachexia. Table 2-1 illustrates the differences between benign and malignant growths. Cancer will be discussed in more depth in Module 5.

2-8 TRAUMA

Trauma results from either a physical injury or a disturbing experience (mental trauma). In this text, we will focus only on physical injury. A physical trauma can occur in many different ways, including motor vehicle accidents (MVAs), gunshot wounds (GSWs), stabbings, burns, and falls. Secondary to a traumatic physical injury, many diseases, such as acute respiratory distress syndrome (ARDS), severe chest trauma, pulmonary embolism, and traumatic brain injury (TBI), can occur, further damaging the body's tissues and complicating the patient's well-being. If trauma is not managed correctly, infection is likely to occur.

Table 2-1 Differences between noncancerous and cancerous growths

BENIGN	MALIGNANT
Noncancerous	Cancerous
Rarely fatal	Can be fatal
Encapsulated cell growth (enclosed in a capsule)	Cells grow in a disorganized manner and have very little to no functionality
Does not invade other tissues (noninvasive) but can interfere with body functions by compressing organs	Metastasizes or spreads by invading other tissues (invasive)
Slow cell growth	Rapid cell growth

LEARNING OBJECTIVE 2.2 Describe the role of immunity against disease.

KEY TERMS

Acquired immunity Immunity developed over time through pathogenic exposure.

Acquired immunodeficiency syndrome (AIDS) Occurs after HIV exposure after the individual's immune system is severely compromised.

Active acquired immunity Immunity occurring when the body is exposed to a pathogen and produces antibodies to defend itself against reexposure.

Allergens Foreign substances to which the body is hypersensitive.

Allergies Bodily reaction to an allergen exposure.

Anaphylaxis reaction A serious, sometimes life-threatening, allergic reaction.

Autoimmunity A situation in which the immune system fights against its own tissues and cells.

Cell-mediated immunity Consisting of specialized white blood cells (WBCs), it is the body's main defender from foreign substances.

Genetic immunity General ability of our body to respond to an invader based on genetic traits we are born with.

Human immunodeficiency virus (HIV) A virus that progressively attacks the body's immune system by destroying specialized cells called helper T-cells.

Humoral immunity A type of acquired immunity from circulating antibodies.

Immune system Specialized cells, tissues, and organs that fight against and protect our bodies from disease.

Immunity Ability to protect from illness.

Immunodeficiency The inability of the body to defend and protect itself from pathogenic organisms.

Inflammation A bodily process used to kill invaders to allow healing.

Maternal immunity Strengthening of a baby's immune system by receiving antibodies from the mother's breast milk.

Nonspecific inflammation A quick response that locates the foreign invader, kills it, and cleans up the remaining debris to allow healing.

Passive acquired immunity The body acquires antibodies for a specific disease from a vaccine.

Specific immune response An immune action that kills the foreign organisms in a selective process by marking the foreign invader.

Wheals Also known as hives or urticaria, are itchy, raised, red-colored circles resembling welts.

2-9 IMMUNITY

Think back to Module 1 when we mentioned hand hygiene. Do you remember the chain of infection? The easiest way to prevent the chain of infection is to wash your hands and rid the skin of potential pathogens. Our skin acts as a barrier to block pathogens from entering our body. However, if the organism gains access to the body through a portal of entry, such as a mucous membrane or an opening in the skin, the body will have to defend itself in other ways. This is made possible because of our immune system. The immune system is an amazing bodily process and we will discuss it in more detail.

Let's start by asking ourselves, what is **immunity**? Immunity means to be excluded from something. In relation to our body, it means to "exclude" or to protect us from illness. Our body is constantly protected by our **immune system**, which consists of specialized cells, tissues, and organs. To function properly, the immune system requires a healthy diet, plenty of rest, and exercise. Our bodies are protected at birth by our genetic immunity.

2-9a Genetic Immunity

Genetic immunity is the general ability of our body to respond to an invader and depends on factors such as sex, race, and other genetic traits. We are born with an immune system to help us fight diseases. Have you ever wondered why physicians claim breastfeeding is better than formula feeding? In addition to personal preference, breast milk contains disease-fighting antibodies that strengthen a newborn's immune system. This is known as **maternal immunity**. If newborns are fed formula, those antibodies will not be present, so the babies will have to develop them on their own, which take about one month.

2-9b Acquired Immunity

Acquired immunity, unlike genetic immunity, is developed over time as the body is exposed to pathogenic microorganisms and learns to combat them. Acquired immunity can be broken down into two types, active and passive. **Active acquired immunity** takes place when the body is exposed to a pathogen and makes antibodies to defend itself against reexposure. This gives new meaning to the old adage, "what doesn't kill you, makes you stronger."

On the other hand, **passive acquired immunity** is achieved by vaccinations. A vaccination administers weakened or dead strains of an antigen that the body recognizes as a threat and develops antibodies for without causing such a disturbance that the individual becomes sick. This is why physicians tell their elderly patients to make sure they receive pneumonia and influenza vaccines so they will be unlikely to become infected with the actual disease. It also should be noted that many vaccinations are a temporary form of immunity. Some vaccines need to be given only once and protect the person for life. Other vaccines are good only for so long, so a booster is needed to remind the body to enable ongoing protection. Some illnesses, such as influenza, are always mutating and have a variety of different strains, which makes it necessary for vaccinations to be given yearly.

2-9c Types of Acquired Immunity

Now that we have established some of the basics of the acquired immune system, let's break it down even further. The acquired immune system has two different types of protection:

- Cell-mediated immunity
- Humoral immunity.

Cell-mediated immunity is the body's chief defender from foreign substances. This is made possible by a certain type of white blood cell (WBC) known as T-cell lymphocytes. T-cell lymphocytes are developed in the thymus gland, hence the name *T-cells*. When responding to a foreign substance, T-cells release sensitized lymphocytes that travel to the area of invasion (where inflammation is occurring) and activate macrophages that also activate helper T-cells. Helper T-cells release antibodies and macrophages to destroy and ingest foreign microorganisms.

Humoral immunity is a type of acquired immunity that comes from circulating antibodies such as immunoglobulins. Humoral means fluids, and you can think of this as specific antibodies circulating within the body's main fluid—blood. The immunoglobulins mark antigens so the body can identify and destroy the foreign invader. The antibodies are derived from B-lymphocytes, which is a type of WBC (see Figure 2-6).

2-9d Autoimmunity

The immune system is an amazing process, but sometimes it too can fail or go awry. **Autoimmunity** occurs when the body's immune system literally turns on itself ("auto" means "self"). With autoimmune disorders, the immune system fights against body's own normal tissues and cells, causing bodily harm. It is not entirely known what causes autoimmune diseases to occur and unfortunately, there is no cure. A few common types of autoimmune diseases are lupus and celiac diseases, Figure 2-7.

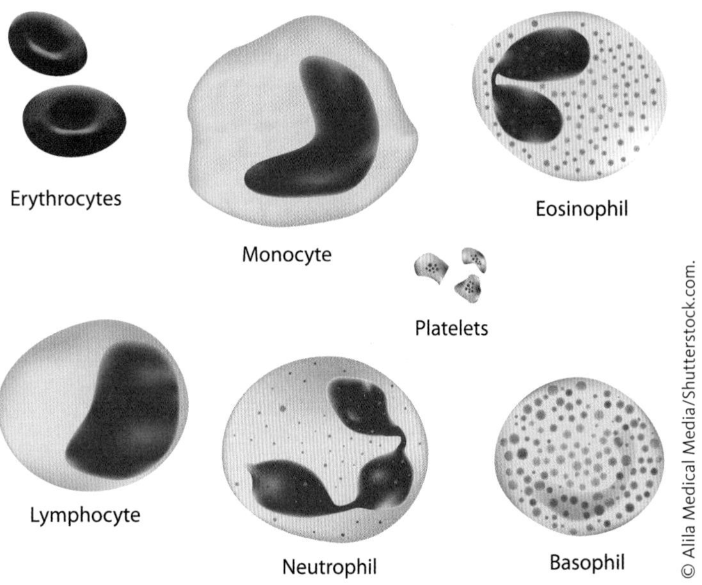

FIGURE 2-6 The cellular components of blood include the erythrocyte or red blood cells for oxygen transport, the platelets to assist clotting, and the various WBCs (monocytes, eosinophils, lymphocytes, neutrophils, and basophils) to fight infection.

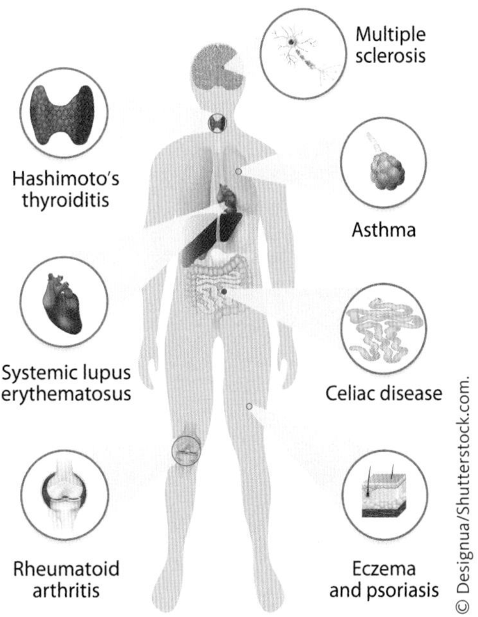

FIGURE 2-7 Various autoimmune diseases and where they are found.

2-9e Immunodeficiency

The immune system also can be affected by **immunodeficiency**, which occurs when the body is unable to defend and protect itself from pathogenic organisms. Patients receiving radiation and chemotherapy suffer from a weakened immune system during treatment, which damages the bone marrow where red blood cells, WBCs, and platelets are produced. The WBCs are needed to help fight infection.

Another example of immunodeficiency is **human immunodeficiency virus (HIV)**, which is the virus that causes **acquired immunodeficiency syndrome** or AIDS. When HIV is introduced to the body, it invades the T-cells, which assist the immune system in fighting infection. However, HIV hijacks these cells and uses them to reproduce. Then the virus leaves the hijacked cell to attack other healthy T-cells. After this process is repeated and repeated, and enough T-cells are destroyed, the person will develop AIDS. Since the immune system is in large part destroyed, those who have AIDS are at greater risk of developing opportunistic infections and often have reoccurring infections. More about HIV/AIDS can be seen in Figure 2-8.

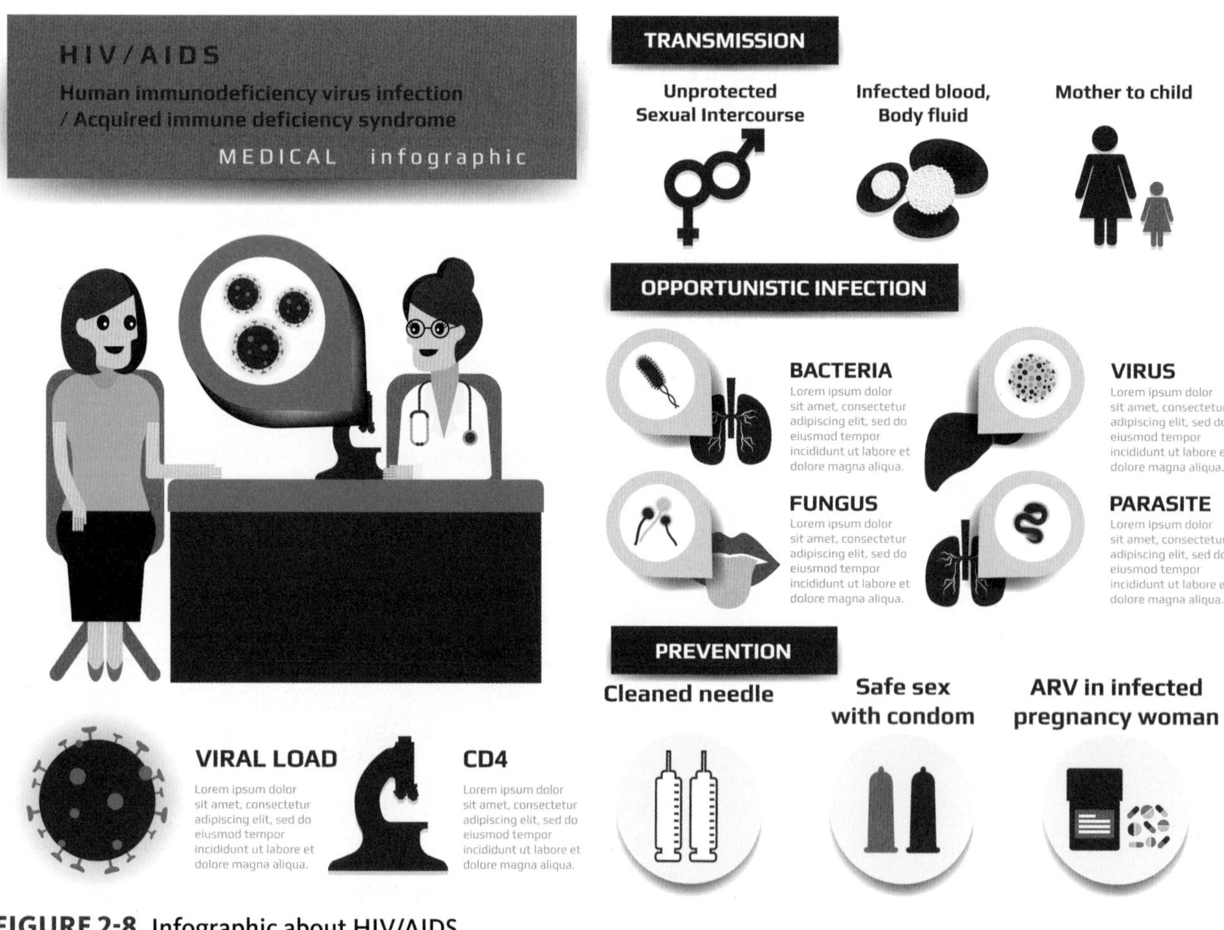

FIGURE 2-8 Infographic about HIV/AIDS.

CLINICAL CONNECTION 2.2

Now that we have talked about the body being attacked by pathogens, resulting in a compromised immune system, we should note that certain procedures used to help a patient regain his or her ability to fight infection require the immune system to be at least partially disarmed. For example, there are occasions when a patient's immune system will be pharmacologically suppressed with high doses of steroids before the patient receives an organ transplant. If the recipient's immune system was not suppressed, it would reject and ultimately kill the transplanted donor organ.

2-9f Allergies

Do you suffer from seasonal **allergies** or know someone who does? Do you know what substance triggers you to have a reaction? Commonly seen **allergens** are pollen, dust mites, pet dander, insect bites, ragweed, and certain foods. Allergic reactions occur when the body's immune system is hyperactive and overreacts to certain types of foreign substances. When this happens, we experience coughing, sneezing, watery eyes, and a runny nose. Other symptoms of an allergic reaction are hives (urticaria), which forms itchy, raised, red-colored circles known as **wheals**. Depending on how the body reacts, hives might be present in a certain area or the entire body. The most serious and life threatening allergic reaction, which results in a loss of blood pressure, is termed an **anaphylaxis reaction**. The patient can use an epinephrine automatic injector to immediately reverse this potentially deadly reaction, Figure 2-9.

Since the potential complications of allergies are dangerous, it is important to figure out what triggers an attack. Triggers (allergens) can be identified by an immunologist or allergist who will diagnose the source of an individual's allergy by examining a blood sample or performing a skin test. Currently, there is no cure, but after the allergen is identified, injections or oral tablets can be given

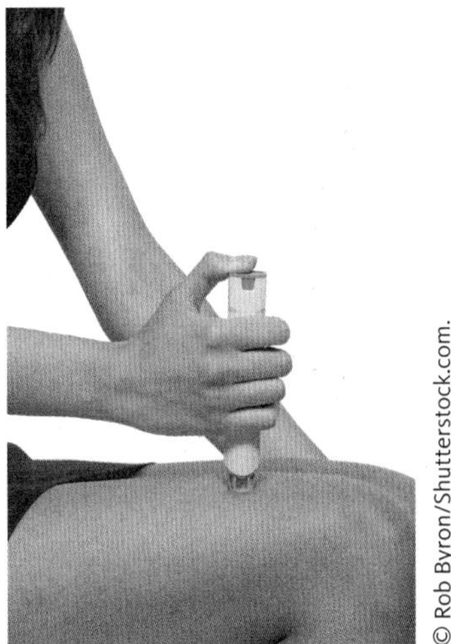

FIGURE 2-9 People with severe allergies should have an epinephrine automatic injector available at all times.

as a form of long-term allergy immunotherapy. Allergic reactions are not only frustrating for many, but can also be severe and even life-threatening.

2-9g Inflammation

Have you ever slammed your finger in a door? Have you ever cut yourself on a sharp object or had a sore throat? Now, what do all of these things have in common? Whether they're caused by a traumatic injury or a pathogenic organism, all incidences will result in inflammation with five cardinal signs:

- Redness
- Pain
- Swelling
- Warmth
- Possible loss of function in the affected location.

Whether you realize it, **inflammation** is a much-needed mechanism of the body. Ideally, before the body has to use its inflammatory mechanism to kill invaders, the microorganism would be caught and blocked by a barrier such as our skin. The surface of the skin is acidic, making it a hostile environment for microorganisms. Glands located just beneath the surface of the skin secrete special enzymes and antibacterial acids, while mucous membranes trap foreign contaminants. However, if a pathogen penetrates this protective barrier, the inflammatory response combats the invasion.

The **nonspecific inflammation** response has many different names, such as *innate* and *native immunity*. We are born with this immunity, and it is permanent. This form of protection does not have a memory or any way of differentiating between pathogens. Therefore, it does not improve with experience. It knows only what does not belong to the body and perceives it as a threat. Therefore, this general response attacks any foreign invader without prejudice by releasing specialized cells to target the affected area and help eliminate and prevent the spread of the foreign invaders. It is followed by another response, known as the specific immune response.

The **specific immune response** or adaptive immunity is developed during the course of one's life, and learns who the pathogens are. As the name implies, this *specific* reaction kills the foreign organisms in a selective process by marking them as foreign antigens. The body then produces specific antibodies that attack and kill the pathogenic cells, and even produces a reserve army of antibodies to prepare the body to seek and destroy the microorganism in the event of another exposure.

But how does this work? Well, for starters, the body can identify cells as "good" or "bad" by the membrane on the outer surface of their molecules. Every organism and human being has their own unique cell surfaces. This distinctive surface allows the body to identify antigens as part of the body (self-recognition) or as a foreign invader (non–self-recognition). The body produces specialized proteins called antigens that attach to foreign invaders and label them as intruding cells, thus marking them to be destroyed by the immune system. Blood proteins called antibodies are then produced to defend the body from the pathogenic antigen.

However, the body can take this mechanism too far (hypersensitive reaction) and actually damage the body to the point of killing the individual. This is typically seen with chronic disease conditions that interfere with the normal way the body functions. People with hypersensitive airways can experience difficulty breathing when they are exposed to an allergen. The body responds with airway inflammation, causing constriction and difficulty breathing. If chronic infection occurs, the airways can actually be remodeled, or permanently disfigured. We will discuss this inflammatory process in more detail later in this module (see Figure 2-10).

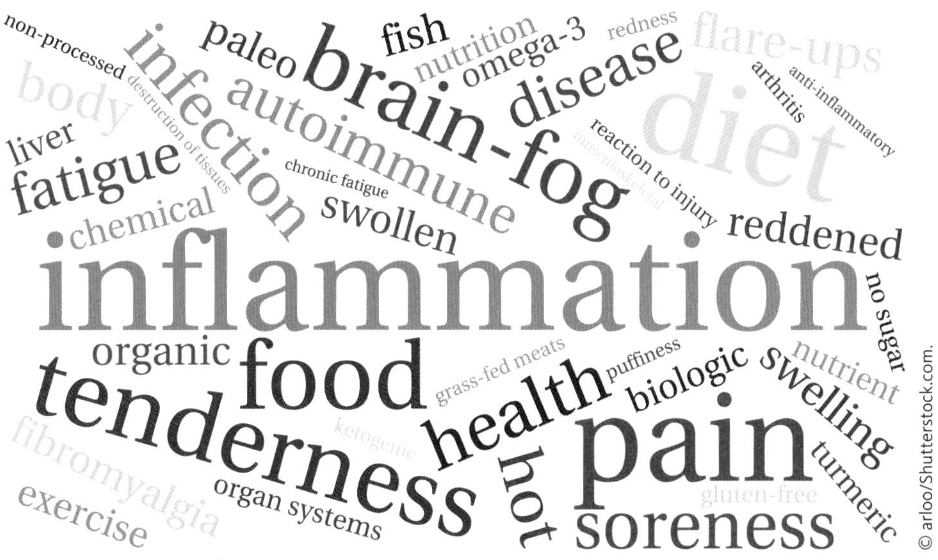

FIGURE 2-10 Words associated with inflammation.

LEARNING OBJECTIVE 2.3 Identify types of infections.

KEY TERMS

Anthelmintics A class of drugs used to treat worm infections.

Antibiotics A class of drugs used to treat bacterial infections.

Antivirals A class of drugs used to treat viral infections.

Bacteria Single-celled microorganisms.

Capsid A virus's outer coating.

Fungus A plant-like organism spread by spores.

Helminths Parasitic worms.

Hookworms Type of parasitic worms, found in tropical regions of the world, that enter the body through the bare feet of those walking on contaminated soil.

Infection Invasion of pathogenic microorganisms.

Methicillin-resistant *Staphylococcus aureus* (MRSA) An antibiotic-resistant strain of bacteria.

Mycosis A disease caused by a fungus.

Normal flora Native bacteria needed for normal body function.

Opportunistic organisms Invade regions of the body causing illness when given the opportunity.

Pinworms The most common parasitic intestinal worm infection in the United States.

Primary infection Infection resulting from first exposure to pathogen.

Protozoa One-cell members of the animal kingdom found in soil and water.

Rickettsiae Nonmotile bacteria.

Secondary infection An infection developing as a result of another illness or injury.

Tapeworms Intestinal parasites found in both humans and animals.

Viruses Microorganisms smaller than bacteria and that require a host cell to reproduce.

2-10 INFECTION

There are many different ways **infection** can occur. We are exposed every day to many pathogens that can cause infection. Even bacteria found in certain areas of our own body can harm us. Known as **normal flora**, these bacteria are needed for normal body function. For example, we have microorganisms that live in our intestines to aid in digestion. However, if something causes these same beneficial organisms to enter our bloodstream, a serious infection can develop.

Sometimes drugs can wipe out the normal flora in our body and other microorganisms can seize this opportunity to occupy that space. These organisms are known as **opportunistic organisms**, and they can invade other regions of the body causing illness.

Even though this is true, we do not fall ill every day because the body's defense mechanism or immune system constantly defends us from exposures. Although on occasion, as discussed in Module 1, a pathogenic organism can gain access to our body through portals of entry. When that happens, the inflammation process occurs in response to the invasion.

CLINICAL CONNECTION 2.3

OPPORTUNISTIC INFECTION

An example of an opportunistic infection seen in patients is the fungus known as *Candida albicans*. This organism is present in our mouth in small amounts. However, our normal flora keeps this fungus in check and prevents it from growing out of control in the mouth. Inhaled steroids, however, can suppress our normal flora, and if the balance is disturbed, the fungal infection known as thrush can take over, as seen in Figure 2-11. This is why it is critical that patients rinse their mouths after taking an inhaled steroid.

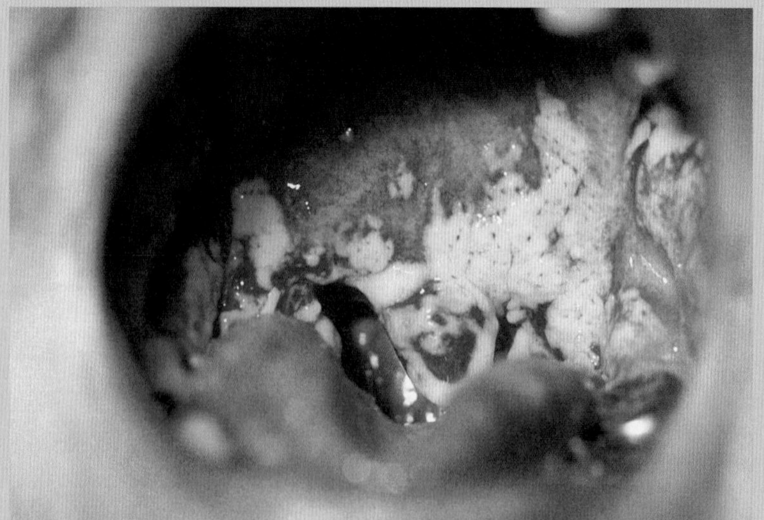

Centers for Disease Control and Prevention

FIGURE 2-11 Thrush found in a patient's mouth.

Infection can occur from many different organisms, such as bacteria, viruses, fungi, protozoa, helminths (worms), and rickettsiae. We will cover these types of infection in greater depth in the following sections.

2-10a Bacterial Infections

Bacteria are single-celled microorganisms that are the major causes of infection. Bacteria, which are larger than viruses, replicate by splitting in half and grow at a very quick rate, in some cases doubling in as little as a half-hour. Therefore, one cell becomes two, then four, then eight, etc. A bacterium does not need a living host to survive. Some bacteria are beneficial and vital for the body to function properly. For example, our intestines have many different bacteria that call that area home, but if it finds its way to another region, an infection will occur.

Bacteria are known to cause both primary and secondary infections. When a person is first exposed to a bacterial pathogen and becomes infected, it is known as a **primary infection**, and if the patient develops an infection as a result of another illness or injury, it is a **secondary infection**. For example, a bacterial pneumonia is a primary infection, but a bacterial pneumonia that develops after a viral pneumonia would be a secondary infection.

Antibiotics are used to treat patients with bacterial infections. Have you ever heard a physician or pharmacist say, "Take your antibiotics until all the medicine is gone, even if you feel better"? The reason is so the bacteria will be completely eliminated and will be unable to sustain their ability to live in the body. If medications are stopped too soon, such as when a patient hoards the remainder of his or her pills for when he or she gets sick again, the bacteria will become harder and more resistant to that antibiotic. Some bacteria such as *Staphylococcus aureus*, which is responsible for causing **methicillin-resistant *Staphylococcus aureus*, or MRSA**, has developed in this manner. MRSA is a commonly found antibiotic-resistant strain, which makes it potentially dangerous. This is why hand hygiene and proper cleaning techniques are so important in the healthcare setting to prevent the spread of this type of infection.

In upcoming modules, we will discuss specific antibiotics that are used to treat various bacterial diseases that can affect different body systems. Bacteria can come in various shapes that help identify the causative microorganism, Figure 2-12.

2-10b Viral Disease

Viruses are smaller than bacteria and spread differently. A virus needs a host to survive, and it cannot reproduce on its own. A virus must hijack a cell to use it as a host cell in order to replicate. The virus contains its genetic coding material within its outer covering, known as a **capsid**. The virus reprograms the host cell to replicate more virus cells, which in turn hijack even more host cells, continuing the process. Viruses can mutate and change over time, so more than one method is needed to fight them. Lymphocytes are a type of white blood cell that is the chief combatant against viruses (see Figure 2-13).

Antibiotics will not kill a virus, instead **antivirals** are used to disable and stop the virus from replicating. An antibiotic might be given to a patient with a primary viral infection because of a secondary bacterial infection.

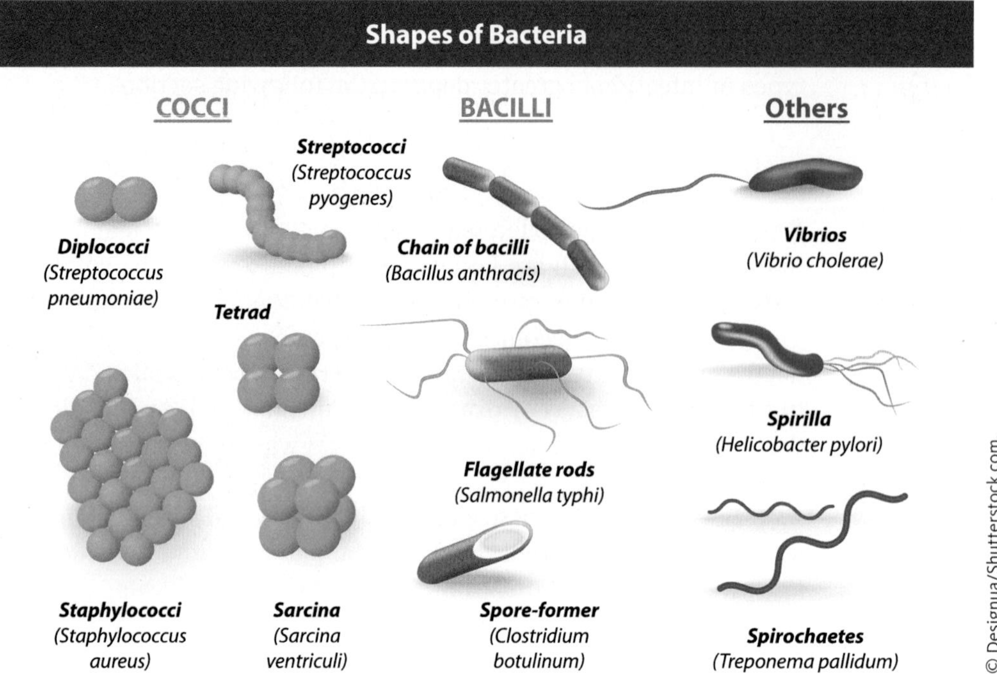

FIGURE 2-12 Bacterial morphology (study of different shapes).

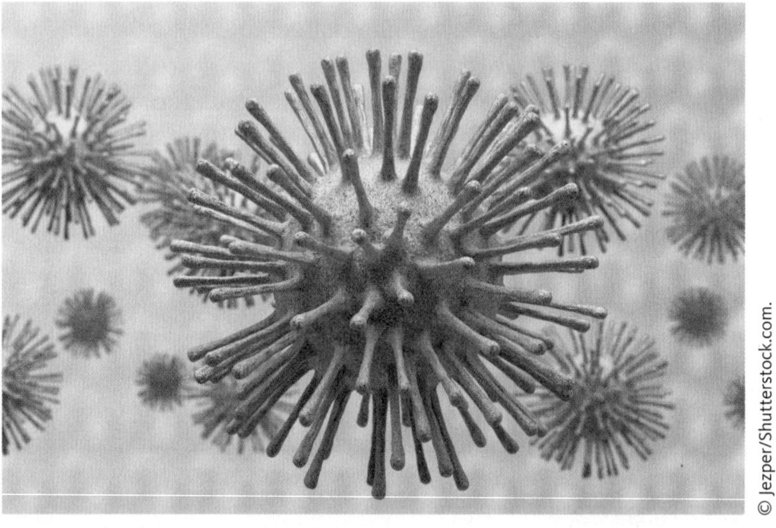

FIGURE 2-13 Illustration of a virus.

Commonly seen infections caused by viruses are influenza, respiratory syncytial virus (RSV) that affects children, and chicken pox. Shingles is derived from the varicella zoster virus that causes chicken pox. It can lay dormant in nerve cells for years, becoming active later in the individual's life. The herpes simplex virus is an example of a virus that is responsible for flare-ups of infections, such as cold sores, a blister-like infection that occurs on the outside of the mouth around the lips.

In upcoming modules, we will discuss specific antiviral agents that are used to treat various viral diseases that can affect different body systems.

In addition, certain viruses can be prevented by vaccination and these will also be discussed in later modules.

2-10c Fungal Disease

The plural term for **fungus**, a plant-like organism, is fungi. Like bacteria, fungi can be harmless. One classic example is the macroscopic edible mushroom, which is a large tasty fungal growth. However, when fungi cause a disease, it is referred to as a **mycosis**. Fungi are spread throughout our environment via spores. Those with a healthy immune system are not affected by fungi. Those with a weakened or compromised immune system from prolonged antibiotic usage or a disease such as AIDS are highly susceptible to fungal growths. In addition, fungal spores can be inhaled, causing many different types of respiratory infection.

Healthy individuals are not completely exempt from fungal infections. Tinea, or ringworm, is shown in Figure 2-14. Unlike its name suggests, ringworm is not actually a worm but is caused by a fungus. Two forms of ringworm are athlete's foot and jock itch. Ringworm is contagious and spread through contact with an infected person.

Individuals who do not rinse out their mouths after using corticosteroid inhalers will kill the normal flora in the mouth. This makes the patient susceptible to a painful fungal infection known as *Candida albicans*, or thrush, that was shown in Figure 2-11. Other common fungal infections are caused by yeast, which are single-celled forms of fungi. Treatment of fungal infections is done

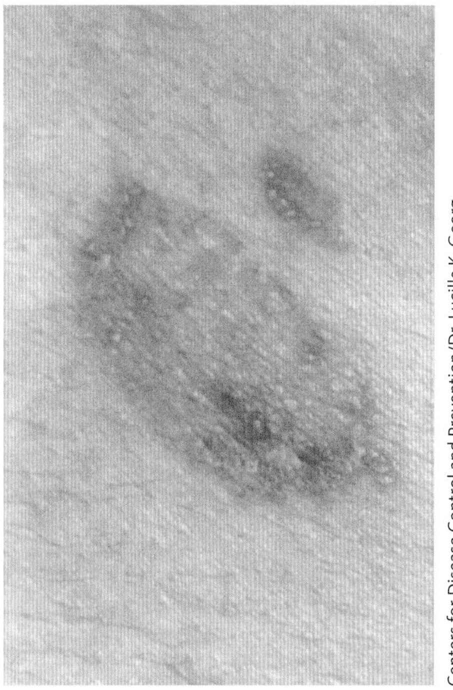

Centers for Disease Control and Prevention/Dr. Lucille K. Georg

FIGURE 2-14 A lesion diagnosed as ringworm as a result of a fungal organism. This itchy infection can occur in almost any area of the body, including the scalp, legs, arms, feet groin, and nails. The skin cracks and becomes scaly with a red, ring-shaped rash.

with antifungal medications, which can be applied directly to the site of the infection. The drugs can also be given orally or injected if the infection is more severe. Specific agents will be discussed in the upcoming modules about body systems.

CLINICAL CONNECTION 2.4

Some patients are more prone to fungal infections than others. However, the type of disease can also depend on where the individual lives. Did you know that some fungal diseases are endemic, meaning they are dependent on specific geographical regions, and this can determine what type of fungal infections a patient is likely to encounter? For example, take a look at three fungal diseases seen in different regions of the United States.

Blastomycosis is a fungal disease that affects people living in the South-Central and Midwestern United States and Canada. Coccidioidomycosis is found in the hot and dry regions of the United States, such as the California, Arizona, and New Mexico. Lastly, the most common fungal disease in the United States is histoplasmosis. Areas with high occurrences of this illness are found along the major river valleys of the Midwest.

2-10d Rickettsiae

Rickettsiae are bacteria that are nonmotile, meaning they do not move on their own. That being said, rickettsia needs a host in order to live and spread, but how is this organism transferred to susceptible hosts? This bacterium spreads by way of types of insects called anthropods such as ticks, lice, fleas, and mites. Infections, which can be life-threatening, are treated with antibiotic therapy. Although Rocky Mountain spotted fever is a rare disease affecting less than 20,000 people a year, it is caused by rickettsia infection. This illness is often transmitted by a tick bite, which causes a rash that looks like spots on the patient's body as shown in Figure 2-15. Other symptoms are a loss of appetite, fever, muscle pain, and headaches. If addressed early with antibiotics, the illness lasts anywhere from days to a few weeks. However, if not treated during its early onset, serious damage can occur to the heart and kidneys.

2-10e Protozoa

Protozoa are one-celled members of the animal kingdom. These microorganisms can be found in the soil and water of our environment. Protozoa can also be found living on decaying or dying organisms and can be acquired if someone drinks water that contains these organisms. Another way these organisms can be spread is through mosquitoes. In Module 1, we learned a mosquito is a biological vector, which in this case means it carries a specific well-known protozoan that causes malaria. Malaria is very deadly because it destroys the red blood cells of those infected, as shown in Figure 2-16. Protozoan infections are treated with antibiotic therapy.

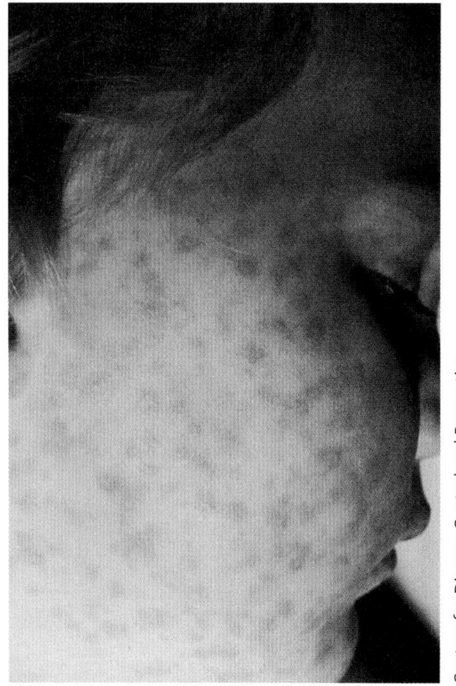

FIGURE 2-15 The rash on the child's face is characteristic of Rocky Mountain spotted fever.

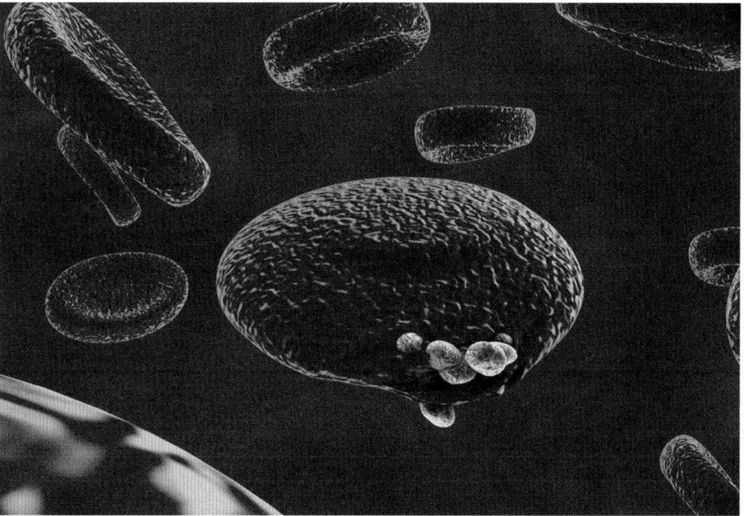

FIGURE 2-16 Red blood cell infected with protozoa in malaria.

2-10f Helminths

Unlike most pathogenic organisms, **helminths** are large enough to be seen without the aid of a microscope. Helminths are parasitic worms that are broadly categorized as flatworms (tapeworms), roundworms (pinworms and hookworms), and flukes. Helminths are commonly found in third-world countries because of poor sanitation and are less likely seen in developed countries. These organisms can survive in both humans and nature, just as a protozoan. There are many different species of parasitic worms, and we will discuss a few that are most common.

Did you know that a tapeworm can live up to 30 years of age? Shown in Figure 2-17, **tapeworms** are an intestinal parasite that can be found in both humans and animals. Animals such as pigs and cows can become infected if the worm is ingested. Humans become infected by eating undercooked beef or pork that has been contaminated by tapeworms. Larvae from the tapeworm have the potential to migrate elsewhere in the host's body, such as the brain or other tissues. Testing individuals for tapeworm is done by examining a stool sample for any worm eggs. Pharmacological intervention is accomplished through a class of drugs used to treat worm infections called **anthelmintics**. Albedazole is an example of a drug used to rid the person of worms.

The most commonly caused parasitic intestinal worm infection in the United States is caused by **pinworms**. Pinworms are white, small, and thin, with a maximum length of about a half-inch, Figure 2-18. Pinworms are transmitted

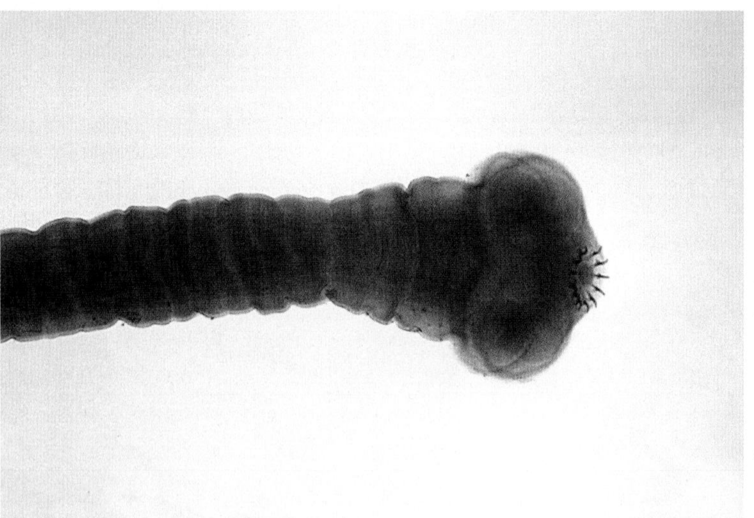

Centers for Disease Control and Prevention/Dr. Mae Melvin

FIGURE 2-17 Microscopic image of the anterior end of parasitic pork tapeworm.

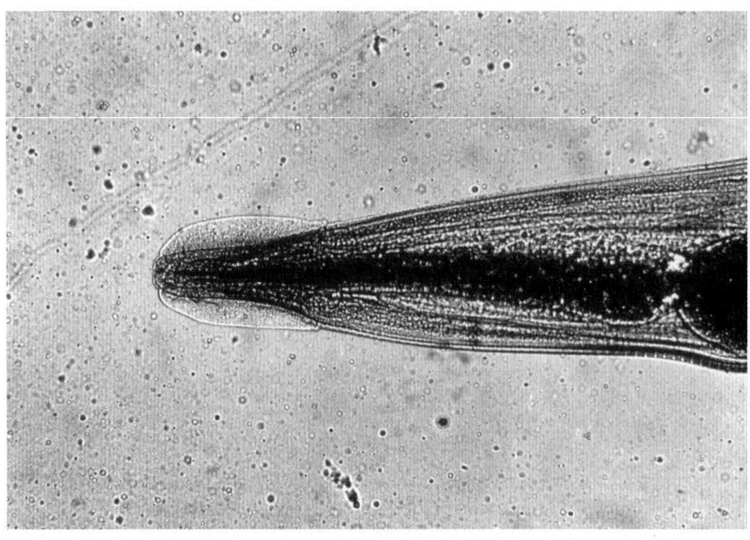

Centers for Disease Control and Prevention

FIGURE 2-18 A microscopic image of a head of a human pinworm.

by ingesting contaminated food or water and are most commonly seen in children. The most common symptom is an itchy anus. A simple test is performed by pressing cellophane tape against the anal area, which is then removed and examined for the presence of any eggs. If the patient is positive for worms, the individual is given an anthelmintic such as Albedazole.

Hookworms are not commonly seen in the United States and are more prevalent in tropical regions of the world, Figure 2-19. Hookworms lay eggs in soil, and the larvae gain access to the body by entering through the bare feet of those walking on contaminated soil. Once in the body, the worm feeds on the host tissues and depletes the body of nutrients and blood by establishing itself in the mucosa of the intestinal wall. Common symptoms that result from this infection are vomiting, nausea, diarrhea, and anemia. Again, anthelmintic agents are used to treat this infection.

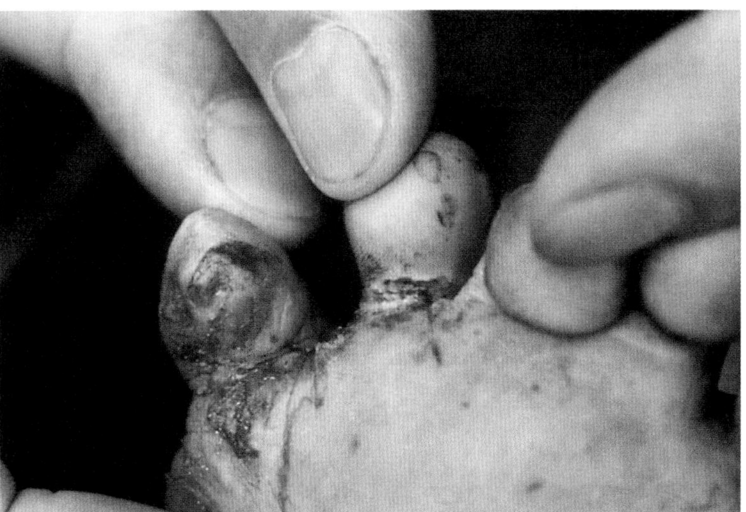

Centers for Disease Control and Prevention

FIGURE 2-19 Hookworm infection involving the toes of the right foot.

LEARNING OBJECTIVE 2.4 Describe inflammation and associated processes.

KEY TERMS

Abscess A collection of pus in an area of the body.

Cellulitis A potentially serious bacterial skin infection.

Chemotaxis The ability of cells to move to a location.

Chronic inflammation Ongoing inflammation of 7 to 10 days.

Diapedesis Movement of cells out of blood vessels during the inflammatory process to assist in the healing process.

Exudates Leakage of cellular debris from the bloodstream to the tissues of the body from an injury or irritation.

Fibrinous exudate Fluid containing fibrinogen that indicates a large injury and inflammation are present.

Granuloma Hardened tissue formed by the calcification of macrophages and fibrous tissues formed by collagen.

Histamines Chemical substances released to cause dilation of vessels in response to injury or irritation.

Hyperemia Increases blood flow to a certain area causing redness and warm sensation.

Inflammatory exudate Cellular debris resulting from inflammation.

Lesion Damaged or defective area on the inside or outside of the body, such as scabs, ulcers, and tumors.

Leukocytes A type of white blood cell.

Neutrophils A specialized WBC that is part of the innate immune response.

Phagocytosis The process of neutrophils escaping blood vessels and entering tissue to surround and attack the foreign invader to destroy it.

Purulent exudate Pus containing cellular and tissue debris.

Pus Viscous fluid containing primarily white blood cellular debris resulting from the inflammatory process.

Serous exudate Thin watery fluid that exudes or escapes from blood vessels into the surrounding tissue.

Transudate Occurs when too much pressure is present, causing fluid to cross the semipermeable membrane of a blood vessel.

Ulcers Cavitous or crater-like sores occurring either internally or externally, causing tissue to slough off.

2-11 INFLAMMATION AND ASSOCIATED PROCESSES

While inflammation was discussed in previous sections, there is a lot more to the story. Let's dive a little deeper into what happens when the body gets injured or attacked. Keep in mind that the inflammatory response is needed and activated to help fight infection and prepares the body for the eventual healing process. Only when the inflammatory response goes too far can it be harmful.

2-11a Inflammation Process

What causes inflammation? Infection from pathogenic microorganisms and physical injury will cause inflammation to occur in the body. The suffix used in medical terminology to express inflammation is *-itis*. For example, tonsillitis means inflammation of the tonsils. What would appendicitis mean? Can you think of more terms that end with *-itis*?

In brief, blood vessels in the affected area are dilated, allowing cells to leave the bloodstream to combat the invasion. As more blood flow enters the tissue, it causes redness and warmth at the affected site. With swelling or edema, pressure increases on the nerve endings, causing pain and loss of function.

When an injury or irritation occurs to the body's tissue, mast cells release **histamines**, which are chemical substances that cause the dilation of vessels such as the arterioles and venules at the site of the irritation. This increases blood flow, which is known as **hyperemia**, leading to redness and a warm sensation (see Figure 2-20). The blood also allows for **leukocytes** (WBCs) to be transported to the region. The major white blood cell is the **neutrophil**, which is part of the innate immune response (nonspecific immunity) or the immune defense we are born with. The neutrophils become active and line the endothelium of the vessels in the affected area. The vessels become semipermeable or leaky because of the stretching of the endothelium cells. Once in position, the neutrophils and **exudates** (stuff that leaks out) begin to cross the semipermeable

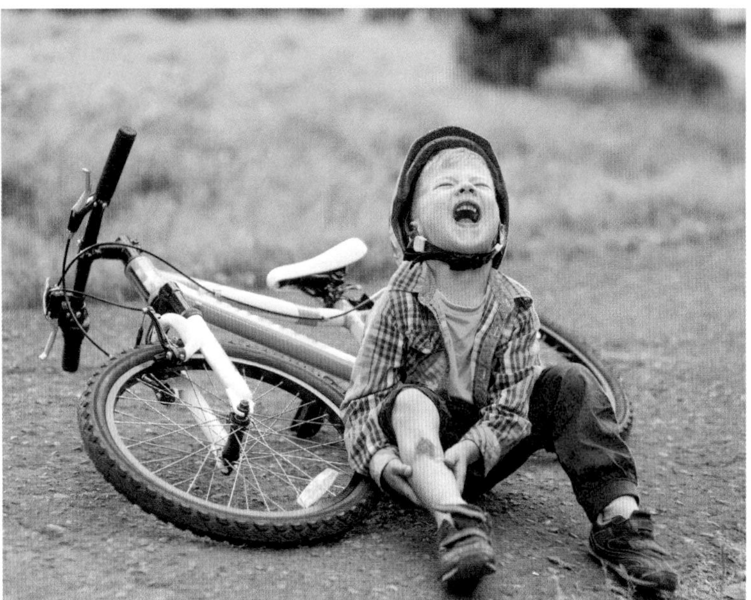

FIGURE 2-20 Pain and redness seen in visible tissue injury on right shin.

membrane of the vessel and then move into the tissue in a process known as diapedesis. At this point, the site is swollen and painful.

Once the neutrophils escape the blood vessels, they enters the tissue, surrounding and attacking any foreign invaders. The neutrophils ingest the pathogen to kill it in a process called phagocytosis. A byproduct of phagocytosis is a yellow- or white-colored fluid containing dead neutrophils known as pus or purulent exudate.

You might be wondering what exudates are and how they are different from transudates. A simple way to remember the difference is that transudate is fluid that crosses a semipermeable membrane of a vessel. The fluid is pushed across (trans = across) the vessel wall because of too much pressure. Exudate is when cellular debris moves from the blood through the vessel and into the tissues of the body as a result of injury or irritation. In short, transudate results from excess pressure with limited amounts of cells found within the fluid. Exudate is from an injury that causes extra cells to breach the area to help kill pathogenic microorganisms so the body can heal.

We've been talking about neutrophils for a while now, but how do they know where to go? The ability of neutrophils to be triggered to arrive to a certain region of the body is called chemotaxis. Neutrophils have the ability to pick up chemical signals sent by invaders from their outer membrane. This attracts many neutrophils to travel to that area.

After the neutrophils do their thing, and kill the invaders, the macrophages arrive at the scene by way of the bloodstream. Macrophages are large WBCs that move slowly as they destroy cellular debris left behind from the neutrophils.

2-12 CHRONIC INFLAMMATION

Chronic inflammation results from a foreign invader that has not been killed after 7 to 10 days. At this time, the immune system will release the "big guns" known as lymphocytes. In an effort to contain the foreign debris and prevent it from establishing itself in other areas of the body, the infected tissue surrounds the microorganism by encapsulating it in a granuloma. The **granuloma** is formed by the calcification of macrophages and fibrous tissues formed by collagen. This tissue becomes hard and can last for the remainder of the individual's life. These calcifications can be seen on the chest X-ray of tuberculosis patients.

2-13 INFLAMMATORY EXUDATE

We briefly mentioned pus in a previous section. Pus is one type of exudate that can occur from injury. However, there are other exudates that are associated with how long an injury was present and to what extent the injury was inflamed. These exudates can be seen by a visual inspection of the patient or with special equipment for an invasive procedure to visualize the lesion. The **inflammatory exudate** can assist the clinician in determining whether it was an acute or chronic infection by the amount of exudate and the contents in the fluid. However, what are the differences seen in exudative fluid and what are the types of exudative fluid?

Purulent exudate is filled with pus containing cellular and tissue debris such as neutrophils and pyogenic or pus-producing bacteria (see Figure 2-21). This can form in a region such as an infected tooth, causing an abscess. Abscesses will be discussed more in the next section.

The fluid in **serous exudate** is clear and consists of small amounts of protein. This fluid is reabsorbed by the body after the healing process starts and the inflammatory process ends. This type of exudate is associated with little tissue damage that has occurred suddenly or acutely. For example, when you touch a hot stove and get a second-degree burn, you get a fluid-filled blister at the affected area. The blister is filled with serous fluid, the clear substance we just mentioned. Now, if you do not pop the blister, the fluid will be reabsorbed by the tissue and the wound will heal on its own.

As its name implies, **fibrinous exudate** contains fibrinogen, which differs from serous fluid. Fibrinogen is a plasma protein required for the clotting

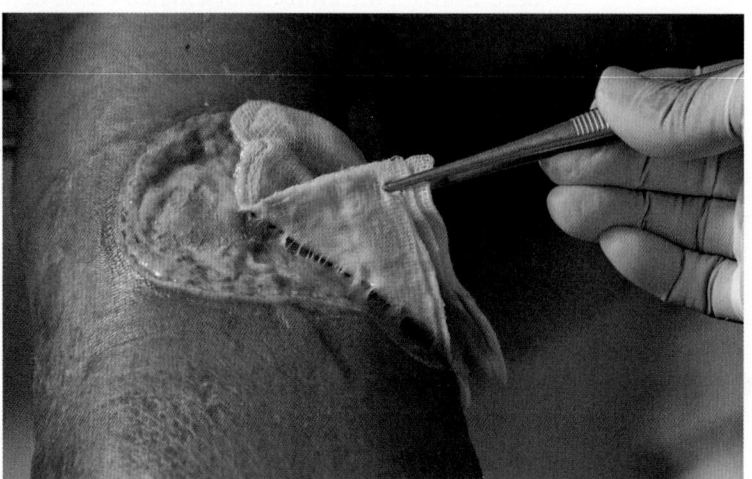

FIGURE 2-21 Pus found in a wound.

process. This type of exudate shows that a large injury is present and has a greater amount of inflammation. The resulting wound can be seen in the form of a **lesion** on the outside of the body known as a scab. A scab is a large mass-like lesion that forms from dried fibrinous exudate, Figure 2-22.

2-14 INFLAMMATORY LESIONS

Let's start off by defining a lesion. A lesion is a tissue wound or abnormality that derives from a disease or physical trauma. Examples of lesions are tumors, ulcers, abscesses, blisters, wheals, vesicles, and the list goes on.

2-14a Abscess

Let's continue our discussion about purulent exudates as our foundation for abscesses. Abscesses are caused by bacteria that cause an infection. In an effort to control the infection and prevent it from traveling elsewhere in the body, it is trapped or encapsulated by the tissue that surrounds the site of infection. This tissue forms a wall around the infection, leading to an **abscess** that contains pus, Figure 2-23. An example that you most likely have seen or possibly experienced yourself is a pimple. Found on the outside of the body, a pimple can be popped to remove the pus. However, if the patient has an empyema, or collection of pus, in a body cavity such as the pleural space in the lungs, it must be drained via medical intervention. Also, please do not pop your pimples.

2-14b Ulcer

Another type of lesion is an ulcer. **Ulcers** are sores that occur either internally or externally and are cavitous or crater-like, and result in tissue sloughing off. Examples of internal ulcers are peptic ulcers that occur in the small intestine, esophagus, and stomach, Figure 2-24. These can be very painful and occur when the protective membrane that lines our digestive tract is damaged by

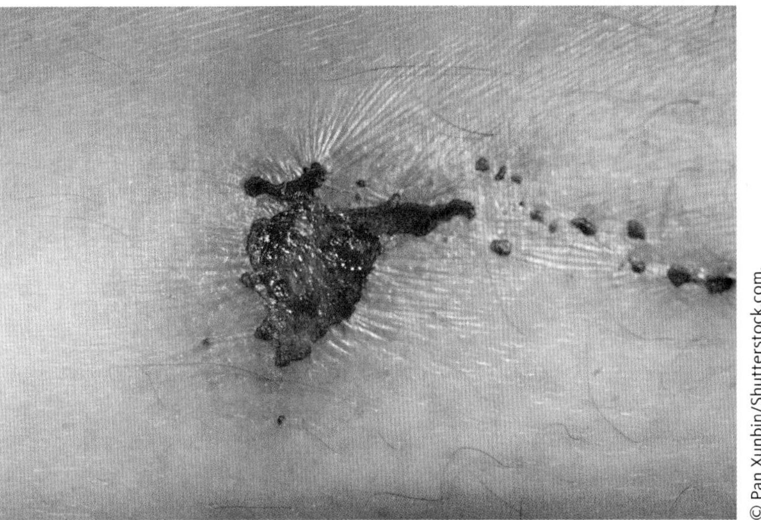

FIGURE 2-22 Scab formation on the skin.

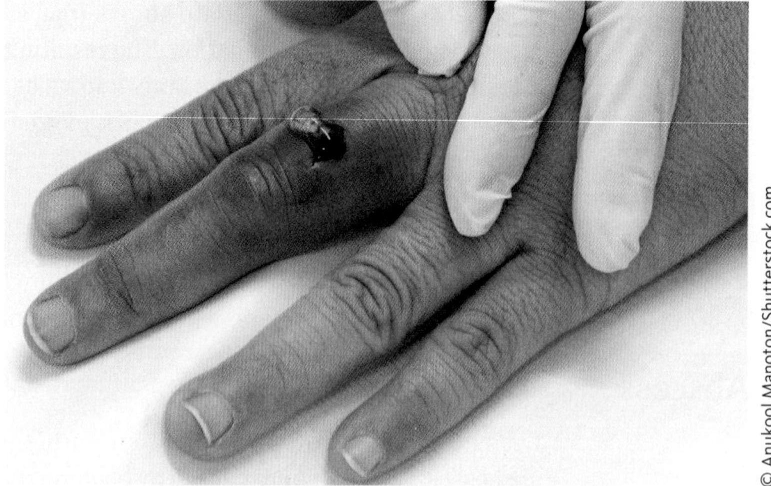

FIGURE 2-23 Finger abscess.

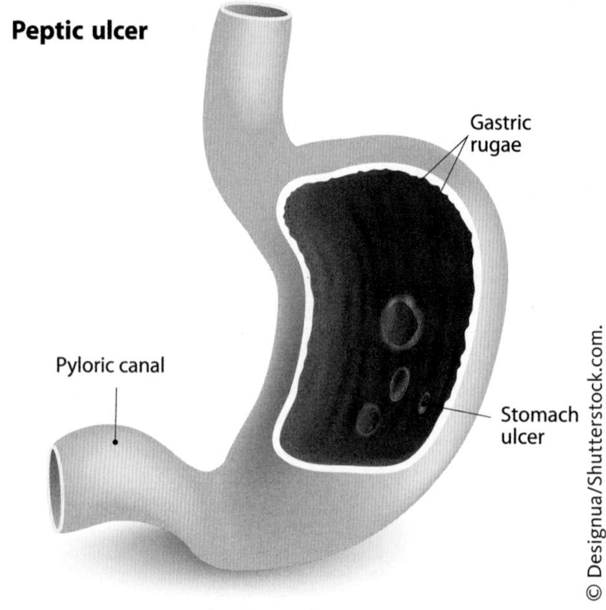

FIGURE 2-24 Stomach or peptic ulcers.

stomach acid. Another type of ulcer is caused by pressure and is known as a bed sore or a decubitus ulcer. This type of ulcer is seen on the outside of the body.

2-14c Cellulitis

Cellulitis is a potentially serious bacterial infection of the skin most commonly caused by *Streptococcus* or *Staphylococcus* bacteria. Cellulitis is an acute inflammation that presents as a red swollen area with a warm and tender sensation, Figure 2-25. This infection does not remain contained to a local area, and it can spread to anywhere in the body through the bloodstream, making it life-threatening. This bacterial infection is successfully treated with a regimen of antibiotics.

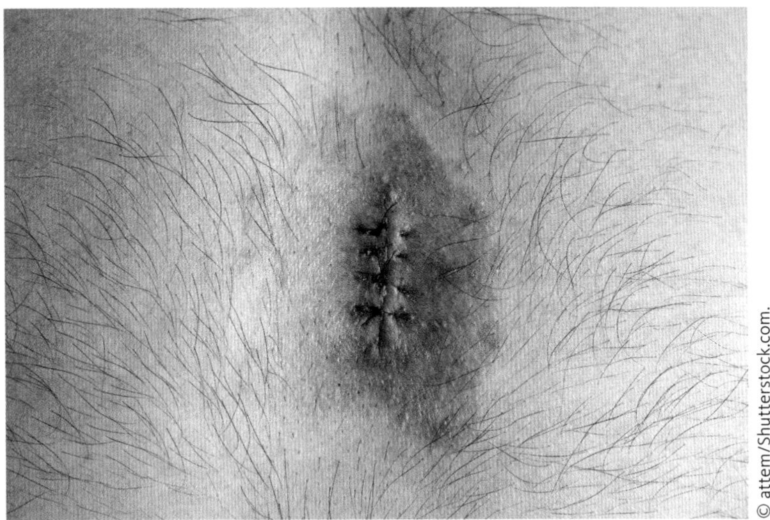
© attem/Shutterstock.com.

FIGURE 2-25 A wound with surrounding infection (cellulitis).

LEARNING OBJECTIVE 2.5 Summarize tissue repair and complications of wound healing.

KEY TERMS

Adhesion A normal scar that develops internally and that can cause structural problems.

Chronic inflammation Ongoing inflammation of 7 to 10 days.

Collagen Fibrous protein in the connective tissue.

Debridement The process of removing foreign material and necrotic tissue from a wound.

Dehiscence The reopening of a wound because of weak scar tissue.

Facultative mitotic cells Cell division process used to replace cells.

Fibroblasts Cells found in connective tissue that fill the deep area of a wound and forms collagen.

Keloid Excessive scar tissue growth.

Mitotic cells A type of cell that always divides and continues to do so throughout our lifetime.

Nondividing cells Cells that do not divide when damaged, resulting in loss of function.

Primary union (first intention) Small wounds with no debris or bacteria present, allowing a quick healing time.

Secondary union (secondary intention) A large wound loaded with debris and/or bacteria making it difficult to heal.

2-15 TISSUE REPAIR

After the body fights off a foreign invader or is physically injured, the body must then heal itself. The healing process begins after the macrophages remove debris from the area. The length of repair depends on the type of tissue cells affected.

The regenerative cell growth or division to heal the damaged tissue can be categorized in three ways:

- Mitotic cells
- Facultative mitotic cells
- Nondividing cells.

2-15a Cellular Reproduction for Tissue Repair

First, let's look at **mitotic cells**. Mitotic cells are found throughout the body. These cells are always dividing and will continue to divide throughout our lifetime. These cells will also repair any cells that might be damaged.

Next are **facultative mitotic cells**. These cells differ from mitotic cells by dividing only when it is necessary to replace damaged cells. These cells are found in certain organs, such as the liver and kidneys, which are repaired only when they are damaged.

Nondividing cells do not divide when damaged, making it impossible for the affected cells to ever regain function after they heal. Examples of organs that contain these cells are the heart, brain, and sensory nerves such as the spinal cord. Have you ever heard the phrase, "time is brain" in regards to a stroke? It means that if cells are deprived of oxygen and die, they can never be revived. As for the heart, once a myocardial infarction or heart attack occurs, the cells lose their function and cannot take part in the heartbeat. This is because the cells become fibrotic or, in other words, they become scar tissue.

Therefore, tissue regeneration occurring with mitotic and facultative mitotic cells will allow the cells to function properly as it did before the injury.

2-16 TISSUE HEALING

Now that we covered tissue repair, we will discuss tissue healing. To get a better idea about this concept, we will draw on some of your own experiences. Have you ever had an operation where surgical incisions were made, or even had a paper cut? These cuts are very thin and clean, in other words, with no debris or jagged edges on the outside of the wound. When the tissue is "clean-cut" and has straight edges, the sides of the wounds stick together nicely and allow the wound to heal quickly. On the other hand, injuries resulting in the tearing of flesh will take longer to heal and will result in visible scarring because the edges don't fit "nicely" back together.

The tissue healing process is based on how the wound heals, whether the edges of the wound come together to close the gap, or if the injury remains separated. In fact, healing is categorized based on the extent of separation from the edges of the wound. This is known as primary and secondary unions. Before discussing the primary and secondary unions, it is important to understand the process of how wounds are healed. The healing process has been broken down into a series of four steps.

STEP 1 The wound starts to fill with serum fluid and then forms a visible scab on top of the wound.

STEP 2 Occurring within the next two days after the injury, the edges of the cut are connected together again with the formation of new capillaries.

STEP 3 The cut develops **fibroblasts**, which fill in the deep area of the wound and forms **collagen**. This new tissue is called granulation tissue and has a pink or paler appearance.

STEP 4 The edges of the wound begin to be pulled together by the newly formed collagen, forming a scar.

Keep in mind that a wound might appear to be healed from the outside. Nevertheless, depending on how deep the wound, it may not be completely healed at the deeper levels. A deep tissue wound can take up to a month or more to completely heal (see Figure 2-26).

2-16a Primary Union

Primary union or first intention is when the edges of the wound are clean and result in minimal damage to the tissue. These wounds are small and do not have any debris or bacteria present, which allow for a quick healing time.

2-16b Secondary Union

Secondary union or secondary intention are larger wounds loaded with debris and or bacteria, which make them difficult to heal. While the healing process is the same as in primary union, it takes longer. More inflammation must be resolved before healing can occur, and the larger surface area of the wound requires more capillaries, fibroblasts, and collagen, which ultimately causes a large scar. If the wound is too large, the body will not be able to properly heal over the area, resulting in the need for a skin graft as shown in Figure 2-27.

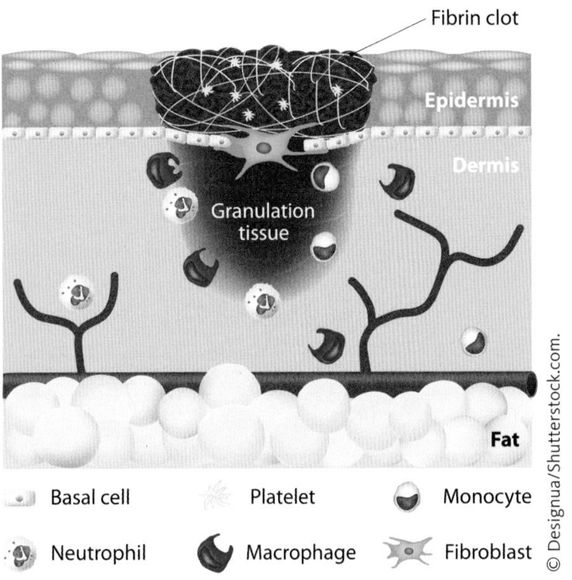

FIGURE 2-26 Image of wound healing.

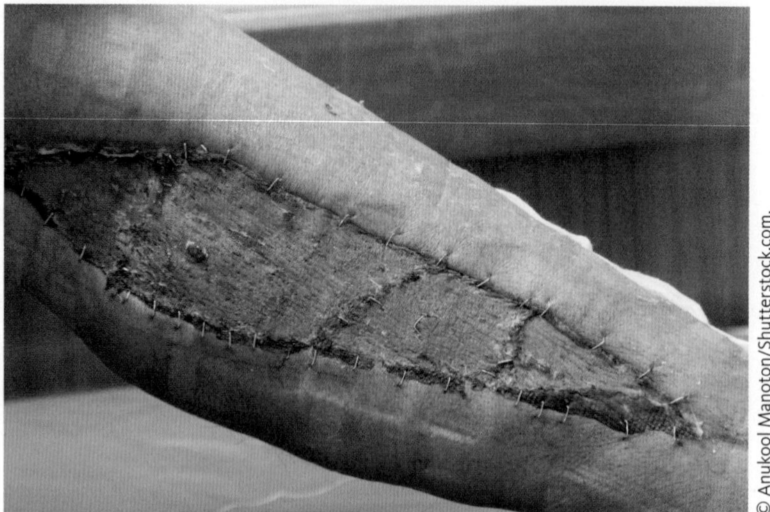

FIGURE 2-27 A skin graft with tissue granulation.

2-17 WOUND HEALING

As we mentioned with secondary union, wound healing can be delayed by the amount of debris that is in the wound. Dead tissue cells have to be removed by the body via phagocytosis, which can take months. Any dead tissue, dirt, and microorganisms can slow down the rate of healing. Medical intervention is needed to speed up the recovery process by washing and removing any foreign material and necrotic or dead tissue. This is accomplished by a process called **debridement**. Many factors affect healing time; Table 2-2 lists the factors and gives a brief reasoning.

Table 2-2 Factors affecting wound healing

FACTOR	REASONING
Age	Wounds heal quicker for younger individuals
Size	Smaller wounds heal faster
Tissue	Epithelial cells heal faster than other tissues
Nutrition	Protein, vitamin C, and other nutrition aid the body in faster healing
Immobility	Wounds heal faster when kept immobile
Circulation	Whether the site can be reached with enough blood supply to allow the healing process to occur
Pathogenicity	Wounds take longer to heal when infected
Steroids	Suppress the body's ability to fight infection and delay the healing process

2-18 WOUND COMPLICATIONS

Other complications can occur during the healing process. Scarring is a normal part of the healing process; however, too much scarring is considered a complication. As shown in Figure 2-28, a **keloid** develops as a result of excess collagen formation. Keloids are smooth, hard, and can be sensitive to the touch. Although these overgrowths might not be a medical problem, they often are a cosmetic concern. On the other hand, **dehiscence** is when the scar is not able to develop enough strength, and the wound reopens or ruptures. Lastly, when a patient has a surgical procedure performed on his or her internal organs, there is a potential for a complication called an **adhesion**. It is a normally developed internal scar, but the organ sticks to the surface of adjacent structures. This is not a serious problem in most cases, unless the adhesion causes an organ obstruction such as intestinal adhesions that would disrupt the flow through the GI tract.

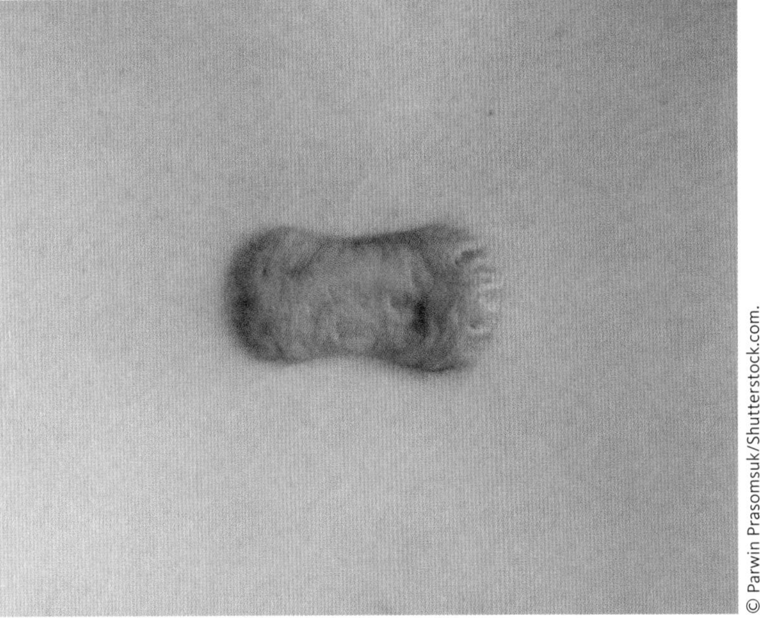

FIGURE 2-28 An overgrowth of scar tissue known as a keloid seen on an individual's skin.

Module 3

Core Concepts of Pharmacology

Module Introduction

This MindTap is titled "Pathopharmacology." In the first two modules, we discussed the *patho* portion concerning the principles of disease. Now that we have laid the groundwork for disease, it's time to dive into the core concepts of the *pharmaco* portion of *pathopharmacology*. After we lay this foundation, we can then put everything together in the upcoming modules to show the interrelationship or pathopharmacology as it relates to each specific body system.

LEARNING OBJECTIVE 3.1 Describe the current drug laws and standards.

KEY TERMS

1906 Pure Food and Drug Act Forces manufacturers that produce drugs for sale in the United States to begin following minimum standards for drug purity, strength, and quality.

1938 Federal Food, Drug, and Cosmetic Act Requires that all new prescription drugs and over-the-counter (OTC) drugs be deemed safe by the FDA before marketing drugs, cosmetics, and therapeutic devices to the public.

1970 Controlled Substances Act (CSA) Categorizes drugs by the acceptable medical uses, the potential for drug abuse, and/or potential for dependency; requires those with prescribing or distributing privileges to have a DEA registration number to prevent fraudulent dispensing of medication.

1983 Orphan Drug Act Gives financial incentives to manufacturers that develop drugs to treat rare diseases.

Acute pain A sudden onset of pain.

Chronic pain Prolonged pain.

Drug Enforcement Agency (DEA) Established to enforce provisions of the 1970 Controlled Substances Act.

Drug legend Statement warning that any distribution without a prescription is prohibited by federal law.

Food and Drug Administration (FDA) Federal agency that ensures drugs and devices are safe to use.

National Formulary (NF) Book of preparations and standards for pharmaceuticals.

Omnibus Budget Reconciliation Act (OBRA) of 1990 Legislation that mandates pharmacies to ask customers if they would like to be educated about their medication at time of purchase.

Over-the-counter (OTC) Any medication bought without a prescription.

Schedule I Listing of drugs not currently used in medical treatment that have a high potential for abuse.

Schedule II Listing of drugs that have usage in medical treatment but with severe restrictions because of a high potential for abuse.

Schedule III Listing of drugs currently used in medical treatment that have less of a potential for abuse than drugs in schedules I and II.

Schedule IV Listing of drugs currently used in the medical treatment but have a slight potential for abuse; less than schedules II and III.

Schedule V Currently used for medical treatment with less potential for abuse than drugs in schedule IV; have a slight possibility for abuse and might cause limited physical or psychological dependence.

United States Pharmacopeia (USP) Collection of drug standards and testing that determines the strength, purity, and quality of a drug.

United States Pharmacopeia and the National Formulary (USP–NF) A reference compiled by combining the USP and NF to form one source.

3-1 DRUG LAWS AND STANDARDS

Before discussing the core concepts of pharmacology, we must understand the importance of the laws and government regulations that have been put in place to protect consumers. If these laws did not exist, how would you know if the drug you just took is actually that particular drug? How could you tell if it is the proper strength? How do you know whether the substance has been altered and not in its purest form, thus decreasing its quality? To put this into perspective, think about illicit street drugs. There is absolutely no way of knowing if the drug purchased illegally is actually the drug desired. The buyer has no idea about the strength and purity of the substance. The drug might be stronger than or possibly weaker than usual, leading to an overdose. Therefore, without regulation, the quality and safety of our medicines suffer.

So how do we keep our legal pharmaceuticals manufactured by big businesses in line with desired expectations? This concept is nothing new. In 1862, President Abraham Lincoln called upon a chemist by the name of Charles M. Wetherill to form the Bureau of Chemistry, which has evolved and transitioned over many decades to become the government agency we know today as the **Food and Drug Administration (FDA)**. The FDA ensures that the drugs are safe to use and that the drugs prescribed will all be the same no matter which pharmacy in the United States fills the prescription (see Figure 3-1).

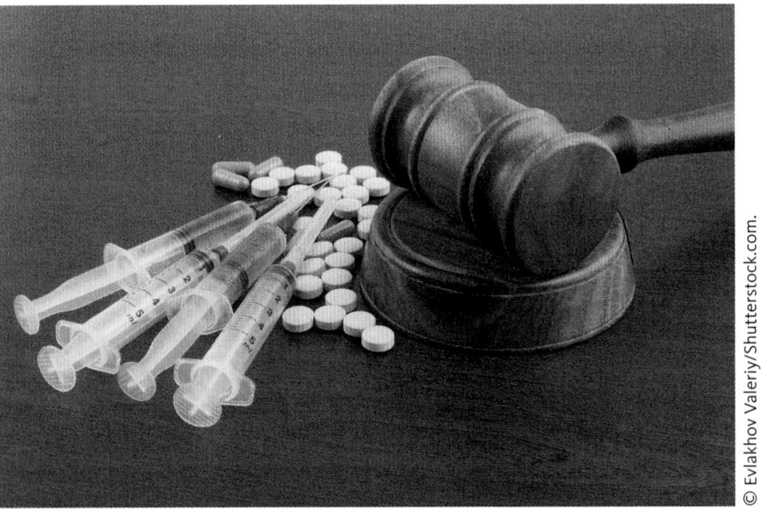

FIGURE 3-1 Laws must regulate drug testing, production, and dispensing to ensure public safety.

3-1a 1906 Pure Food and Drug Act

The United States had no laws regulating the manufacture and sales of drugs until the **1906 Pure Food and Drug Act**. This act was the first real step toward actually establishing consumer protection in drugs and foods. The law required manufacturers producing drugs for sale in the United States to begin following minimum standards for drug purity, strength, and quality. Drug labels were mandated to display whether the drugs were made using any dangerous ingredients. Figure 3-2 illustrates not only the display of active ingredients but other drug facts now required for drug labeling.

This law brought about the need for an official publication pertaining to the drug standards. Actually, two publications originally became the official written resource of US drug-making standards, the **United States Pharmacopeia (USP)** and the **National Formulary (NF)**. Today, these two sources have been combined into one, known as the **United States Pharmacopeia and the National Formulary (USP–NF)**, which is conveniently available online.

3-1b 1938 Federal Food, Drug, and Cosmetic Act and Amendments of 1951 and 1962

Another important law to mention is the **1938 Federal Food, Drug, and Cosmetic Act** and Amendments of 1951 and 1962. This law required that all new drugs, including **over-the-counter (OTC)** drugs, be deemed safe by the FDA before being marketed to the public. The protection also extended to cosmetics and therapeutic devices. The medication labeling must state whether the drug can be sold with or without a prescription and *warning labels* had to be placed on medications such as "Do not operate heavy machinery," "Do not drink alcoholic beverages when taking medication," and "May cause dizziness" (see Figure 3-3).

CLINICAL CONNECTION 3.1

Often warning labels come after a large lawsuit filed in the wake of a tragic incident. For example, someone might have taken a drug and then been injured while operating heavy equipment when the drug affected his or her ability to operate it. One of the author's favorite examples is the warning label on hemorrhoidal creams that state "Do not take internally." Think about it.

3-1c 1970 Controlled Substances Act

Some drugs have a great potential to be abused and therefore need to be more tightly controlled. Indeed, the problem was so drastic that an entire agency was formed to enforce the controls for this potentially dangerous group of medications.

In 1973, the **Drug Enforcement Agency (DEA)** was established to enforce provisions of the **1970 Controlled Substances Act (CSA)**. The

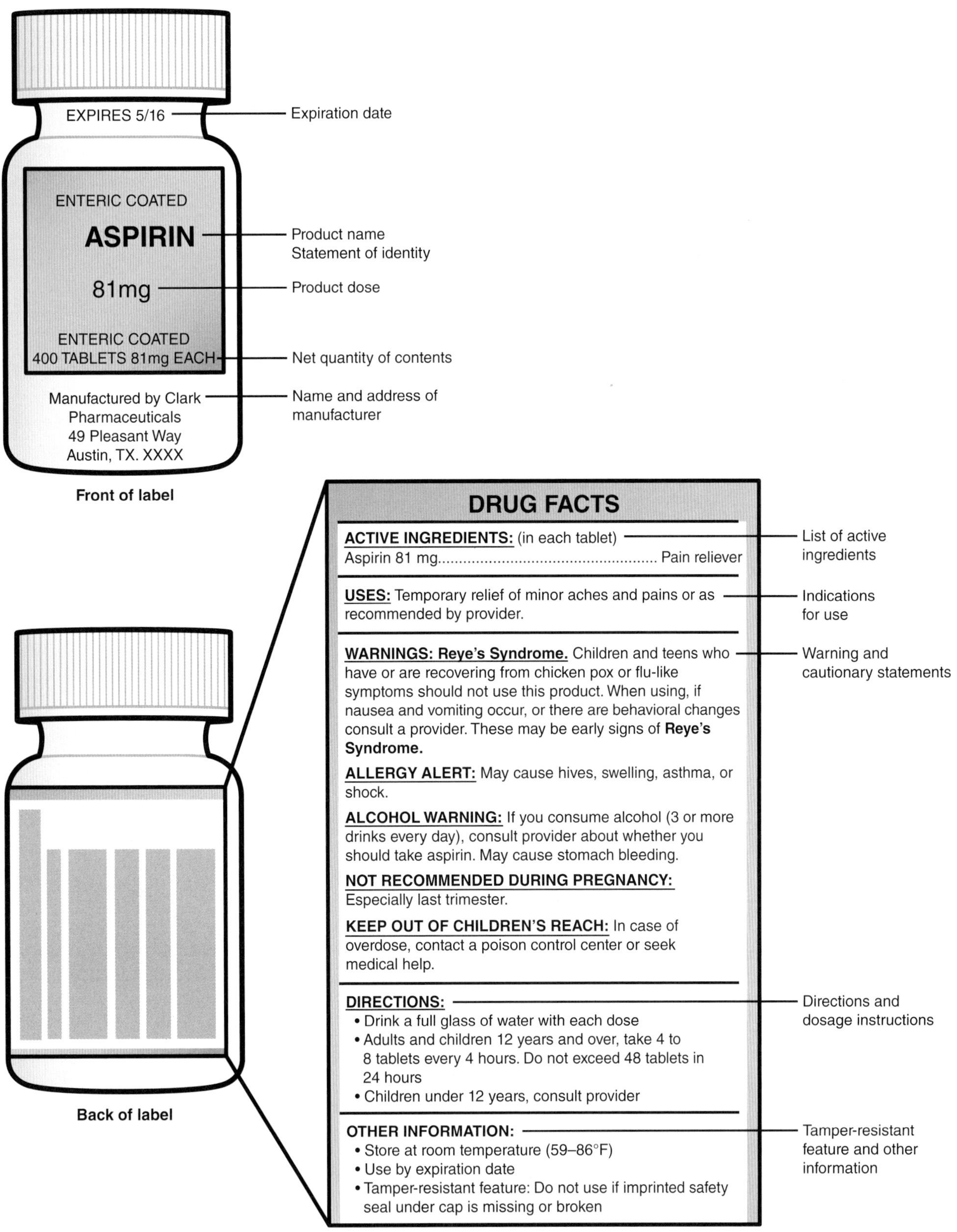

EXPIRES 5/16
Expiration date
ENTERIC COATED
ASPIRIN
Product name
Statement of identity
81mg
Product dose
ENTERIC COATED
400 TABLETS 81mg EACH
Net quantity of contents
Manufactured by Clark
Pharmaceuticals
49 Pleasant Way
Austin, TX. XXXX
Name and address of manufacturer
Front of label
DRUG FACTS
ACTIVE INGREDIENTS: (in each tablet)
Aspirin 81 mg.. Pain reliever
List of active ingredients
USES: Temporary relief of minor aches and pains or as recommended by provider.
Indications for use
WARNINGS: Reye's Syndrome. Children and teens who have or are recovering from chicken pox or flu-like symptoms should not use this product. When using, if nausea and vomiting occur, or there are behavioral changes consult a provider. These may be early signs of Reye's Syndrome.
Warning and cautionary statements
ALLERGY ALERT: May cause hives, swelling, asthma, or shock.
ALCOHOL WARNING: If you consume alcohol (3 or more drinks every day), consult provider about whether you should take aspirin. May cause stomach bleeding.
NOT RECOMMENDED DURING PREGNANCY: Especially last trimester.
KEEP OUT OF CHILDREN'S REACH: In case of overdose, contact a poison control center or seek medical help.
DIRECTIONS:
• Drink a full glass of water with each dose
• Adults and children 12 years and over, take 4 to 8 tablets every 4 hours. Do not exceed 48 tablets in 24 hours
• Children under 12 years, consult provider
Directions and dosage instructions
OTHER INFORMATION:
• Store at room temperature (59–86°F)
• Use by expiration date
• Tamper-resistant feature: Do not use if imprinted safety seal under cap is missing or broken
Tamper-resistant feature and other information
Back of label

FIGURE 3-2 Example of a drug label containing important drug facts.

Controlled Substances Act schedules or categorizes drugs by the acceptable medical uses, the potential for substance abuse, and addiction or potential for dependency. The lower the number is, the greater will be the risk of abuse and dependence. For example, drugs that are schedule I have more risk of dependency than schedule II; while schedule II is more addictive than schedule III; and so on. The schedule can be illustrated as a C with a roman numeral after it indicating its schedule, Figure 3-4. Drugs with the greatest potential for psychological and physical dependence and considered the most dangerous are listed as schedule I narcotics. Table 3-1 lists the five drug schedules and examples of drugs included in each category.

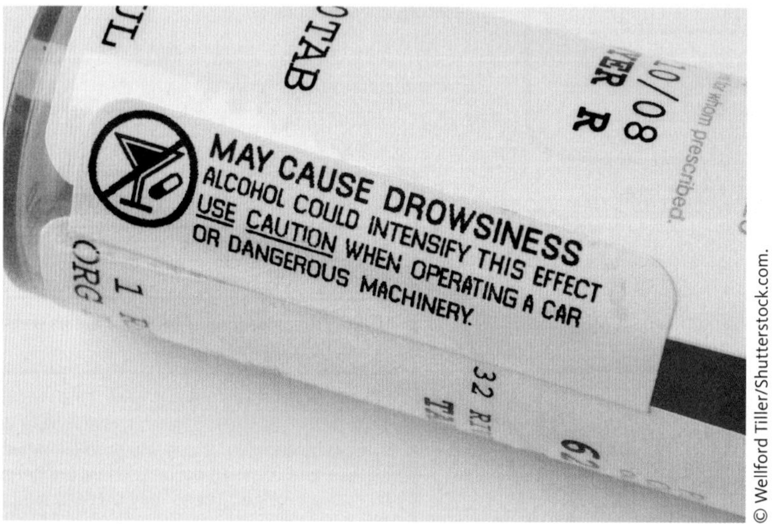

FIGURE 3-3 Example of a warning label.

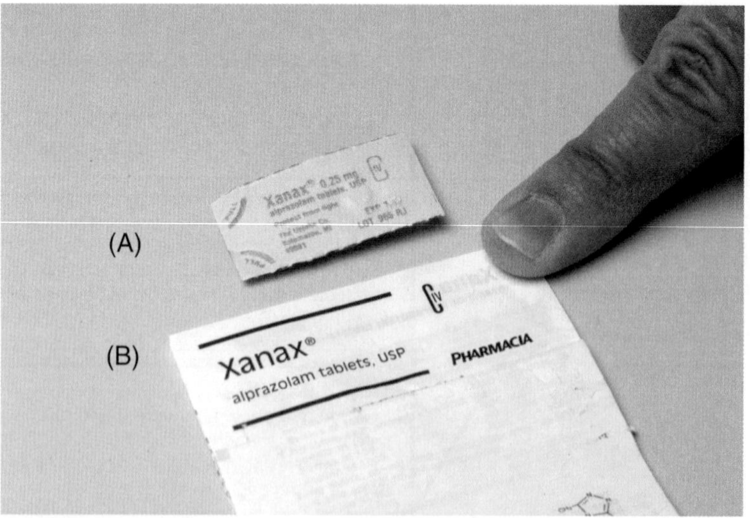

FIGURE 3-4 Controlled substance schedule numbers appear in a variety of drug information resources, including (A) drug packages and (B) drug inserts. Schedule numbers are also found in drug reference sources.

Table 3-1 Controlled Substances Act schedule and drugs

CONTROLLED SUBSTANCES ACT SCHEDULE	COMMON EXAMPLES OF DRUGS
Schedule I: High potential for abuse No current usage in medical treatment	Heroin Bath salts LSD Marijuana Ecstasy Quaaludes Peyote
Schedule II: High potential for abuse Has current usage in medical treatment with severe restrictions Abuse can cause a major psychological or physical dependence	Dilaudid Methadone Percocet OxyContin Fentanyl Morphine Codeine Cocaine Hydrocodone with Tylenol
Schedule III: Less potential for abuse than drugs in schedules 1 and 2 Used currently in medical treatment Abuse can cause a high psychological dependence or low to moderate physical dependence when compared to the drugs in schedule II	Amphetamines Anabolic Steroids Ketamine
Schedule IV: Less potential for abuse than drugs in schedule III Currently used in medical treatment Slight possibility abuse might cause a physical dependence or psychological dependence when compared to the drugs in schedule III	Alprazolam Xanax Soma Darvocet Valium Ativan Ambien Tramadol
Schedule V: Less potential for abuse than drugs in schedule IV Currently used for medical treatment Slight possibility abuse might cause limited physical dependence or psychological dependence when compared to schedule IV	Lomotil Motofen Lyrica Parepectolin Cheratussin AC Promethazine with codeine

Note: All healthcare professionals who have the ability to prescribe or distribute drugs are required to have a DEA registration number that must occur on any prescription of controlled substances. All controlled substances must be locked and secured.

CLINICAL CONNECTION 3.2

PAIN AND ADDICTION

Analgesics or painkillers are very addicting and should be taken only as prescribed by the physician. Pain is any hurtful discomfort, and it is not a normal process of aging. Two types of pain are acute and chronic. Acute pain is a warning signal that something is not normal with our body. Acute pain occurs suddenly, lasting only a day or two. **Acute pain** can be associated with an infection, procedure, inflammation, etc. Once the cause of pain has been identified, it can be treated and relieved in a relatively timely fashion. However, **chronic pain** is prolonged pain, lasting much longer than its acute stage.

What do we do when we are in pain? We want to take a pill to make it go away, right? It is common practice for people to rush to their physician's office for a pain pill prescription. It is vital to treat the underlying cause of the pain to prevent the patient from masking it with analgesics. Opioids are narcotics used to treat pain, but they can be addicting when they are used to produce an intoxicating high and reduce anxiety. This drug classification is one of the most abused drug classes in the United States.

3-1d 1983 Orphan Drug Act

It is no secret that pharmaceutical sales are a multi-billion-dollar, profit-driven business. Common diseases affecting millions of people have an array of drugs produced by pharmaceutical companies that all want to get their share of the pie and make a significant profit. But, what about rare diseases that are contracted by only a few people? Do we just let them suffer because there is virtually no money to be made?

By the time a drug is produced, from start to finish, a company spends millions and millions of dollars. So, what incentives can drug companies be given to pursue the development of medicinal products for these rare conditions? The **1983 Orphan Drug Act** provides financial incentives for pharmaceutical companies to develop drugs for these otherwise poor money-making projects.

3-1e Omnibus Budget Reconciliation Act (OBRA) of 1990

Have you ever purchased prescription drugs from a pharmacy and had to check a box stating that you decline any and all drug counseling at this time? Have you ever wondered why you are asked if you need an overview of the medication? It is not just a common courtesy; it's the law. The **Omnibus Budget Reconciliation Act (OBRA) of 1990** requires that pharmacies ask if people desire to be educated about their medication. This law also states that all nonprescribed or over-the-counter (OTC) drugs taken by a patient must be written down in the patient's medical record. OTC drugs, even though easily found and purchased, can still be dangerous if not used properly and have many interactions with prescribed drugs.

3-2 HEALTHCARE PRACTITIONERS AND THE LAW

No matter what your profession, if you work around pharmaceuticals, you have a great responsibility, especially when dispensing drugs to patients or working in an environment containing vast quantities of medications. When administering medications, accurate records must be maintained for all controlled drug substances and kept available for 2 years. After that point, any old records must be shredded and properly disposed.

It is also important to stay current with all news regarding FDA and DEA regulations. If you are employed at a physician's office, monitor the expiration date of the DEA registration number of the physician, to ensure everything is up-to-date.

Some duties might include calling in prescriptions to pharmacies. If that is the case, we urge you to make an attempt to establish a good relationship with the people who work there. Pharmacists can be invaluable sources of information when you face any uncertainties about a drug or if any legal responsibilities are in question. Also, an up-to-date drug reference should be kept on hand to help identify unknown medications.

Keeping an organized inventory of all pharmaceuticals and supplies is essential. It might take some time getting organized, but knowing exactly how much of any drug is on hand or what is going to expire soon will save a lot of time in the long run. Any drugs that have expired must be properly discarded so they are not accidently dispensed to a patient or fall into the wrong hands.

All controlled substances must be locked up, and, in most cases, require a double-lock, meaning a lock on the door to get into the "med room" and a lock on the cabinet or drawer in which they are stored (see Figure 3-5). Speaking of locking up items, all prescription pads must be kept out of the public's eye and in a locked drawer. This precaution will decrease the likelihood of any someone attempting to illegally write prescriptions to obtain a controlled substance.

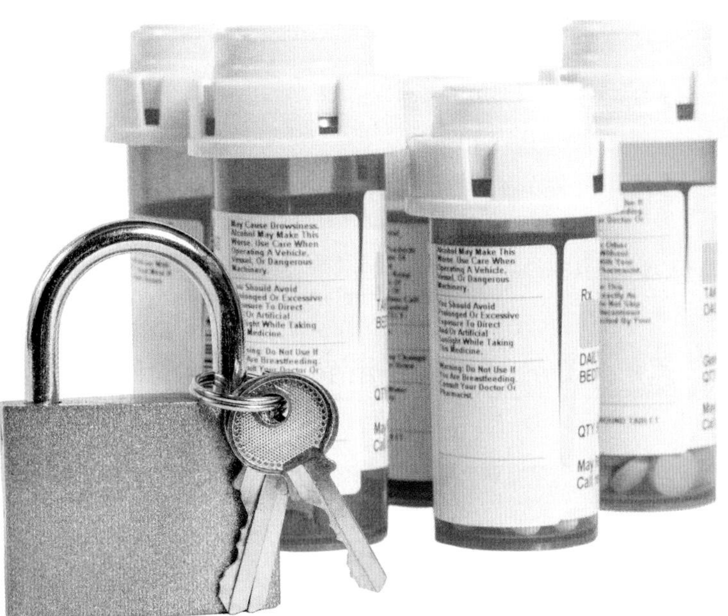

FIGURE 3-5 Lock up medications.

3-3 LEGAL TERMS REFERRING TO DRUGS

Before moving forward, we are going to further develop a few legal terms that we have previously mentioned. It is important to become familiar with these terms since they deal with the legal availability of medications.

Over-the-counter medications can be purchased without a prescription. Even though these drugs are readily available, OTC drugs should be respected because they too can be hazardous, especially when too much is taken or if they are not taken as directed. Therefore, care should be taken when using these medications, just as if they were prescribed drugs.

To stop the alarming epidemic of methamphetamine use in the United States, President George W. Bush signed the Combat Methamphetamine Epidemic Act of 2005. This law was integrated into the Patriot Act and limits how much a person can purchase of OTC medication that can be used to make illegal methamphetamine. Purchase of any OTC drugs containing pseudoephedrine such as Sudafed, as shown in Figure 3-6, is closely monitored and requires a photo ID and a signature in a logbook.

Drug legend Bob Marley . . . wait, wrong topic. A **drug legend** is a cautionary label stating "federal law prohibits dispensing without a prescription." The term drug legend means that the drug is approved by the FDA and requires a person with appropriate licensing, such as a physician, to prescribe the medication, and another licensed person, such as a pharmacist, to dispense it to the public.

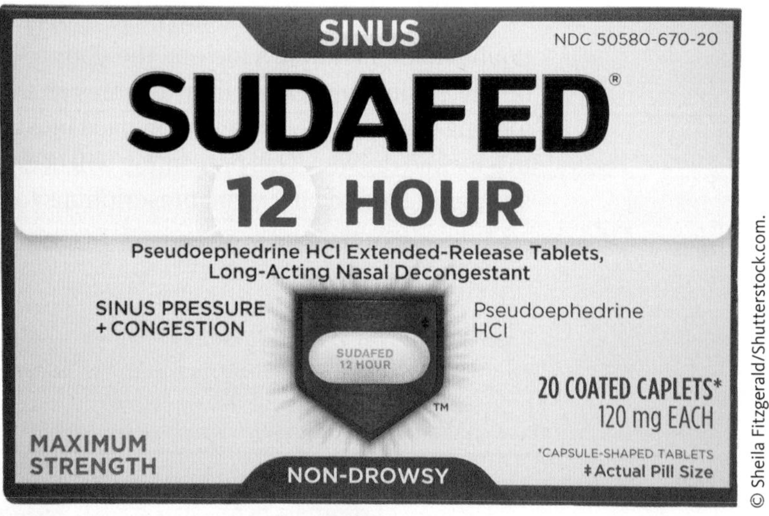

FIGURE 3-6 The purchase of Sudafed is regulated so it cannot be bought in large quantities to manufacture illegal street drugs.

LEARNING OBJECTIVE 3.2 **Describe terminology associated with pharmacology.**

KEY TERMS

Brand names Proprietary drug name owned by a company.

Chemical name The drug name used to describe the anatomic or molecular structure of a substance.

Drug classification A method used to group drugs in a meaningful way.

Formulary A list of medications offered in a particular hospital or healthcare system.

Generic name A name not owned by any particular pharmaceutical company.

Official name Name given by the USP/NF, after the drug has been approved for use.

Pharmacist Individual licensed to prepare and distribute medications.

Pharmacogenetics Pertains to genetic differences that can cause a drug to affect us in different ways, whether therapeutically or adversely.

Pharmacogenomics Analyzes human genes to better understand how an individual's genetics affects the way drugs affect his or her body.

Pharmacology The study of the origin, uses, effects, and actions of chemicals in living organisms.

Pharmacotherapy The act of giving drugs targeted to treat disease.

Pharmacy Dispenses medications to the public.

Pharmacy technicians Individuals who assist and work under the direct supervision of pharmacists.

Prescription Written orders for a certain therapy or medication; also called scripts.

Prototype A drug that typifies a certain drug classification.

Therapeutic level Preferred level of a drug required to treat disease.

Toxicology The study of a chemicals and pharmacologic actions on the body with poisons and antidotes.

Trade name Proprietary name owned by a pharmaceutical company to market its creation to the public; also known as a brand name.

United States Adopted Names (USAN) Council Group that gives names to generic medications.

3-4 BASIC PHARMACOLOGIC TERMS

Now that we have discussed the legal aspects of pharmacology, let's discuss what exactly is pharmacology? **Pharmacology** is the study of the origin, uses, effects, and action of chemicals in living organisms, such as our body. While pharmacology is the "study of drugs," **pharmacotherapy** is the application or use of medications to treat diseases. Ideally, drugs are used to achieve a **therapeutic level**, which is the desired level needed to treat disease. Drugs (and other chemicals) can also act as poisons within the body. The study of pharmacologic actions on the body with poisons and their resultant antidotes is termed **toxicology**.

We all have genetic differences that can cause a drug to affect us in different ways, whether it is therapeutically or adversely. This was known as **pharmacogenetics**, but is now called **pharmacogenomics** and will be discussed later in the module.

To receive any prescribed medications, one must go to a **pharmacy**, which prepares and dispenses drugs under the supervision of a pharmacist. A **pharmacist** is a person who has acquired the education and state licensing required to prepare and distribute medications. **Pharmacy technicians** work closely under the direct supervision of pharmacists to perform their duties. Both positions require a heightened sense of detail.

3-5 PRESCRIPTIONS

A **prescription** is a written order for a patient to receive a certain therapy or medication, Figure 3-7. Not all healthcare professionals are given the legal authority to write prescriptions. Prescriptions can be written by physicians, dentists, nurse practitioners, and veterinarians, as well as a few other practitioners, but not chiropractors, for example. After an authorized individual writes a prescription, the next step is for it to be filled at a pharmacy. The prescription, also called a script, has certain areas that must be filled out.

- The patient's name, address, and date prescribed
- The prescription (Rx), which is a written authorization by the prescriber for a certain medication or other therapy
- The name and quantity of the drug being prescribed
- Transcription, which is the information the pharmacist must put on the label as instructions to the patient, such as how much and how frequently to take the medication
- Signature of prescriber
- Name of prescriber
- DEA number

Each pharmacy has a certain listing of drugs they keep in stock, and this is known as their **formulary**. The list of medications offered in a particular hospital or healthcare system also is called a formulary. Each healthcare setting will stock the most commonly needed and prescribed medications they encounter. If a drug is not in their formulary, they have access to a network to obtain that drug quickly.

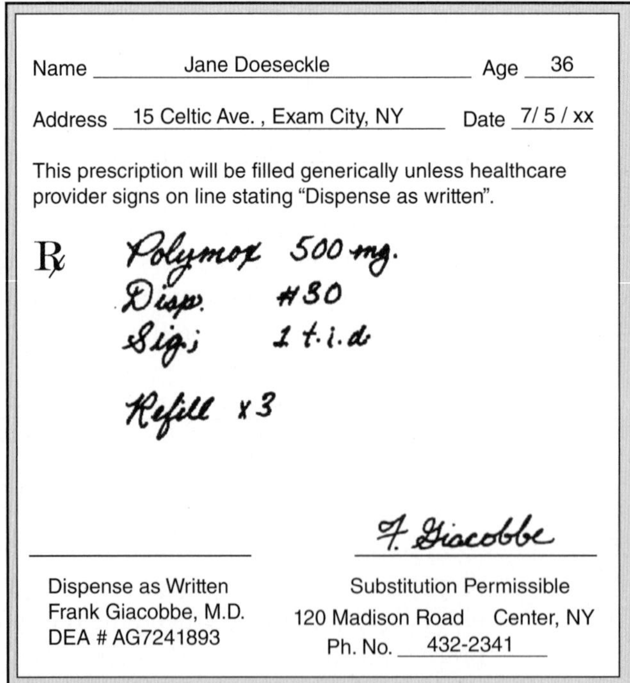
Name Jane Doeseckle Age 36

Address 15 Celtic Ave. , Exam City, NY Date 7/ 5 / xx

This prescription will be filled generically unless healthcare provider signs on line stating "Dispense as written".

℞ Polymox 500 mg.
Disp. #30
Sig: 1 t.i.d.

Refill x3

F. Giacobbe

Dispense as Written | Substitution Permissible

Frank Giacobbe, M.D.
DEA # AG7241893

120 Madison Road Center, NY
Ph. No. 432-2341

FIGURE 3-7 Sample prescription.

3-6 DRUG CLASSIFICATIONS

There are many different kinds of drugs that are on the market, and those drugs can be grouped in many different ways, such as chemical structure, and body system targeted. A meaningful grouping for healthcare professionals is by therapeutic usage, known as **drug classification**. See Table 3-2 for examples.

Some drugs are used to treat many different ailments, so they are found in more than one category or classification. For example, aspirin is an analgesic used to treat pain, an anti-inflammatory used to treat inflammation, an antithrombotic agent for its blood thinning abilities, and lastly, an antipyretic agent to reduce fevers. No wonder aspirin was called a "wonder drug" when it was first discovered.

CLINICAL CONNECTION 3.3

When a new car is being designed, a prototype is developed to represent the vehicle model, and other models can be derived from that prototype. So too when a drug is developed from which alternate forms can be made, it is referred to as the drug **prototype** of a new classification. For example, atropine was the prototype drug for a classification of drugs used to block the parasympathetic response, and now several drugs fall under this drug category.

Table 3-2 Examples of different drug classifications

CLASSIFICATION	THERAPEUTIC USAGE	DRUG EXAMPLES
Antiemetic	Prevent vomiting	Emend (aprepitant) Inapsine (droperidol)
Antacid	Neutralize stomach acidity	Maalox (aluminum/magnesium) Mylanta (calcium carbonate/magnesium carbonate)
Beta blockers	High blood pressure	Tenormin (atenolol) Zebeta (bisoprolol)
Decongestants	Relieve nasal congestion by vasoconstriction of vessels in mucosa	Sudafed (pseudoephedrine) Neo-Synephrine (phenylephrine)
Nonsteroidal anti-inflammatory drugs (NSAIDS)	Reduce inflammation	Motrin (ibuprofen) Naprosyn (naproxen)
Diuretic	Increase urinary output	Lasix (furosemide) Edecrin (ethacrynic acid)

3-7 IDENTIFYING TRADE (BRAND) AND GENERIC NAMES

The list of drugs that are marketed keeps expanding. We see television and magazine advertisements for all that the pharmaceutical companies have to offer. Most people have seen commercials for drugs that will help you combat obesity, decreased libido, high cholesterol, risk of heart attack from blood clots, sleeplessness, and the list goes on and on. These marketing campaigns usually mention the drug by its trade name. What is the difference between a trade name and generic name? Why don't drugs have just one name? It can be daunting to new healthcare students to have to become familiar with all these different names. Learning drug names can be a "bitter pill to swallow," but the task can become easier when you understand the various types of names.

Medications do not magically appear on the market for use. A company must first develop a promising drug and submit it to the FDA for approval. The new drug then must be given a name by which it can be tracked. This name is called the **generic name**. Generic names are provided by the **United States Adopted Names (USAN) Council**. A generic name is a nonproprietary name that is not owned by any particular pharmaceutical company.

A **trade name** is a catchy name that is developed by pharmaceutical companies to market their creations to the public. A trade name often has a hidden meaning, or one that is not so hidden, as to what the medication does. Some examples include:

- Prevacid (prevents acid)
- Ambien (good morning)
- Plan B (an emergency backup plan to prevent pregnancy)
- Flomax (maxing urinary flow).

Trade names and **brand names** are synonymous, and imply ownership. The trade or brand drug names are owned by the company, which has spent hundreds of millions of dollars and many years in researching and developing the drug to become effective and approved by the FDA. Just as you might recognize brand-name clothing with ease and might even associate it with quality, drug companies want you to recognize and to buy their medications. It is only fair that the company that first came out with the drug be allowed to profit from its work without competitors, who potentially could siphon away profits by selling the drug at a lower cost. Therefore, the developing drug company gives a catchy brand name to its officially approved *generic named* drug. The patent protection of a drug is 20 years, but many years go by while the company waits for final FDA approval to sell the drug on the market.

After the patent expires, other companies are free to produce the same drug. Therefore, generic drugs will not be produced until the patent protection has expired. A generic drug is the bioequivalent or the same as a brand-name drug except it costs less money.

How can we tell the difference between a brand name and generic name? Well, usually you can tell the difference just by looking at the drug name. A brand name will often have a registered trademark symbol after its name and usually begins with a capital letter. Generic names are always written in all lowercase letters (unless they begin a sentence) and always

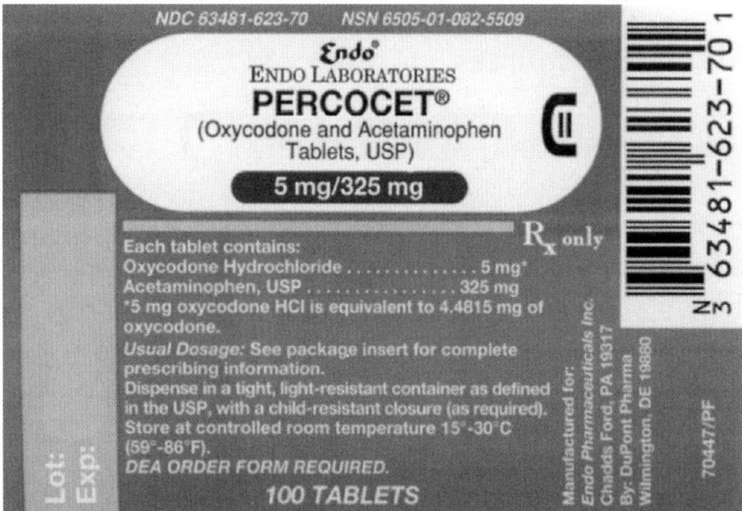

FIGURE 3-8 Trade name and generic name found on Percocet label. Note that the generic names on this label begin with capital letters but do not in texts or readings.

lack a trademark symbol. For example, acetaminophen is the generic name for Tylenol®. The label in Figure 3-8 shows both the brand name and generic name. In this MindTap, we will capitalize all trade names and will not use the trademark symbol.

CLINICAL CONNECTION 3.4

Many states in the United States have generic substitution laws. These laws allow pharmacists to substitute prescriptions with generic drugs from other manufacturers. However, pharmacists are not permitted to change the strength of the medicine prescribed. If physicians do not wish for their patients to receive any generic substitutions for whatever reason, a "Dispense as written" or "Do not substitute" order must accompany the script.

3-8 OFFICIAL AND CHEMICAL NAMES

Just when you thought the same drug had enough names, there are even more. Medications also receive an **official name** given by the USP/NF, after the drug has been approved for use. The good news that this name is usually the same as the generic name.

Each drug also has a **chemical name** that is important in the drug manufacturing process. This name describes the molecular structure of a substance. These names are rarely, if at all, used in a clinical setting or marketing campaign because of their shear complexity. Can you imagine receiving a prescription or an order for 8-chloro-1-methyl-6-phenyl-4H-s-triazolo [4,3-α] [1,4] benzodiazepine? This chemical structure is for Xanax (alprazolam). Thankfully, we need only to know the brand and generic names, which does not seem too bad after considering the chemical names.

LEARNING OBJECTIVE 3.3 Compare terms indicating drug actions and drug reference sources.

KEY TERMS

Absolute contraindication Medication or procedure is life-threatening and the benefits do not outweigh the risks; should not be administered.

Adverse reactions Can occur suddenly or over time and range from patient discomfort to possible death; also known as side effects.

AHFS Drug Information (American Health-System Formulary Service) A book primarily for pharmacists that covers such topics as drug stability and chemical information.

Cautions A list of certain patients for whom or conditions under which a drug should be used with close supervision.

Contraindications A list of reasons why a certain drug should not be given.

Drug actions The interactions between a drug and body at the cellular level.

Interaction List of items that can interact and change a drug's effect.

Labeled indications Uses for what the drug is intended to treat.

Nonlabeled indication When a drug or medication is used to treat a condition for which it is not approved; may be used if enough research proves it beneficial.

Physician's Desk Reference (PDR) Collection of specific drug information required by the FDA from drug manufacturers that includes photos of medications.

Relative contraindication A drug or procedure that is only done if the benefits outweigh the risks.

Side effects Undesirable experiences of medication that can occur quickly or over time; also known as adverse reactions.

3-9 INDICATIONS

Did you ever receive a medication with a folded drug insert with all kinds of information in small type with what seemed to be complex terminology? Being a good consumer, you immediately read and understood the entire packet—yeah, right. Don't worry; hardly anyone does, but after completing this objective it will make much more sense, and you will be able to focus on the more meaningful sections.

One of the most important sections is the indications, which list the diseases the drug is used to treat, such as insulin is indicated to treat diabetes. Drugs can also have more than one use. There are two types of indications, labeled uses and nonlabeled uses. **Labeled indications** of a drug means its use has been widely proven to be effective in treating certain conditions.

Nonlabeled indication of a drug means the medication is not approved for a specific ailment, but might be used if enough research proves it beneficial. It also means the manufacturer has not applied for approval by the FDA for that particular condition.

3-9a Contraindications

Contra means *against* so obviously this section will look at reasons why a drug should not be administered or its **contraindications**. Keep in mind that drugs are not the only therapy that might be harmful to a patient. If any surgeries,

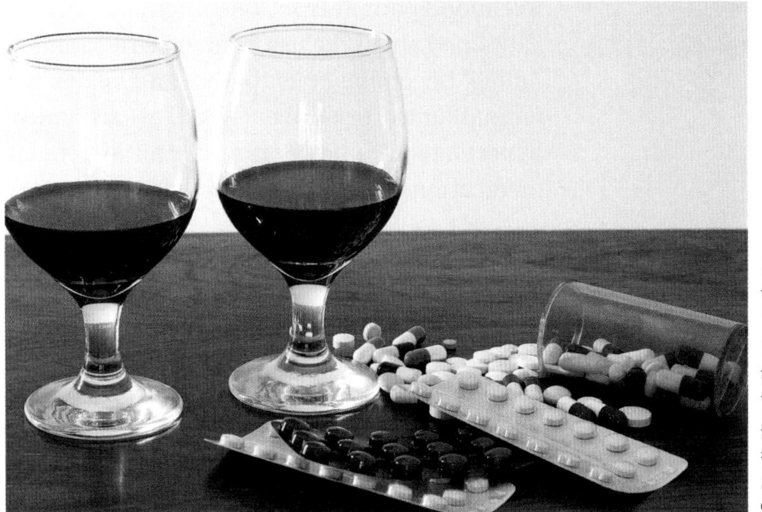

© GiselleFlissak/Shutterstock.com.

FIGURE 3-9 Drugs and alcohol do not mix.

procedures, or other treatments might harm a patient if they were done, they also are considered to be contraindications. When a patient is taking a blood thinner such as Coumadin, it is contraindicated for the patient to take aspirin, which also thins the blood. Another commonly seen warning on drug labels is the consumption of alcohol while taking medication (see Figure 3-9).

Contraindications can have different levels. For example, a **relative contraindication** means the drug should not be used in this situation UNLESS the benefits outweigh the risk. For example, a drug is contraindicated for people with heart disease because it might cause some irregular beats. In one case, however, the physician believes the patient will die if the drug is not taken. Obviously, although the drug is contraindicated, the benefits outweigh the risks.

However, if the medication or procedure will be life-threatening, and the benefits do not outweigh the risk then it is an **absolute contraindication**, and it should not be given at all. For example, according to the FDA, children under 2 years of age should not take any OTC cold and cough medicines. Not only will these not help relieve symptoms in the child, but they can also be dangerous and should be avoided. The active ingredients can cause an increased heart rate, convulsions, unconsciousness, and death.

3-10 DRUG ACTIONS

Drug actions are defined as how a drug interacts with the body at the cellular level. In simpler terms, it is how a drug does what it is supposed to do. Drugs can increase and decrease the body's ability to slow down or speed up certain processes. For example, we can give Lasix to remove fluid from the body by increasing urination. Another example is Flomax, which is used to relax muscles in the neck of the bladder and prostate to make it easier for men to urinate.

3-11 CAUTIONS

Cautions are a list of certain patients or conditions with which a drug should be used under close supervision. Patients with certain conditions such as pregnancy must be closely monitored as a precaution when there is a greater likelihood certain reactions might occur. Adults older than 65 years of age are cautioned about the use of muscle relaxants because of the increased chance of falling, becoming constipated, and issues with urination. Certain nonsteroidal anti-inflammatory drugs (NSAIDS) are known to potentially cause pulmonary hypertension in newborns, so cautions must be taken when suggesting these medications to pregnant women.

3-12 SIDE EFFECTS

Side effects or **adverse reactions** are not only undesirable experiences, but also possible deadly events. Side effects are classified as mild, moderate, severe, or life-threatening. These adverse events can occur quickly or over time, and the patient should stop taking the medication and notify his or her physician if any adverse reactions occur.

Side effects are found not only in prescription drugs but also in over-the-counter pharmaceuticals. Since all drugs have some possible side effects, why does the FDA approve drugs that are potentially deadly? Well, think of it this way. Why do we do open-heart surgeries or place stents in closed arteries during a cardiac catheterization, when these procedures can kill the patient?

The answer is that the benefits have to outweigh the risks. Some drugs are known to be carcinogenic, or cancer-causing. For example, the drug Tamoxifen is used to treat breast cancer; however, it has been discovered that it can cause uterine cancer. Again, the benefit has to outweigh the risk. Side effect warnings are listed in medication inserts.

Take a look at the many possible side effects of Lipitor, a commonly prescribed pill used to lower high cholesterol:

tenderness	jaundice	muscle pain
confusion	clay-colored stools	weakness drowsiness
problems with memory	diarrhea	blurred vision
fever	swelling	weight loss
dark-colored urine	increased thirst	nausea
increased urination	dry mouth	upper stomach pain
little or no urinating	dry skin	loss of appetite
	itching	hunger
	sweet fruity-like breath	weight gain

3-13 INTERACTIONS

A drug's **interaction** is a list of foods, drugs, and supplements that can interact with and change the effect of certain medications. Interactions can occur when taking more than one type of drug, possibly increasing or decreasing their effectiveness. The more drugs a patient is administered, the greater will be the likelihood of this occurrence. For example, antibiotics can decrease the effectiveness of oral contraceptives to prevent pregnancy. Thankfully, physicians do not have to rely solely on memory to know the drug interactions of the ever-increasing numbers of new drugs being introduced to the market every year. Instead software programs are now used to flag any possible drug interactions.

3-14 DRUG REFERENCES

With all the different and continuously evolving medications available today, there is no shame in looking up a drug in one of the many drug references available. No matter what healthcare setting you work in, a reference of some sort should be within reach. It is highly important to keep up-to-date on all the latest information to maximize care and minimize error.

3-14a Book References

The **Physician's Desk Reference (PDR)** is a collection of specific drug information required by the FDA from the drug's manufacturers. This reference is updated every year and has three different versions for physicians, nurses, and consumers. Found within the PDR is product information such as dosage, indications, common brand names, administration, contraindications, warnings and precautions, adverse reactions, and drug actions. The negative aspects of the book are that it contains the names of only the drugs that manufacturers paid to be included and that the standard edition contains no OTC drugs. If you wish to have OTC drugs in a PDR format, then the PDR OTC text must be purchased. The drugs that are listed have pictures of the medications to assist in identifying a drug. Traditionally, this very thick reference was only in book form. However, it is also available online and can now be accessed from a smartphone.

Another drug reference source available is the United States Pharmacopeia and the National Formulary (USP-NF) book. In the United States, the FDA considers the USP-NF to be the official standard for drugs on the market. This reference contains standards not only for pharmaceuticals but also for medical devices and dietary supplements. The USP-NF is a combination of two books that have been blended together to enhance its usage. This book can be confusing to use and does not come with pictures of medications because it is directed toward laboratories and manufacturers.

The **AHFS Drug Information (American Health-System Formulary Service)** is a paperback book that is more geared to pharmacists and contains information not necessarily needed by healthcare professionals, such as drug stability and chemical information. Also, there are no pictures that can be used for drug identification purposes. This resource organizes the drugs by classifications and also has off-label drug uses (see Figure 3-10).

3-14b Internet References

Internet references are popular for easy access and ease of use. However, it is important to use only trusted Web sites from reputable organizations. Otherwise, the information might be incorrect and jeopardize a patient's care. Pay close attention to the date the article was published. It might be outdated and

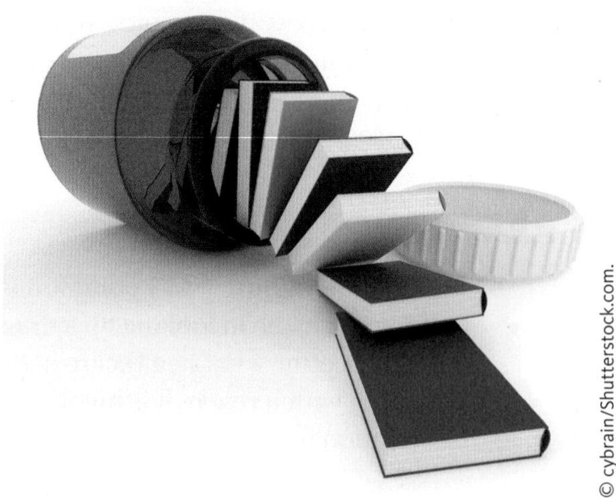

FIGURE 3-10 Every medical facility or practice should have up-to-date drug references available.

no longer a standard practice. Also, keep away from biased Web sites listing testimonials and other medication forums. A few professional sources include:

http://www.pharmacist.com

http://www.fda.gov

http://www.safemedication.com

http://www.usp.org

http://www.cdc.gov/vaccines/

http://www.nlm.nih.gov/medlineplus/

LEARNING OBJECTIVE 3.4 Summarize pharmacognosy and contrast local and systemic effects of drugs.

KEY TERMS

Chemoinformatics The usage of analytical data about the properties, structure, and molecular activities of chemical compounds used to design a drug.

Investigational new drugs (IND) Three-step process for a drug to be approved by the FDA for clinical use.

Local effect Stimulation of a certain part or region of the body.

Pharmacognosy Studies the natural sources of pharmaceuticals.

Semisynthetic Drug having a natural origin with a chemically altered variation.

Synthetic Chemically manufactured drug.

Systemic effect Effect of a drug on the entire body.

3-15 DRUG SOURCES

Whether intentionally or accidentally discovered, drugs are derived from many different sources. The discipline that studies the natural sources of pharmaceuticals is known as **Pharmacognosy**. When it comes to medicine, we consumers see the drug in its finalized form, such as a capsule, syrup, or injection. The medicine has a processed appearance that in most cases in no way resembles its origin, so consumers have no way to identify its origin. Drugs can come from plants, minerals, animals, chemicals (synthetics), and recombinant DNA technology.

3-15a Plants

Plants have been used to cure ailments for centuries. Plant leaves, flowers, roots, stems, seeds, fruits, and barks often can be used to produce a pharmacologic effect, whether it be for medicinal or illicit use. Examples are willow bark, which is used to make aspirin, and foxglove leaves, which are used to make digoxin (see Figure 3-11).

Opium is used to make morphine, and coca leaves produce cocaine. Plants can have a powerful effect on the body, and it is important to tell your physician if you are taking any herbal supplements because they might cause an unwanted drug reaction. Just because a label says "natural" does not mean that it is always a healthy choice. For example, garlic supplements are used for the potential effects of decreasing high blood pressure and hardening of arteries. However, if a person takes garlic supplements with medication with anticoagulation properties, such as aspirin and warfarin, the chances of bleeding are increased as a possible side effect.

3-15b Animals

This may shock vegans, but another source for medication is from animal products, such as pictured in Figure 3-12. Hormone medications used to treat hypothyroidism might be derived from animals. Some substances might state it is a bovine derivative, meaning it came from a cow. If the drug is from a porcine origin, then it came from a pig. Premature babies can benefit from the harvest of surfactant from the lungs of cows and pigs. Surfactant is a natural phospholipid substance produced by the body that lines the alveolar surface of the lungs

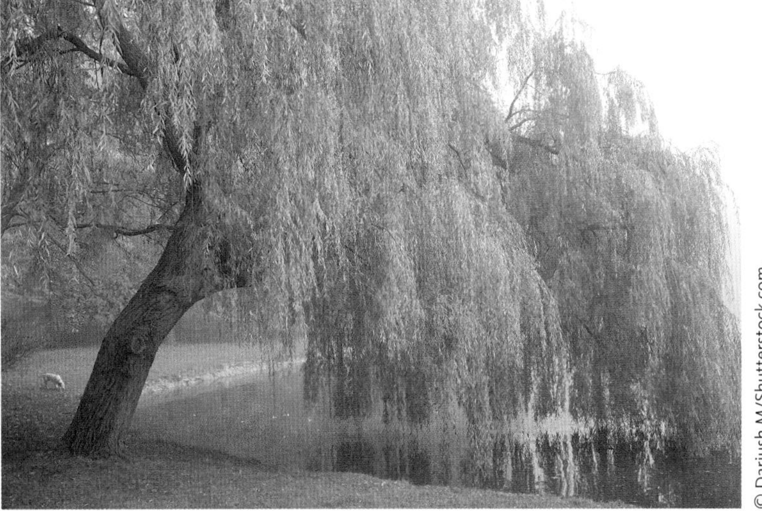

FIGURE 3-11 The bark of a willow tree contains the active ingredient in aspirin.

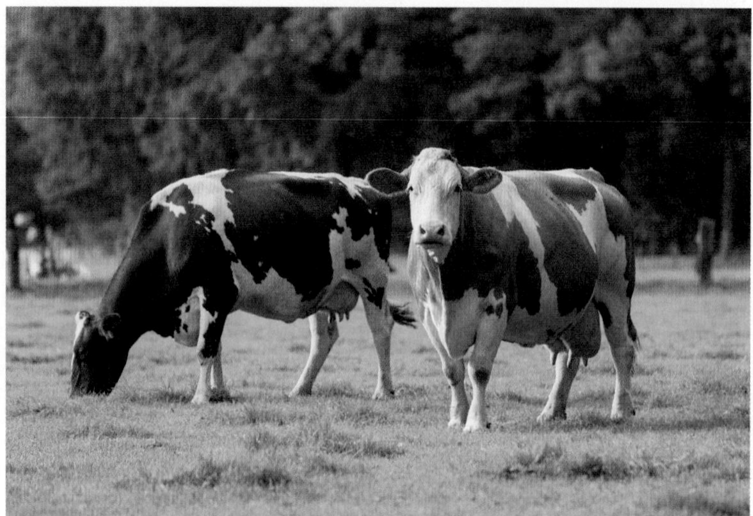

FIGURE 3-12 Bovine derivatives from cows can be used to make a variety of medicines, including the life-saving substance surfactant for premature infants.

and prevents alveolar collapse. Premature infants often have not developed enough surfactant to keep their lungs open as this substance is developed late in pregnancy. Surfactant is instilled into the lungs to help the patient breathe better. You are probably also familiar with fish oil products that are used to lower cholesterol.

3-15c Minerals

Gold, which has anti-inflammatory abilities, is used to treat rheumatoid arthritis. Iodine is used as an antiseptic, and zinc is used as a topical ointment for skin conditions such as eczema or in creams such as sunscreen. Heartburn can be relieved with antacids that contain calcium, magnesium, and aluminum as their active ingredients. If constipation is the issue, there is a mineral for that, too. Magnesium hydroxide is the active ingredient found in laxatives. Mineral oil is a lubricant laxative, meaning that it does not allow the intestines to pull water from stool so it remains within the stool instead, causing the stool to soften (see Figure 3-13).

3-15d Synthetic

The drugs derived from plants and animals are *natural drugs*. However, many drugs are **synthetic**, which means they are made with materials not found in nature. They are built intentionally with altered chemical structures to achieve a new beneficial property.

You can also have a hybrid of natural and synthetic materials to make a drug. If a drug is **semisynthetic**, its origin is natural, but the chemical structure was changed. For example, the cancer drug paclitaxel starts out with an extraction of liquid from the needles of the yew tree. Then the liquid undergoes chemical changes to get the final product.

This is all possible because of highly trained staff and well-equipped laboratories with advanced technologies. Companies are researching with various chemicals to develop synthetic drugs that might one day cure today's incurable

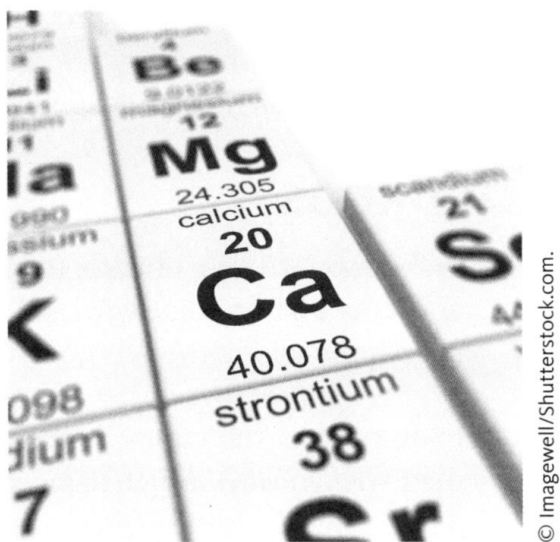

© Imagewell/Shutterstock.com.

FIGURE 3-13 Many minerals can be used for medicinal purposes.

conditions. **Chemoinformatics** is a process that uses analytical data about the properties, structure, and molecular activities of chemical compounds to design a drug (see Figure 3-14).

3-16 INVESTIGATIONAL NEW DRUGS

Developing a new drug is by no means a simple endeavor. However, once a new drug has been developed and passed through animal trials, it must prove itself to the FDA to be a safe medication before it goes to market. This process is very much involved and lengthy. **Investigational new drugs (INDs)** enter a three-phase process:

- Phase one: The drug is given to a small group of healthy human subjects.
- Phase two: The drug is administered to a small group of people suffering from the condition the drug is intended to treat.
- Phase three: The drug is given to a large group and a multicenter study is done, which means the study is done at more than one facility.

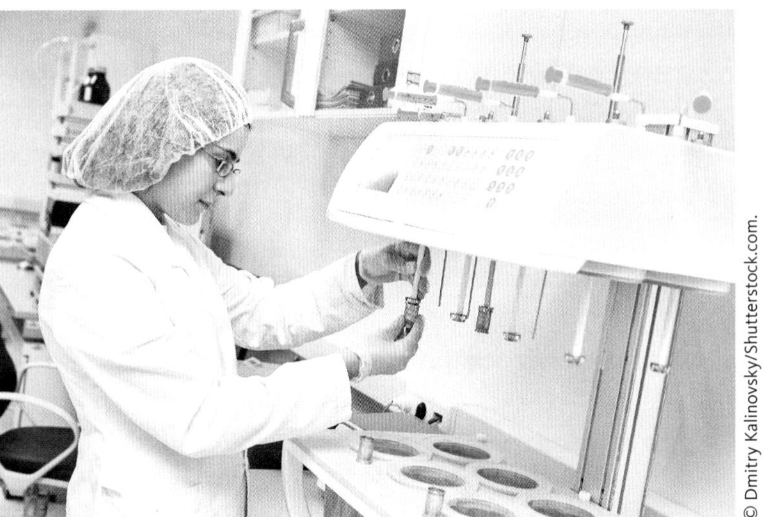

© Dmitry Kalinovsky/Shutterstock.com.

FIGURE 3-14 Pharmaceutical researcher.

After this three-step process is finished and the FDA concludes the drug is safe, the agency approves the drug for general clinical use and the manufacturer can complete a new drug application.

3-17 EFFECTS OF DRUGS

The reason we take drugs is to have some sort of a result or an effect. All drugs affect the body in some way, and the effect can be confined to one area or spread out over the entire body.

A **local effect** is just that, a stimulation of a certain part or region of the body without the entire body being affected. Examples include a local anesthetic (Novocain), which is injected to numb a specific area as in dental procedures; topical steroids and creams (Cortizone-10) that are applied directly to an affected area; and respiratory inhalers (Combivent) and nebulizers (Duoneb), which promote airway dilation when inhaled directly into the lungs.

A **systemic effect** is when the drug has an effect on the entire body. An example is a drug that is taken to relieve pain, such as ibuprofen, which is taken by mouth and broken down by the body to reach the affected site via the bloodstream.

LEARNING OBJECTIVE 3.5 Explain the process of pharmacokinetics.

KEY TERMS

Absorption Drug dissolution into the patient's bloodstream.

Additive Effect that occurs when two drugs are taken separately, but at the same time together, summative affect when two drugs are taken together.

Agonist Substance that binds to a receptor site and causes a response.

Antagonist Blocks a desired effect; when two drugs are given and they cancel out the desired effect.

Bioavailability The measurement of how much of a drug is found in our bloodstream.

Biotransforms The chemical changes of a drug in the body as a result of metabolism.

Cumulative effect Occurs when a drug is not eliminated from the body and the drug level accumulates.

Excretion Stage at which the drug has been broken down to be eliminated from the body.

Ionized A charged state in which drugs will not be absorbed until they reach a certain environment that allows them to become nonionized; then they can be absorbed.

Lipid (fat) solubility Ability to dissolve in lipids (fats); substances with low-fat solubility are absorbed at a slower rate, while those with a high-fat solubility are absorbed faster.

Metabolized When a drug is broken down or biotransformed, primarily done in the liver.

Nonionized Noncharged state during which drugs can be absorbed through the membranes of the body and into the blood.

pH In regards to drugs, it is the range from acidity to alkalinity in the GI tract.

Pharmacodynamics Actions from a drug in the body.

Pharmacokinetics The movement of a drug through the body from absorption to elimination.

Placebo effect Fake pill or sugar pill that the patient believes is medicine to treat his or her condition.

Potentiation When two or more drugs have an increased response or a prolonged effect when given together.

Prodrugs Drugs that only become active as they are broken down into metabolites.

Selective distribution Occurs when drugs have a greater affinity to reach a certain area than others, such as a cell or organ in the body.

Synergism Effect when two drugs work together to reach an increased effect much greater than if either drug was given alone.

Therapeutic range Amount of a drug present in the blood that gives the desired effect without causing any toxicity or side effects.

Volume of distribution (VD) Areas where a drug can be distributed in the body.

3-18 OVERVIEW

Before we begin to talk about the somewhat complicated process of pharmacokinetics, please view this animation, which will set the scene for our discussion.

3-19 PHARMACOKINETICS

Pharmacokinetics is the study of how the body processes drugs. Let's start by learning exactly what pharmacokinetics means. *Pharmaco-* means *drug* and *-kinesis* means *to move*. Therefore, pharmacokinetics is the movement of a drug through the body, from the time it enters until it exits. All drugs go through this process, which consists of the following phases:

- Absorption
- Distribution
- Metabolism
- Excretion

3-20 ABSORPTION

Absorption takes place after the drug has been broken down and dissolved into the patient's bloodstream. If the drug is in solid form, absorption occurs after it is dissolved into a liquid. For example, if you swallow a pill, it must be broken down first before moving into the bloodstream.

However, this step can be skipped if the drug is in a solution that can be injected directly into the blood. You'll learn more about the various routes by which a drug can be administered in the next module. Keep in mind that the faster the drug is absorbed, the quicker it can have an effect. That is why an oral pill takes longer to have an effect than getting an injection.

Also, keep in mind that all of the drug administered will not make its way into our bloodstream. The measurement of how much of a drug is found in our bloodstream and therefore able to have an effect is known as the **bioavailability**. The bioavailability can be measured by taking a blood sample and assessing how much drug is within the bloodstream. Several factors can affect the level of the bioavailable drug. When drugs are taken orally, the stomach acidity levels and stomach contents can affect bioavailability.

3-20a pH of the Gastrointestinal Tract

pH is the measure of the acidity or alkalinity of a substance. We should all know our stomach is very acidic to break down food (and drugs) to a soluble form that can then be dissolved. However, did you know the pH changes along the gastrointestinal (GI) tract? The GI tract is illustrated in Figure 3-15.

Our stomach has an acidic environment of about 1–2 pH, while the remainder of the GI tract becomes more alkalotic, such as in the intestines, where the pH is 4–5. So what does this have to do with bioavailability? We have to add one more chemistry concept to explain. For a drug to have an effect, it must be able to pass through a cell membrane. In order to do this, it must be in a noncharged state, meaning it has no electrical charge that would repel it from the cell membrane.

Chemically speaking, drugs that are **nonionized** do not have a charge or are neutral. The nonionized state is when drugs can be absorbed through the membranes of the body and into the blood. On the other hand, **ionized** drugs will not be absorbed until they reach a certain environment that allows them to become nonionized.

pH affects how much of the drug will be in its ionized form and how much will be nonionized. Therefore, drugs such as aspirin that are more likely to being

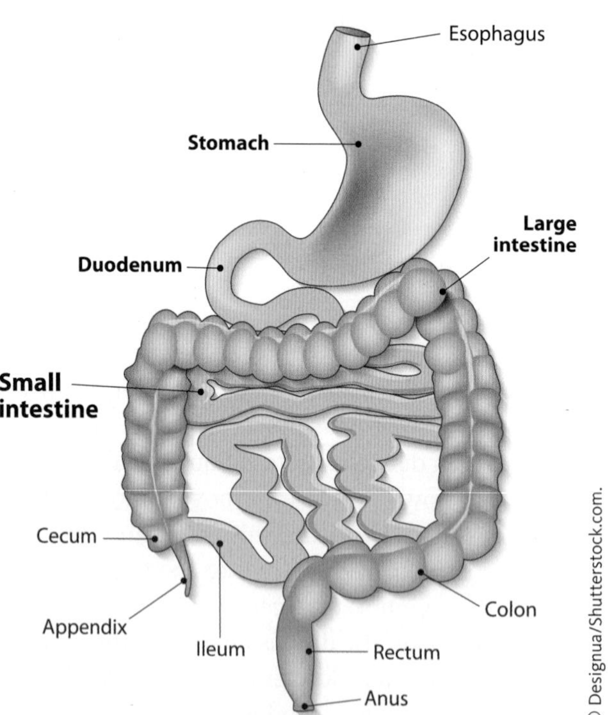

FIGURE 3-15 The stomach has a low pH, making it very acidic. As the medication travels through the GI tract, the pH increases and it becomes more alkalotic in the intestines. Absorption also occurs in the stomach and small intestine, while elimination is done via the large intestine.

nonionized in an acidic pH will be absorbed through the acidic stomach environment. In contrast, alkalotic favorable drugs are absorbed in the lower GI where a more alkaline environment exists.

How does this all apply to medications? What we eat can have an effect on the rate of absorption. Dairy products such as milk can affect the rate of absorption because they decrease acidity, making it difficult for acidic drugs to be readily absorbed. That is why the instructions of some drugs are that they are not to be taken with milk. Some drugs such as quinidine need to be absorbed in the intestines and not in the stomach. Therefore, it is a more alkaline favorable medication.

3-20b Lipid Solubility

Lipid (fat) solubility can also affect drug absorption. The cell membrane through which the drug must pass is composed of lipids, so it makes sense that lipid soluble (able to dissolve through lipids) drugs would be absorbed better.

Drugs with high-fat solubility are absorbed through the stomach mucosa, while substances with low-fat solubility are absorbed at a much slower rate. Drugs with low-fat solubility are not often given by mouth for that reason. However, there are instances where you can use this to an advantage. For example, neomycin is a low-lipid drug used to treat intestinal infections. Here, you do not want it to be absorbed in the stomach but wait until it reaches the intestines to begin its work. Therefore, neomycin can be given orally but will not start to be absorbed until it reaches the intestinal tract, where it can then combat the infection.

3-20c Stomach Contents

Another factor that can cause disturbances in the rate of absorption is the presence or absence of food in the stomach. It is possible for a drug to absorb slower in the stomach if food is also present, since the body has to process those contents as well. This is not always an unwanted situation, and is useful for drugs that would be too harsh on the stomach and might otherwise result in nausea or even an ulcer (see Figure 3-16).

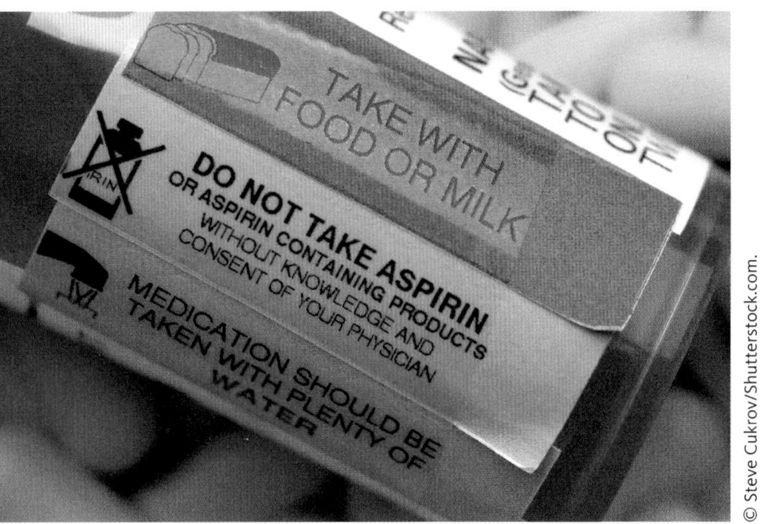

© Steve Cukrov/Shutterstock.com.

FIGURE 3-16 Drug label emphasizing to take with food or milk.

3-21 DISTRIBUTION

After the drug has been given and is absorbed into the bloodstream, the substance must now travel via the circulatory system to the tissues and fluids where it is needed (see Figure 3-17). The regions where a drug can be distributed in the body is known as the **volume of distribution (VD)**.

What factors determine where a drug will be distributed? We already discussed a very important one. Drugs that are lipid- or fat-soluble have the ability to pass more easily through the phospholipid cell membrane.

Therefore, lipid-soluble drugs can also have a greater effect in obese patients because of their higher fat content. Another variable to consider in drug distribution is **selective distribution**. Selective distribution is the term applied when drugs have a greater affinity to reach a certain area and target a specific cell or organ in the body. For example, the human chorionic gonadotropin hormone has selective distribution to the ovaries. This is quite advantageous since this is used as a fertility drug.

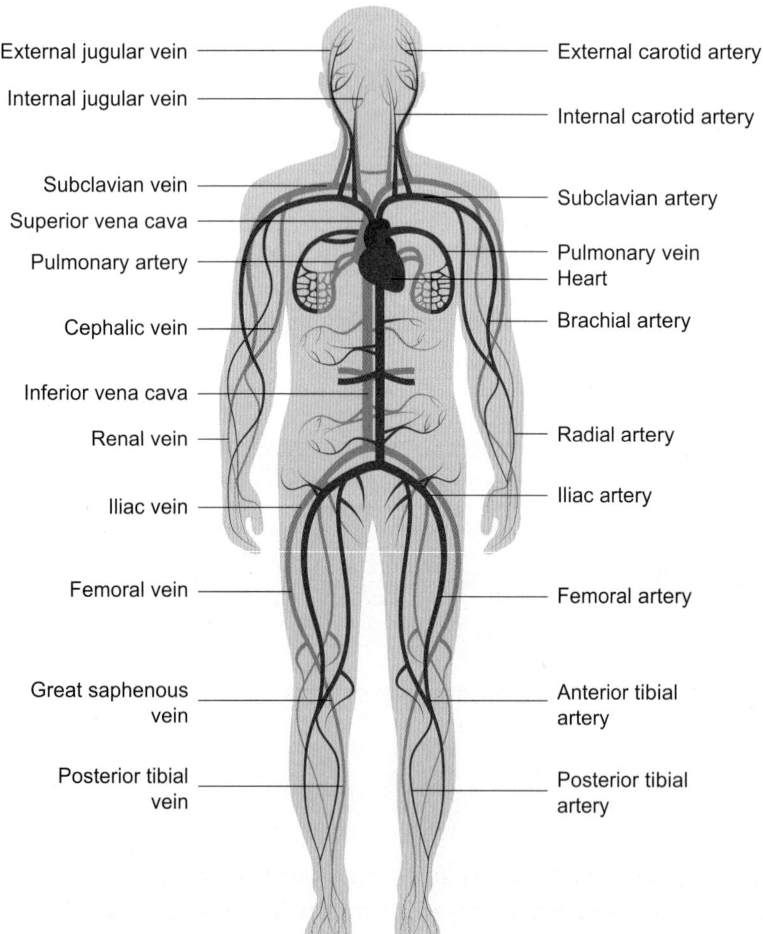

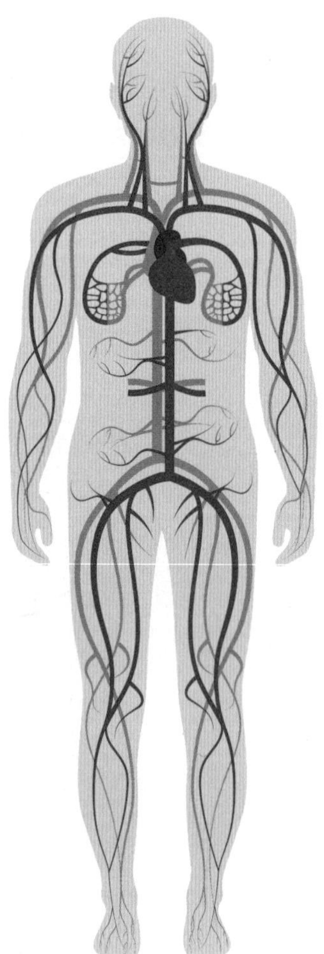

FIGURE 3-17 A drug is distributed throughout the body after it reaches the bloodstream.

3-22 METABOLISM

When we take medication, it is, to us, just a drug to make us feel better. However, to our body, it is a foreign substance that it wants to break down and remove. While this might sound harsh, essentially a drug is a controlled poison used to get our body back to homeostasis.

After a drug has been absorbed, and distributed, it is then **metabolized** by the body so the substance can be excreted. The liver is the organ that breaks down or **biotransforms** (metabolizes) pharmaceuticals into water-soluble metabolites or byproducts that can then be eliminated by the kidneys, feces, sweat glands, or even our breath. People with liver diseases will not be able to properly metabolize drugs, so careful monitoring must take place to ensure proper dosages (see Figure 3-18).

In most cases, a drug becomes inactive after it is broken down into smaller chemical molecules (metabolites). However, there are always exceptions to rules. Some drugs are engineered to be inactive until they are metabolized and then the metabolites become active and have an effect. These drugs are called **prodrugs**, and the drug Plavix is one example.

CLINICAL CONNECTION 3.5

Have you ever wondered why some medications warn their users not to consume grapefruit or other citrus fruit? The prohibition includes extracts used to flavor drinks and fruits crossed with a grapefruit. This might seem like it's not a big deal, but it is potentially life-threatening. The problem is that citrus fruit chemicals can interfere with the body's enzymes and its ability to metabolize a drug to excrete it from the body. Depending on the medicine, a drug taken with grapefruit juice might be in the body too long and build up to toxic levels.

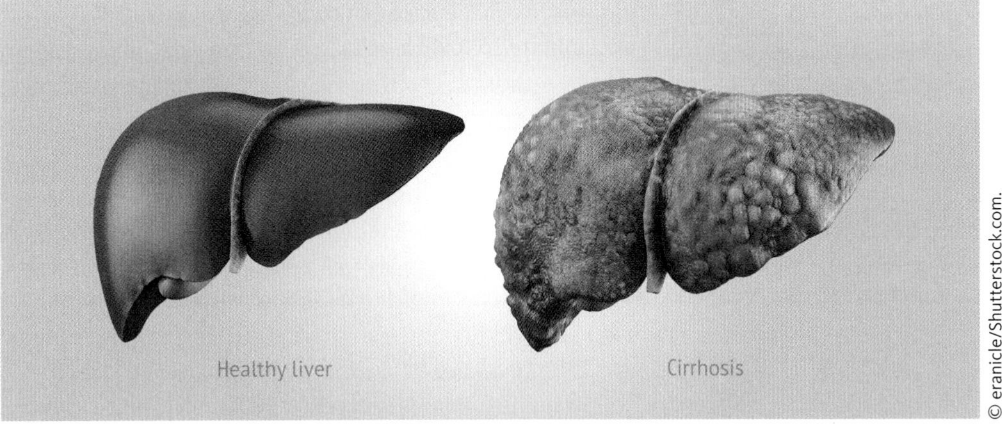

FIGURE 3-18 The liver is the organ that metabolizes drugs. Any diseases that affect this organ will decrease its ability to metabolize a drug and therefore the drug can "stay around" longer and have a greater than expected effect. A diseased liver is shown on the right.

3-23 EXCRETION

The last stage in the pharmacokinetic process is the **excretion** stage. At this point, the drug has been broken down to be eliminated from the body via feces, urine, breast milk, and even our breath. The kidneys are the main organ that removes drugs from our body via urine. Patients with renal diseases must be closely monitored for proper drug levels in their body. If unable to be eliminated from the body, drugs can accumulate in excessive quantities in the blood because of the **cumulative effect** (see Figure 3-19).

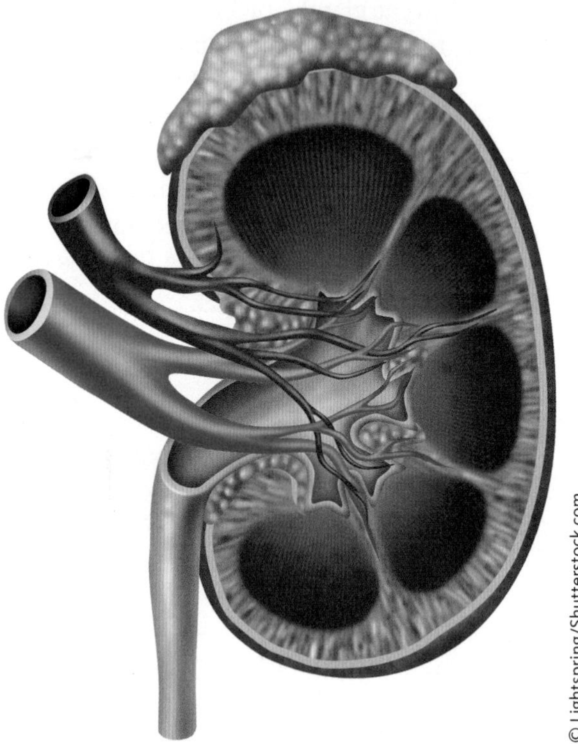

FIGURE 3-19 While excretion occurs in different ways, the chief way this occurs is through the kidneys. Renal disease can cause the drug to accumulate to toxic levels.

CLINICAL CONNECTION 3.6

To see if an individual used drugs, a drug test can be done in different ways, such as blood, saliva, urine, and hair follicle samples. However, since the kidneys filter and clean the blood of toxins and waste products, traces of excreted drug metabolites (drug ruminants broken down by the body) can be found in a person's urine.

The test used will depend on how long a drug can be found in the body. Drugs can be detected in a urine sample anywhere from a few days to a month, while a test used to examine hair follicles can trace drugs trapped in the hair up to 90 days. Although the hair follicle test is better for detecting chronic usage, it is more expensive than a urinalysis, making a urinalysis more commonly used.

CLINICAL CONNECTION 3.6 (*Continued*)

Whether the drug test is scheduled or at random, every test is conducted by a certified laboratory to ensure accuracy and dependability. You might have heard the term drug panel but, what exactly is it? A panel is a group of drugs the drug screen looks to discover in an individual's specimen sample. An employer or police, for example, can choose which panel or group it would like to test. The higher the panel is, the more groups of drugs can be found. For example, a four-panel drug screen tests for four categories of drugs while a nine-panel drug screen looks for traces of nine drug categories. Both illegal and prescription drug use can be reflected in a sample. A lab will ask you to list the medications you are currently prescribed because if the test is "flagged" as positive, the lab will know it is a legally prescribed substance.

The **therapeutic range** is the amount of a drug that needs to be present in the blood to have the desired effect without causing any toxicity or side effects. This range is found by examining a sample of blood from the patient with each drug having its specific therapeutic level.

3-24 OTHER VARIABLES AFFECTING DRUG ACTION

Age can have a huge impact on a drug and its effects. Older patients have a slower metabolism, which means it takes longer for their bodies to process a drug. The elderly do not urinate as frequently as do younger people, which can cause an increase in the drugs in their body. If they do not eliminate the drug before receiving more dosages, it will add up in the bloodstream and could increase the side-effects. Children, on the other hand, might not have a fully developed system to eliminate drugs from their bodies as efficiently as adults. These are some reasons the clinician must pay close attention to dosages.

Another variable is the weight of the user. Drug dosages are calculated by the patient's weight. When administering dosages, generally the larger the person is, the larger will be the dose.

Gender also plays a role in drug dosing. Women and men do not respond in the same manner. Generally speaking, women are smaller than men and have a different body mass. Pregnant women must be extra cautious about what they put into their bodies because substances can cross the placental barrier and affect the developing fetus. Even harmless drugs can have undesired consequences in unborn babies. Drugs the mother takes also can be passed onto her child through breastfeeding. Men tend to metabolize drugs faster than females. Their hormones differ, and the woman has an ability to become pregnant.

The **placebo effect** is another drug action variable that needs mentioning. The placebo effect occurs when a patient is given a fake pill or sugar pill and told is it is medicine that will help his or her condition. But because it is an inactive substance, it will have only a psychological effect. This phony pharmaceutical is used in research trials to see whether a drug is working for a patient population by giving one group the actual drug and a control group the placebo. No one knows if they are taking the actual drug or placebo and therefore this is termed a "blind study" to see if this drug is truly effective in treating this disease.

CLINICAL CONNECTION 3.7

Polypharmacy poly = many, or the over-prescribing of medications can occur in different ways and is a critical concept to keep in mind when treating patients, particularly elderly patients. Pharmacokinetics can be affected by age, especially if any impairment of the kidneys and liver is present. If the body cannot efficiently manage medications, the drug will remain in the patient's system longer, potentially building up to toxic levels causing adverse effects. Below are a few examples of how polypharmacy can occur in a clinical setting.

- When a physician orders multiple medications for a patient who is also being prescribed medication by another medical practitioner.
- When a patient is being treated for more than one ailment.
- Poor communication between treating physicians.

To prevent polypharmacy from occurring, a patient should have a list of all current medications so the physician can review the drugs the patient is currently taking.

3-25 PHARMACODYNAMICS

Pharmacodynamics are the actions of a drug in the body. While pharmacokinetics described what the body does to the drug, pharmacodynamics focuses on what the drug does to the body. In each of the system modules, you will learn about the specific pharmacodynamics of the drugs used to treat a specific disease. For now, remember that for a drug to work, it must reach a receptor site and cause or block an action. If a drug binds to a receptor site and causes a specific action, such as speeding up the heart, it is called an **agonist**. If the drug blocks a specific response, it is known as an **antagonist**. For example, a beta antagonist (also called a beta blocker) will block the action of the heart and slow its rate and force of contraction.

3-26 DRUG INTERACTIONS

Drug interactions within the body are increased when a patient is taking multiple drugs. These interactions can increase or diminish the desired effect of a drug. There are several terms to describe how these potential multidrug interactions can occur.

Synergism occurs when two drugs work together to achieve an increased effect greater than if either one drug was given alone. Think of it as if each drug that is given to a patient is a piece of a puzzle. With the addition of other drugs or puzzle pieces, the bigger picture or the desired response can now be seen (see Figure 3-20). Any drug that has this ability is referred to as a synergistic drug. For example, ibuprofen is an anti-inflammatory drug, and this classification

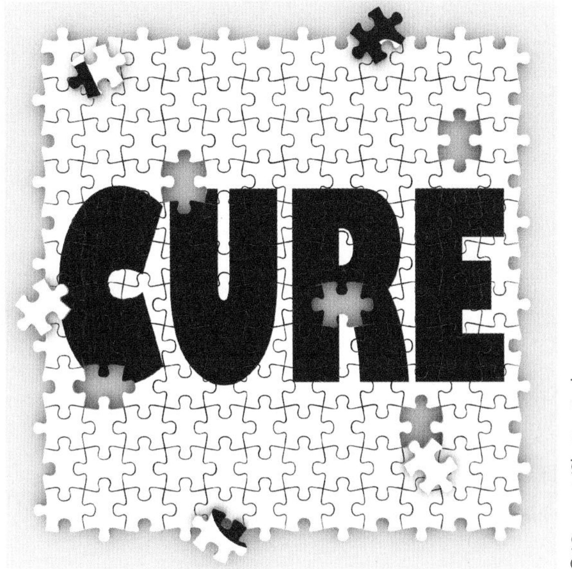

FIGURE 3-20 Synergistic drugs work together to achieve the desired outcome and response.

has synergism with opioids, since both classes are used to treat pain in different ways. Opioids reduce the signals being sent to the brain, which then reduces the message of pain being received. Anti-inflammatory drugs decrease special enzymes that the body uses to release prostaglandins, which if not stopped increase the pain and inflammation experienced by the patient. So by using these drugs together, one can tag-team both pain and inflammation more efficiently when the occasion arises.

While not mathematically correct you can think of synergism as $1 + 1 = 4$, whereas the ibuprofen might decrease the pain a little, and the opioid a moderate amount if given separately, however the combination greatly reduces or eliminates the pain.

Also, often seen with pain medications, **potentiation** is when two or more drugs have an increased response or a prolonged effect when given together. The difference with synergism is that one drug alone would have no effect. For example, antihistamines such as Benadryl, which do not reduce pain, can potentiate the effect of a pain-reducing opioid such as Demerol. This would increase the effect of Demerol by taking it in conjunction with Benadryl so a patient could have less of the narcotic to achieve the desired effect. To keep with the crazy math theme, this would be $1 + 0 = 3$ where 0 represents the drug with no effect on pain.

Additive is when two drugs are given separately but at the same time. The sum of two drugs adds up to give the desired effect. Therefore, two smaller doses of a drug can be given to get the desired effect while decreasing the side-effects. Now, the math analogy actually is correct with $1 + 1 = 2$.

Antagonism occurs when two drugs are given and they cancel each other's actions or decreases the desired effect. For example, Narcan (naloxone) is an opioid antagonist, used to partially or completely reverse a narcotic overdose. The math example here would be $1 - 1 = 0$.

CLINICAL CONNECTION 3.8

CLINICAL USE OF ANTAGONISM

Antagonism can be a very good thing as the case of using an antagonist to block or reverse a narcotic overdose. For example, naloxone (Evzio) is the first auto-injecting device used for narcotic overdoses. This device is intended to be kept at home or with a caregiver to prevent an overdose. If the occasion arises, the medication is administered by an injection in the victim's outer thigh, with or without clothes on. Once placed at the targeted site, the needle will inject the antidote into the patient and then retract into the device to prevent accidental needle sticks.

LEARNING OBJECTIVE 3.6 Compare dosing types and adverse reactions.

KEY TERMS

Anaphylactic reaction A severe and potentially life-threatening allergic reaction to a drug.

Booster dose Given to maintain the desired immune response of a primary immunization.

Dependence Occurs when a person has a desire or a need for a drug.

Half-life (T 1/2) The time for a drug dose to decrease by half after it is administered.

Hypersensitivity When a patient has an allergic reaction to a substance.

Idiosyncratic reaction Type of adverse drug reaction that is uncommon in response to a drug.

Lethal dose A drug dose causing death.

Loading dose Larger initial dose given to quickly establish the desired therapeutic effect.

Maintenance dose Drug dose given to maintain a desired dose of drug in the blood.

Maximum dose The largest dose without causing a toxic effect.

Minimum dose The smallest dose of a drug required to obtain the desired therapeutic effect.

Paradoxical reaction Drug reaction that does the opposite of what was intended.

Pregnancy category A Category of drug that has been studied and shown to have no adverse fetal effects.

Pregnancy category B Category of drug tested on animals with no adverse effects but not tested on pregnant women.

Pregnancy category C Category of drug with no convincing studies done on animals or pregnant women to determine adverse effects.

Pregnancy category D Category of drugs showing adverse effects to fetus and given only when benefits to mother outweigh fetal risk.

Pregnancy category X Category of drugs showing adverse fetal effects and not to be used under any circumstances.

Steady state Method of drug administration where the same amount of drug is eliminated as administered therefore giving a predicable effect.

Teratogenic effect Drugs that can cause physical malformations in a fetus.

Therapeutic dose Is the dose needed to obtain the desired effect.

Tolerance Process that occurs when a dose of a drug is taken repeatedly and has less effect on the person, so a larger dose is required to reach the desired effect.

Toxic dose Side effects that can result in poisoning the patient.

3-27 DOSAGE

The type of dosage depends on the desired therapeutic effect in regards to the drug's onset, duration, and effect on the body. Too little or too much of a drug will not give the patient the desired effect. If too much of the substance is given, it can become toxic and be deadly.

Since a drug is a poison and foreign substance in the body, the body tries to eliminate it as soon as possible. The **half-life (T 1/2)** of a drug is the time it takes for the dosage of a drug to decrease by half after it is administered. Some drugs have a short half-life so they will not stay in the body long, while drugs with long half-lives will stay in the body for a long time. Ideally, the drug dosing is monitored to achieve a **steady state** of drug delivery, meaning that the same amount of a drug is eliminated as administered so the drug can have a consistent and predicable effect.

There are several dosing types depending on the given patient's condition or needs. Table 3-3 contrasts these various dosing strategies.

3-28 PHARMACOGENOMICS

Previously called pharmacogenetics, pharmacogenomics uses cutting-edge technologies to analyze human genes to understand better how an individual's genetics affects how specific drugs affect his or her body. The idea of this concept is to custom design drugs specifically for a person's body to maximize safety and efficacy, which means to produce the desired effect with the lowest dose (see Figure 3-21).

Table 3-3 Types of dosages

DOSAGE	DEFINITION
Minimum dose	The smallest amount of a drug given to obtain the desired therapeutic effect
Maximum dose	The largest dose that can be given without a toxic effect
Therapeutic dose	The dose needed to obtain the desired effect
Booster dose	Given after a primary immunization to maintain the desired immune response
Loading dose	An initial dose that is larger dose given to quickly establish the desired therapeutic effect
Maintenance dose	The drug amount needed to maintain a certain consistent level of drug in the blood
Toxic dose	Dose that produces serious adverse effects that result in poisoning the patient
Lethal dose	Dosage that causes death to occur. Although it may be a sensitive subject, some state governments use lethal injections to humanely euthanize those convicted of a crime and given the death penalty

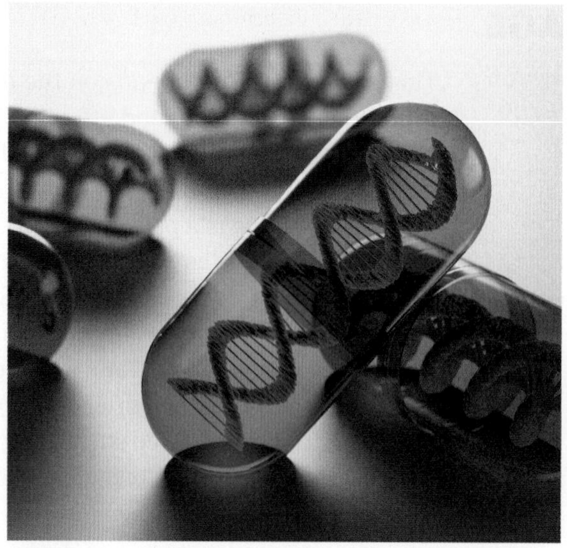

© iStockphoto/ktsimage.

FIGURE 3-21 Drugs might soon be genetically tailored for each individual to choose the best drug and dosage based on the person's genetic make-up.

Until drugs can be specially made for every patient, we must be on alert for any possible adverse reactions. It is critical to monitor patients for any unexpected response to drugs. As mentioned in a prior section, adverse reactions are unpleasant responses that occur from taking a drug and can happen to anyone at any age. Adverse reactions assume a variety of different forms, which will now be discussed.

3-29 TYPES OF ADVERSE REACTIONS

When a drug is found to have a potentially harmful effect on a developing fetus, it is termed to have a **teratogenic effect**. When a pregnant woman takes a teratogenic medication, the pregnancy has a significant chance of becoming compromised. Not only can physical malformations occur in the fetus, but the pregnancy itself can even be stopped. Table 3-4 presents more teratogenic drug categories put forth by the FDA.

There are other terms to describe potential drug reactions. An **idiosyncratic reaction** is an adverse drug reaction that is an uncommon and unpredicted response to a drug, which results from mechanisms that are not well understood. Examples are jaundice, hearing loss, and kidney damage.

A **paradoxical reaction** is a drug reaction that is the opposite of what was intended. For example, a paradoxical response would occur if a patient is given a sedative, but instead becomes anxious instead of tranquil.

Tolerance is when a dose of a drug is taken repeatedly and has less effect on the person over time. This means that a larger dose is now needed to achieve the desired effect or the drug that has the tolerance effect needs to be replaced by another drug.

Dependence occurs when a person has a desire or a need for a drug, and when it is discontinued, the patient might exhibit physical and/or psychological withdrawal symptoms. Physical dependence occurs when the body's cells have

Table 3-4 FDA drug pregnancy categorization and risk factors

PREGNANCY CATEGORY	EXPLANATION
Pregnancy Category A	Research studies on drugs in this category did not show risk to the fetus
Pregnancy Category B	Studies were done on animals and did not show any risk; not tested on pregnant women
Pregnancy Category C	Convincing studies have not been done on either pregnant women or animals
Pregnancy Category D	Studies show that the drug will cause adverse reactions to the fetus and should be used only if the mother benefited from the drug prior to the pregnancy and benefits to the mother outweigh the risks
Pregnancy Category X	Drugs that will cause teratogenic effects and should not be used during pregnancy

a need for the drug and cause symptoms such as sweating, nausea, shaking, even pain when the drug is withdrawn. Psychological dependence is when the person mentally craves the drug without exhibiting any physical symptoms other than anxiety.

CLINICAL CONNECTION 3.9

When out in public, you can see many people "doing drugs" in plain view for everyone to see. Although cigarette smoking is harmful and frowned upon by nonsmokers to the point where it has been banned in many public places, such as restaurants and even bars, cigarettes are used to administer a drug called nicotine.

Nicotine is found in all tobacco products, including both smoke and smokeless varieties. Nicotine creates an addiction that is very difficult to break, but how does this addiction occur? When a cigarette is lit and inhaled, the nicotine makes it into the blood within 10 seconds. Then the drug goes to the brain, where it stimulates the release of adrenaline. This adrenaline release causes the person to feel enjoyable effects.

The experience feels great, but it does not last long, and the person craves the return of the desirable effect. So, the person smokes another cigarette to get back to what he or she perceives as an enjoyable experience. As with any drug, a tolerance can be built, causing the person to increase the amount or frequency of tobacco usage to reach the same desired effect.

When a person decides to quit, he or she will go through withdrawal symptoms. Even though the physical withdrawal symptoms—headaches, irritability, hunger, and anxiety—last about a week, the psychological craving for another cigarette lasts much longer, and is the major factor of why people fail to quit.

3-30 HYPERSENSITIVE REACTIONS

Hypersensitivity to a drug is when a patient has an allergic reaction to the substance. The severity varies with each case. While most likely to happen in those with known allergies, an individual might experience hives or a rash after using the drug for a few days as shown in Figure 3-22. A reaction can also occur even after using the drug in the past without any allergic responses.

An **anaphylactic reaction** is the most severe and potentially life-threatening reaction one can have to a drug. This response, which causes a loss of blood pressure or shock, can commonly be seen in certain antibiotics such as penicillin, dyes used for imaging, even food such as peanuts and shellfish, and insect stings. Those aware of the possibility of a severe reaction often carry an epinephrine automatic injector to immediately inject epinephrine causing blood vessels in the body to constrict and heart rate to increase to prevent the blood pressure from dropping. Epinephrine also dilates the airways preventing bronchoconstriction, which causes wheezing and difficulty breathing. Other signs and symptoms such as itching and hives also are alleviated.

If the person does not have an epinephrine injector and stops breathing and/or does not have a heartbeat, CPR must be performed until help arrives. After the patient is in the care of medical professionals, fluids and epinephrine (Adrenalin) will be given to increase blood pressure.

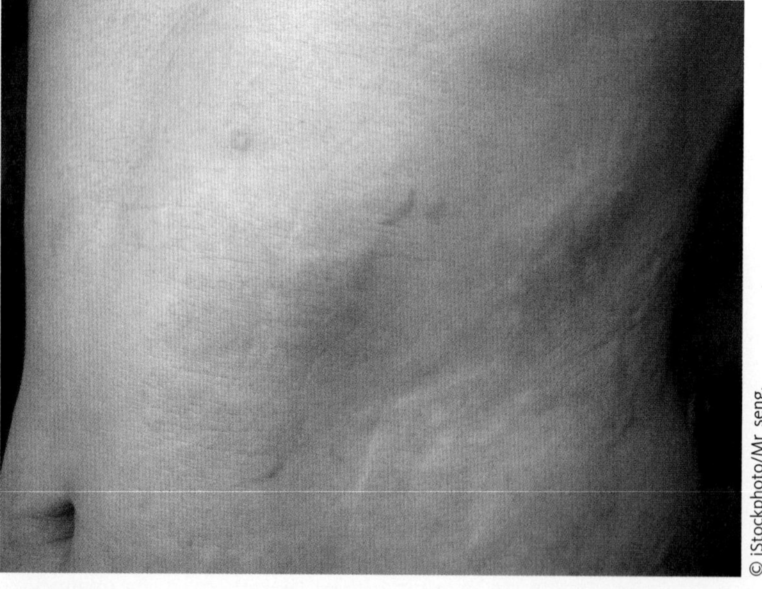

FIGURE 3-22 Presentation of hives on skin from an allergic reaction.

Module 4

Drug Administration and Dosage Forms

Module Introduction

The previous module introduced many different concepts and principles of pharmacology. To set those principles in motion, we must first administer a drug. The amount, dose, and route the substance is delivered makes a great difference on what effect it will have on the patient's body. In this module, we will develop an understanding about the various methods available to administer medications. Routes will vary from common to rarely used methods of delivery. We will also take a look at the supplies used to administer drugs, medication orders, and the abbreviations associated with those orders. This module will also discuss dosing to various patient populations as well as mentioning the steps to error reporting and reconciliation.

While we discussed pharmacokinetics in Module 3, this principle relates directly to the routes of administration that will be learned in this module.

LEARNING OBJECTIVE 4.1 Differentiate the enteral routes of administration and the available dosage forms.

KEY TERMS

Capsule (cap) A pill with a gelatin coating, making it easier to swallow.

Elixir (elix) Liquid drug mixed with an alcohol base.

Emulsion Liquid drug preparation containing fats and oils in water.

Enema Liquid solution instilled into the rectum with an applicator bottle.

Enteral route Giving drugs by way of the GI tract.

Enteric-coated tablet Coated pill that prevents disintegration by gastric juices.

Lozenge (troche) Flavored tablet held in the mouth, where it slowly dissolves.

Nasogastric tube (NG) Narrow tube passed through the nose to the stomach.

Nothing by mouth (NPO) No food, beverage, or medication to be given orally.

Oral route (PO) Taken by mouth.

Rectally (PR) or (R) Administering a drug by inserting into the rectum.

Solution Usually clear in appearance, the drug is in liquid form that is completely dissolved within the fluid.

Suppository (supp) Drug is suspended in a solid substance and inserted into the rectum.

Suspension (susp) A liquid drug form that must be shaken before using to mix the drug in the fluid.

Sustained-release capsule or tablet Medication with a coating to deliver a dose over an extended period time.

Syrup Sweetened, colorful liquid drug often masked with palatable flavors.

Tablet (tab) Form of compressed drug that comes in a variety of colors and shapes.

4-1 INTRODUCTION

Each route of administration has its own advantages and disadvantages. How quickly the drug will take effect depends on the route chosen. Drugs are given in different forms because:

- A drug might only come in a certain form, which will limit how it can be administered to a patient.
- A physician is looking for a desired effect in a patient such as a local versus systemic effect or a fast versus slow drug response. For example, if the physician wants the drug to take effect quickly, it can be given by an injection instead of a pill. Pills take longer to act because the body has to metabolize the drug before it can enter the bloodstream and be distributed throughout the body.
- The absorption characteristic of the drug.

Drugs come in a wide array of forms in addition to the various delivery routes. We will discuss these concepts more in depth throughout this module.

4-2 ENTERAL ROUTE

The term **enteral route** means through the gastrointestinal (GI) tract. When a drug is taken by mouth, also known as **the oral route (PO)**, a drug is swallowed and passes through the esophagus, into the stomach, and then through the small intestine, where it is absorbed into the blood, and through the large intestine where it is eventually excreted. Drugs administered through this route take longer to take effect since the body has to process the substance before getting it into the bloodstream. This route also includes medication given via a **nasogastric tube (NG)**, and **rectally (PR) or (R)**. Let's now examine the different forms of medications that can be administered via this route.

4-3 ORAL DRUG FORMS

Oral medications are the easiest and, in most cases, the cheapest drug forms. They cannot be used in all situations, such as emergencies when the drug must bypass the GI tract and is injected directly into the blood for immediate action. Oral forms cannot be used if the patient has difficulty swallowing, or a physician has ordered, **nothing by mouth (NPO)**. All forms discussed in this section can be seen in Figure 4-1.

A **tablet (tab)** is a compressed drug that comes in many different colors, sizes, and even shapes. Tablets often have lines down the center of the pill. These score marks are used to evenly break the pill in half or at times into thirds. This line or scoring on the pill ensures equal dosing if the pill is required to be broken. Often a pill has an outer coating that makes swallowing easy, but that is not always the case. Have you ever swallowed a vitamin or pill that seemed to stick to the back of your tongue and throat? It is likely that the pill did not have a coating on it.

An **enteric-coated tablet** is a coating on a pill that does not allow the tablet to be disintegrated by gastric juices. The drug can then pass though the stomach without being absorbed and will be broken down and absorbed farther

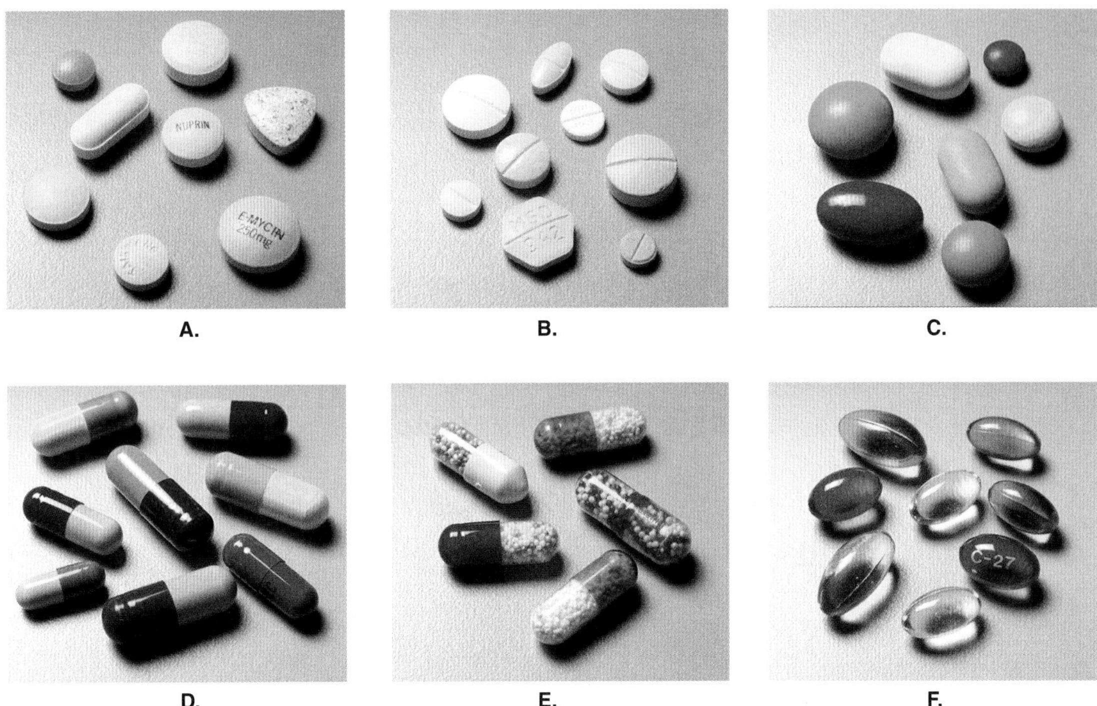

FIGURE 4-1 The oral drugs pictured come in many different colors, shapes, and sizes. (A) Tablets, (B) Scored tablets, (C) Enteric-coated tablets, (D) Capsules, (E) Sustained-release capsules, and (F) Gelatin capsules.

down the GI tract. This coating is useful for drugs such as aspirin that can irritate the stomach. It is important to keep in mind that the coating will not be effective if it is damaged from chewing or crushing.

A **capsule (cap)** is a pill that has a gelatin coating on the outside that acts like a container. This coating makes it easier to swallow than pills without the coating. Unless specified otherwise for absorption purposes, the gelatin-coating container can be pulled apart and added to food such as applesauce or drink if the patient has difficulty swallowing a pill.

A **sustained-release capsule or tablet** comes in many different coatings and colors and differs in the amount of time it takes for the coating to be dissolved. This type of coating is used to deliver a dose over an extended time period, thus decreasing the amount of times or frequency a drug has to be taken. Inside extended-release capsules are little round balls or pellets, which must not be crushed or altered. If they are, instead of the drug releasing in the body at certain time intervals, the drug will be absorbed all at once, potentially causing an overdose. Therefore, these types of capsules should remain intact or kept whole.

4-3a Other Oral Drug Forms

A **lozenge (troche)** is a tablet that is usually flavored to have a pleasant taste. The lozenge is held in the mouth where it slowly dissolves. To be effective, the patient should avoid drinking any fluids for 15 minutes after administration to prevent the effect from being washed away. Used for a sore throat, lozenges can have a soothing or even numbing effect, as seen with Chloraseptic lozenges.

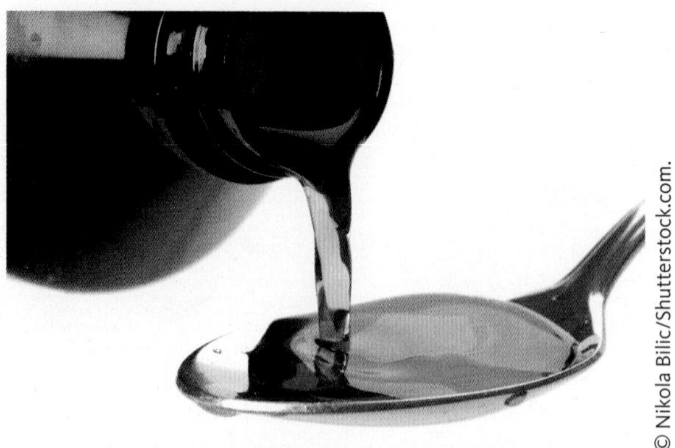

FIGURE 4-2 Pouring cough syrup onto a spoon.

A **suspension (susp)** is a liquid form of a drug that must be shaken before use to suspend the drug in the fluid. The drug particles settle at the bottom of the bottle so they are not dissolved evenly throughout the liquid until it is shaken. An antibiotic given to children called cephalosporin (cephalexin) is an example of a liquid medication that has to be shaken to suspend the drug in the liquid.

An **emulsion** is a type of drug preparation that is a liquid containing fats and oils in water.

An **elixir (elix)** or fluid extract is a liquid drug mixed with an alcohol base and should not be administered to alcoholics for that reason. In addition, because alcohol evaporates quickly, the lid must be kept on the medication securely.

A **solution** is a drug in a liquid form that is completely dissolved in the fluid. It is usually clear in appearance. A solution differs from suspension because the drug does not settle at the bottom of the bottle.

A **syrup** is a sweetened, colorful liquid drug form often with palatable flavors such as orange, grape, or cherry (see Figure 4-2). An easy way to remember this is to think of maple syrup, which is also a sweet liquid.

CLINICAL CONNECTION 4.1

Codeine is a narcotic that is used in cough syrup to suppress a cough. This should be used only for a dry, nonproductive cough. If the patient has a productive cough, and it is stopped, the mucus could settle in his or her lungs and the patient might develop pneumonia.

4-4 RECTAL DRUG FORMS

A less-desirable way to receive and administer medication is the rectal route. Rectal drug forms do serve a purpose, however, such as for a patient who can take nothing by mouth (NPO). Infants and young children who can't swallow pills can be given rectal suppositories. Drugs that can be given this route are sedatives, laxatives, antipyretics, and analgesics. Even though the drug does not travel through the entire GI tract, it is still an enteral route drug because the rectum is part of the GI tract, and the drug is absorbed in the rich blood supply in that area. These methods of delivery include suppositories and enemas.

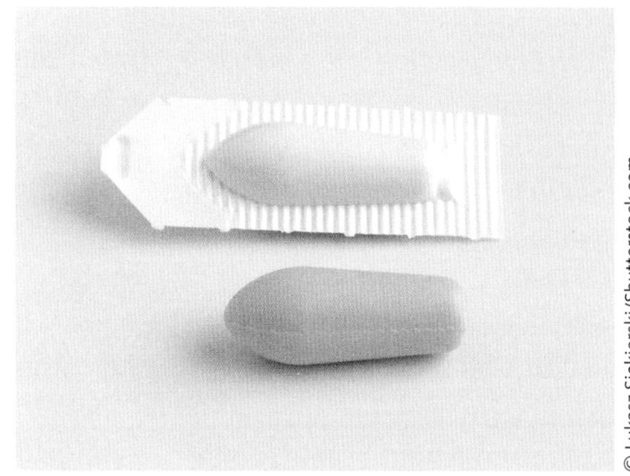

FIGURE 4-3 Rectal suppository shown inside and outside of wrapper.

A **suppository (supp)** is inserted directly into the rectum with a finger. The drug itself is suspended in a solid substance that resembles a bullet shape, Figure 4-3. The pointed end is inserted first, while the flat end is used as a surface to push the suppository into the rectum. Once inserted, the substance melts at body temperature, releasing the drug into the mucous membrane where it is absorbed.

An **enema** is a liquid drug that might be either a solution where no shaking is needed or a suspension drug where the fluid must be shaken to mix the drug. The liquid is instilled into the rectum with an applicator bottle.

LEARNING OBJECTIVE 4.2 Explain the parenteral routes of administration and related dosage forms.

KEY TERMS

Breath-actuated nebulizer (BAN) A type of nebulizer able to deliver an aerosol continuously or on inspiration only.

Buccal tablet A tablet that is kept between the cheek and gum.

Creams Thin semisolid topical drug form applied to the skin.

Dermal patches (transdermal patches) Deliver medication externally through the skin.

Douche solution A solution used to irrigate the vaginal canal.

Drops (gtt) Liquid drops of medication that can be instilled in eyes, ears, and nose.

Dry powder inhaler (DPI) A device used to administer a dry powder inhalant aerosol to lungs.

Epidural Injection into the epidural space of the spinal cord.

Eye ointment Semisolid substance used for ophthalmic purposes.

Injectable routes The ways in which a substance can be injected directly into the body.

Intracapsular (intra-articular) Injection into the joint.

Intradermal (ID) Injection right below the skin.

Intramuscular (IM) Administering a drug directly into a muscle.

Intraosseous Injecting medication into the patient's marrow of the long bones for immediate systemic effect.

Intraspinal Injection into the spinal cord.

Intravenous (IV) Directly injecting into a blood vessel.

Intraventricular route Medications are given through a catheter into the ventricle of the brain.

Liniment Medicated preparation used to soothe aches and muscle pains.

Lotion Topical cream that comes in both medicated and nonmedicated forms.

Metered dose inhaler (MDI) Uses a propellant to propel the aerosolized drug from a canister into the airways; this form can be used to give both maintenance and rescue doses.

Ointments Thick semisolid drug form applied on skin or mucosal membranes.

Parenteral route Any route that does not go through the GI tract, but term is commonly used for an injectable route.

Powder drug form Drug in powdered form that must be mixed with fluid for oral or injection. In addition, fine powdered drugs can be administered via the inhalation route.

Reconstituted Act of mixing fluid with a powdered drug form to create a solution.

Small volume nebulizer (SVN) Deliver a continuous aerosolized solution to the airways.

Solution form Solution that does not need shaken and the drug is uniformly distributed within the mixture.

Spacer Reservoir that can be added to an MDI to assist in treatment administration.

Subcutaneous (subcu) Injection of a drug into the fatty tissue layer located just below the skin.

Sublingual tablet Placed under the tongue to slowly disintegrate and absorb into the mucosa under the tongue.

Suspension form Occurs when a drug is suspended in a solution mixture and must be shaken up to mix the particles sitting on the bottom of the bottle.

Vaginal creams Medicated creams inserted into the vagina.

Vaginal suppositories Drugs suspended in a substance that melts at body temperature after being inserted into the vagina.

4-5 PARENTERAL ROUTES

Para can mean *outside* and literally the **parenteral route** means any route outside of the GI tract. There are many other ways to administer medication besides the enteral route, the most commonly thought of being the various injections, or "shots and IVs" that patients are given. However, since parenteral means any route outside of the GI tract, you will soon learn there are several parenteral routes other than injectable routes. We will begin with the injection routes, however, because they usually come to mind first. **Injectable routes** are among the fastest ways to deliver a drug. The medication is injected directly into the bloodstream, skipping the lengthier processing of the GI tract. Drugs given this route are more invasive and have a greater risk for causing an infection than with other, less invasive, routes.

4-5a Injectable Drug Forms

A liquid drug form for injection comes in two different forms:

a. **Suspension form** occurs when a drug is suspended (not dissolved) in a solution such as sterile water or oil mixture. The drug must be shaken up to mix the particles sitting on the bottom of the bottle.

b. In a **solution form**, the drug will not need shaken since it is dissolved in the solution. If the drug is in a sterile water form, it is known as an *aqueous solution (aq)*. If the drug is in an oil base, the oil makes the solution thicker or more viscous, causing the drug to have a longer absorption time than if it were mixed with water.

A **powder drug form** cannot be injected directly in the dry powder form. It first must be **reconstituted** by mixing it with a liquid such as a sterile water or saline solution.

4-6 INTRAVENOUS INJECTION ROUTES

Not all injections are the same; it depends on which tissue is injected and how the drug will be absorbed by the body. One of the most common types in the acute care setting because of its quick action is to inject directly into the bloodstream. **Intravenous (IV)** means within or to administer into a vein. Drugs administered in this manner have direct access to the bloodstream and immediate availability to vital organs, making it quick acting but potentially very dangerous. This means a lesser drug dose is needed to achieve the desired effect than if the drug were given orally. Therefore, only trained professionals should ever administer drugs via this route. Various forms of intravenous injections are the IV push, IV infusion, and IV piggyback.

The *IV push* is when a small volume of a drug called a bolus is injected into a peripheral saline lock known as a PRN adapter that is connected to a catheter already inserted into a vein. An IV push can also be given by injecting a drug into a port of a continuous IV line (again the catheter is already in the vein). See Figure 4-4.

You have probably seen an IV bag hanging in a patient's room. An *IV drip* or *IV infusion* is used to administer a large volume of fluid or fluid mixed with medication, delivered continuously into the vein at a set rate, Figure 4-5.

Sometimes you want to deliver a large amount of fluid with an IV bag and give medication on an intermittent schedule and not continuously. Another bag can be set to deliver the desired medication at a specific intermittent dosing schedule. An *IV piggyback (IVPB)* is a way to give a moderate amount of medicine via 50 to 250 mL bags. The primary IV bags usually range from 500 to 1000 mL. The piggyback IV bag needs to be given slowly and intermittently, about every 6 to 8 hours, which is why it is not mixed with the primary bag and given all at once. Therefore, the secondary bag or piggyback is hung above the primary bag, Figure 4-6.

4-7 OTHER INJECTABLE ROUTES

Another injectable route is the **intramuscular (IM)** route, in which the drug is administered directly into a muscle. This can be used for smaller doses of drugs than given IV. This injection differs from others in that it is given by a needle inserted at a 90-degree angle from the skin. A drug is quickly absorbed into the blood because of the many blood vessels in the muscle tissue.

A **subcutaneous (subcu)** injection is absorbed slower by the body than with IV or IM injections since the drug is administered into the fatty tissue

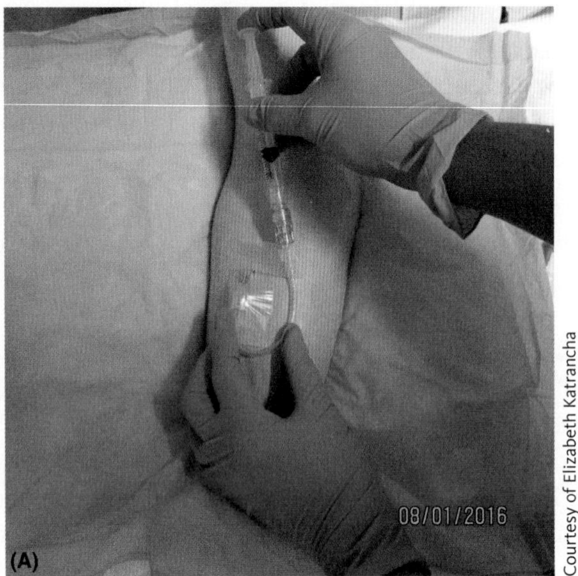

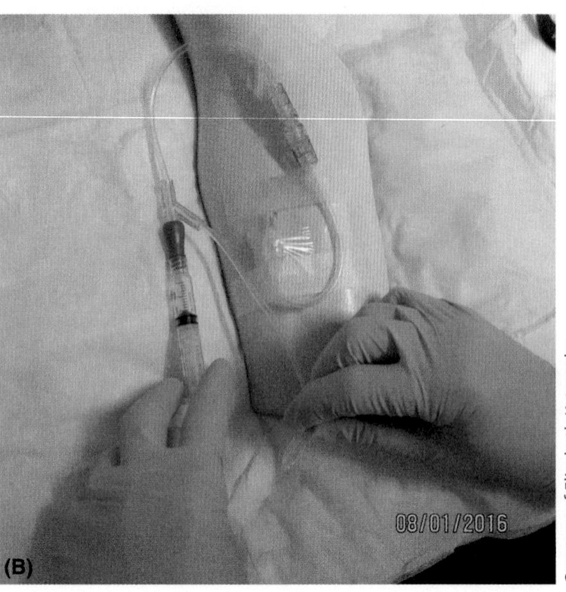

FIGURE 4-4 Intravenous administration. Different forms of IV injection include (A) IV push, injecting a bolus of medication into a peripheral saline lock; (B) pinch closed the IV tubing of a primary infusion line to administer an IV push medication.

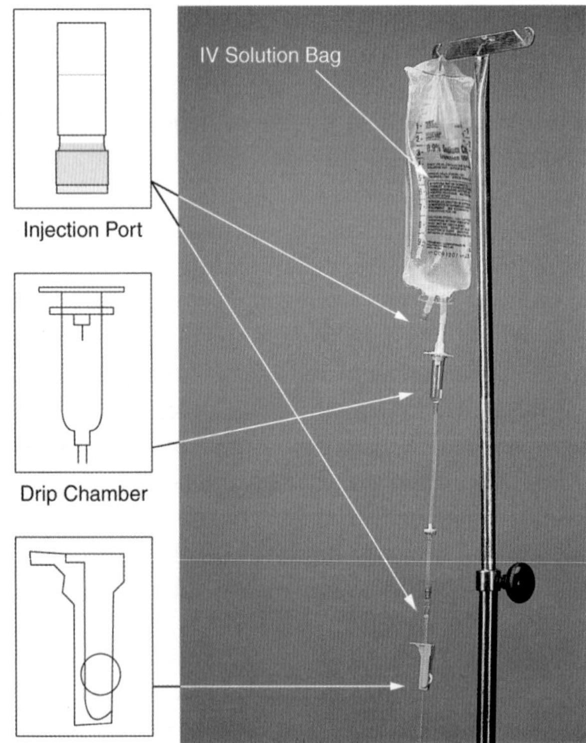

FIGURE 4-5 IV infusion (continuous). The roller clamp is used to make the IV tubing narrower to slow the IV fluid or to widen the IV line to increase the amount of fluid moving though the IV tubing. The drip chamber is kept half full so there is enough room to count how many drops is falling, called the infusion rate. The injection port is used to administer medication into the IV bag.

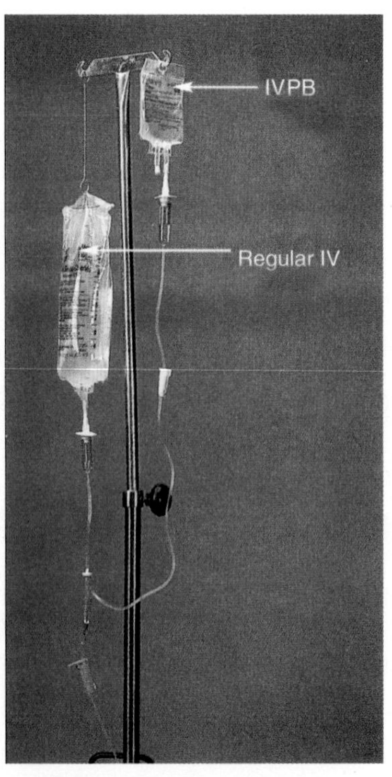

FIGURE 4-6 IV piggyback (IVPB) intermittent.

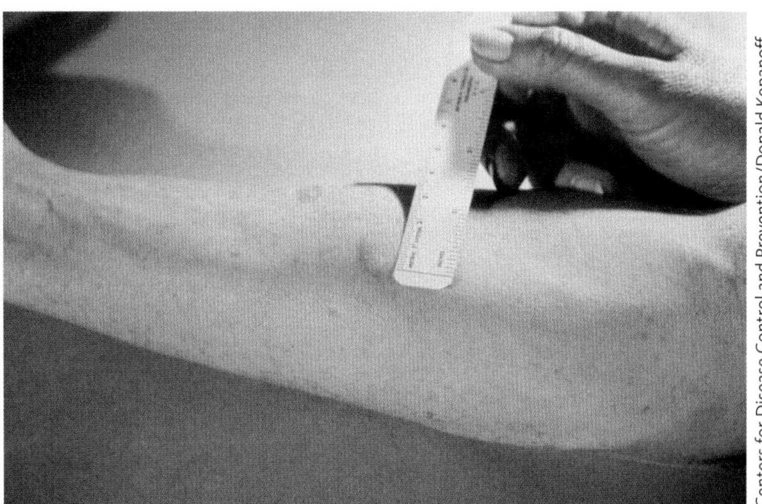
Centers for Disease Control and Prevention/Donald Kopanoff

FIGURE 4-7 Individual measuring a positive induration.

layer located just below the skin. This injection is delivered by inserting the needle at a 45-degree angle. However, if the patient is self-injecting, a shorter needle is usually used and the patient is instructed to insert the needle at a 90-degree angle.

Intradermal (ID) injections are placed below the skin, where few vessels are located, causing a slow absorption rate. This type of injection causes the delivered substance to have a localized effect rather than systemic.

This route is the best one for allergy and tuberculosis testing. As for the technique used to deliver the substance in this area, the needle is angled at 10 to 15 degrees with the bevel up and a small amount (0.1 to 0.2 mL) is injected. For allergies, the amount of redness shown is examined to determine if an allergic reaction has occurred to the injected substance.

For tuberculosis testing, the injection is given and then examined 48 to 78 hours later and the wheal or hive known as an induration is measured, if one is present. If the result is a red mark with no raised bump (no induration), the result is negative for TB. However, if an induration is present, it is measured in millimeters to see if the bump indicates a positive reading as shown in Figure 4-7. For protocols on positive PPD test results, check with your local Public Health Department.

4-8 EPIDURAL INJECTIONS

Performed by an anesthesiologist, an **epidural** is an injection that travels through a catheter into the epidural space of the spinal cord (see Figures 4-8, 4-9, and 4-10). The injection is used to control pain or to block nerves, thereby causing complete loss of movement. Medication can be given either in a bolus or continuously. There are two different types of epidural:

- *Epidural analgesia* is used to control pain without losing feeling or muscle movement. This form might be used postsurgery.
- *Epidural anesthesia* is used to control pain by blocking the nerves completely, resulting in no pain or muscle movement. This type might be used during a Caesarian childbirth, better known as a C-section.

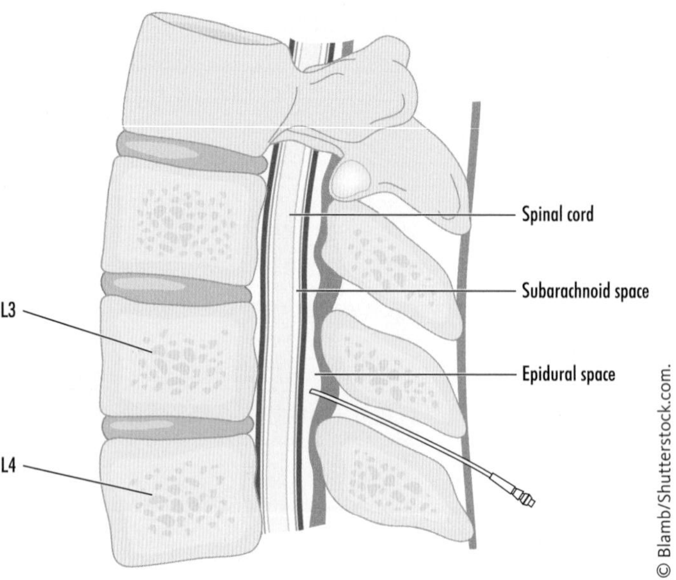

FIGURE 4-8 Cross-sectional image of the spine showing the epidural space with catheter insertion.

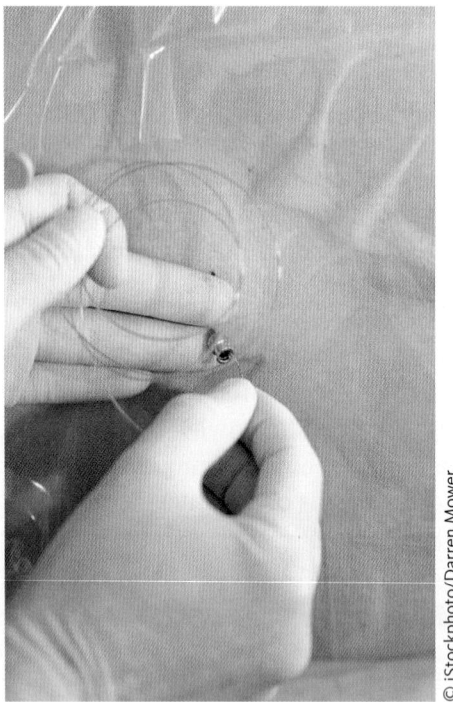

FIGURE 4-9 Epidural catheter being placed into injection site.

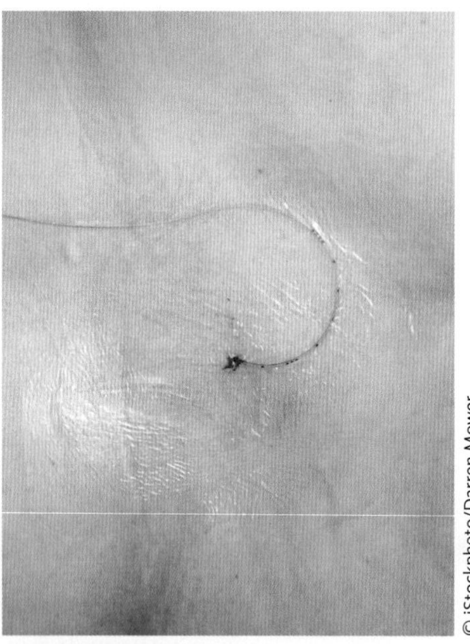

FIGURE 4-10 External view of an epidural catheter line.

CLINICAL CONNECTION 4.2

When injecting a patient with any needle, the bevel tip should be up. This means that the very sharp tip of the needle should penetrate the skin first.

4-9 LESS COMMON INJECTION ROUTES

Less commonly used parenteral injection routes are usually given by a physician and these forms are as follows:

The **intraosseous** route was discovered in 1922. This form of injection is done by actually injecting medication into the marrow of the patient's long bones, where the drug can have an immediate systemic effect. It can be used to administer medications into systemic circulation when the patient's blood vessels would collapse or could not be found such as during a cardiac arrest.

Intraventricular route route, which is used to inject medication into the brain, is not commonly used. Medications given by this route are delivered by a catheter called a ventriculostomy tube, which is placed into the brain ventricle.

Intraspinal is an injection into the spinal cord. The drug is administered into the subarachnoid space and into the cerebral spinal fluid surrounding the spinal cord. This route is mostly used to give anesthetic agents that cause a loss of feeling in regions distal or away from the injection site.

Intracapsular (intra-articular) is an injection used to decrease the inflammation of a joint. Antiinflammatory agents are injected into the capsule of a joint such as a shoulder, elbow, wrist, knee, hip, or ankle to provide relief for those suffering from arthritis or bursitis.

4-10 OTHER NONINJECTABLE ROUTES

Now that we have covered the various injectable routes, there are other routes outside of the GI tract and therefore technically could be called parenteral routes. However, in medicine, these routes have now become specialized enough to stand on their own, and parenteral routes are usually associated only with injectable routes. The other specialized routes include inhalational, topical, and mucosal routes.

4-10a Inhalation Drug Forms: The Metered Dose Inhaler

Inhalers are both portable and convenient for patients, but require good patient effort and coordination. The patient inhales an aerosolized form of a drug directly into the respiratory system. This route has a fast onset of action because the lungs have a large surface area and a tremendous blood supply. Drugs administered in this route are given to treat acute or chronic lung conditions that cause constriction of the airways such as asthma or COPD (chronic pulmonary obstructive disease). Several types of devices are used to generate aerosolized medication, and the most familiar one being the **metered dose inhaler (MDI)** as shown in Figure 4-11.

MDI inhalers use a self-contained propellant to deliver a dose of medication. This device is convenient to use and carry, as it does not require any external gas sources. An MDI does require patient cooperation and coordination, in which case a reservoir or **spacer** (shown in Figure 4-12) can be added to an MDI to assist in administering the dose to the patient. A handy feature some spacers have is that they will whistle and sound like a harmonica if the

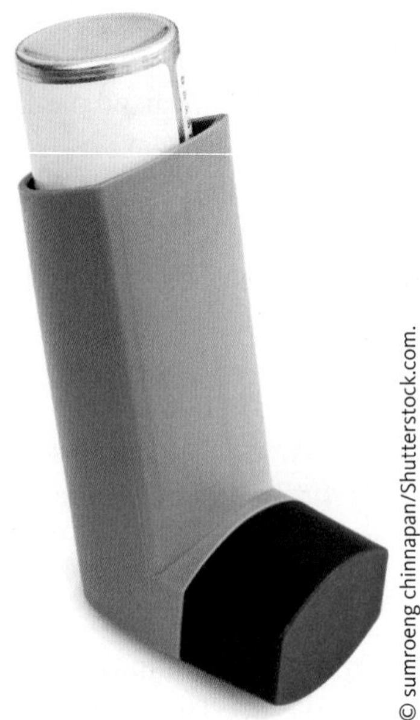

FIGURE 4-11 Metered dose inhaler.

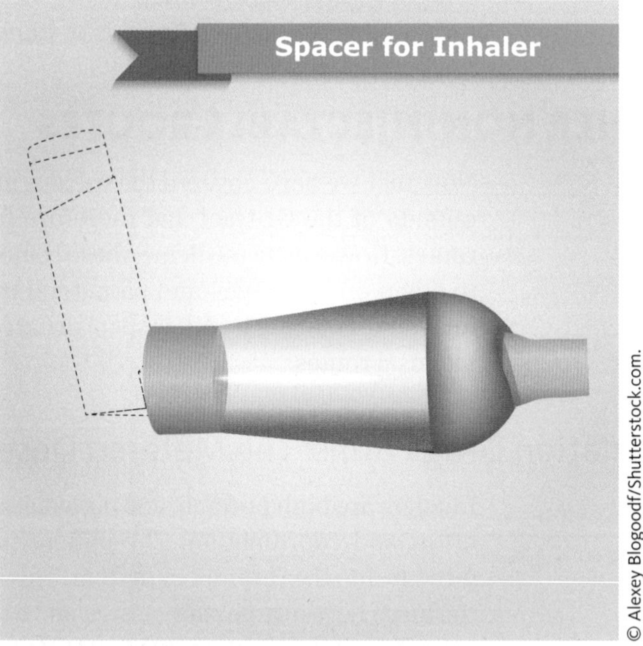

FIGURE 4-12 Spacer for MDI to help deliver a more effective dose to the lungs.

patient inhales too fast. When the patient actuates the canister, the metered dose, commonly referred to as a "puff," moves into the reservoir, from which the patient can slowly and deeply inhale the drug, maximizing its distribution throughout the lungs. If prescribed to a pediatric patient, a mask can be added to the end of the MDI to help administer the dose. For MDI patient education, see Table 4-1.

Table 4-1 MDI administration technique

Patient Education: How to use an MDI
1. Ensure the patient is sitting in an upright position or standing
2. Assemble the inhaler and dispense a waste dose if it has not been used within 24 hours to ensure consistent dosing
3. Remove dentures if loose
4. Check to ensure no debris is in the mouthpiece of the inhaler
5. Exhale slowly to completely remove air form the lungs
6. Place the mouthpiece between the lips to form a tight seal around the inhaler or mouthpiece of the spacer
7. Push down on the canister while taking a slow deep breath, inhaling to full capacity
8. Hold the breath for 5–15 seconds to give the aerosol time to deposit into the smaller airways
9. Exhale through pursed lips to effectively remove all of the air inhaled

Note: If the patient is ordered to take more than one puff, the patient should rest 1–2 minutes before the next dose. In addition, if a patient is also ordered to take an inhaled corticosteroid at the same time, make sure to give the bronchodilator first. The patient must rinse out his or her mouth after the steroid to avoid getting an oral fungal infection commonly referred to as thrush. Thrush, which looks like white fuzz, causes painful sores in the mouth and throat.

CLINICAL CONNECTION 4.3

Believe it or not, many patients have difficulty self-administering their respiratory medication. This is another reason why patient education is so crucial, especially when sending a patient home with a drug. The reason behind this particular struggle is that both inhalers and nebulizers are effective only if they are properly administered. Unlike taking a pill or a teaspoon of cough syrup, a specific technique should be used when taking inhaled medication. Many patients complain that the medicine has not helped their condition. When this occurs and the patient does not require a dose, give the patient a placebo inhaler and ask him or her to demonstrate how he or she takes the drug at home. You might be surprised with what you see. One of the authors had an older patient who complained his MDI inhaler wasn't working. When asked to show how he used the inhaler, he activated the inhaler, and then blew into it. No wonder he did not feel any relief from the drug. Some patients, especially the elderly, require more attention and reinforcement, especially if the drug is newly prescribed.

4-10b Dry Powder Inhaler

Dry powder inhaler (DPI) crushes capsules filled with a dry powder that is then inhaled forcefully (fast and deep breath). Because this inhaler does not use a propellant (see Figure 4-13), this method is used to give medication to a range of patients from children to the elderly. The catch is that since there is no propellant or gas source, the patient must be able to generate enough inspiratory force to "suck in" all of the powder. It also requires patient coordination and participation. For patient education, see Table 4-2.

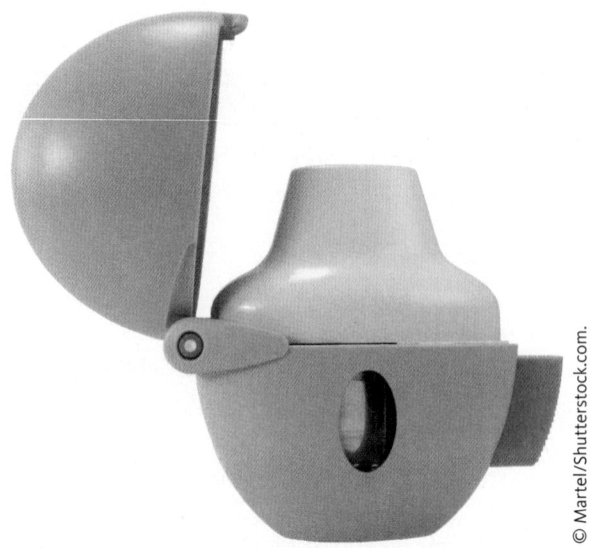

FIGURE 4-13 Image of Spiriva (tiotropium bromide) inhalation powder inhaler.

Table 4-2 DPI administration technique

Patient Education: How to use a DPI
1. Ensure the patient is sitting in an upright position or standing
2. Break open the capsule inside the inhaler (this action varies per inhaler)
3. Remove dentures if loose
4. Check to ensure no debris is in the mouthpiece of the inhaler
5. Exhale slowly to completely remove air form the lungs
6. Place the mouthpiece between the lips to form a tight seal around the inhaler
7. Inhale fast and deep to capacity
8. Hold your breath for at least 5–15 seconds
9. Exhale through pursed lips to effectively remove all of the air inhaled

Note: These devices are not used in an emergency situation and should be used only on patients with the ability to generate high inspiratory flows. Medications that come in this form are used as maintenance therapy or as prevention of acute episodes.

4-10c Nebulizers

Nebulizers are used to deliver an aerosol to the patient's airways. This can be done with a variety of different nebulizers. We will focus our attention on two types.

A **small volume nebulizer (SVN)** is used to deliver an aerosol to a patient (Figure 4-14). To function, this device requires a gas source, which can be provided as piped-in oxygen in medical facilities or a portable air compressor unit for medication delivery at home. The patient must be instructed and coached to take in slow deep breaths with a breath hold. This will help prevent dizziness, which is a common side effect caused by patients inhaling too quickly (hyperventilating).

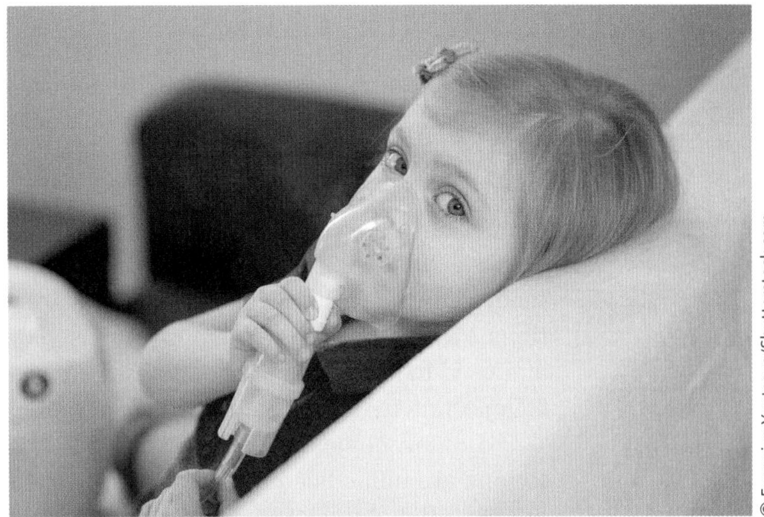
© Evgeniya Yantseva/Shutterstock.com.

FIGURE 4-14 SVN with a facemask.

Breath-actuated nebulizer (BAN) differs from SVNs by having the ability to be set on two different modes. This nebulizer can deliver a drug continuously like an SVN or it can be switched over to the breath-actuated setting so the nebulizer will give a breath only when the patient inhales through his or her mouth. Therefore, if the patient is on a face mask, the breath-actuated setting will not work. However, when used properly, this nebulizer prevents the drug from being wasted because it will nebulize on only inspiration and not continue to nebulize on exhalation. See Table 4-3 for more information about the advantages and disadvantages of aerosol medications.

Table 4-3 Pros and cons of inhalation therapy

ADVANTAGES OF INHALATION THERAPY	DISADVANTAGES OF INHALATION THERAPY
Local drug effect on the body (airways and lungs), not systemic; therefore, lower doses can be given to produce desired effect on lungs	Requires patient cooperation
Rapid onset	Can cause bronchoconstriction or airway irritation if not given correctly
Painless/noninvasive	Patients with chronic lung diseases might become dependent on inhalation therapy
Convenient	Because of the quick onset of action, adverse effects can occur rapidly
Potent drugs can be given at lower doses to minimize side effects	Device must be cleaned or replaced regularly to prevent possible infection

4-11 TOPICAL (TOP) DRUG FORMS

Topical agents are administered externally by applying a drug directly to the skin or mucosal membrane. These will produce a local affect at the site of application.

Creams and **ointments** might seem as if they are the same thing, but actually they are not. Although both are topical and in a semisolid form, creams are thinner in consistency and have a more liquid base, making them absorb more quickly. Ointments are thicker and more concentrated with an oil base, giving them a stickier feeling. Not all ointments are used solely for treating skin conditions. Vicks VapoRub is a menthol oil-based ointment that is rubbed on the body and used in humidifiers to treat nasal congestion, Figure 4-15. Keep in mind it is important to use the medication as directed by your physician or pharmacist.

Lotion comes in both medicated and unmedicated forms. Many hand lotions are unmedicated, and therefore could be rubbed all over the area of dry skin. But, if the lotion being used is medicated, such as calamine lotion for poison ivy, it should be patted only onto the affected area.

Liniment is a medicated preparation with active ingredients used to soothe aches and muscle pains. Have you have ever pulled a muscle and used some Bengay or Icy Hot? If so, you felt the cool, tingly, warm sensation of a liniment.

Dermal patches (transdermal patches) were first used in space in the 1990s to deliver nausea medication to astronauts. Today, these patches are used to deliver several other medications. Typical examples of drugs provided in this manner are nicotine for smoking cessation, nitroglycerin for chest pain, and fentanyl for chronic pain.

The rate of delivery of a drug depends on the size and shape of the drug molecules. Therefore, unlike other routes, patches vary in the duration of delivery, some lasting hours while others can last for days. Patches are easy to use and cause minimal, if any, discomfort, such as an undesirable taste associated by taking a drug by mouth. Another advantage to using a patch rather than taking a pill is that the drug is continuously delivered to the body with a patch, which

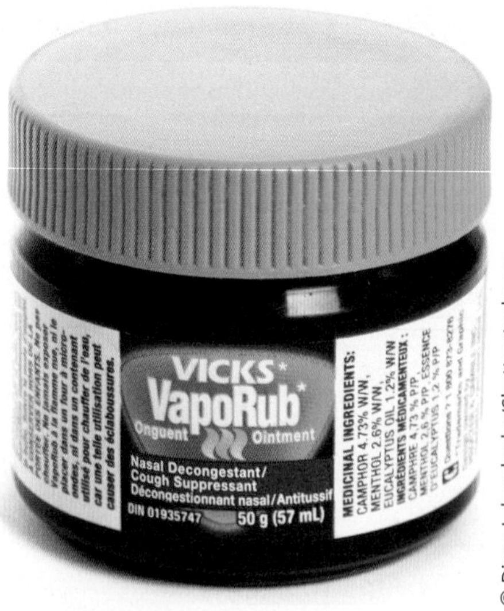

FIGURE 4-15 Ointment used for nasal decongestion.

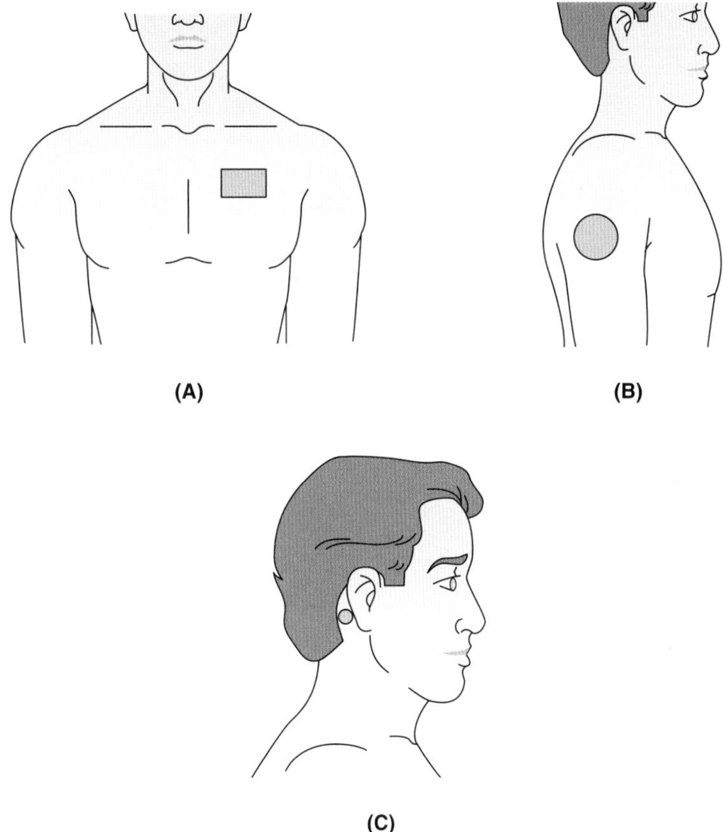

FIGURE 4-16 Dermal patches come in a variety of different shapes and sizes. Both A and B can be used to prevent chest pain (angina pectoris), while image C is the placement used for motion sickness.

allows the therapeutic level in the blood to remain constant, whereas with a pill the drug concentrations in the body will fluctuate.

Did you know glaucoma can be treated with a patch? It is not placed on the skin like most patches, but it is placed in between the eye and eyelid. This might seem uncomfortable but reports of any discomfort are minimal. Figure 4-16 shows common placement areas and types of transdermal drugs delivered.

CLINICAL CONNECTION 4.4

Robert has been a smoker for 10 years, but now that he is 32 years old and has a child, he is more motivated than ever to quit smoking. He has tried to quit cold turkey but has failed. Desperate for help, his friend recommended him to try nicotine patches. He picked up a box of OTC patches from his local drug store. Ignoring the warning labels on the back of the box, stating "keep away from children," he put a patch on his arm and left the box on his nightstand. After using the patches with success, he was on the third and last step of the nicotine patch containing the lowest dose of nicotine.

One day after work, his 3-year-old daughter began to cry, and Robert went to see what was wrong. His daughter complained of

CLINICAL CONNECTION 4.4 (*Continued*)

having a "belly ache" and feeling what he interpreted as dizzy, and she started to vomit. He noticed that she had put a nicotine patch on one of her legs, so she could "be like daddy." In a panic, he took the child to the hospital, where he explained what his daughter had done.

After medication was given for nausea and the child's vital signs remained normal, the physician reassured Robert that his daughter would be all right. The physician proceeded to educate Robert about the dangers of nicotine patches and that he must keep them out of his daughter's reach. The physician explained that mild symptoms of nicotine poisoning include nausea, vomiting, dizziness, sweating, and high blood pressure, while severe symptoms could result in seizures. Had she ingested the patch, the physician said, she would have needed more than medicine for nausea. The physician said that her stomach would need to be lavaged, which is done by having a tube placed into the stomach to wash it out. The physician said, "Let this be a learning experience."

4-12 MUCOSAL DRUG FORMS

Mucosal membranes are located in certain regions of the body, such as the nasal and oral mucosal linings. Have you ever been told not to touch your face during flu season? It is because whatever is on your hands can be transferred to mucosal membranes, such as your mouth and nose, causing you to become sick. The same method of transport can be used for medication that is absorbed by mucosal linings.

Drops (gtt) are used to provide the mucosal linings of the eye, ear, and nose with medication by instilling sterile drops directly into that location.

Eye ointment is a semisolid substance, just like the ointment previously mentioned. However, instead of applying the ointment to the skin, it is placed in the eye to provide it with medication, such as an antibiotic. This is not your average tube of antibiotic ointment, though; it is solely intended for ophthalmic use.

Vaginal creams are most commonly used antifungal or antibiotic medicated creams. Often these medications come with an applicator to assist the user with inserting the medicine into the vagina.

Vaginal suppositories use a substance that releases a drug. Once the suppository is inserted into the body, it begins to melt and release the medication into the vaginal mucosa to be absorbed systemically by the body.

A **douche solution** usually consists of sterile water and povidone-iodine, which is used to wash or irrigate the vaginal canal; while some home remedies call for a douche solution of water and a mild vinegar. The American College of Obstetricians and Gynecologists (ACOG) does not consider this process to be a safe practice. Douching can cause not only bacterial infections, but some research suggests it can also be linked to pregnancy complications and cervical cancer. Instead, it is recommended to use soap and water and allow your body to balance itself out, or allow nature to take its course.

A **buccal tablet**, although not commonly used today, is one that is not to be swallowed but should be kept between the cheek and gum. The tablet

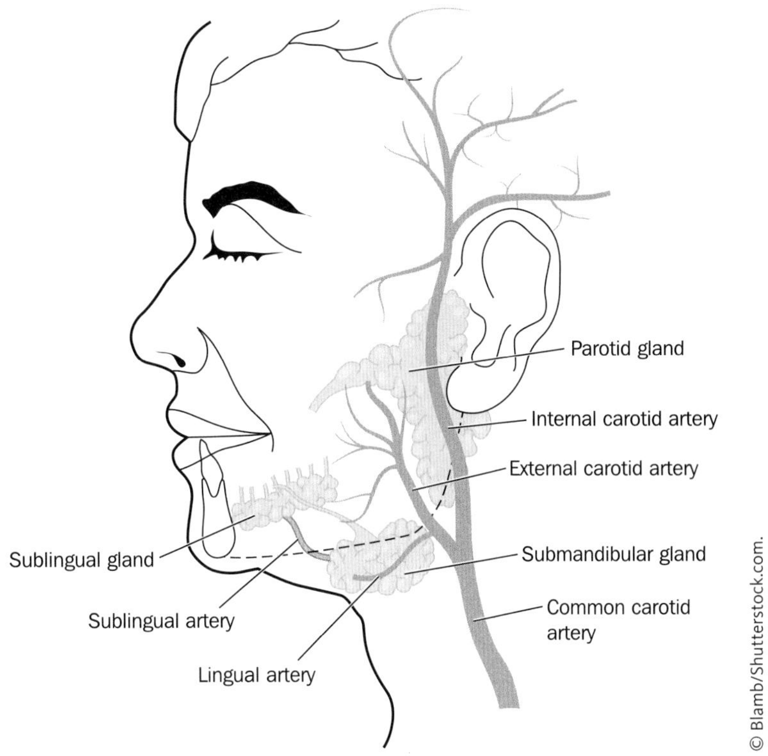

FIGURE 4-17 This image shows the vasculature of sublingual and buccal routes.

will slowly dissolve and be absorbed by the mucosa in the mouth and into the bloodstream.

A **sublingual tablet** is similar to a buccal tablet, but is a more preferred method of administration. Like the buccal tablet, it is not to be swallowed, but is placed under the tongue where it will slowly disintegrate. The drug is then absorbed into the mucosa under the tongue, which has a rich blood supply. The drug is absorbed through these many vessels, which provides a very quick drug response. The most common drug administered via this route is nitroglycerin, used to treat chest pain (angina). Typically, the angina will be relieved within 1–5 minutes after tablet placement. See Figure 4-17.

LEARNING OBJECTIVE 4.3 Describe equipment and supplies used to administer medication.

KEY TERMS

Ampules A glass bottle that is fused closed and must be broken to open.

Gauge The diameter or width of a needle.

Hypodermic syringes Commonly used to inject medication.

Insulin syringes Special syringes used only to give insulin preparations to diabetics.

Mortar and pestle Used to crush pills into a powder.

Oral syringes Needleless syringe used to deliver medication orally.

Paper medicine cups Disposable containers used to hold pills, tablets, and capsules.

Pill crushers Used to crush tablets into powder.

Pill splitter Used to split a pill in half.

Plastic medicine cups Disposable containers used to give liquid medications orally.

Prefilled syringes Used to deliver a premeasured amount of a substance.

Syringes Devices used to inject substances into or withdraw substances from the body.

Tuberculin (TB) syringes Used to deliver a small quantity of a substance intradermally.

Vial Glass container with a lid and rubber stopper to hold one dose or many doses depending on bottle size.

4-13 TABLET AND SYRUP DISPENSING SUPPLIES

To administer drugs, you must be familiar with the supplies used to administer them. One common supply is the medicine cup. Medicine cups come in two different forms, both of which are used in the healthcare setting.

- **Paper medicine cups** are used to hold pills such as tablets and capsules
- **Plastic medicine cups** are used to orally administer liquid medications

Pill crushers are not used for any sustained-release pills because it would alter the pharmacokinetic ability of a drug. However, if authorized by a physician, nonsustained-released tablets and capsules can be crushed. A few common reasons why a drug might be crushed are to administer the drug through a feeding tube or to mix it in food or a beverage if a patient has difficulties swallowing a pill.

To crush a drug, simply place the pill within the device and push down until the pill is sufficiently crushed, Figure 4-18A.

A **pill splitter** is used if a scored table is required to be split in half, Figure 4-18B.

Mortar and pestle, shown in Figure 4-19, is another method used to crush pills. The tablets are placed in the glass bowl or cup, known as the mortar, while

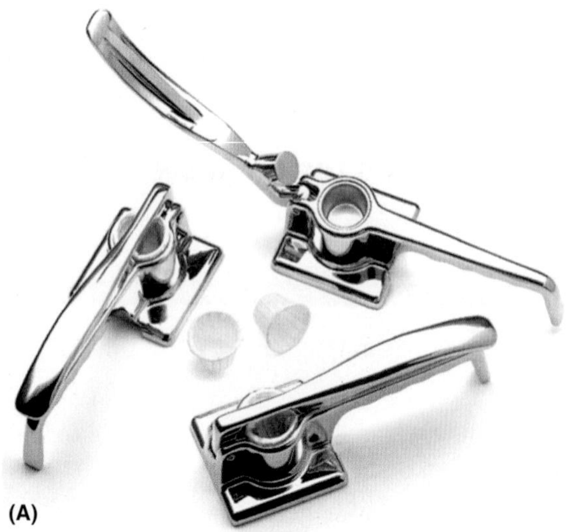

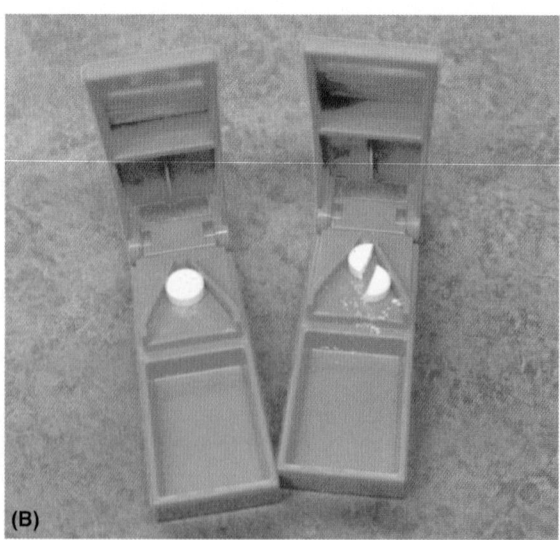

FIGURE 4-18 (A) Pill crusher. Place the pill within the device and push down until the pill is sufficiently crushed. (B) Scored tablets can be cut in half, if necessary.

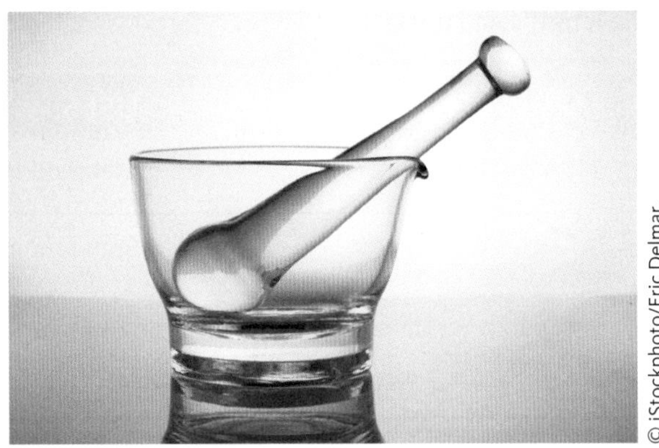
© iStockphoto/Eric Delmar.

FIGURE 4-19 A mortar and pestle.

the pestle is the cylindrical glass tool with a rounded bottom used to crush the medicine. This device can also be seen in kitchens, although commonly constructed from marble or wood.

4-14 SUPPLIES ASSOCIATED WITH INJECTIONS

Medication given to a patient by an injection is dispensed by an ample, vial, or prefilled syringe. These act as containers that hold the medication. There are also differences in needles used to inject medications.

Ampules hold a measured amount or single dose of sterile solution that is to be injected. The glass container differs from a vial in the way it is sealed. The glass bottle top of an ampule is fused or melted together and must be broken to open. This is why it holds a single dose, since it cannot be reclosed.

A **vial** can hold one dose or many doses, depending on the size of the bottle. What gives this glass container the ability to do this is that it has a lid with a rubber stopper. The needle can be passed through the stopper numerous times to fill a syringe. Another way a vial differs from an ampule is that it comes in either liquid or power drug forms. If the medication is a powder, however, it must be mixed with sterile liquid (a process known as reconstitution) before it can be injected.

4-14a Needles

Needles come in a variety of sizes or gauges and lengths and have different parts with which practicing clinicians must be familiar. First let's discuss the lengths and gauges, and then follow up with the parts of a needle.

- Lengths of needles vary depending on where they are going to be injected, Table 4-4.
- The **gauge** is the diameter of a needle. Gauges commonly used in health care range from 16 to 27 gauge. The larger the gauge number is, the smaller will be the diameter. Smaller gauge needles look thicker in appearance than larger gauge numbers, Figure 4-20.

4-14b Components of Needles and Syringes

Now, when you think of a needle, you might think about only a piece of sharp metal used to pierce flesh, but there is more to it. There are actually three parts to a needle.

Table 4-4 Needle lengths and uses

NEEDLE	LENGTH	USES
Short	3/8 inches	Standard injections
Medium	1–1½ inches	Standard injections
Long	2–5 inches	2–5 inches used for intra-articular injections 5 inches intraspinal and intraosseous

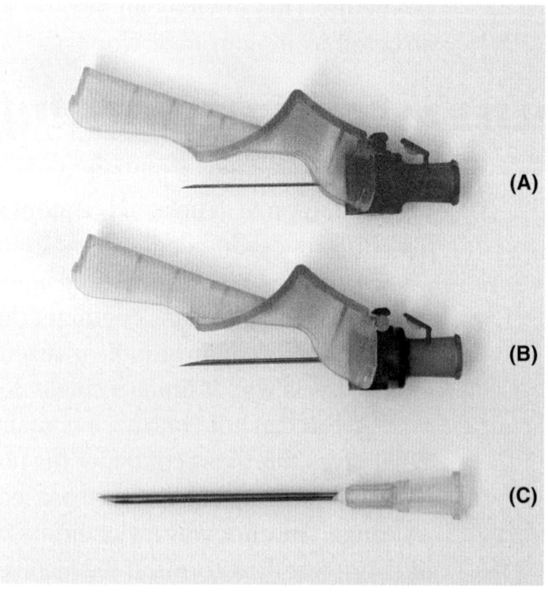

FIGURE 4-20 Example of needle gauges. (A) 25 gauge, (B) 21 gauge, and (C) 18 gauge.

- Beveled tip
- Shaft
- Hub

Let's start at the tip and work our way up the needle. The tip of a needle is the "business" end and has a slanted portion called a bevel, making the needle into a point. The shaft, or body of the needle, comes in different lengths and is connected to the hub. The hub connects the needle to the syringe tip, Figure 4-21.

Syringes come in many different varieties, all of which consist of a hollow tube or barrel that has a tip on one end where a needle hub can be connected and an opening on the other end where the plunger is inserted. Syringes are usually made of disposable plastic, but some syringes are glass and are reused after sterilization. Before delving into the different types of syringes, we will discuss the three parts of a syringe, Figure 4-21.

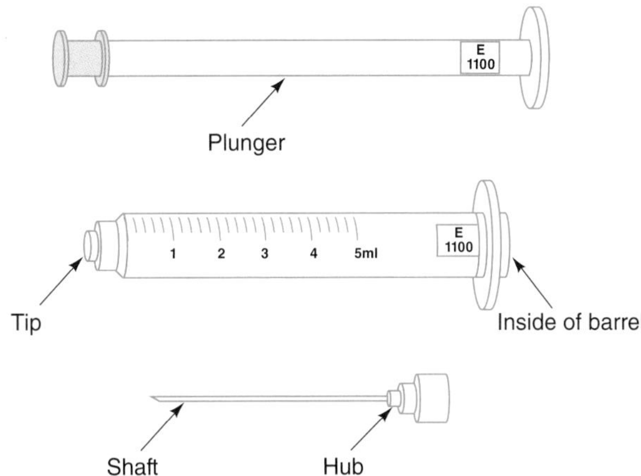

FIGURE 4-21 Parts of a needle and syringe.

- The *tip* is the end of the barrel that seats the needle hub. While some tips are plain, others have a Luer-Lok, which is a screw-on tip that is used to lock the needle in place.
- The *barrel* is a hollow tube used to hold medication or blood, if a sample is being taken. On the outside of the barrel, there are numbers used to measure the contents being held in the tube.
- The *plunger* is a solid, inner shaft with a rubber tip that fits tightly into the barrel. The plunger is pulled back away from the needle to draw or "suck in" fluid and pushed toward the needle to evacuate the contents.

4-14c Syringe Types

Different syringes are used for certain purposes. The three most commonly used disposable syringes are tuberculin, hypodermic, and insulin.

Hypodermic syringes, meaning *under the skin*, usually has a capacity of 2–3 mL. Outfitted with the proper needle gauge and length, this syringe is commonly used to inject medication subcutaneously or intramuscularly. All hypodermic needles are marked on the barrel in 10 calibrations per milliliter (mL), with each small line measuring 0.1 mL. Therefore, when preparing an injection, it should be measured to the closest 0.1 mL.

Insulin syringes are used only to give insulin preparations to diabetics. Those administering insulin should have a great understanding about how to do so before attempting to deliver a dose.

Insulin needles vary in size to fit a patient's body type, so an obese person might require a longer needle to properly penetrate to a suitable depth to administer the insulin efficiently. The most common insulin syringe is the U-100 (units per milliliters) syringe. When looking at this syringe, located on the side of the barrel are two sets of measurements. One side is measured in even numbers while the other is in odd numbers, Figure 4-22.

When preparing a dose of insulin for a child, another type of insulin needle is used, such as the Lo-Dose insulin syringe that comes in 50-unit and 30-unit syringes, as shown in Figure 4-22(B). These provide a more accurate measurement of smaller doses. It should also be pointed out that each calibration on a Lo-dose syringe is one unit. Ideally, before administering insulin, the dose should be double-checked before injecting.

Other types of syringes are:

- **Tuberculin (TB) syringes** are calibrated in tenths of a milliliter (1 cc or 1 mL). Therefore, this syringe is used to deliver a small quantity of a substance via the intradermal route. This syringe is used for tuberculosis testing or to deliver an allergen during an allergy test. However, since only 1 mL can be held in this syringe, it can also be used to deliver small doses of medication subcutaneously to a neonate or pediatric patient.
- **Prefilled syringes** are used to deliver a premeasured amount of a substance, Figure 4-23.

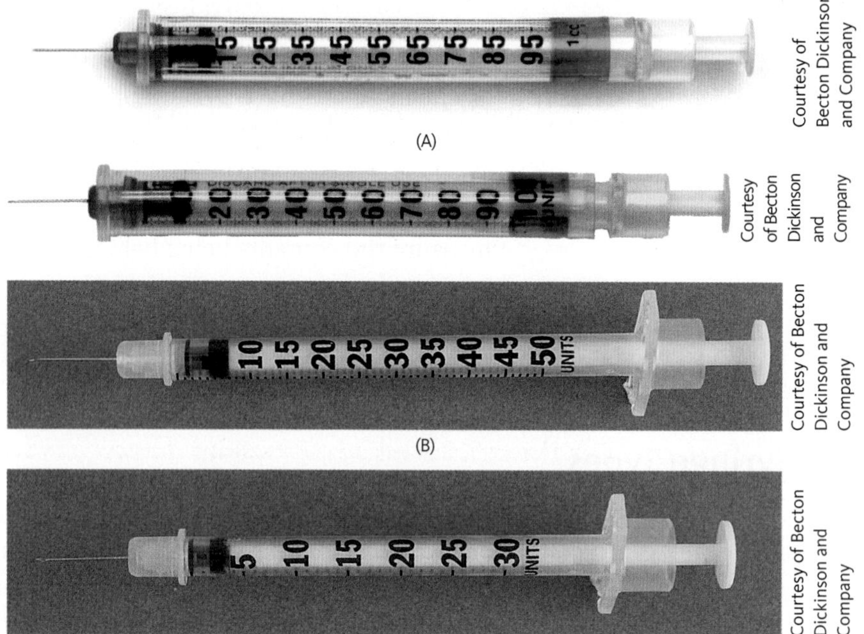

FIGURE 4-22 (A) is an image of U-100 syringes from both sides to show even numbers on one side and odd numbers on the other. (B) shows Lo-dose 30-unit and Lo-dose 50-unit syringes.

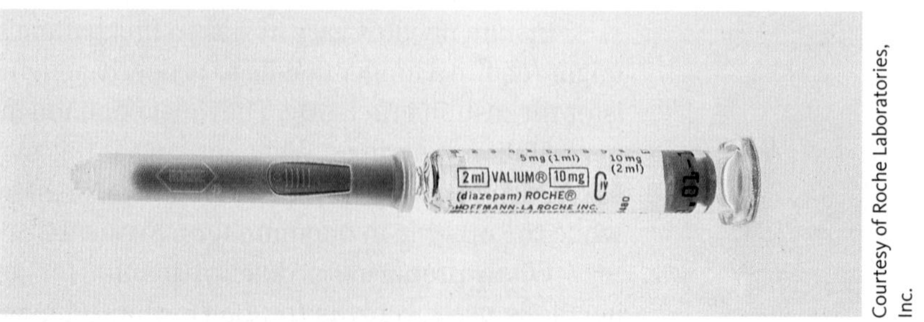

FIGURE 4-23 Prefilled, single-dose syringe.

- **Prefilled cartridges** consist of a premeasured dose that is in a cartridge that can be given through an IV line if the needle is not attached.
- **Oral syringes** deliver medication orally without a needle. These syringes come capped, prefilled with medication labeled by the pharmacy with "not for injection" or "for oral use only."

LEARNING OBJECTIVE 4.4 Summarize the principles, rights, abbreviations, and medication orders associated with drug administration.

KEY TERMS

Medication error A preventable mishandling of medication.

Medication reconciliation Comparing the patient's medications to the drugs currently ordered by the physician when a change of care occurs.

Telephone order repeated back (TO/RB) Verbally repeating the physician's order over the phone; used to increase accuracy and reduce error.

Telephone order (TO) Used to receive physician orders via telephone when the physician is not present.

4-15 PRINCIPLES AND RIGHTS OF ADMINISTRATION

Before administering medications to your patient, you should be familiar with these important principles.

1. Cleanliness
   a. The clinician should always wash his or her hands before and after making contact with a patient. This includes washing hands before preparing medication.
2. Organization
   a. Drugs should be prepared in the medication room and any drugs used should be recorded to be sure they can be replenished. This has become easier because many facilities use automated dispensing machines, which keep track of amounts available and allow the pharmacy to restock used medications.
3. Preparation area
   a. Medications should be prepared in a well-lit private area free from distractions to prevent errors.

While these principles should be employed in preparing the medication, six rights are commonly cited to make sure potential errors are avoided. The Six Rights of Medication Administration is a guideline to use when administering medication to patients. Each of the six steps is used to prevent a medication error from occurring, Figure 4-24.

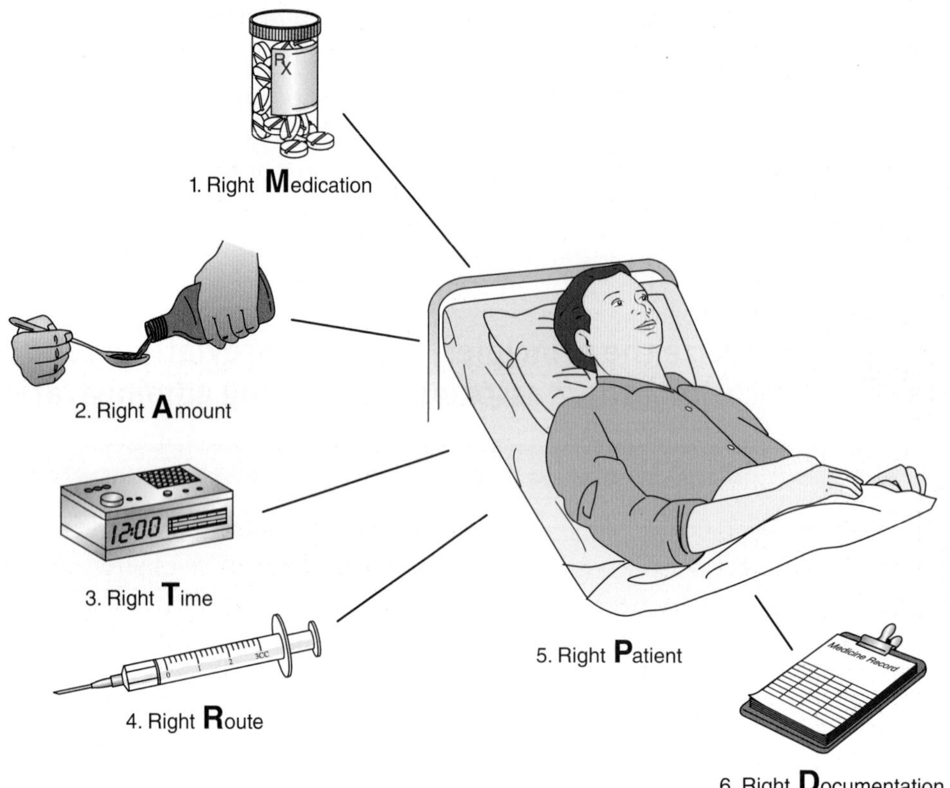

FIGURE 4-24 Illustration of the Six Rights of Medication Administration.

1. Right Drug

   It is your responsibility to make sure the medication and dosage are the same as ordered by the physician. Since many drugs look the same and begin or end in the same letters, be sure that the medication name is visible and not partially missing. If you are ever in doubt, you must question the pharmacist before administering. If someone asks you to give a dose he or she has prepared, it is in your and the patient's best interest to decline. If you dispense such a medication, and an issue occurs, you would be the one at fault.

2. Right Amount

   When administering medication, it is crucial to be as accurate as possible and to double-check that the medication you have is the one ordered on the patient's medical records. If the dose does not seem correct, call the physician to verify the correct dosage.

3. Right Time

   A drug should be given during the prescribed time to allow for the proper therapeutic drug range in the bloodstream. It is important to become familiar with drug frequency abbreviations to ensure accurate dosage times, since some drugs might be ordered to be given every 4 hours, before meals, on a full stomach, or before bed. The upcoming medical abbreviation section will help you with this. Before the patient is discharged home or leaves the office, it is important to educate him or her not only on how to take his or her medication, but when.

4. Right Route

   Many drugs can be administered in numerous ways, each having a different effect on the drugs' absorption, possible side effects, and speed of onset. Again, if you are the person giving the medication, you are responsible to ensure the medication is given via the correct route. If you are concerned that the route chosen might not be best for the patient for any reason, or if there is a change in the patient's status such as if the patient is vomiting or nauseated, contact the physician. You cannot change the route on your own. If it needs changed, for whatever reason, a physician's order is required.

5. Right Patient

   You MUST properly identify your patient before administering a drug. Your organization should have its own protocol about how to accurately identify a patient. Patient identification is done by asking the patient his or her name and date of birth, then checking the patient's wristband to verify the patient's name, date of birth, and medical record number. This is still done today even with the evolution of technology in health care. Currently, hospitals are converting to electronic medication administration records (MARS). Here the patient's ID wristband is scanned, then the medication is scanned, along with asking the patient's name, all of which must match exactly before the drug is administered.

6. Right Documentation

   Every organization might have different methods governing a patient's charting, which should be followed. Once the dose has been given, you must accurately document the dose, time, route, and location (if it was given by an injection or dermal patch). In addition, the MAR must be initialed and signed with the approximate time the drug was given. When documenting by hand, the clinician should always use either a black- or blue-colored ink pen. If an error occurs, never use whiteout, instead put one line through the mistake and write error and initial it. If something out of the ordinary occurs, such as an adverse effect or patient refusal, that too must be documented by annotating exactly what happened. It is important to be specific, because any documentation can be subpoenaed into a court of law. Therefore, what you documented might be very beneficial to the outcome of a malpractice lawsuit. Remember, if it was not documented, it did not happen.

4-16 MEDICATION ADMINISTRATION ABBREVIATIONS

It is imperative that abbreviations are read correctly and that the clinician understands the appropriate routes of administration. For example, could you imagine giving a pill or inhaler rectally? If you saw albuterol PR on the MAR sheet or computer system, you would know that means to give albuterol per rectum, and it is never given that way. The order was supposed to be PRN (as needed) but the "N" was omitted. Always pay close attention for any mistakes. If you have the power to give a medication, you should be well versed in how to recognize a mistake, and make corrections through the appropriate channels.

When you are in a clinical setting, you will be interpreting physician's orders and following them accordingly. It is your responsibility to have the proper understanding and knowledge about how to prepare and administer medications. However, to ensure the orders are being followed correctly, health-care professionals must have a strong background in medical terminology and abbreviations. Tables 4-5 and 4-6 focus on a few commonly seen and used abbreviations in health care. Note that if you are not sure or it is unclear about what is expected, be sure to ask before giving the medication to avoid any medication errors. Medication errors will be discussed in an upcoming section.

4-17 MEDICATION ORDERS

Whether in a physician's office or medical center, medication orders must contain the following six parts:

Part 1: Time and date of order

Part 2: Name of patient

Table 4-5 Common dosage abbreviations

ABBREVIATION	MEANING
cap	Capsule
tab	Tablet
L	Liter
ml	Milliliter
IV	Intravenous
IM	Intramuscular
ut dict	As directed
sig	Directions
Rx	Take
NPO	Nothing by mouth
PO	By mouth

Table 4-6 Common frequency abbreviations

ABBREVIATION	MEANING
ac	Before meals
pc	After meals
prn	As needed
q	Every
q2h	Every 2 hours
q3h	Every 3 hours
q4h	Every 4 hours
qid	Four times daily
tid	Three times a day
bid	Twice daily
w/a	While awake
Hs	Hours of sleep
Stat	Immediately

Part 3: Name of medication name (brand or generic)

Part 4: Dosage and/or amount of medication

Part 5: Route of administration

Part 6: Directions for use including time and frequency to be given.

To avoid medication errors, if the order is in question or is missing a part, the physician must be contacted to correct the absence of information. When this occurs and the physician is not present, you might have to write the order in the patient's medical record or chart. If such a scenario occurs and the order is given over the phone, you must use the appropriate designated protocols and abbreviations when charting. If not, the order you wrote will not be recognized as a legitimate order. After a verbal order is written, the prescriber has 24 hours to personally sign the verbal order for it to remain in effect.

To write an order, make sure you are authorized to do so by your organization's protocols and policies. If you are indeed allowed to write an order for a patient, there are a few things to keep in mind.

1. When writing a **telephone order (TO)**, always make sure to get the prescriber's name and write it next to the medication or procedure.
2. When receiving an order from the prescribing practitioner, make sure to:
    - Repeat the drug name
    - Repeat the dosage
    - Repeat the frequency
    - Repeat the route of administration
    - Repeat the time the order was taken
    - Write down your name since you are the one receiving the phone call.

This is known as a **telephone order repeated back (TO/RB)** and is done to increase accuracy and decrease any opportunity for an error. If an error or discrepancy occurs and a lawsuit is filed, the order can be used as evidence. Therefore, proper documentation not only protects the patient, but you as well.

4-18 DRUG DOSAGE CALCULATIONS

It is evident that dosing is not the same for every patient because people come in all different heights, weights, ages, and so on. Furthermore, special considerations should be taken into account especially when dealing with pediatric and geriatric patients. A pediatric dose is based on the child's weight, age, or body surface area (BSA). Notably, neonatal patients do not have fully developed renal systems and some enzyme systems, interfering with drug absorption and metabolism, which is responsible for a decrease in the body's ability to eliminate drugs from their system. Dosages are usually referenced in milligrams per unit of body weight, per unit of time. For example, a drug dose might present as 5 mg/kg/12 h. This means 5 mg of the drug is given for each kilogram the patient weighs every 12 hours.

For appropriate dosing of children and adults, these areas must be taken into consideration:

- Age
- Sex
- Weight
- Metabolic condition
- Pathological condition
- Psychological condition.

As with children, drug dosages are often reduced in the elderly. When drugs accumulate and remain in the body, side effects are likely to occur. Common factors that increase the risk of adverse reactions or even accidental overdoses in elderly patients include:

- Slower metabolism
- Poor circulation
- Decreased function of:
  - Central nervous system
  - Kidneys
  - Liver
  - Lungs

Therefore, a good approach to use when dosing the elderly is to "start low and go slow." This will help to reach safely the desired therapeutic level needed to treat the patient while avoiding complications such as mental status alteration or even potentially deadly interactions. To help avoid dangerous situations, ensure the patient is properly assessed and monitored for chronic diseases, dehydration, electrolyte imbalances, and physical weakness resulting from an illness because all of these can all have an effect on how a drug works.

While most drugs come premixed or as unit doses to be administered directly as is, sometimes drugs dosages might need to be calculated and modified. While dosage calculations is a subject that you would need more in-depth study to master.

4-19 RESPONSIBLE DRUG ADMINISTRATION

Being a healthcare professional, you have a great responsibility to uphold.

1. Patients are entrusting you with not only their care, but their lives. First, you must be *up to date* in all areas of your clinical capacity. Being knowledgeable in your field and understanding the medications you administer is vital. Being current on the latest drug information includes drug indications, routes of administration, potential side effects, interactions, cautions, and contraindications is critical.
2. Clinicians need to have the *wisdom* to understand what medications are appropriate for their patient's needs based on clinical evidence, even though they are not ordering the medication. Healthcare workers need the skills necessary to properly assess the patient's response to medication, and have the ability to plan any actions to improve the quality of life or patient condition.
3. You must possess the *skills* needed to deliver medication to the patient in a proper manner. This includes both administering and charting any medications or procedures.
4. You must provide good *patient education.* Another reason you must know everything possible about the medications and care you provide is to educate patients and their family members. Think of it as a quiz. The patient's family will be concerned about the health of his or her loved one and will want to know what exactly is going on. "What are

the side effects?" "How long will she need this medicine?" When asked a question you must provide an accurate and appropriate answer as long as it is within your scope of practice. If it is not within your scope, it is best to defer the question to someone who can provide an answer.

If you were a family member asking caregivers about what procedure or medication they are administering to your loved one and they could not answer your question, you might feel uneasy and not trust them with the care of yourself or your family member.

Remember you must be true in your obligation as a healthcare professional to uphold your duty to care for your patients. You must remain true to your scope of practice and not take on roles that are not licensed or part of your training. This is known as *role fidelity*.

It is very important that a patient understands what is being done to, or given to him or her. When responding to a patient or family's question, always keep the medical jargon to a minimum and speak in layman's terms. If you don't, the patient might become confused, scared, or possibly agitated.

4-20 MEDICATION ERRORS

Unfortunately, sometimes healthcare professionals experience the strain of fatigue from working long hours, understaffing, misinterpretation of illegible handwritten orders, but they are not an excuse for medication errors. A **medication error** is a preventable mishandling of medication regardless of whether harm has occurred. When an error occurs, it must always, always, always be reported to the individual in charge, so the proper steps can be done to correct the mistake, which will be discussed further in this section. Remember, it is better to come clean immediately and own your mistake than to cover it up or place blame on someone else. If not, the patient's well-being might be jeopardized, as well as your future in health care.

The possible types of error include:

1. Administering a drug to the wrong patient
2. Administering the wrong drug
3. Administering the drug via the wrong route
4. Administering a drug at the wrong time
5. Wrong documentation on a patient's chart

4-21 MEDICATION ERROR REPORTING (MER)

With today's technology, computerized charting and automated medication dispensing systems are used in many healthcare facilities. To access medications or patient charting, you have to use a password, fingerprint, or some other means of identification so the computer system can verify that you have the authority to do so. After you are granted permission, every medication you remove from a dispensing machine will be traced back to you. Therefore, if an error occurs, the system will identify you as the one who removed it from the system. Therefore, if the drug was removed and the healthcare professional said they did not give it to the patient, then why was it not returned? Why was it found in the patient's system?

If the error is severe enough to land in court, it would have been best to have been honest than to have lied. If you have taken an ethics class you probably have discussed the term "nonmaleficence" meaning "First, do no harm." Therefore, as a healthcare professional, you must do everything you can within your scope of practice to ensure the patient is not harmed in your care.

To ensure medical errors are reported and corrected, the U.S Pharmacopeia (USP) created the Medication Errors Reporting (MER) Program. In addition, the Agency for Healthcare Research and Quality (AHRQ) has federally certified the Institute for Safe Medication Practices (ISMP) as a Patient Safety Organization (PSO) to operate a national error-reporting program for both vaccine and medication errors. Healthcare professionals and the public should be encouraged to report errors to ISMP because PSO confers with both privilege and confidentiality to the information reported. Error reporting by healthcare professionals and hospitals is necessary to develop safety alerts and quality improvement programs.

4-22 MEDICATION RECONCILIATION

Medication reconciliation is done every time there is a change in the patient's care to prevent any potential medication errors. For example, if a patient is admitted to a hospital from a skilled nursing facility, the patient's medications are compared to the drugs currently ordered by the physician. Medication reconciliation is a five-step process:

1. Develop a list of current medications
2. Develop a list of medications to be prescribed
3. Compare the medications on the two lists
4. Make clinical decisions based on the comparison
5. Communicate the new list to appropriate caregivers and to the patient

Module 5

Cancer and Antineoplastic Pharmacology

Module Introduction

Your body needs various types of cells to perform many different functions. Not only does the body need to reproduce these cells, but it must also grow them in a healthy and orderly manner. Several factors related to healthy growth include proper growth rate, size, shape, and even how they align with other cells. Normal cellular reproduction is a multistep process and if even one of these steps is adversely affected, wild, uncontrolled growth can happen. In fact, you will soon learn that cancer is just that—wild, uncontrolled cellular reproduction.

LEARNING OBJECTIVE 5.1 Explain the normal anatomy and physiology concepts associated with cellular growth and reproduction.

KEY TERMS

Apoptosis Cellular death.

Asexual reproduction Cellular division producing identical copies without the involvement of another cell.

Benign Noncancerous.

Binary fission Asexual cellular reproduction forming two identical cells.

Cell cycle Is the total life span of eukaryotic cells; two major phases are known as interphase and the mitotic phase.

Cellular reproduction Is the process of one cell dividing into two cells, also known as cellular division.

Cytokinesis The division of the cellular cytoplasm.

Eukaryotic cells Cells having a true nucleus bounded by a nuclear membrane and containing cellular organelles.

Interphase Where the majority of the cell cycle is spent on normal functioning and stockpiling needed materials for cellular division.

Malignant Cancerous.

Metastasize To spread from original site.

Mitosis Cellular division used for tissue growth where daughter cells have same number of chromosomes as original mother cell.

Mitotic phase Phase of actual cell division.

Neoplasm A new growth that results from overproduction of cells forming a lump or tumor.

Oncologist Specialist who treats cancer.

Prokaryotic cells Cells that lack a nucleus such as bacteria.

5-1 COMMON CANCER TERMINOLOGY

Many internal body conditions and even external factors such as the environment can trigger changes in the way the cells reproduce and grow. If cell growth becomes uncontrolled, too many cells can be produced resulting in a new lump, or tumor. This is also termed a **neoplasm**, which literally means "new growth." Tumors can be classified as either **benign** (noncancerous) or **malignant** (cancerous). The specialist who treats cancer is an **oncologist**; *onco* refers to *tumors* so oncology literally means the study of tumors (see Figure 5-1).

As noncancerous neoplasms, benign tumors generally are non–life-threatening, but they can grow rapidly and push aside healthy tissue or cause dangerous obstructions. Malignant tumors are cancerous and will actually invade healthy cell tissue. Cancer means "crab" just like the Zodiac sign because it can spread out into healthy tissue like the legs and pinchers of a crab.

Cancerous tumors also differ from benign tumors in that parts of a cancerous tumor can **metastasize**, or break off and travel through the blood system or the lymphatic network, and start new tumors in other parts of the body.

5-2 CELLULAR REPRODUCTION AND CELL TYPES

We learn in anatomy that cells group together to form tissues, making cells the building blocks of the body. Cancer is the No. 1 type of cellular disease and can have devastating effects throughout the body. Before we talk about abnormal cell growth, it is important to understand how cells should make "good copies" of each other. **Cellular reproduction** also known as *cellular division* is the process of one cell dividing into two cells. When cells divide and make identical copies of themselves without the involvement of another cell, this is called **asexual reproduction**. Most cells are able to reproduce themselves asexually whether they are animal cells, plant cells, or bacteria.

The cells that make up the human body are called **eukaryotic cells**. Eukaryotic cells have a nucleus, cellular organelles, and usually several chromosomes in the nucleus. The chromosomes contain the cellular instructions

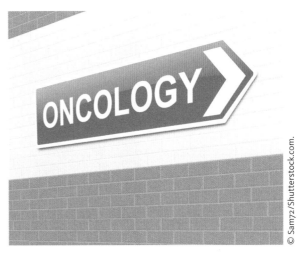

FIGURE 5-1 Oncology is the department where cancer is diagnosed and treated.

and therefore must be copied exactly for proper cellular function. It doesn't matter whether the cell has only one chromosome as in bacterial cells or 46 chromosomes as in human cells; all the chromosomes must be copied before the cell can divide.

Bacterial cells are much simpler and classified as **prokaryotic cells** or organisms. Prokaryotic cells do not have a true nucleus or nuclear membrane and their reproductive process is much simpler. Bacteria reproduce through a much simpler two-step process called **binary fission** as shown in Figure 5-2. In Step 1, when the cell is ready to divide, it makes a copy of its DNA. Step 2 is dividing the liquid internal environment known as the cytoplasm, and then splitting in half into two new cells.

CLINICAL CONNECTION 5.1

Through the process of binary fission, bacteria have the potential to double their population every 30 minutes. You can now appreciate how fast a bacterial infection can grow and spread if not properly treated.

5-2a Mitosis

When it comes time for the eukaryotic cells of our body to divide, the process is more complex because they have 46 chromosomes and many organelles that must be copied exactly.

The process of sorting the chromosomes, so that each new cell gets the right number of copies of all the genetic material, is called **mitosis**.

Why do we need mitosis? Cells can become damaged, wear out, or die and need to be replaced with healthy cells. Many body tissues, which are made up of many cells, need to be replaced on a regular basis. Types of tissues that need regular replacement include bone, skin, and epithelial tissue. Our blood cells also need to be replaced on a regular basis because they have a certain life cycle. For example, the red blood cells, whose vital function is to carry oxygen, wear out in 120 days.

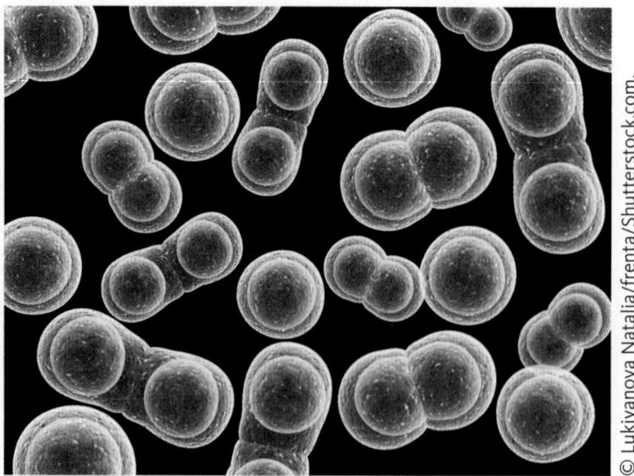

FIGURE 5-2 Binary fission reproducing prokaryotic bacterial cells.

Tissue also needs to repair and regenerate when damaged, and mitosis is the vital process for forming new cells for this purpose. For example, think what would happen if you cut yourself and you did not have mitosis. The wound would remain forever. Luckily through mitosis, the skin is replaced, first by collagen, then eventually by the original tissue.

A broken bone requires healthier bone cells (osteocytes) to be formed to repair and rebuild the break. Mitosis is also vital for growth such as the lengthening and broadening of the bones as you grow. All the organs and vessels must also increase in size along with all your other body tissues. Growth would be impossible without mitosis of cells in the individual tissues or organs. All this means that asexual reproduction of body cells or mitosis is needed for growth and replacement of old or damaged cells.

LEARNING HINT: MITOSIS VERSUS MEIOSIS

The words *mitosis* and *meiosis* sound and look alike and describe similar processes, so they are often confused. Meiosis produces gametes or sexual cells, commonly called sperm and eggs, each of which contains half the complement of chromosomes. The sexual union of male and female gametes makes a full complement of chromosomes. Meiosis is therefore *sexual* cellular reproduction. Mitosis is *asexual* and produces exact copies of the cell, with each containing the full complement of chromosomes.

5-3 THE CELL CYCLE

Apoptosis refers to cellular death; it is estimated that approximately 300 million body cells die every minute. Cell types have varying life spans. Certain white blood cells live for only a few hours, intestinal cells last 2 to 3 days, and muscles cells can last for up to 15 years. Nerve cells win the longevity contest, because they can last a lifetime.

During its life span, a cell can divide many times and cycles back and forth between normal functioning and asexual reproduction. The total life span of eukaryotic cells can therefore be divided into two major phases known as the **cell cycle**. The majority of the cell cycle, known as the **interphase** portion, is spent on normal functioning and stockpiling needed materials in preparation for division and by copying DNA and making new organelles. Only a brief portion of the cell cycle, the **mitotic phase**, is devoted to actual cell division when the need arises. The mitotic phase is subdivided into two major portions, with mitosis being the division and sorting of the *genetic material*, and the final phase, **cytokinesis**, being the division of the *cytoplasm*. See Figure 5-3.

5-4 TYPES OF GROWTH (PLASIAS)

Cellular growth and reproduction has many steps. *Plasia* is the medical term for *growth* and there are many similar terms that can be confusing. **Hyperplasia** means an increase in growth that can be caused by a number of stimuli. For example, body builders tear down muscle by lifting weights, and the hyperplasia that results builds larger muscles. If you get a callus on your hand from working

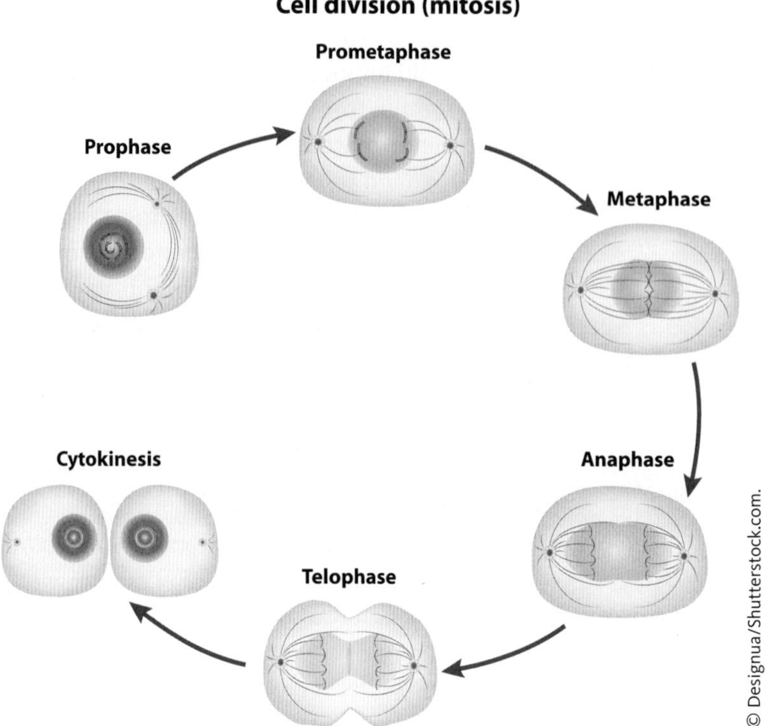

FIGURE 5-3 Mitosis, or division of the genetic material in a eukaryotic cell, produces identical daughter cells with the exact number of chromosomes and same organelles as the original cell. The various phases of mitosis are based on the position of the chromosomes relative to the new cells.

LEARNING OBJECTIVE 5.2 Describe the terminology related to neoplasms.

KEY TERMS

Angiogenesis Formation of new blood vessels.

Cachexia Weakened and frail state because of nutrient deprivation, often seen in cancer patients.

Cancer General term for malignant growth.

Carcinoma General term for cancerous tumor.

Carcinoma in situ A cancer that is "just sitting there" in the particular tissue and hasn't broken through the basement membrane and invaded other tissues or sites.

Dysplasia Abnormal tissue development.

Hyperplasia Excessive growth of normal cells.

Leukemia Malignant neoplasms of the blood and blood-forming organs.

Lymphomas Malignant neoplasms of the lymphatic system.

Malignant growths Neoplasms whose cells are uncontrolled and have no function and an irregular structure.

Neoplasia New growth formation.

Sarcoma Cancerous tumor found in the connective tissue of bone, fat, or muscle.

Tissue necrosis The death of healthy tissue.

without gloves, the skin was irritated or stimulated to produce more growth, in this case, a callus. It is important to note that when the stimulus is removed, the hyperplasia stops and the callus goes away. That is also why you lose muscle tone if you do not work them regularly.

Hyperplasia can also occur because of hormone stimulation. For example, a deficiency of the thyroid hormone causes the thyroid to enlarge (hyperplasia) to produce more cells to attempt to make up the deficiency. Some hyperplasias can be formed from unknown stimuli such as prostatic hyperplasia in older men. The bottom line is that hyperplasia is an increase in the growth of tissue because of excess cellular reproduction, and when the stimulus is removed, the growth stops.

Dysplasia means "bad or difficult growth." This is an alteration in the size or shape of cells, or even how the cells are arranged, and is caused by an irritant or stimuli. Dysplastic cells can return to normal, but often they can progress to neoplasia.

Neoplasia literally means "new growth," but it also means the cells are developing in an *uncontrolled manner*. Neoplasms differ from hyperplasias in their cause, extent of growth, and their ability to remain (and even continue to grow) even after the stimuli is removed. One other very important difference is while both neoplasms and hyperplasias increase in cell numbers, the cells in hyperplasia remain identical, whereas in neoplasms the reproduced cells change appearance and do not look like the original cell (mother cell) from which they divided. This difference in cellular appearance helps the pathologist contrast a neoplasm from a hyperplasia growth.

5-5 NEOPLASM CLASSIFICATIONS

The uncontrolled growth of neoplasms leads to a lump or tumor. If they are benign tumors, they usually grow slowly and are confined to a specific area. Benign tumors do not spread and are generally harmless unless they obstruct blood flow, compress nerves, or are found in a contained area such as the brain, where they can cause an increase in pressure (see Figure 5-4). Malignant or

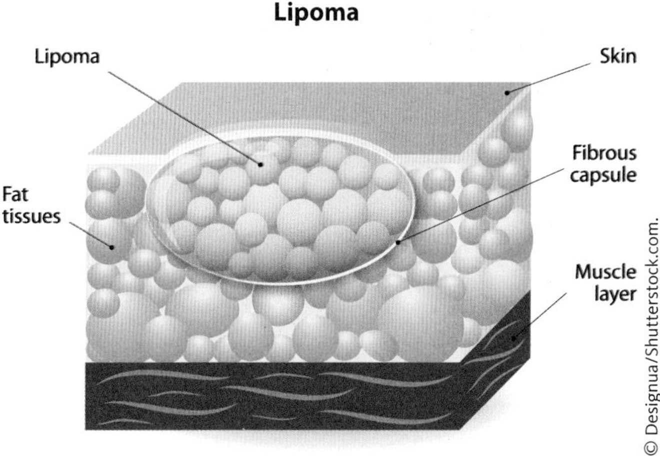

FIGURE 5-4 Lipomas are usually benign fatty tumors. Notice the cells are normal and simply overproduced to form tumor.

cancerous tumors grow very rapidly and can invade surrounding tissue and spread or metastasize to other areas of the body. The general term for any malignant neoplasm is **cancer**.

5-5a Tissue of Origin Classification

Oma is the medical term for *tumor*, and after the tumor has been classified as benign or cancerous, the second step is to classify it according to the tissue type where it originated. If it is cancerous, and found in skin epithelial tissue or glands, the term **carcinoma** is added to the original tissue. For example, an adenoma is a benign tumor of a gland, and an adenocarcinoma would be the name of a cancerous tumor of a gland. **Sarcoma** is the term used if a cancerous tumor is found in the connective tissue of bone, fat, or muscle. For example, an osteoma would be a benign bone tumor, and an osteosarcoma would be a cancerous bone tumor. A lipoma is a benign fatty tumor, and a liposarcoma would be cancerous.

Cancer can also be found in the lymphatic system or within the blood stream. **Lymphomas** are malignant neoplasms of the lymphatic system. All lymphomas are malignant and have no benign counterpart. **Leukemia** is the term for malignant neoplasms of the blood-forming organs. Table 5-1 contrasts benign and malignant neoplasms.

CLINICAL CONNECTION 5.2

HEMATOMA

Did you ever get a bad bruise that became swollen and turned red and purple? Since this is a swelling because of inflammation, it is technically a tumor. The medical term is hematoma, because "heme" refers to blood, and this is a swelling produced by excess blood. Of course, it is a benign tumor and the blood will reabsorb and the bruising will go away in time.

Table 5-1 Benign and malignant neoplasms

CELL OR TISSUE OF ORIGIN	BENIGN NEOPLASM	MALIGNANT NEOPLASM
Squamous epithelium	Epithelioma	Squamous cell carcinoma
Glandular epithelium	Adenoma	Adenocarcinoma
Adipose (fatty tissue)	Lipoma	Liposarcoma
Bone	Osteoma	Osteosarcoma
Blood	None	Leukemia
Lymphatic	None	Lymphoma

5-6 MALIGNANT NEOPLASM

Malignant means "bad" and **malignant growths** are neoplasms whose cells are uncontrolled and grow excessively with no regulatory factors, such as contact inhibition with normal cells, stopping their growth. Malignant cells have no function and their structure is not uniform like other reproducing cells. Malignant cells have surfaces that look like a crab, with extensions projecting out in all directions, which can help it to invade normal tissue. Figure 5-5 shows a breast cancer tumor and its invasive nature.

Malignant cells are therefore called cancer cells and are extremely fast growing. While cancer cells serve no physiological purpose, their metabolism is geared exclusively for growth and reproduction, which requires a lot of nutrients and oxygen. Therefore, to meet this hyperreproductive need, new blood vessels are needed to supply the oxygen and nutrients. The development of new blood vessels is termed **angiogenesis** and this is why bleeding is often a sign of cancer. In addition, the need for nutrients for hyperreproduction of the cancer cells draws nutrients from normal cells and deprives them of needed nutrients. This is why cancer patients lose weight and become frail and weak. This weakened state is called **cachexia**.

5-7 CANCER METASTASIS

Carcinoma in situ refers to cancer that is "just sitting there" in the particular tissue and hasn't broken through the basement membrane and invaded other tissues or sites. Cancer first begins at the *primary site* as a local invasion of the surrounding tissue with its tentacle-like projections entangling normal tissue structures. As it grows, the malignant tumor can block blood flow and cause the death of healthy tissue, which is termed **tissue necrosis**. Cancer can then spread from this primary location to *secondary sites* through the process of metastasis.

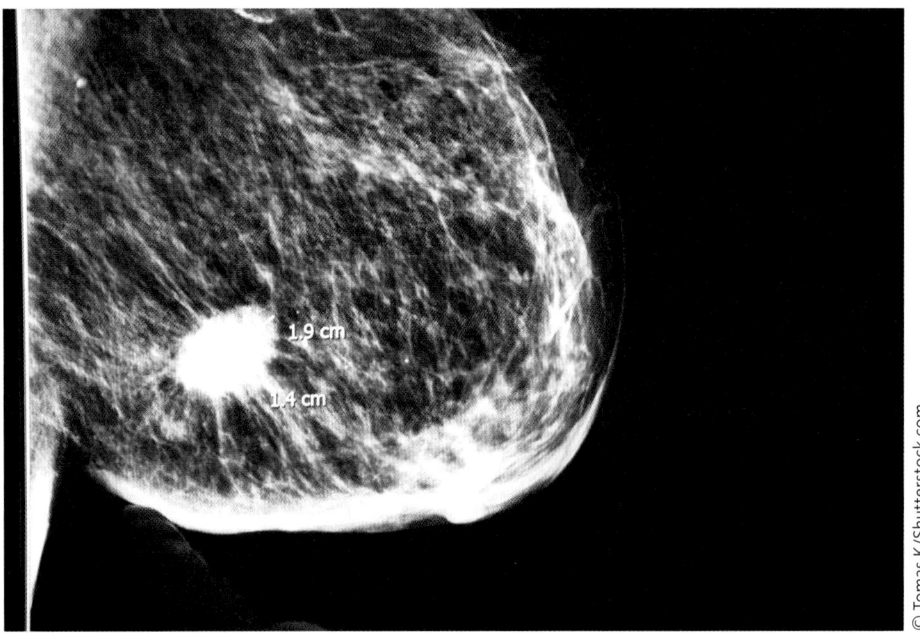

FIGURE 5-5 Breast cancer tumor showing the tentacle-like spread.

Often cancer spreads through the lymphatic system, where lymph nodes attempt to filter the abnormal cells. When the lymphatic system is overwhelmed by the cancerous cells, the filters can become blocked and spill out the cancerous cells into the bloodstream, which basically runs parallel to the lymphatic system. After cancerous cells are in the blood circulatory system, they can spread to secondary sites. This is why close proximity or sentinel lymph nodes are removed or biopsied to determine if the cancer has entered the lymphatic system.

Cancer cells can also be seeded by invasion and implantation within serous (watery filled) cavities such as the pleural cavity. *Hematogenous spread* occurs when cancer cells invade the blood vessels.

While all the body systems can be ravaged as shown in Figure 5-6, common secondary sites of cancer include the brain, lung, bone, and liver. Often it is unfortunate for the patient that the secondary site is discovered first.

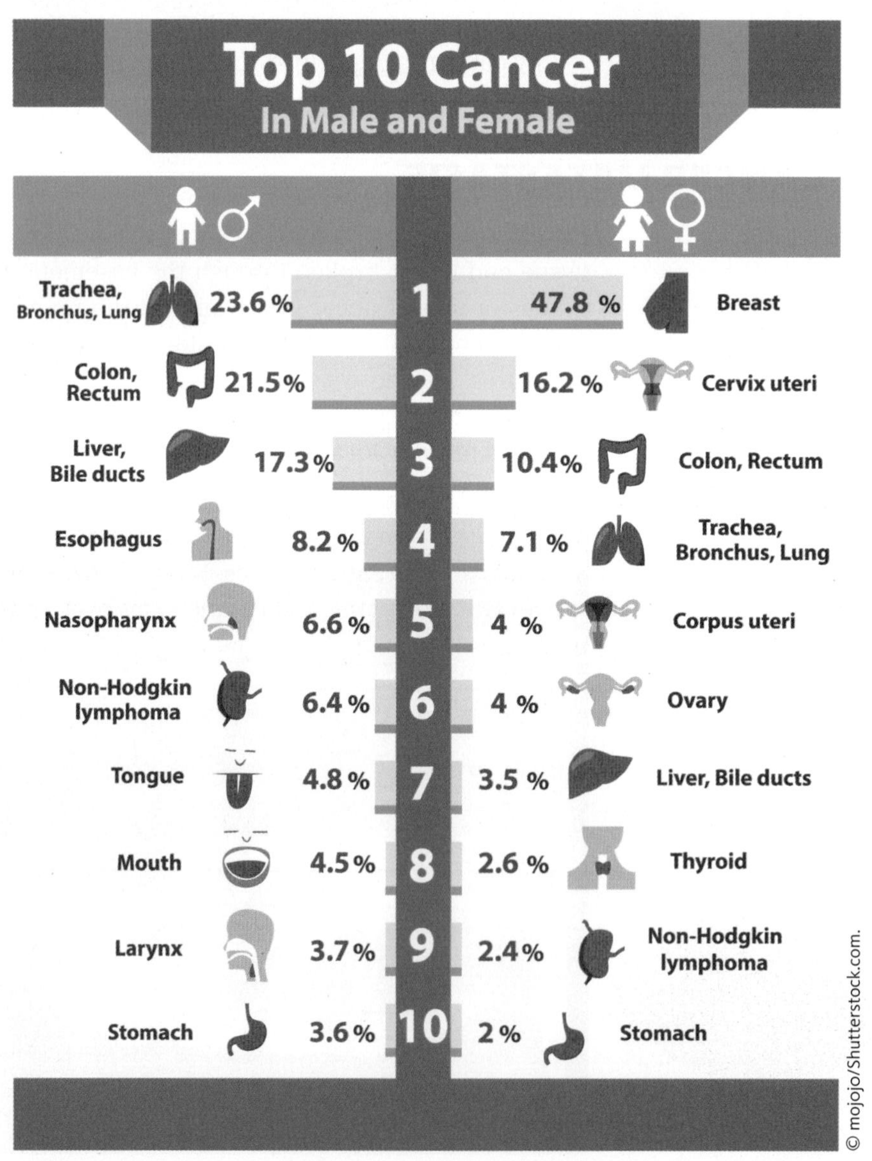

FIGURE 5-6 Various locations where cancer can exist.

LEARNING OBJECTIVE 5.3 **Differentiate the causes and risk factors associated with cancer.**

KEY TERMS

Carcinogenic Potential to cause cancer.

Human papilloma virus (HPV) A sexually transmitted virus associated with cervical cancer.

Ultraviolet (UV) radiation High-energy radiation from the sun or from tanning beds that can be carcinogenic with excessive exposure.

5-8 CAUSES OF CANCER

Often the cause of most cancers is unknown. However, it is known that genetic alterations within the cellular DNA are the foundational cause of cancerous cells. It is thought that these genetic mutations occur rather frequently, but an intact and healthy immune system destroys the abnormal cells before they can reproduce. However, if the body is overwhelmed by triggers that cause the genetic mutations and/or the immune system is weakened, cancer can develop.

Genetic alterations can be triggered by many situations, including the patient's genetic make-up or genes. For example, a blood test can tell if a woman has the BRCA1 or BRCA2 gene mutation, which can indicate a higher risk of breast cancer. Other triggers include radiation, sunlight exposure, smoking, fatty foods, viruses, and chemical exposure. Some of these triggers, such as genes or some viruses, are difficult to avoid; however, others, such as smoking, sunlight, radiation exposure, and fatty foods, can avoided be pretty easily by smart lifestyle choices.

Many chemicals or even biological agents can cause cancer and are termed **carcinogenic**, which literally means producing cancer (Figure 5-7). Continued exposure to a carcinogen such as asbestos can increase abnormal cells and the likelihood of developing cancer. Cancer might take years to develop and can have many different outcomes, with the worst being progression and spread. However, cancer might start and stop over time or might go into complete remission.

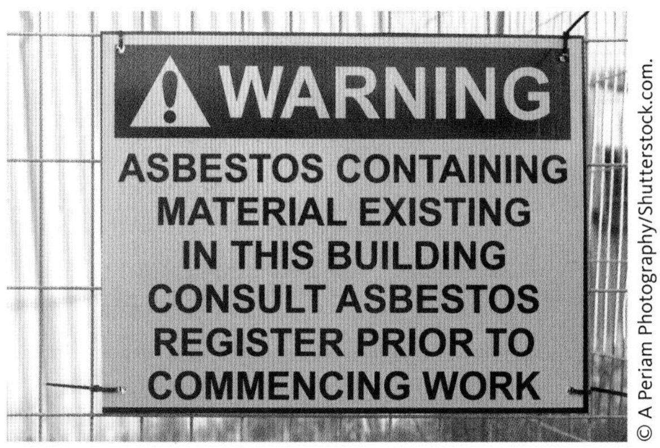

FIGURE 5-7 The carcinogen asbestos is still contained in many old buildings.

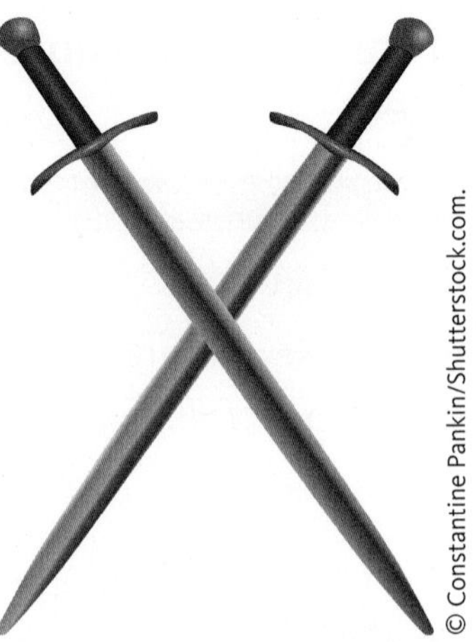

FIGURE 5-8 Hormones can be a double-edged sword, both causing and treating cancer.

5-8a Cancer and Hormones

Hormones are a double-edged sword (Figure 5-8). At times, they can cause cancer such as the excessive production of estrogen in females leading to breast or uterine cancer. However, in some cases, hormones can actually treat cancer. For example, prostate cancer can be stimulated by the male hormone testosterone. One potential treatment is to slow the growth with the female estrogen hormone to counteract testosterone's effects.

5-8b Cancer and Radiation

Radiation can come in several different forms and from several sources. **Ultraviolet (UV) radiation** from the sun or from tanning beds can be a carcinogen, leading to approximately one million cases of skin cancer each year (see Figure 5-9). Excessive exposure to X-rays or radioactive materials or not being properly protected can lead to the development of cancer. Again, radiation is another double-edge sword, because radiation can also be used in cancer treatment.

5-9 RISK FACTORS

One of the keys to cancer prevention is a personal risk factor evaluation. For example, smoking is the leading cause of lung cancer, increasing a person's risk to 15 times more than a nonsmoker. In addition, smoking has a correlation to bladder and pancreatic cancer, and has been associated with cardiovascular and other system problems. Simply put *do not smoke*, and if you do, you should quit as soon as possible, or STAT as they say in the medical profession. Module 11 covers smoking cessation programs and the pharmacologic aids to stop smoking.

Another risk factor is diet. Obesity and a high consumption of fat in the diet is a risk factor for colon and breast cancer. Many food additives

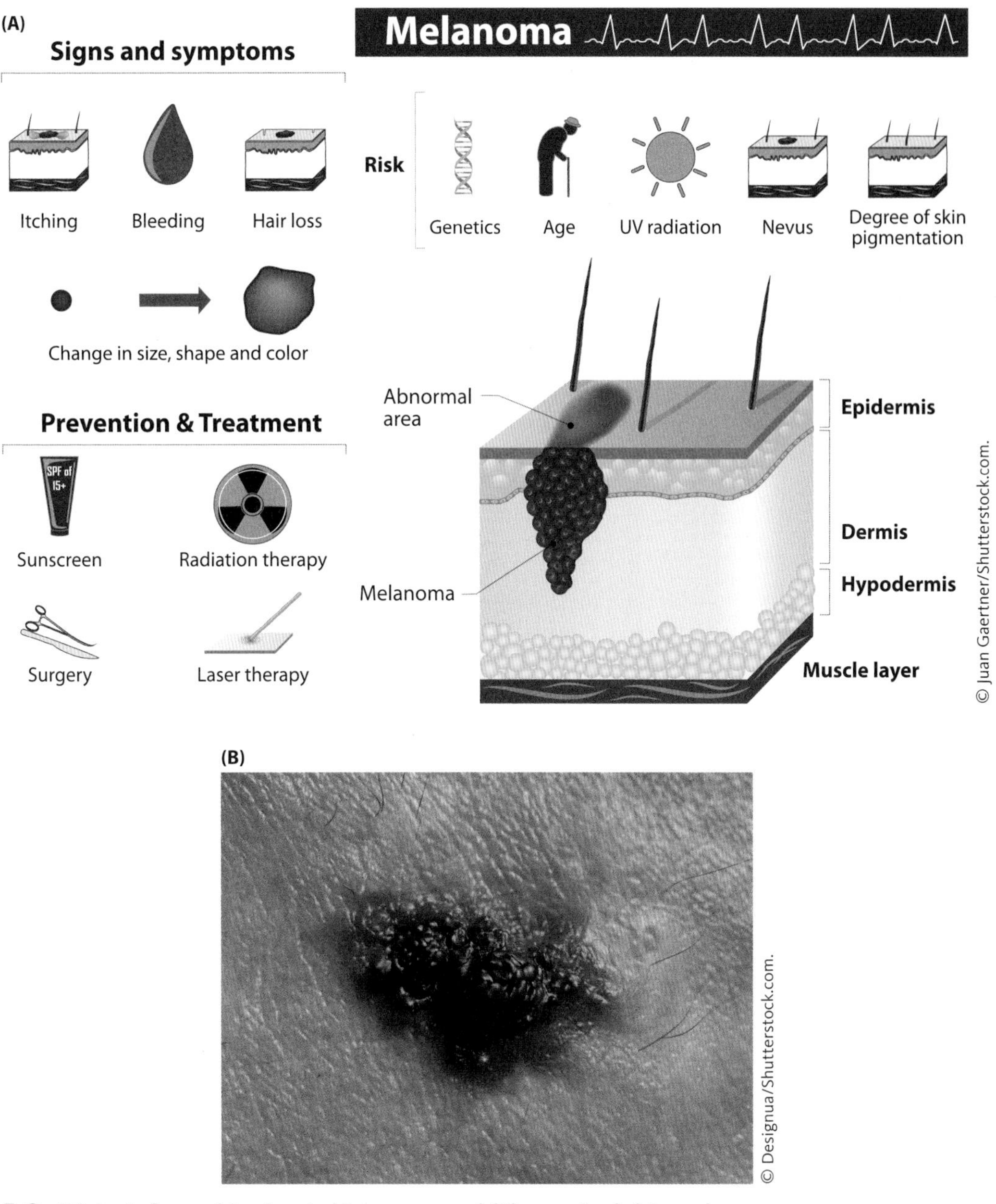

FIGURE 5-9 (A) An infographic about skin cancer and (B) an actual skin melanoma.

such as nitrates used as meat preservatives and sugar substitutes have been shown to cause cancer in laboratory animals, but the findings in humans are still controversial.

Excessive alcohol use has been associated with cancers of the mouth, throat, and esophagus, and women who are moderate drinkers have a higher incidence of breast cancer. Viruses also have been associated with cancer development. Hepatitis B virus has been associated with liver cancer, and **human papilloma virus (HPV)** is associated with cervical cancer. HPV transmission can be prevented with protected sex and routine HPV vaccination for both young girls and boys.

CLINICAL CONNECTION 5.3

CANCER VACCINE

Gardasil is the one FDA-approved vaccine to prevent HPV (Figure 5-10). Keep in mind that it will not treat an existing infection, so it is imperative that it be given prophylactically.

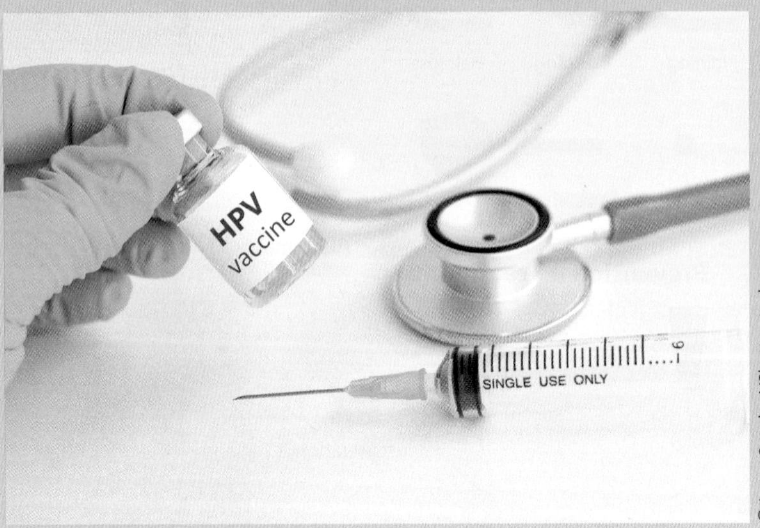

© Jarun Ontakrai/Shutterstock.com.

FIGURE 5-10 The HPV vaccine to help prevent cervical cancer.

LEARNING OBJECTIVE 5.4 Explain the process of cancer diagnosis and staging.

KEY TERMS

Anemia Low hemoglobin commonly seen as a result of hemorrhage or a decrease in red blood cells.

Biopsy Procedure during which a tissue sample is obtained for testing.

Cancer staging Objective measurement system to determine the severity of the cancer based on the size and spread of the original or primary tumor.

Endoscopy Viewing of internal portions of body and/or body passageways through use of flexible fiber optic scopes through which tissue biopsies also can be taken.

Forceps Set of surgical pinchers that can be advanced through an endoscope to sample a portion of a tumor for testing.

Occult stool Fecal test for blood in stool.

Pap tests Named after the founder Dr. George Papanicolaoua; stain the cells from the body sample (usually cervical smear) and look for abnormal cells.

Tissue biopsy Removal of small portion of a suspicious tissue for microscopic examination by a pathologist.

5-10 CANCER FACTS AND STATS

Before discussing cancer diagnosis, it is important to understand the scope of this dreaded disease. According to National Cancer Institute, the following statistics illustrate cancer's widespread occurrence.

- In 2016, there were an estimated 1,685,210 new cases in the United States, with 595,690 cancer deaths.
- The most common cancers in 2016 were breast, lung, prostate, colon, rectal, bladder cancers, melanoma of the skin, non-Hodgkin's lymphoma, thyroid cancer, kidney cancer, leukemia, endometrial cancer, and pancreatic cancer.
- The national expenditure on cancer in the United States was $125 billion in 2010 and could reach $156 billion in 2020.
- Cancer is the leading cause of death worldwide.

According to the American Cancer Society, the warning signs for cancer can be remembered by the acronym CAUTION:

Change in bowel or bladder habits

A sore that does not heal

Unusual bleeding or discharge

Thickening or lump in breast or elsewhere

Indigestion or difficulty swallowing

Obvious change in wart or mole

Nagging cough or hoarseness.

5-11 CANCER DIAGNOSIS

Routine check-ups and screenings are critical to cancer diagnosis and especially for early detection. Screenings for women can include monthly self-breast exams, regular **Pap tests**, and mammograms. **Occult stool** examination after age 40 for both sexes tests for blood in stool. Of course, any tumor discovery should be fully investigated. Often tumors are found or further investigated by imaging examinations such as X-rays, CT scans, positron emission tomography (PET) scans, or MRIs, which can give more details about exact tumor location and size.

Cytology is the study of cells, and tumor cells are among those that can be examined under a microscope. In a Pap test, named after the founder Dr. George Papanicolaoua, the cells from the body sample are stained and abnormal cells can be seen with a microscope. The Pap test is mainly taken from cervical smears, but it also can be used to test urine and other fluids for abnormal cells.

While cytology studies cells obtained from a sample of body fluids, histotechnology examines actual tissue samples. A small portion of suspicious tissue can be removed in a process known as a **tissue biopsy**. The tissue sample can then undergo microscopic examination by a pathologist.

Tissue sampling can be done by needle or aspiration **biopsy**. During a needle biopsy, a needle is inserted into the tumor or suspicious tissue and a sample

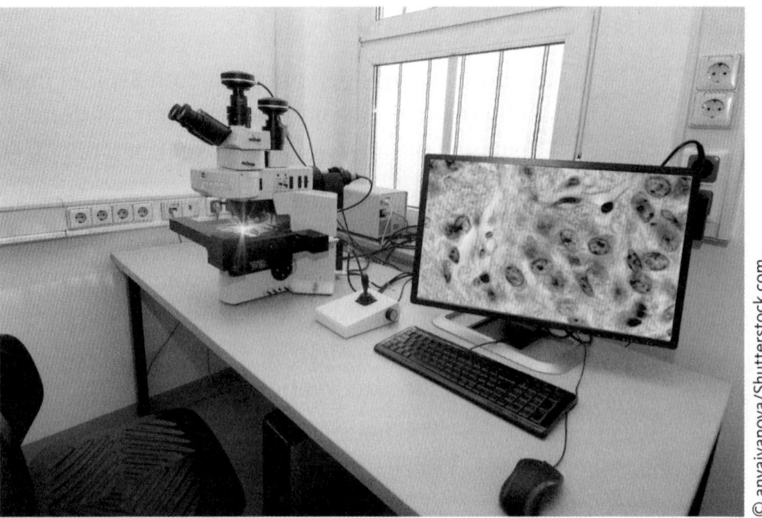
© anyaivanova/Shutterstock.com.

FIGURE 5-11 Modern microscope with a tissue sample displayed on a viewing screen.

is removed from the lumen (hollow opening) of the needle for testing (see Figure 5-11). Aspiration biopsy also uses a needle, but it is attached to suction device to remove part of tumor.

5-11a Endoscopic Sampling

Surgical biopsies can also be performed by surgically removing a portion of the tumor's tissue or removing and testing the entire tumor. Surgery is very invasive but is often needed, depending on the location of the tumor. Tumors within body passageways present another option for removal and/or sampling by using **endoscopy**.

The word "endo" means within and "scope" is an instrument used for viewing. Therefore, an endoscope is an instrument that can view inside your body. Endoscopes are usually flexible fiber optic scopes that can snake their way through body passageways such as the gastrointestinal tract or the respiratory bronchial tree. Not only can you view the internal structures for possible tumors, but if found, you can advance **forceps** (set of surgical pinchers) that can sample a portion of the tumor for testing. Endoscopes can view and sample your airways (bronchoscopy), colon (colonoscopy), or stomach (gastroscopy) as some examples. Figure 5-12 shows the components of an endoscope.

5-12 SIGNS AND SYMPTOMS

Often cancer is asymptomatic (without symptoms) until late in its development, which is why early screening so important. Even when symptoms present, they can be highly variable according to the site and the type of malignancy.

Pain is usually a late symptom because the tumor has grown to size that obstructs an opening, presses on a nerve, or occludes a blood vessel. Hemorrhage can be caused by an ulceration, along with the angiogenesis that occurs as the tumor makes new vessels to survive. Hidden blood in stool can be tested with occult stool test. **Anemia** or low hemoglobin is common as a result of hemorrhage or a decrease in red blood cells because of cancer treatment. Since the

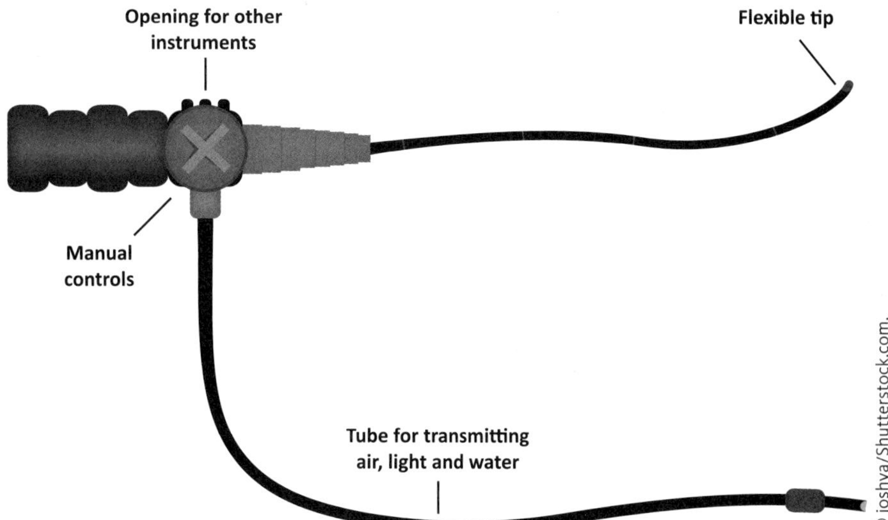

FIGURE 5-12 Endoscope showing flexible portion that can enter body for viewing. The opening for other instruments is where forceps can be advance through the tube to sample tumors.

red blood cells carry oxygen, the patient will often be short of breath because of decreased oxygen-carrying capability.

With bone cancers, bones can weaken and can fracture. Infection is also common, especially when immunity is decreased with cancer treatments such as chemotherapy. Systemic infections can occur and be life-threatening if not treated quickly. Cachexia is the weakened frail health associated with malnutrition often seen in terminal patients as the needed body nutrients are being fed to rapidly growing cancer cells.

In addition to the general signs and symptoms discussed, each type of cancer, such as skin cancer as shown in Figure 5-13, can have specific signs and symptoms. More details about cancer signs, symptoms, and treatment for specific cancer types, such as breast or colon cancer, will be covered in the respective upcoming system modules.

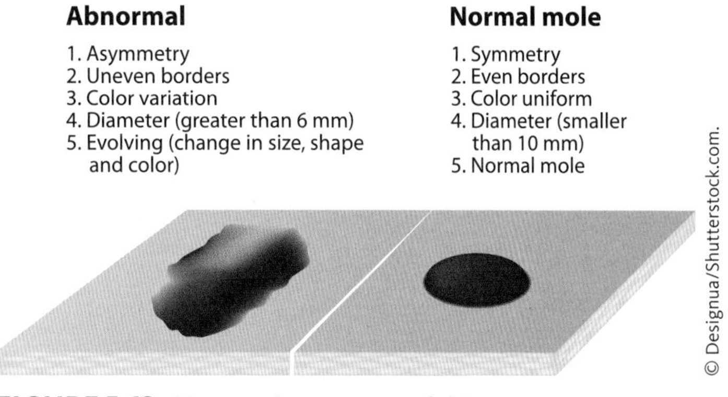

FIGURE 5-13 Signs and symptoms of skin cancer.

5-13 CANCER STAGING

The first question usually asked after the shock of being diagnosed with cancer resides is how bad is it? **Cancer staging** is done to objectively measure the severity of the cancer. It is based on the size and spread of the original or primary tumor. This can help determine the extent of the cancer and plan proper treatment and give the patient a prognosis.

All cancers are staged when diagnosed. Staging includes the site of the primary tumor, cell type (for example, squamous cell), tumor size, or extent. In addition, staging can include the number of tumors and if there is regional lymph node involvement.

The most widely used system is the TNM system in which:

T = size and/or extent or reach of the primary tumor

N = amount of spread to nearby lymph nodes

M = spread or metastasized

Some examples of the scoring system include:

T0 score means no evidence of primary tumor

Tis stands for carcinoma "in situ," which means abnormal cells are present but have not spread; or it's not cancer yet but might become cancerous (pre invasive cancer)

T1–T4 grades the tumor from small to large, respectively

N0 means no lymph node involvement

N1, N2, N3, … gives the number of lymph nodes involved

M0 means no metastasis

M1 means distance metastasis is present

So a score of T1, N0 would mean a small tumor with no lymph node involvement and therefore no spread.

Note: Not all cancers have TNM designation. This system is not used for cancers of blood, bone marrow, and brain.

LEARNING OBJECTIVE 5.5 Compare the various types of cancer treatments to include pharmacotherapy.

KEY TERMS

Adoptive cell transfer Cancer treatment using patient's own selectively grown T-cells.

Angiogenesis inhibitors (AIs) Biological response modifier therapy that targets and destroys cancer-feeding blood vessels. Drug example: bevacizumab (Avastin).

Antiandrogens Medications that suppress the production and effects of testosterone and can be used to treat prostate cancer. Drug examples are Eligard and bicalutamide (Casodex).

Antiemetics Classification of drugs to treat nausea often given in conjunction with cancer treatment.

Antiestrogens Drugs that modify or block the cancer-causing effects of the hormone estrogen on breast tissue. Tamoxifen is an example of a selective estrogen receptor modifier.

Antimetabolites Cancer medications that interfere with cellular metabolism and thus interfere with cellular repair and reproduction. Drug examples are methotrexate and fluorouracil.

Antineoplastic agents Medications that counteract the growth and spread of malignant cells.

Biological response modifier therapy This "targets" the cancer by manipulating the immune system to hunt down and specifically kill the cancer cells.

Chemotherapy Use of chemical substances or drugs to treat a disease, usually in reference to cancer.

Colony-stimulating factors (CSFs) Biological response modifiers that stimulate the bone marrow to develop red and white blood cells and platelets, which are often deficient in many cancers. Example drug is Erythropoietin (Epogen and Procrit).

Immunotherapy Use of natural or synthetic substances to stimulate or suppress immune system.

Interferons Biological response modifier therapy that actively stimulates the body's immune response to fight cancer.

Mitotic inhibitors Chemotherapeutic agents derived from natural substances used to inhibit cellular reproduction of cancer cells. The drug paclitaxel derived from the bark of the Pacific yew tree is an example.

Monoclonal antibodies (MABs) Biological response modifier therapy that uses genetically engineered antibodies that are too large to enter the targeted cell but can attach to the outside surface of the cancer cell thus tagging it for destruction by immune system.

Palliative therapy Therapy aimed at alleviating symptoms such as pain or obstructions to improve the quality of life.

Signal transduction inhibitors (STIs) Targeted cancer therapy agents that block specific enzymes and growth factors in cancer cells. Imatinib (Gleevec) is an oral STI that is approved for chronic myelogenous leukemia and some rarer types of cancers.

Targeted therapy Precision medicine that targets the desired abnormal cell (usually cancerous) for treatment and does not affect normal cells.

5-14 CANCER TREATMENT: BEGIN WITH PREVENTION

Many types of cancer can be prevented or managed with a healthy diet and exercise. Even genetic susceptibility to cancer can be lessened by preventative measures. Testing, such as mammograms (for breast cancer), colonoscopy (for colon cancer), and Pap tests (for cervical cancer), can improve survival rates by detecting cancers early, before they have metastasized, or even allowing the removal of abnormal cells before they become cancerous.

Lifestyle changes should be considered key tools in cancer prevention. Since smoking is estimated to cause 30% of all cancers, the obvious lifestyle change is to never start smoking, and quit if you do. Also limit your alcohol consumption. A cancer-protective diet is low in fat and high in fiber-rich foods such as whole grains, fresh fruits, and vegetables. Moderate and regular exercise has been shown to be cancer protective.

Protect your body from harmful environmental carcinogens. Get only needed X-rays, and make sure you are protected when having any imaging exam. Protect yourself around potentially harmful household products, such as insecticides, solvents, cleaners, pesticides, and pool chemicals. Avoid harmful chemicals if possible, or wear proper masks to prevent breathing them in and wear proper clothing to prevent contact with your skin.

Melanoma is one of the most widespread and deadliest forms of skin cancer, produced by hyperreproduction of the pigment-producing skin cells called melanocytes. Genetic factors also can cause melanoma, but high exposure to UV sunlight and sunburns are the key risk factors by far. That is why it is important to limit sun exposure and wear protective clothing and a sunblock SPF 15 or higher.

Since prevention and screening are critical, review Table 5-2, which gives recommendations from the American Cancer Society.

The prognosis of cancer is greatly enhanced by catching it early, before it becomes invasive and spreads. Other factors that can affect the prognosis are the type of cancer, age of patient, immune status, and efficacy of treatment.

5-15 TYPES OF CANCER TREATMENT

Treatment of cancer can be preventive as discussed in the previous section or can become curative or palliative after a diagnosis is established. **Palliative therapy** is aimed at alleviating the symptoms and improving the quality of life. An oncologist can recommend several options depending on the type and staging of cancer, including surgery, chemotherapy, radiation, hormone therapy, or some combination of these treatments.

CLINICAL CONNECTION 5.4

COMPLEMENTARY MEDICINE

Complementary medicine can be integrated effectively with traditional cancer therapy to lessen side effects and improve the patient's quality of life. These can include exercise, nutritional therapy, yoga, meditation, and hypnosis.

Table 5-2 Cancer screening

TYPE OF CANCER	RECOMMENDED SCREENING
Breast	• Perform monthly breast self-examination • Annual mammography for woman older than 45–54
Cervical/uterine	• HPV vaccination for presexually active girls; note: boys should also receive to prevent transmission and spread of HPV to females • Pap test at age 21 or within 3 years of first sexual intercourse
Colorectal	Fecal blood test or colonoscopy at age 50
Prostate	Prostate specific antigen test at age 50; men at risk at age 45

5-16 SURGERY

Cancer treatment usually involves surgical removal of the cancerous cells if possible, along with some form of treatment to kill any cells remaining in the body. Surgery can be curative, palliative, or preventive. Curative surgery would remove the entire tumor leaving no trace of the cancer remaining. Preventative surgery would remove suspicious growths for testing. Palliative surgery is used when a cure is not possible but the surgery will alleviate obstruction, stop bleeding, or lessen the patient's pain.

5-17 RADIATION

Radiation is often used to treat tumors that are inoperable. Radiation uses energy waves to shrink tumors and can be used as palliative therapy to relieve an obstruction or pain. The radiation therapy can be delivered by a targeted external ray as shown in Figure 5-14 or given internally in forms of radioisotope implanted beads or capsules.

Radioactive isotopes can be injected at the cancer site or can even be administered PO. For example, radioactive iodine is given orally to treat thyroid cancer since thyroid cells naturally absorb iodine. Again, the goal of radiation is to destroy as much of the tumor as possible without affecting normal tissue. Side effects of radiation therapy include nausea, vomiting, anorexia, hair loss, and impaired immunity.

5-18 CHEMOTHERAPY

Chemotherapy utilizes powerful medications that can be used in conjunction with surgery and radiation therapy (see Figure 5-15). These powerful **antineoplastic agents** (against new formation) counteract the growth and spread of malignant cells. However, often the cytotoxic (cell killing) effects are not limited to the cancer cells and can also affect other *normally* proliferating (rapidly producing) cells such as bone marrow, skin, and hair follicles.

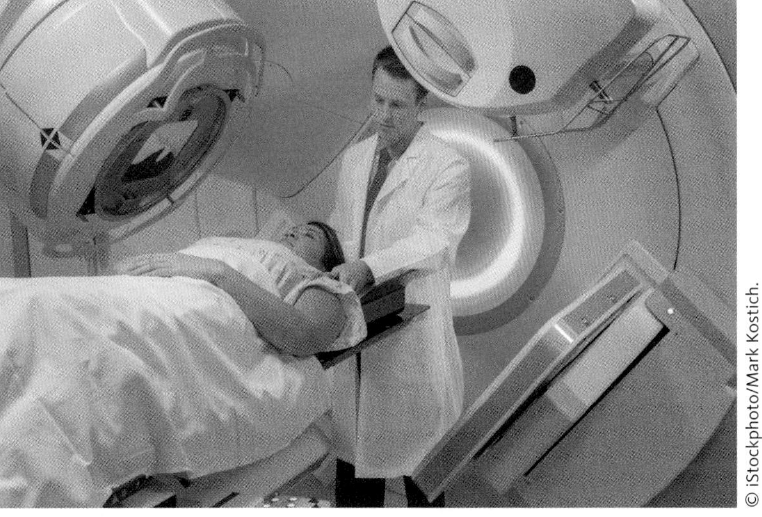

FIGURE 5-14 Radiation therapy in the treatment of cancer.

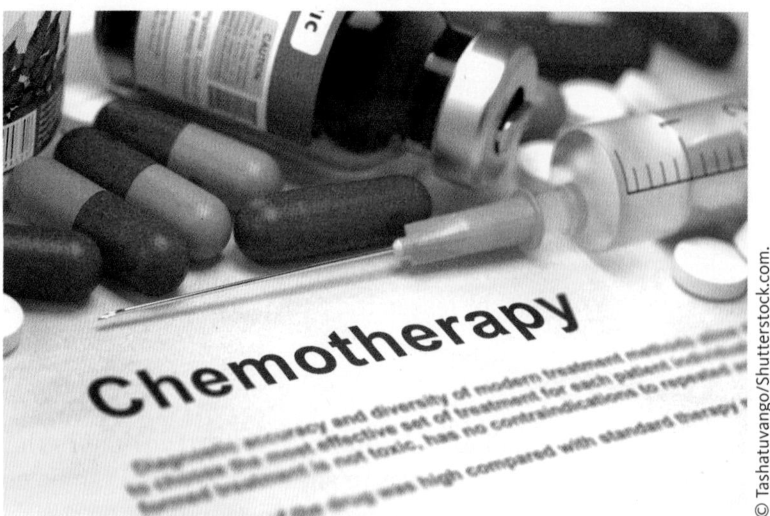

FIGURE 5-15 Chemotherapy utilizes powerful combinations of medications to treat cancer.

This is why there are often numerous side effects with chemotherapeutic agents. Ideally, chemotherapy is used on rapidly growing cancer cells with hopefully minimal effects on normal cells. This has led to the evolving development of **targeted therapy**. Targeted therapy is precision-type medicine that targets the changes in the cancer cells that help them reproduce. This will be further explained in the upcoming section concerning specific pharmacologic agents used for targeted therapy.

Antineoplastic drugs are often administered in high doses on an *intermittent schedule*. Since normal tissue has a greater regenerative capacity than malignant cells, this intermittent drug-free period can allow the normal tissue that suffered collateral damage to repair.

Chemotherapy is a very individualized complex treatment and is constantly monitored for modification according to patients' response and side effects. Since nausea and vomiting is a major and common side effect, the classification of drugs to treat nausea, called **antiemetics**, are often given in conjunction with chemotherapy.

There are many different groups of antineoplastic agents with many drugs under each group. The upcoming sections will explain how each group of antineoplastic medication works and give a representative medication for each category. If you work with cancer patients, the National Cancer Institute's Web site will give a complete listing of all the latest drugs available.

5-18a Antimetabolites

Cellular metabolism results in DNA synthesis that helps the cell to repair and reproduce. **Antimetabolites** interfere with cellular metabolism and thus interfere with cellular repair and reproduction. Two examples of antimetabolites include the drugs:

- methotrexate
- fluorouracil

Methotrexate can be given orally or injected. Fluorouracil can be given parenterally or comes in the topical cream Efudex for the treatment of skin cancer. Certain normal tissues that have high rates of metabolism such as hair follicles, bone marrow, and GI linings are most susceptible to collateral damage, and the following side effects can be found:

- Nausea, vomiting, and diarrhea
- GI bleeding and ulceration
- Bone marrow suppression causing leukocytopenia and anemia
- Alopecia (hair loss)

Closely related to the antimetabolites are *alkylating agents* that specifically damage the DNA needed for cellular reproduction. An example of an alkylating agent is the drug cisplatin.

5-18b Mitotic Inhibitors

As discussed in the beginning of this module, mitosis is the process of cellular reproduction, and since cancer is uncontrolled cellular reproduction, mitotic inhibitors can be an effective treatment. **Mitotic inhibitors** are derived from natural substances found in plants and trees. For example, the drug vinblastine is derived from the periwinkle plant.

The drug paclitaxel is derived from the bark of the Pacific yew tree and is used to treat breast and ovarian cancer. A form of paclitaxel called Abraxane is mixed with albumin nanoparticles (one billionth of a meter), which act as a biological carrier molecule to deliver and target the medication right to the site of action (see Figure 5-16). Side effects of mitotic inhibitors include peripheral neuropathy, bone marrow suppression, nausea, vomiting, diarrhea, and alopecia.

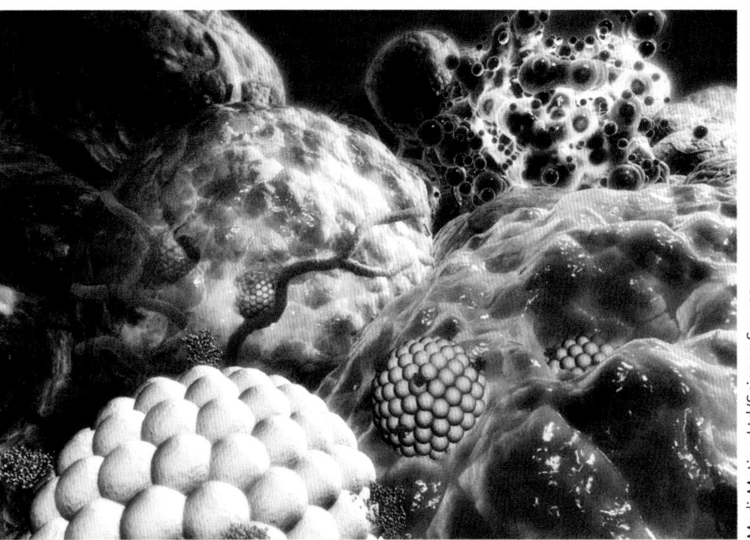

Medi-Mation Ltd/Science Source

FIGURE 5-16 Illustration of nanoparticles (blue) containing cytotoxic drugs and targeting the tumor cells (purple). The orange cells represent dead and dying tumor cells.

5-18c Hormones and Hormone Modifiers

Corticosteroid hormones are used to suppress the immune system specifically in leukemia and lymphoma. They are also used in combination with other chemotherapeutic agents to prevent the severe allergic reactions that can occur with these powerful cytotoxic medications. The two corticosteroids most commonly used in cancer treatment are:

- prednisone
- dexamethasone

Side effects listing of steroid use are very long, but the most common are:

- Fluid retention and edema (Cushing's syndrome)
- Osteoporosis
- Steroid-induced diabetes
- Nausea, vomiting, and diarrhea
- Electrolyte imbalance

Another group of drugs can be used to modify the effects of hormones. **Antiestrogens** will block estrogen's effects that can cause cancer and even osteoporosis. Tamoxifen is a selective estrogen receptor modifier that treats breast cancer by blocking the effects of estrogen on breast tissue.

Antiandrogens, which suppress the production and effects of testosterone and can be used to treat prostate cancer. Eligard and bicalutamide (Casodex) are examples of antiandrogens. Side effects include impotence and hot flashes.

5-19 BIOLOGICAL THERAPIES

Biological therapy or **immunotherapy** "targets" the cancer by manipulating the immune system to specifically hunt down and kill the cancer cells (see Figure 5-17). This therapy is also known as **biological response modifier therapy** because it does just that. Several types of biological modifications can occur.

Interferons actively stimulate the body's immune response to fight the cancer. Interferon alfa (Intron A) is used to boost the immune system to fight certain leukemias, melanoma, Kaposi's sarcoma, and non-Hodgkin's lymphoma. Interferons are also used to treat hepatitis and multiple sclerosis. Common side effects of interferons include flulike symptoms, nausea, vomiting, diarrhea, cough, sleep disturbance, and neuropathy.

Colony-stimulating factors (CSFs), which stimulates the bone marrow to develop red and white blood cells and platelets, are often deficient in many cancers. This is especially true since many antineoplastic medications suppress the bone marrow function. The Erythropoietin drugs Epogen and Procrit are two commonly prescribed CFS agents.

Another clever biological modification occurs with **monoclonal antibodies (MABs)**, which can mark cancer cells to alert the immune system where to concentrate the fight. Monoclonal bodies are genetically engineered antibodies that are too large to enter the targeted cell, but they can attach to the surface of the cancer cell, thus tagging it for destruction by immune system. Monoclonal

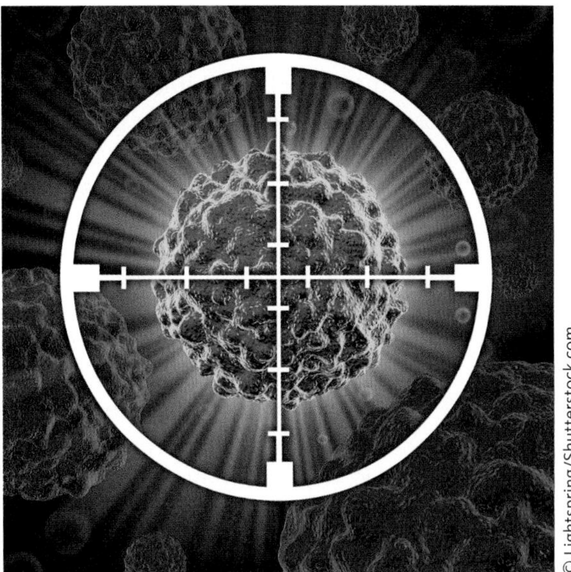

FIGURE 5-17 Biological therapy or immunotherapy "targets" the cancer by manipulating the immune system to specifically hunt down and kill it without affecting the surrounding normal cells.

antibodies such as trastuzumab (Herceptin) are administered IV and usually combined with other chemotherapeutic drugs or radiation to seek out and kill cells. Side effects of MABs are fever, headache, rash, nausea, and vomiting. Interestingly, side effects can be minimized by pretreating with acetaminophen (Tylenol) or diphenhydramine (Benadryl).

We previously mentioned how cancerous tumors develop their own proliferative blood supply through angiogenesis to supply nutrients for their hypermetabolic growth. A group of drugs can actually target these cancer-feeding blood vessels and are aptly named **angiogenesis inhibitors (AIs)**. Bevacizumab (Avastin) is a commonly used AI-type medication. AI side effects can include angioedema, hypotension, dyspnea, cardiac disturbances, and GI bleed.

5-19a Latest Targeted Therapies

Signal transduction inhibitors (STIs) represent one of the newest forms of targeted cancer therapy. These agents block specific enzymes and growth factors in cancer cells that cause the cancer to be so proliferative. Imatinib (Gleevec) is an oral STI that is approved for chronic myelogenous leukemia and some rarer types of cancers.

Adoptive cell transfer is also being investigated and employed in the arsenal of cancer therapies. Here T-cells are removed from the malignant tumor and isolated and grown in the lab. The T-cells are then tested to see which ones are best at attacking the tumor. The best or strongest T-cells are then grown in large numbers and reintroduced to fight the cancer.

New treatments are constantly under development and you will undoubtedly see more drug categories over time. Future therapy most likely will be individualized, since cancerous tumors can now be tested to see if a drug exists that can target that specific type of cancer cell.

5-20 VACCINES

Vaccines boost the immune system's ability to protect against foreign invasion. Cancer vaccines can either be preventative (prophylactic) or therapeutic to treat an already existing cancer. The FDA has approved two vaccines (Gardasil and Cervarix) to protect against forms of the human papilloma virus (HPV) that causes approximately 70% of cervical cancer cases worldwide.

These vaccines will not protect against all forms of HPV so regular cervical exams are still required. Most importantly, these are prophylactic and will not treat an existing HPV infection, so it is imperative that they be administered prior to the onset of sexual relationships.

Sipuleucel-T (Provenge) is the first vaccine approved for the treatment of metastatic prostate cancer. This is a form of adoptive cell therapy in which the patient's own white blood cells are used to stimulate the immune system.

Module 6

Pathopharmacology of the Musculoskeletal System

Module Introduction

The first portion of this chapter introduces the anatomy and physiology of the skeletal muscle system so you will have a normal reference point for the pathologies and treatments of this critical system of movement and protection. To provide movement, our muscles are groups of contractile tissue that contract and relax because of nerve impulses. This is why we will discuss this important neuromuscular connection later this chapter.

Muscles support our body's framework of bones, provide us with movement, and even help to produce body heat. The origin of the term muscle comes from the Latin word *mus*, which means mouse. Believe it or not, the idea behind the name is that when a muscle contracts it resembles a mouse running under the skin. Now that you are grossed out with the thought of vermin under your dermis, let's discuss the three different types of muscles found throughout the body as well as the purpose of each.

LEARNING OBJECTIVE 6.1 Explain the normal anatomy and physiology of the skeletal muscle system.

KEY TERMS

Actin Thin myofilaments mainly constructed of a protein.

Agonist muscle Muscle that causes other muscle to move.

Antagonist muscles Muscles that inhibit certain movement and return a muscle contraction back to its original resting position by opposing the muscle contraction.

Bone Mass Density (BMD) Diagnostic test using X-rays to measure the amount of minerals (especially calcium) in a bone.

Cardiac muscle Involuntary muscle found only in the heart.

Compact bone Hard, very dense, and tightly compact bone tissue that covers the outer layer of bones.

Contractility Ability of the muscle to shorten or contract.

Dual energy X-ray absorptiometry (DXA) Testing that uses X-rays to measure the amount of minerals (especially calcium) in a bone.

Elasticity Muscle's ability to return back to its original length after contracting.

Electromyography (EMG) Testing used to examine muscle disorders by inserting a small needle into the patient's muscle tissue and recording its electrical activity.

Endomysium Sheath of connective tissue around myofibrils.

Excitability Ability to respond to certain stimuli such as electric signals.

Extensibility Ability for a muscle to be stretched.

Flat bones Bones that have a plate-like structure.

Involuntary muscle Muscles that move without conscious effort.

Irregular bones Bones that are in many different shapes and sizes.

Irritability (see excitability).

Long bones Bones that are longer than they are wide.

Myofibrils Tiny strands of muscle fiber that makes up muscles.

Myopathy General term for muscle disease (*myo* = muscle).

Myosin Thick myofilaments of protein.

Osteocytes Mature bone cells found in the area surrounding the blood vessels in the bone.

Osteons Holes found in compact bone tissue.

Primary mover muscle Main muscle causing movement.

Sarcomeres Protein threads of small contractile units of striated muscle.

Short bones Bones that are cube-like in appearance since they are similar in width and length.

Skeletal muscle Voluntary muscle fiber looks like striated, long cylinder-like strands and is found attached to bones.

Smooth muscle (visceral muscle) Involuntary muscle found within the lining of hollow organs such as the intestines and blood vessels and airways.

Spongy bone Porous, sponge-like appearing bone.

Synergistic muscles Move to help assist the primary muscle's movement.

Trabeculae Irregular holes or pores come from the bars and plates that make up the bones' spongy structure.

Voluntary Muscle that requires conscious effort to move.

Z lines Myofilaments striations (dark bands) repeated throughout the muscle.

6-1 NORMAL MUSCLE STRUCTURE AND ANATOMY

When we think of muscle, often we think of the external muscles such as our biceps and triceps. However, we also have important internal muscles that also assist in movement, such as the muscles in our digestive system and blood vessels to keep internal fluids moving. And even though the Tin Man thought he didn't have a heart, we can't forget about the vital cardiac muscle. The three types of muscles are as follows:

- Skeletal
- Cardiac
- Smooth

Skeletal muscle is **voluntary** muscle that requires conscious effort to move. It is called skeletal because it attaches to the bones of our skeleton. The skeletal muscle fiber looks like a striated (striped), long cylinder-like strand attached to our bones. We use our skeletal muscles for our everyday external movement such as walking, running, and lifting.

Cardiac muscle is a type of **involuntary muscle** meaning that it moves without conscious effort. In appearance, this specialized muscle has slight stripes or striations and is only found in the walls of the heart. It contracts the heart to provide circulation of the blood. As an involuntary muscle, it moves on its own and does not require you to consciously think to move it. How tiring and all-consuming would it be to have to consciously tell your heart to beat each time?

Smooth muscle also known as **visceral muscle** is another type of involuntary muscle found in certain regions of the body. Unlike skeletal and cardiac muscle, this muscle is nonstriated, hence the name "smooth."

This muscle is found within the lining of hollow organs, such as the intestines, blood vessels, and airways. Smooth muscle is responsible for the ability to constrict or dilate the diameter of blood vessels, which changes the flow of blood in our circulatory system. It is also found in the airways and digestive tract, where it can alter the diameter of the "tubes" to modify the flow of air in our airways, and food through our gastrointestinal tract. Could you imagine having to make a conscious effort to tell your body to digest food or open up your airways to breathe? Figure 6-1 illustrates these muscles.

6-2 MUSCLE CONTRACTION AND RELAXATION AND ASSOCIATED TERMINOLOGY

Before getting into contraction and relaxation of muscles, let's first take a look at how our muscles are attached to our skeletal system. After all, our skeletal muscles would not be very useful if they were not tied into our skeletal framework. The body has connective tissue that holds our muscles together as well as *tendons*, which attach our muscles to our bones. The difference between tendons and ligaments is that *ligaments* connect bone to bone.

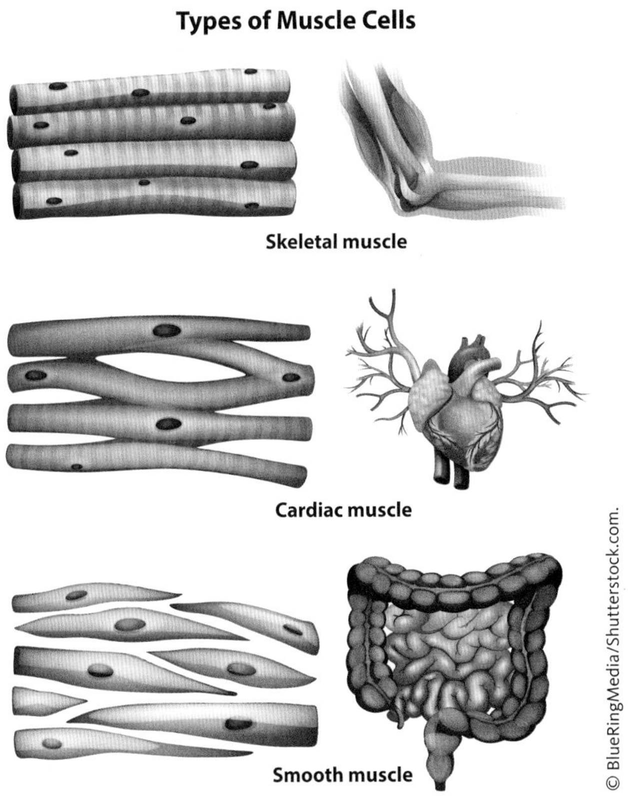

Types of Muscle Cells

Skeletal muscle

Cardiac muscle

Smooth muscle

FIGURE 6-1 Types of muscles and examples where found.

Our muscles are made up of tiny strands of muscle fiber called **myofibrils**, which have a sheath of connective tissue around them known as **endomysium**. Each myofibril is made of **sarcomeres**, which are actual protein threads of small contractile units of striated muscle. Sarcomeres come in two different types of myofilaments. These filaments of myofibrils are made of thick or thin protein threads. The thick myofilaments are made of protein called **myosin**, while the thin myofilaments are mainly constructed of a protein called **actin**. These myofilaments are repeated throughout the muscle strand and are separated by striations (dark bands) called **Z lines**. It is the sliding of these filaments and the forming of actin–myosin bridges that cause the muscle to contract,relaxation occurs when the bridge connection is broken and the muscles returns to their resting relaxation state.

This all requires energy. The energy source for muscle movement can be attributed to the metabolism of adenosine triphosphate (ATP) in the muscle cell and calcium. Both ATP and calcium are needed for contraction and muscle relaxation. The calcium is stored in the sarcoplasmic reticulum when the muscle is relaxed and is released to allow actin and myosin to connect when a contraction occurs. While this might sound complicated, the thing to keep in mind is calcium is needed for muscular contraction. Figure 6-2 illustrates the anatomy.

Muscle movement consists of several characteristic: contractility, extensibility, elasticity, excitability, and irritability. **Contractility** is the ability of the muscle to shorten or contract (forming those cross bridges). **Extensibility** is the ability for a muscle to be stretched. **Elasticity** is the muscle's ability to return

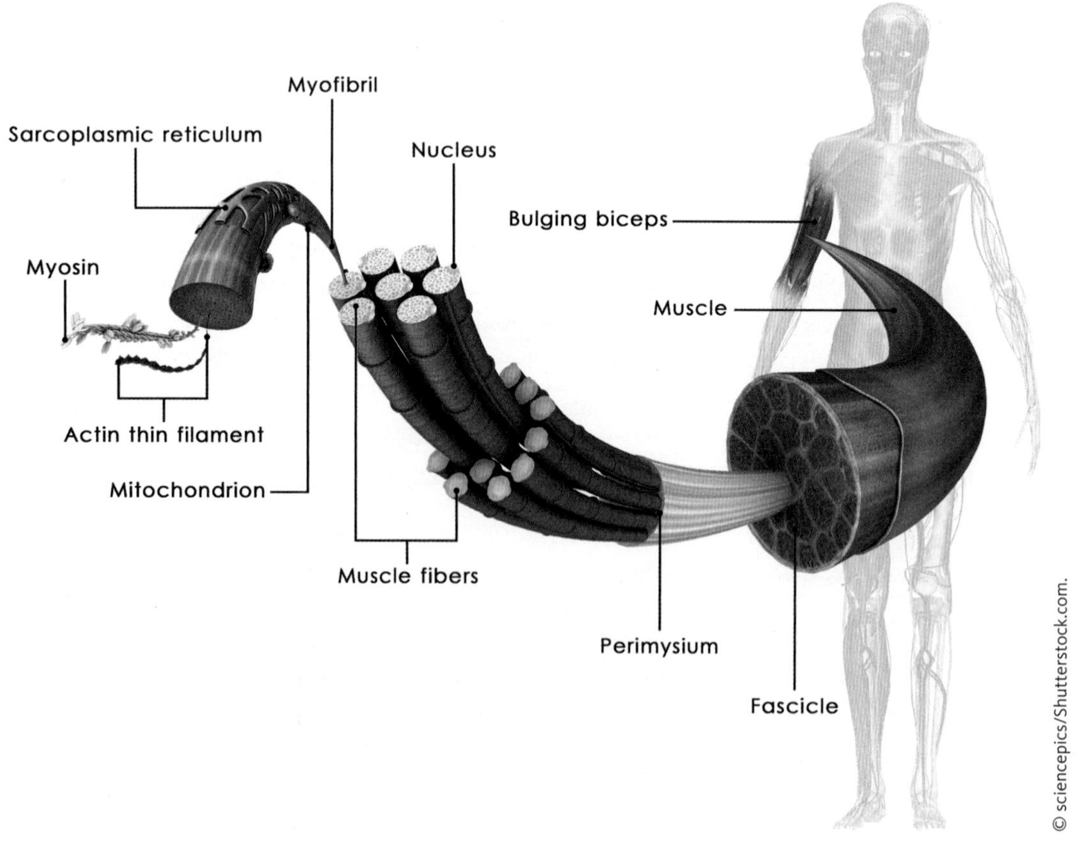

FIGURE 6-2 Muscle anatomy.

back to its original length after contracting (breaking the bridges), while **excitability** and **irritability** mean that muscles have the ability to respond to certain stimuli, such as the creation of electric signals (the neuromuscular connection).

Our muscles can move either by themselves or in conjunction with others. The main muscle causing movement is called the **primary mover** or **agonist muscle** because it causes movement to occur via its own contraction. **Antagonist muscles** returns a muscle contraction back to its original resting position by opposing the muscle contraction. Muscles that move to help assist the primary muscle's movement are called **synergistic** muscles.

6-3 NORMAL BONE STRUCTURE AND ANATOMY

Our bones are the framework of our body, giving it structure and acting as an internal armor to protect vital organs such as the heart, lungs, and brain. For example, our rib cage helps to protect the heart and lungs located in the thoracic region. Our bones also perform certain jobs that are vital to sustain life. Bones make blood cells within the bone marrow and distribute those new cells throughout our body where they mature and support life.

When looking at bones in textbooks or hanging in a classroom, you might get the impression that bones are nothing but dried up and hard tissue. In fact, the term skeleton comes from the Greek meaning "dried-up body," because early studies of bones were done after the body had decomposed to the point where nothing was left but the bones. However, our bones are very much alive. Bones are vascular, allowing blood to move through them through a network of blood vessels, and they create new blood cells used by our circulatory system. Our bones also store minerals such as calcium, sodium, phosphorous, and magnesium needed for growth and repair. In fact, 50 percent of our bones weight actually comes from these stored minerals.

Bones are classified according to their shape. **Short bones** are cube-like in appearance since they are similar in width and length. These types of bone can be found in our ankles and wrists. **Long bones** are longer than they are wide and are found in our arms and legs. For example, our femur (thigh bone) is the longest bone in our body. **Flat bones** have a plate-like structure that comes in flat and curved varieties. Examples of flat bones are the ribs and sternum. Lastly, **irregular bones** come in many different shapes and sizes, such as vertebrae or the pelvis, that connect with other bones.

6-3a Microanatomy of Bone

Now, let's take a look into our bones at a microlevel. Our bones are made up of two types of bone tissue, spongy and compact. **Spongy bone** resembles a sponge, as it is very porous. The irregular holes or pores come from the bars and plates that make up the bones spongy structure called **trabeculae**. Spongy bones allow a space for red bone marrow to produce red blood cells, as well as reducing the weight of the bone. Yellow bone marrow also can be found in a bone to produce cartilage, fat, and actual bone.

Compact bone is hard and very dense tissue that covers the outer layer of bones. While compact bone is dense, it does have tiny holes called **osteons** that resemble rings of a cut tree trunk. Osteons contain blood vessels that

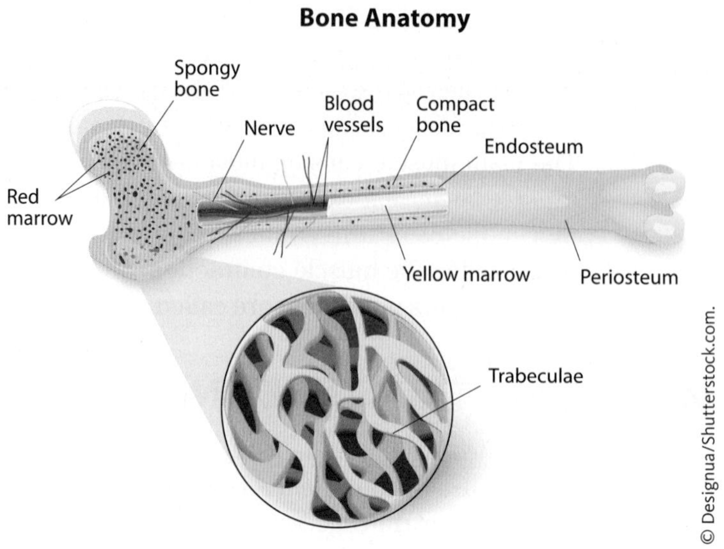

Bone Anatomy

Spongy bone
Red marrow
Nerve
Blood vessels
Compact bone
Endosteum
Yellow marrow
Periosteum
Trabeculae

FIGURE 6-3 Bone anatomy.

penetrate into the bones to supply them with oxygen and nutrients. The area surrounding the blood vessels in the bone house mature bone cells called **osteocytes**.

Many different bumps and grooves project and depress along the outside surface of bones. These unsmooth surfaces allow bones to be connected to muscle by ligaments and tendons (see Figure 6-3).

6-4 NORMAL JOINT FUNCTION AND ANATOMY

Our bones are connected together by joints, without which we would not be able to move. Joints are classified according to their movement and structure. The functional classification of joints includes those that can move freely, those that slightly move, or those that remain stationary. Our skull and its associated joints are stationary joints, while the elbows are freely moving, and the pelvic joints provide a small amount of movement. Joint structure includes fibrous, cartilaginous, and synovial joints. As we age, our joints begin to show wear and tear and disease, all of which will be discussed later in this chapter (see Table 6-1).

Figure 6-4 contrasts a healthy joint with a joint with rheumatoid arthritis.

6-5 DIAGNOSTIC TESTING FOR THE MUSCULOSKELETAL SYSTEM

While patient history and physical exam is vital in assessing the musculoskeletal system, imaging diagnostics give us a picture of what is going on beneath the surface. The main imaging tools used to diagnose joint and bone disorders are X-rays. A CT scan or MRI is used instead of a standard X-ray when a higher resolution image is needed. Review Chapter 1 for more information regarding X-rays, CTs, and MRIs.

Diagnostic testing can test for bone hardness. A **bone mass density (BMD)**, also referred to as a **dual energy X-ray absorptiometry (DXA)**, uses X-rays to measure the amount of minerals (especially calcium) in

Table 6-1 Joint structures

JOINT STRUCTURE	DEFINITION	EXAMPLE
Fibrous	Consists of short strands of connective tissue that holds this type of joint together and are stationary or move slightly.	Skull
Cartilaginous	Holds bones together with cartilaginous disks.	Connection between the sternum and ribs
Synovial	Many different types of synovial joints move freely in different ways. Each of these joints consists of a joint cavity that is lined with a synovial membrane and filled with synovial fluid to reduce friction during movement.	Knee, elbow

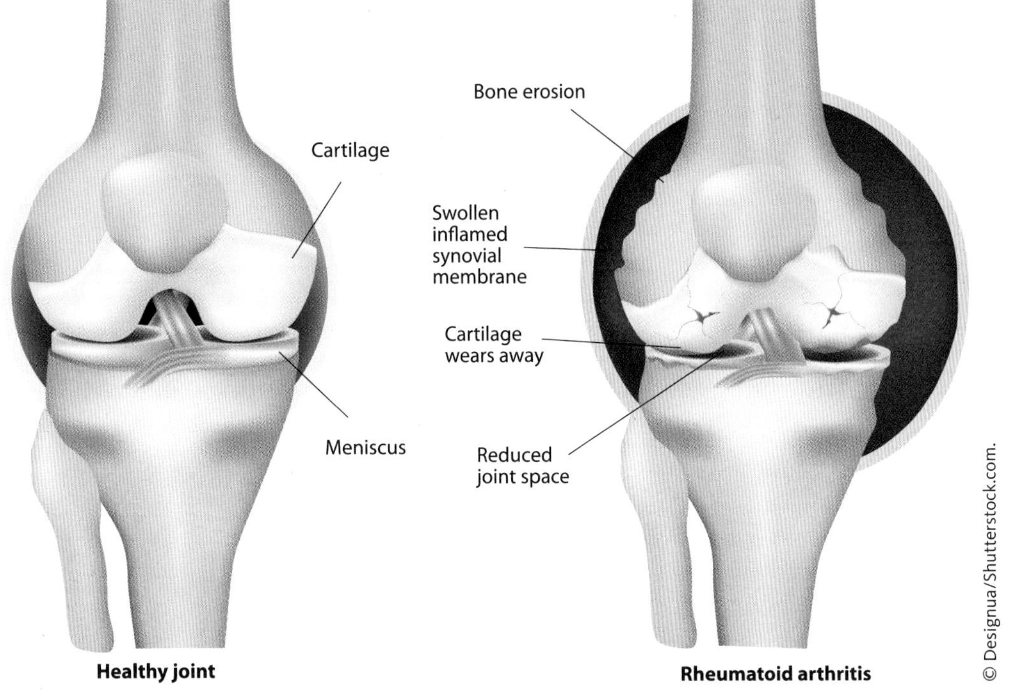

FIGURE 6-4 Contrasts of a healthy joint with a joint with rheumatoid arthritis.

a bone. This test screens for low bone mass, as seen with osteoporosis (see Figure 6-5). DXAs are relatively quick, painless, and do not require any medications or dyes. Typically, this diagnostic can be done as an outpatient procedure, meaning the patient does not need to be hospitalized. There are two types of DXA procedures: peripheral and central tests. The peripheral DXA looks at the body's periphery, such as the bones in the patient's feet, legs, hands, and arms. Depending on the results, a central DXA might be needed to check the bones in the torso, hips, and spine. The values used for interpreting the image results can be seen in Table 6-2.

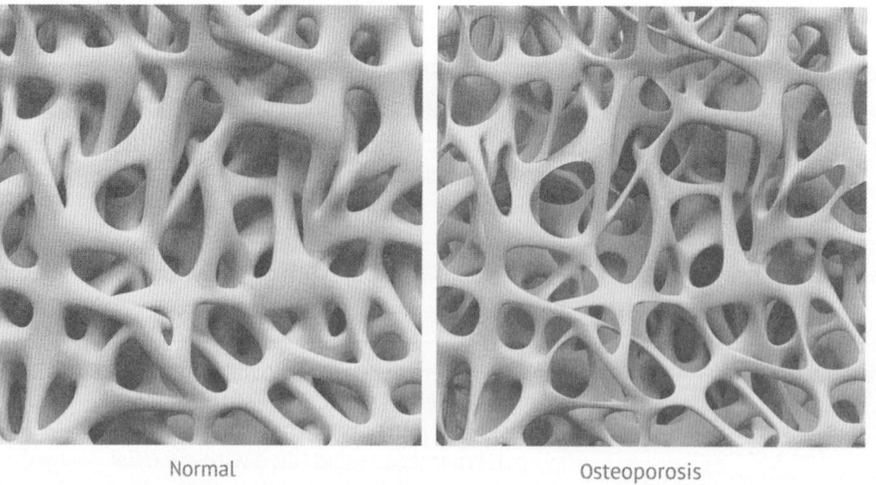

FIGURE 6-5 This image contrasts the differences between healthy bone tissue and that of osteoporosis.

Table 6-2 DXA interpretations

CONDITION	VALUES
Normal	Above −1
Osteopenia (penia = lack)	Between −1 and −2.5
Osteoporosis	Below −2.5

When a muscle has a disease it is known as **myopathy**. An **electromyography (EMG)** is used to examine muscle disorders by inserting a small needle into the patient's muscle tissue and recording the electrical activity of the muscle. The purpose of this exam is to figure out whether the disorder is neurological or muscular. Another way to understand what is happening to the patent's muscle is to perform a biopsy. This allows the physician to get a tissue sample, so it can be tested to determine the root of the problem.

LEARNING OBJECTIVE 6.2 Describe pathopharmacology of the musculoskeletal system due to use and misuse.

KEY TERMS

Adhesive capsulitis Also known as a frozen shoulder, the shoulder becomes stiff and painful to move due to the lack of movement over time.

Bursitis Inflammation of the fluid-filled sac found in joints.

Carpal tunnel syndrome Inflammation pressing on the median nerve in the wrists from strenuous or repeated movement.

Cruciate Ligament Tear Tear in the ACL (anterior cruciate ligament) or PCL (posterior cruciate ligament).

Dislocation Total or complete separation of a bone from a joint.

Eversion Ankle has moved or rolled outward.

Herniated nucleus pulposus (HNP) Herniated vertebral disc.

Inversion Ankle turns inward.

Meniscal tear Tear in the semilunar pads in the knees that are a cushion between the femur and the tibia.

Muscle strain A pulled muscle.

Plantar fasciitis Condition of pain and inflammation occurring from small tears in the plantar fascia ligament from activities causing repeated pressure on the bottom of the foot such as running or walking long distances.

Sprain Complete or partial damage done to the ligaments such as tearing or stretching.

Subluxation A partially separated bone from a joint injury.

Tendonitis Inflammation of the tendon.

Torn rotator cuff Stress injury in which a tear occurs in a tendon within a collection of muscles that hold the head of the humerus into the shoulder socket.

6-6 SPRAINS, STRAINS, AND OTHER PAINS

The conditions in the following section are not congenital or neuromuscular, but rather caused by our own actions or the result of another's doing. In other words, this section will describe wear and tear conditions caused by an accident, improper lifting, and over-usage of an appendage. You might be more familiar with the conditions in this section than others since these ailments commonly happen to young and active people. For example, you might have experienced a sprain, strain, dislocation, or even shin splints, but how do they differ? This section will discuss that.

Before getting into the specific conditions, since pain obviously is one of the major symptoms, a review of pain medications is in order. Let's discuss a little about the previously mentioned analgesic drug classes from Chapter 2. The word analgesic means "without feeling." An analgesic alters the way the brain perceives pain. For example, Tylenol (acetaminophen) is a widely used analgesic commonly used to treat pain by deadening the pain receptors. Other commonly used over-the-counter analgesics can treat both acute and chronic pain and come in various forms. Powerful analgesics containing opiates are used to control severe pain. They require a prescription and are more likely to cause an addiction so they are more tightly controlled (again see Chapter 2). These drugs have a quick onset and can last for hours. Table 6-3 is a list of common analgesics containing opioids.

Nonsteroidal anti-inflammatory drugs (NSAIDS) also relieve pain, but also decrease inflammation to the injured area. When injured, our body releases several chemicals related to the inflammatory response, with prostaglandins being one that causes swelling and pain at the damaged area.

NSAIDS such as Advil or Motrin (ibuprofen) and Aleve (naproxen) do not work the same as acetaminophen. Instead, NSAIDS inhibit the body's response to injury to release hormone-like substances called prostaglandins, which cause inflammation to occur.

Table 6-3 Common analgesics containing opioids

DRUG	ONSET	DURATION
Codeine	5 minutes via IV 30 minutes by mouth	3 to 6 hours
Hydrocodone	Given only orally, 10–20 minutes	4 to 8 hours
Fentanyl	Given only by IV, almost instantly	30 minutes to two hours
Morphine	5 minutes via IV 30 minutes by mouth	3 to 6 hours

If NSAIDs are not enough to control inflammation, more powerful anti-inflammatory steroids can be used. Steroids do not work the same way as NSAIDs to control inflammation. Instead, corticosteroids resemble cortisol, which is a steroidal hormone naturally produced by the adrenal glands that sit above our kidneys. Steroids help relieve inflammation by decreasing the overall body's immune system. This is what makes steroids so valuable in treating conditions such as asthma and even arthritis. Steroids can be given in many different ways, including orally (tablets and inhalers), intranasally (nasal spray for allergies), topically (ointments and creams for skin conditions), and for the purpose of this chapter, injected directly into the joint or muscle to reduce inflammation. Common steroids include cortisone, hydrocortisone, and prednisone.

Muscle relaxants are used only after failed attempts to control pain with analgesics and NSAIDs. Muscle spasms are often associated with the overuse of muscles or injury, such as in the lower back. Muscle relaxants depress the nervous system to stop uncontrolled spasms. However, these drugs are only used for a short time to avoid possible addiction and serious side effects, such as seizures, paralysis, and loss of vision. Other less severe adverse reactions are headache, tremors, nausea, and insomnia. Table 6-4 lists commonly used muscle relaxants and their uses.

Table 6-4 Muscle relaxants

BRAND NAME (GENERIC NAME)	USES
Soma (carisoprodol)	Alleviates muscle spasms caused by muscle conditions (shortterm)
Flexeril (cyclobenzaprine)	Treats pain associated with fibromyalgia as well as other muscle conditions causing pain
Valium (diazepam)	Treats muscle spasms, seizures, even anxiety

6-6a Sprain

Have you ever sprained your ankle badly enough that you temporarily lost function? This traumatic event is very painful, but what exactly is a **sprain**? When a sprain occurs, either complete or partial damage has been done to the ligaments, such as tearing or stretching. Other tissues that might be injured are tendons and the muscles located in that specific area. Remember, a ligament is connective tissue that attaches bone to bone, and tendons connect muscle to bone. The intense pain that follows such injury requires an anti-inflammatory or analgesic. Other symptoms are swelling, redness, and a warm sensation. If blood vessels have been broken, a purple discoloration might appear. Two words that you might come across when dealing with a sprain is **inversion** and **eversion** as shown in Figure 6-6. An inversion means the ankle went inward, while eversion means the ankle has moved or rolled outward.

Usually, you can tell you have a sprain based on the appearance and history of the injury. However, if you choose to go to a medical facility, an X-ray might be taken to check for any broken bones. As for treatment, the acronym PRICE is often used, especially for the first 48–72 hours.

- (P) Protection: Prevent from further damage/injury by using braces and bandages
- (R) Rest: Keep weight off the injury
- (I) Ice: Place an ice pack onto the site with a small barrier such as cloth between skin and ice to protect the skin from the cold
- (C) Compression: Use a wrap to help decrease the amount of swelling occurring in the site
- (E) Elevation: Keep the injury above the level of the heart to reduce swelling.

To prevent a sprain, it is important to stay fit, and strength train. Even wearing proper equipment, such as high top sneakers for basketball, can help prevent this painful event.

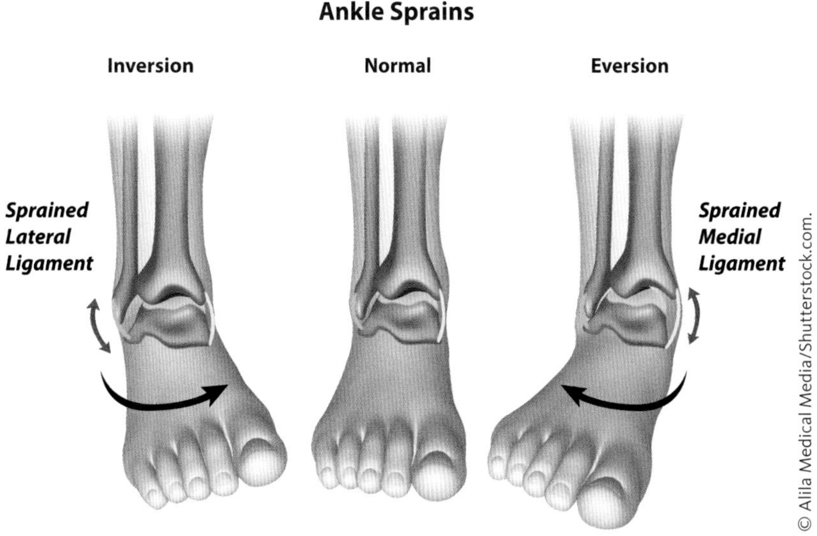

FIGURE 6-6 Types of ankle sprains.

6-6b Strain

Most people have experienced a **muscle strain** at some point in his or her life. This can be caused by overexerting yourself when lifting or having a weekend crammed full of physical activity, such as yardwork. These pulled muscles are tender and sore for the next few days. This type of injury can be diagnosed by a physical exam and the history of the injury. Strains are commonly treated by applying a pain relief cream and moist heat.

Some people often choose to use an analgesic or anti-inflammatory drug as well. As previously discussed, the analgesic Tylenol (acetaminophen) can be used for pain and nonsteroidal anti-inflammatory drugs (NSAIDS) for pain as well as to decrease inflammation to the injured area. However, if the injury is severe, physical therapy might be needed for the individual to regain normal functionality.

6-6c Dislocations and Subluxations

Dislocations and **subluxations** are both painful injuries. A dislocation is a total or complete separation of a bone from a joint, while a subluxation is a partially separated bone from joint injury. These injuries are commonly associated with motor vehicle accidents, falls, and sports-related injuries. The act of putting a bone back into the correct position is called *reduction*. Since inflammation will occur rapidly, it is best to place the dislodged bone back into its correct location as soon as possible. If a person has recurring dislocations or subluxations, they should be taught how to properly put the bone back into place. If the bone keeps popping out of place, strength training might be an option to prevent further issues. However, surgery might be required to strengthen the injured area to actually tighten the ligaments to prevent a bone from leaving a joint. To prevent either injury, strength training and wraps can be done (see Figure 6-7).

Another issue that can occur is the locking or freezing of a joint. For example, **adhesive capsulitis** is a condition that causes shoulder stiffness and pain. Typically, this condition arises when the shoulder has been injured causing a lack of or limited movement. To treat this condition, the patient may be injected with corticosteroids or numbing agents. Range of motion exercises are also performed to regain normal shoulder movement.

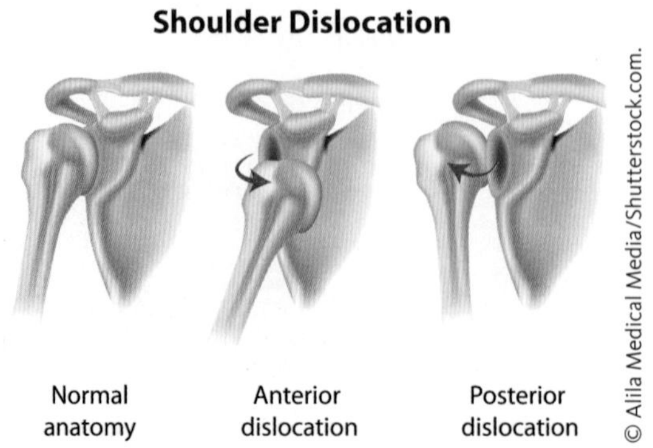

FIGURE 6-7 Types of shoulder dislocations.

6-6d Lower Back Pain (LBP)

The lower or lumbar region of the back is susceptible to injury because of preventable factors, such as poor lifting techniques and obesity, or unavoidable factors, such as spinal diseases, deformities, osteoporosis, and bone cancer. These injuries can be acute or chronic in nature.

X-rays, MRIs, and CTs can be performed to aid in a diagnosis. Treatment consists of many of the previously mentioned healing methods, such as analgesics, anti-inflammatory agents, and muscle relaxants. The muscle relaxants prevent muscle spasms and cramping of muscles, which are very painful for the patient.

To prevent back injuries from occurring in the future, the back needs to be strengthened with proper exercise to tone the lumbar muscles. Of course, proper lifting techniques and even a lifting belt to prevent future injury is a major preventative measure, coupled with weight loss if needed.

6-6e Herniated Nucleus Pulposus

Have you ever heard of a person complaining about a herniated or ruptured disc? These terms are commonly thrown around, but if you ask someone, odds are that they would not be able to explain what this condition is nor know the official medical term: **herniated nucleus pulposus (HNP)**.

To understand the pathology, we must briefly discuss what a disc is. Our discs are cushions between our vertebrae that absorb energy from our everyday movement, acting just like small shock absorbers for our spine. These discs are hard on the outside and soft in the center. As a result of an injury, the hard exterior portion of the disk can be damaged, which allows the softer interior to leak out and compress spinal nerves or even the spinal cord (see Figure 6-8). Those affected can have symptoms of pain that radiates down the back of his or her leg. This is caused by the herniated disc compressing on the sciatic nerve.

Diagnostic tests used to diagnose such condition are an MRI and CT scan. Also, a myelogram can be performed, which involves injecting a dye into the subarachnoid space of the spinal canal. The dye highlights the nerves in a radiopaque fashion to give the examiner a better view of the nerves and spinal cord to see if any compression exists. This exam is also used to check for other problems such as infection, spinal stenosis (narrowing) from arthritis, and even spinal tumors.

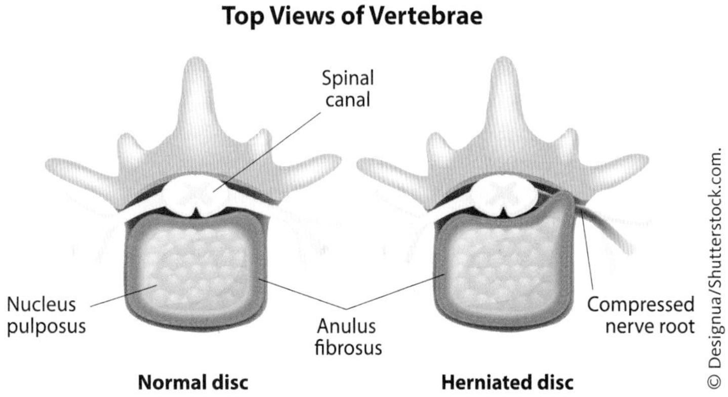

FIGURE 6-8 Comparison of a normal and herniated disc.

A few treatment options exist. To alleviate pain, a noninflammatory agent such as ibuprofen (Advil, Motrin) should be given to decrease swelling that is further compressing any nerves. If inflammation is severe, steroids can be administered. If the pain is bearable, the patient might benefit from exercise therapy to decrease the size of the herniation. Other methods used to decompress the nerves involve invasive procedures:

- *Laminectomy*, to remove a portion of the vertebrae to decrease the pressure in the herniated region, thus diminishing the pain
- *Discectomy*, surgically removing the damaged disc.

For herniated discs, prevention is key. Exercising and proper lifting techniques are great ways to prevent back injuries.

6-6f Bursitis

As shown in Figure 6-9, we have fluid-filled sacs called bursae in our joints. This fluid reduces friction during movement. Often times, you might hear about a shoulder (the most common site) or an elbow (tennis elbow) being the site of pain. However, **bursitis** can occur in any joint. The pain can be so bad that it limits the patient's mobility. The cause of this condition is contributed to the repeated movement of a joint. Patients with bursitis are diagnosed by learning the history of the condition and also an X-ray, if needed. A diagnosis of tennis elbow can be made by pushing the patient's middle finger backward against resistance. It will hurt.

Treatment for bursitis can include resting the sore joint and treating with analgesics and anti-inflammatory medications. If these methods do not work, the patient might have to undergo more invasive procedures, such as a corticosteroid injection and possibly draining the site with a surgical incision. After surgical intervention, physical therapy will be used and the patient will be instructed to perform range-of-motion exercises to regain mobility of the joint. To prevent this form of injury, you should avoid repetitive motion activities that cause pain. Proper exercise and strength training also can help.

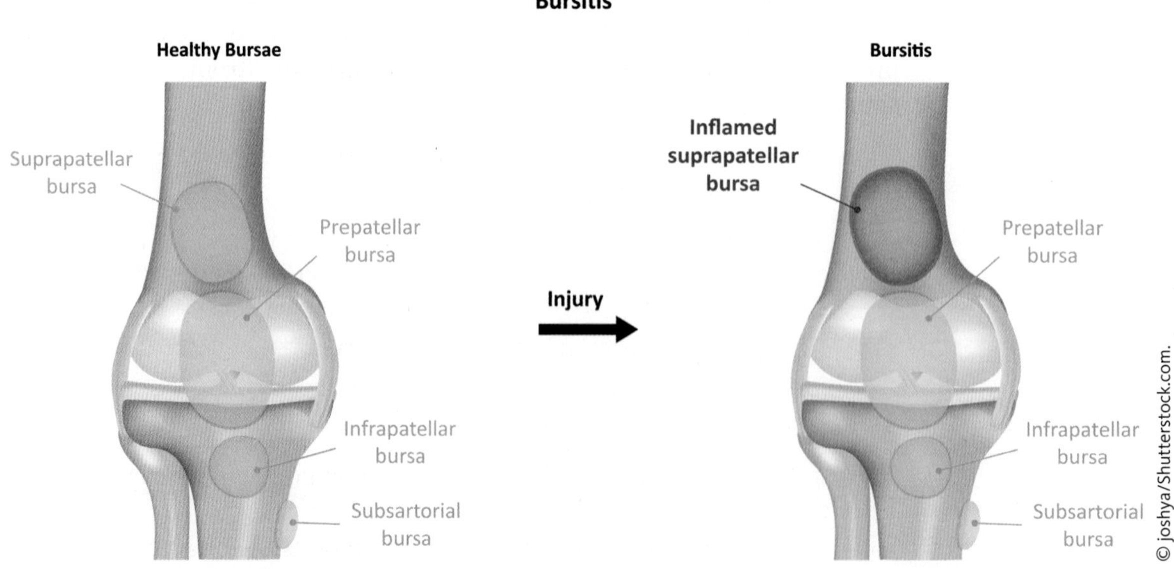

FIGURE 6-9 Image of bursa sacs found in the knee.

6-6g Tendonitis

Tendonitis is an inflammation of the tendon, a piece of connective tissue that attaches muscle to bone. Like bursitis, tendonitis often occurs when there is a recurrent motion; however, this condition also can be caused by calcium deposits. In addition, tendonitis and bursitis even can occur together.

The most common site for this condition is the shoulder, and it is most often seen in athletes. The dominate symptom associated with this injury is pain, which can be severe in nature and can occur over time or immediately after an activity. A physical exam can determine whether there is any tendon tenderness, especially when resistance is added.

Rest is needed for the joint to recover, and ice can be applied during the first day of the injury. Other care includes taking analgesics and anti-inflammatory agents to relieve pain and inflammation, respectively. The patient might undergo physical therapy and perform range-of-motion exercises to regain movement. If the patient does not move the joint because of soreness and inflammation, adhesion can occur, making it difficult to move. Preventative measures include routine exercising and avoiding overexertion and repeated movements.

Table 6-5 provides a summary of the conditions and medications discussed thus far.

6-7 CARPAL TUNNEL SYNDROME

Another commonly occurring condition resulting from repetitive movement, such as typing on a keyboard, is **carpal tunnel syndrome**. Located in your wrist or carpus is a small passageway that runs from the wrist to the forearm called the carpal tunnel. The median nerve and tendons to manipulate your fingers are located in this narrow passageway. Repeated or strenuous use of your hands can cause inflammation. This inflammation presses on the median nerve, causing pain and discomfort. This results in poor gripping ability, numbness, weakness, burning, and tingling sensations. Methods to diagnose include:

- *Tinel sign*, a positive sign is indicated when light tapping is done over the median nerve causing a tingling (pins and needles) sensation.
- *Phalen's maneuver*, a positive sign is indicated by instructing the patient to flex his or her wrist as far as possible causing numbness to occur within 60 seconds.

Treatment consists of avoiding poor posture and repetitive hand movements. Physical therapy might be required and NSAIDs can be administered to reduce inflammation. If the condition does not improve, surgical intervention might be needed to decompress the median nerve (see Figure 6-10).

6-8 PLANTAR FASCIITIS

Plantar fasciitis, also called a heel spur, is a condition of the bottom of the foot. More specifically, it deals with the plantar fascia, a ligament that goes from the heel to the toes and helps form the arch of our foot. When this connective tissue becomes strained from activities causing repeated pressure on the bottom of

Table 6-5 Summary of conditions for sprains, strains, and other pains

DISEASE/ CONDITION	ETIOLOGY	MAJOR SIGNS/ SYMPTOMS	DIAGNOSTIC TESTS	MAIN PHARMACOLOGIC TREATMENT
Sprain	Traumatic event	Pain	Physical exam	Analgesics
	Sports activity	Swelling Redness Warm Sensation	X-ray	NSAIDs
Strain	Overexertion Lifting	Pain Stiffness Swelling	Physical exam	Analgesic NSAIDs
Dislocation and subluxation	Associated with motor vehicle accidents, falls, and sports-related injuries	Pain Swelling Bone keeps popping out of place	Physical exam X-ray	Analgesic NSAIDs
Lower back pain (LBP)	Poor lifting Techniques Obesity Spinal diseases and deformities	Pain	X-ray MRI CT scans	Analgesics NSAIDs Muscle relaxants
Herniated nucleus pulposus (HNP)	Improper lifting Falls Car accidents	Radiating pain	MRI CT scan Myelogram	NSAIDs Ibuprofen (Advil, Motrin)
Bursitis	Repeated movement of a joint	Pain	Physical exam X-ray	Analgesics Corticosteroids NSAIDs
Tendonitis	Recurrent motion Calcium deposits	Pain Tenderness	Physical exam	Analgesics NSAIDs

the foot, such as running or walking long distances, small tears in the ligament cause pain and inflammation.

People who are obese or are pregnant are likely to encounter this condition. Those affected notice stiffness and pain in his or her feet in the morning or after sitting for extended periods of time. A diagnosis can be made after patient history, physical exam, and X-ray. Treatment involves rest, ice, and NSAIDs. Orthopedic pads can help decrease pressure on the feet.

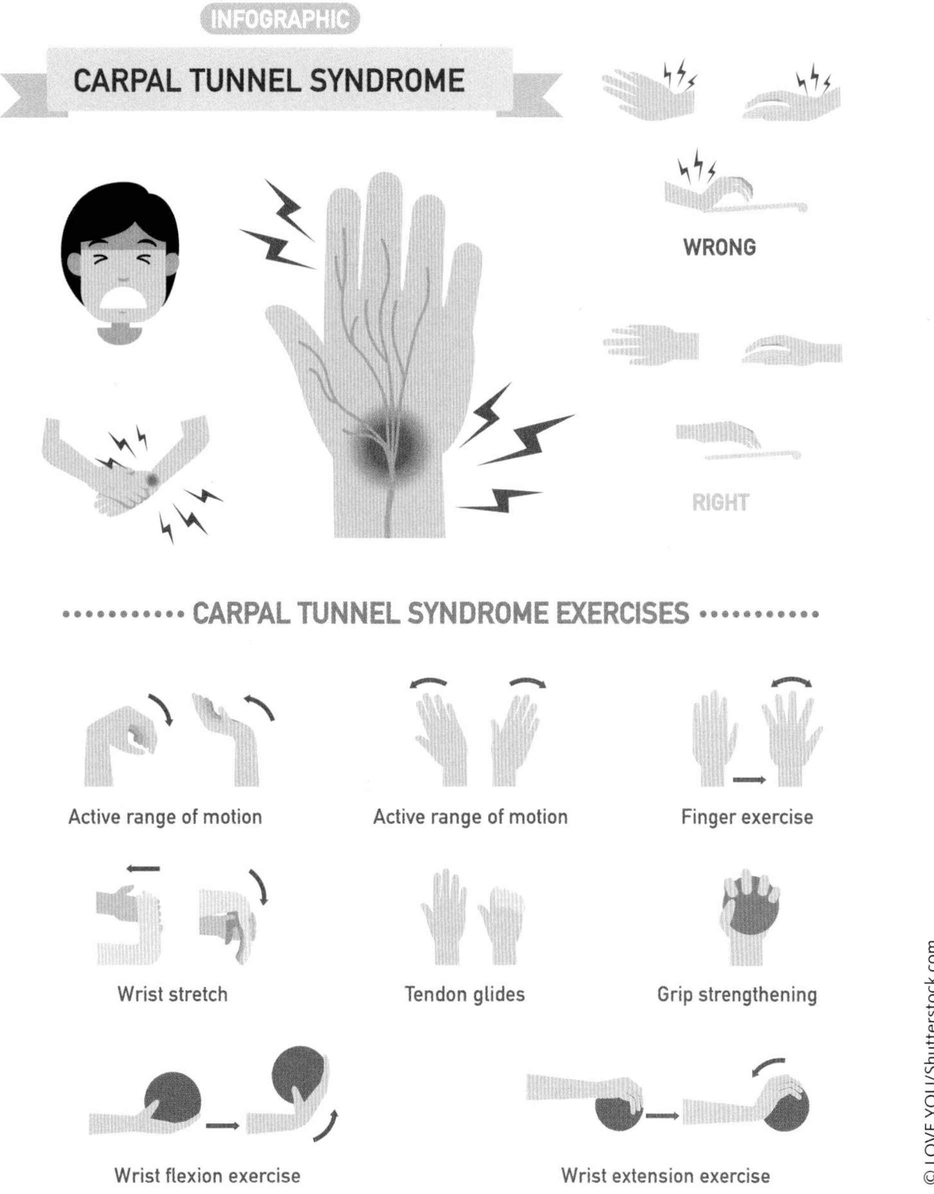

FIGURE 6-10 Carpal tunnel syndrome infographic.

After the pain is under control, usually with NSAIDs, the patient can do exercises to strengthen the feet and prevent a reoccurrence. Although corticosteroids could decrease inflammation, they are not likely to be used because they can lessen the strength of the fascia. If a severe heel spur develops, surgery might be required. To prevent this type of injury, it is recommended to wear shoes that support the arch of the foot and limit walking barefoot (see Figure 6-11).

6-9 TORN ROTATOR CUFF

In our shoulders, we have a collection of muscles that hold the head of the upper arm bone or humerus into the shoulder socket. A **torn rotator cuff** occurs when a tendon within this muscle group tears. The patient might notice

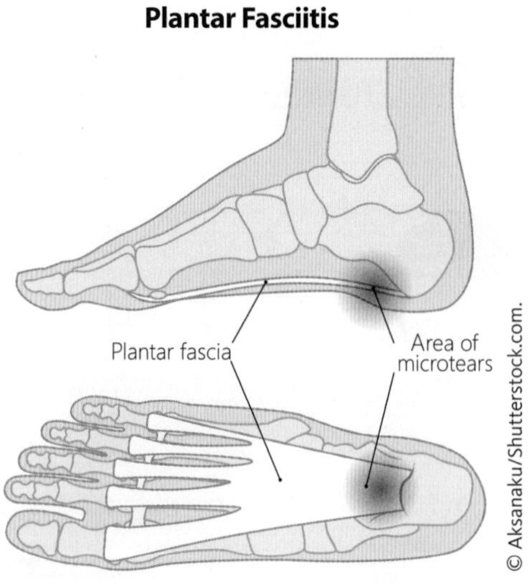

Plantar Fasciitis

Plantar fascia

Area of microtears

© Aksanaku/Shutterstock.com.

FIGURE 6-11 Illustration of plantar fasciitis.

a snapping sound, accompanied by sudden pain, and will find it difficult to raise (abduct) his or her arm. This condition is typically associated with sports-related injuries, such as baseball and tennis.

To confirm a diagnosis of a torn rotator cuff, a CT scan or arthroscopy (a long fiber optic scope inserted into the joint) can be performed. Medications such as anti-inflammatory and analgesics can be used to relieve pain and inflammation. Surgery is often needed to repair the damage, and the patient will be required to keep his or her shoulder immobilized for three to four weeks after the surgery. Physical therapy will be needed to regain strength and mobility. To prevent this type of injury from occurring, an individual should exercise regularly and strengthen this area along with flexibility exercises.

6-10 MENISCAL TEAR

The lateral (outside) and medial (inner) meniscus is cartilaginous, semi-lunar pads in the knees that are a cushion between the femur and the tibia bones. A **meniscal tear** injury happens when the knee is bent, and the leg moves suddenly. Symptoms associated are general stiffness and pain upon applying weight to the effected knee. Depending on the location of the tear, a feeling of looseness in the knee or locking may be felt. An MRI is needed to confirm the diagnosis and differentiate it from other injury.

Immediately after injury, the knee should be rested and elevated while applying ice. Surgery will be required to repair the tear, and physical therapy will be needed to regain mobility. Exercising on a regular basis can help prevent this type of injury. Analgesics and anti-inflammatory agents can be taken to alleviate pain (see Figure 6-12).

6-11 CRUCIATE LIGAMENT TEARS

Also located in the knee are cross-shaped ligaments, known as cruciate ligaments. We often hear about people injuring his or her ACL or PCL. If so, they injured one or both of these ligaments that work in conjunction with one another.

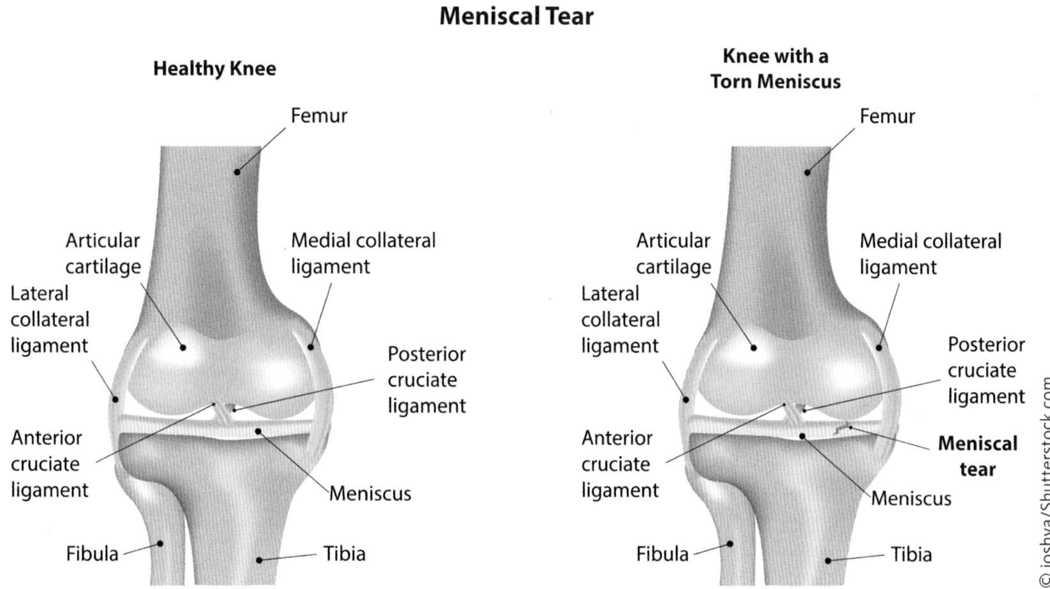

FIGURE 6-12 Healthy knee contrasted to a meniscal tear.

An ACL is the *anterior cruciate ligament*, while the PCL is the *posterior cruciate ligament*. Upon injuring one or both ligaments, a popping sound might be heard, accompanied by inflammation, pain, and knee instability. To diagnose **cruciate ligament tear**, the physician might order an MRI or CT scan following the physical exam.

Treatment types are dependent upon the severity of the injury. If severe, surgery will be required to repair the tear. However, an individual with a small tear might recuperate with rest and immobilization. Medications used for this injury are NSAIDs and anti-inflammatory agents. As with other preventative measures, the risk of ACL or PCL tears is minimized with regular physical exercise.

6-12 SHIN SPLINTS

Many injuries can be prevented by exercising; however, shin splints are primarily experienced after prolonged exercise, such as running. People who are not accustomed to exercising or who have suddenly increased activity level also might experience shin splints. Shin splints are not only caused by the amount of movement, but also the surface on which the individual is running. Shin splints are caused by running on hard surfaces, such as pavement, or overexertion of the lower portion of the leg. Those who are affected experience a sharp, aching pain in the inside region of the tibia. When resting, the pain goes away, but returns when the patient resumes exercising. A physician can conclude the condition is shin splints after taking the patient's history. An X-ray can be taken to ensure that the pain is because of shin splints and not a different condition, such as a fracture. Resting the legs with the application of ice and moist heat is helpful in decreasing the pain. Common types of medications used to treat are anti-inflammatory and pain medications.

See Table 6-6 for a summary of the conditions and medications in the wear and tear conditions discussed.

Table 6-6 Summary of additional wear and tear conditions

DISEASE/ CONDITION	ETIOLOGY	MAJOR SIGNS/ SYMPTOMS	DIAGNOSTIC TESTS	MAIN PHARMACOLOGIC TREATMENT
Carpal tunnel syndrome	Repeated/ strenuous use of hands	Pain Discomfort Poor gripping ability Numbness Weakness Burning and tingling sensations	Tinel sign Phalen's maneuver	NSAIDs
Plantar fasciitis	Activities causing repeated pressure on feet	Stiffness Pain in morning or after sitting for extended periods of time	Physical exam X-ray	NSAIDs Corticosteroids
Torn rotator cuff	Usually associated with sports-related injuries	Possible a snapping sound Sudden pain Difficulty raising the arm	CT scan Arthroscopy	Analgesics NSAIDs
Meniscal tear	Occurs when the knee is bent and the leg moves suddenly	Stiffness Pain Looseness or locking of knee	MRI Physical exam	NSAIDs Analgesics
Cruciate ligament tears	Often sports related	Popping sound Inflammation Pain Knee instability	MRI or CT scan Physical exam	NSAIDs
Shin splints	Prolonged exercise	Sharp, aching pain	X-ray Physical exam	NSAIDs Analgesics

LEARNING OBJECTIVE 6.3 Discuss the Pathopharmacology of the Bones.

KEY TERMS

Avulsion fracture Fracture causing a small bone fragment to separate from the bone where the tendon or ligament is attached.

Closed reduction Required when fracture does not require a surgery and needs only a cast to fixate the fracture.

Colles' and Pott's Fracture A fracture at the end of the radius of a bone, typically seen in wrist and ankle injuries.

Comminuted fracture Fracture in which the bone breaks into two halves with many bone fragments at the site of the break.

Complete fracture Fracture that goes completely through the bone.

Compression fracture Collapsing of the vertebrae in the spinal column.

Displaced fracture Bone fragments are not in the original correct position.

Extracapsular fracture Break that occurs in the outside of a joint capsule.

Femoral neck fracture Crack in the neck of the femur near the hip joint.

Greenstick fracture Classification of bone fracture in which one side of the bone breaks while the other side is bent, just as if it were a green tree limb.

Hairline fracture Very thin fracture line that resembles a strand of hair on an X-ray.

Impacted fracture Bone fracture that is forced into the end of another bone.

Incomplete fracture Break that does not completely separate the bone.

Intertrochanteric fracture Describes fractures in the trochanter of the femur.

Intracapsular fracture Fracture occurring inside a joint capsule.

Kyphosis Humpback curvature of the spine.

Longitudinal fracture Vertical crack that goes the length of a bone.

Lordosis Anteroposterior curvature of the lumbar of the spine.

Oblique fracture A transverse pattern of bone fracture.

Open fracture Classification of broken bones that protrude through the skin at the site of injury.

Open reduction Fracture requiring surgical correction such as the insertion of pins, screws, plates, and rods.

Osteomalacia Softening of the bones.

Osteomyelitis Inflammation of bone tissue caused from a bacterial infection.

Osteoporosis Condition causing gradual decrease in bone density, causing the bones to become porous.

Satellite fracture Cracks in bone that appear to be in a star-like pattern.

Scoliosis Condition where spine appears to be in an S-shape from the lateral or sideways curvature of the spine.

Simple fracture Classification of bone fracture that does not break the skin surface.

Spiral fracture Crack that twists around a bone.

Subcapital fracture Describes a break in the femur at the proximal end.

Transverse fracture Horizontal lines spanning across a bone at a 90-degree angle.

6-13 OSTEOPATHY (BONE DISEASE)

Before delving into the different types of bone diseases, we will discuss the many different types of fractures and how bone repairs itself after being damaged. Bone injury is often caused by trauma, but some diseases can cause our bones to deteriorate so that even minor bumps or sudden movements can cause breakage to fragile bones. Cancer and osteoporosis are two causes of bone deterioration.

6-13a Bone Fractures

A fracture (fx) is a crack or break in a bone. There are many different types of breaks, and clinically they are grouped in different categories to aid identification and treatment.

Broken bones that protrude through the skin at the site of injury are known as an **open fracture** or *compound fracture*. The reasoning behind its name is that not only has a bone broken, but the opening of the skin worsens the injury and risk of infection. When open fractures occur, medical attention must be sought immediately because of the greater risk of an infection, and the patient must undergo debridement (removal of dead or severely damaged tissue) to clean out the wound, which will require surgical intervention. If the skin is not broken; however, it is a **simple** or *closed fracture*, even though it might not feel like a simple break to your patient.

Another classification system helps to be more specific on the type of fracture. A **greenstick fracture** is named after, well, a green stick. A branch on a live (green) tree is hard to break, and often a piece will remain connected to the tree. This is how a greenstick fracture appears when looking at the patient's X-ray film. If the bone fracture goes completely through the bone, it is known as a **complete fracture**, but if the break does not completely separate the bone, it is called an **incomplete fracture**.

Other ways to describe a fracture is by the number or the position of the bone fragments. In a **displaced fracture**, the bone fragments are not in the original correct position. A **comminuted fracture** is when the bone breaks into two, but many bone fragments can been seen at the site of the break. Bone splinters often are embedded in the tissue surrounding the site of the break (see Figure 6-13). A **compression fracture** commonly involves the collapsing of the vertebrae in the spinal column. An **impacted fracture** is when the bone fracture is forced into the end of another bone. If a fracture causes a small bone fragment to separate from the bone where the tendon or ligament is attached, this is known as an **avulsion fracture**.

Tables 6-7 and 6-8 list other terms used to describe a specific type of fracture line and location.

6-13b Treatment of Bone Fractures

Treatment depends on the type of fracture. A patient will be in pain, and the muscles in the affected area might be tensed up. The patient might be given an analgesic or muscle relaxant to control the pain. The site of the injury must be immobilized by splinting the break to prevent further damage. Do not attempt to realign or push a bone back into place because that will cause more damage and pain.

Reduction of the fracture can begin after the patient is admitted for treatment. If the fracture does not require a surgery and needs only an external cast to fixate the fracture, it is called a **closed reduction**. If the injury requires surgical correction, such as the insertion of pins, screws, plates, and rods, it is an **open reduction** (Figure 6-14). After the fracture is reduced or set, traction is applied to the site of injury, to keep the fracture stable so it can properly heal.

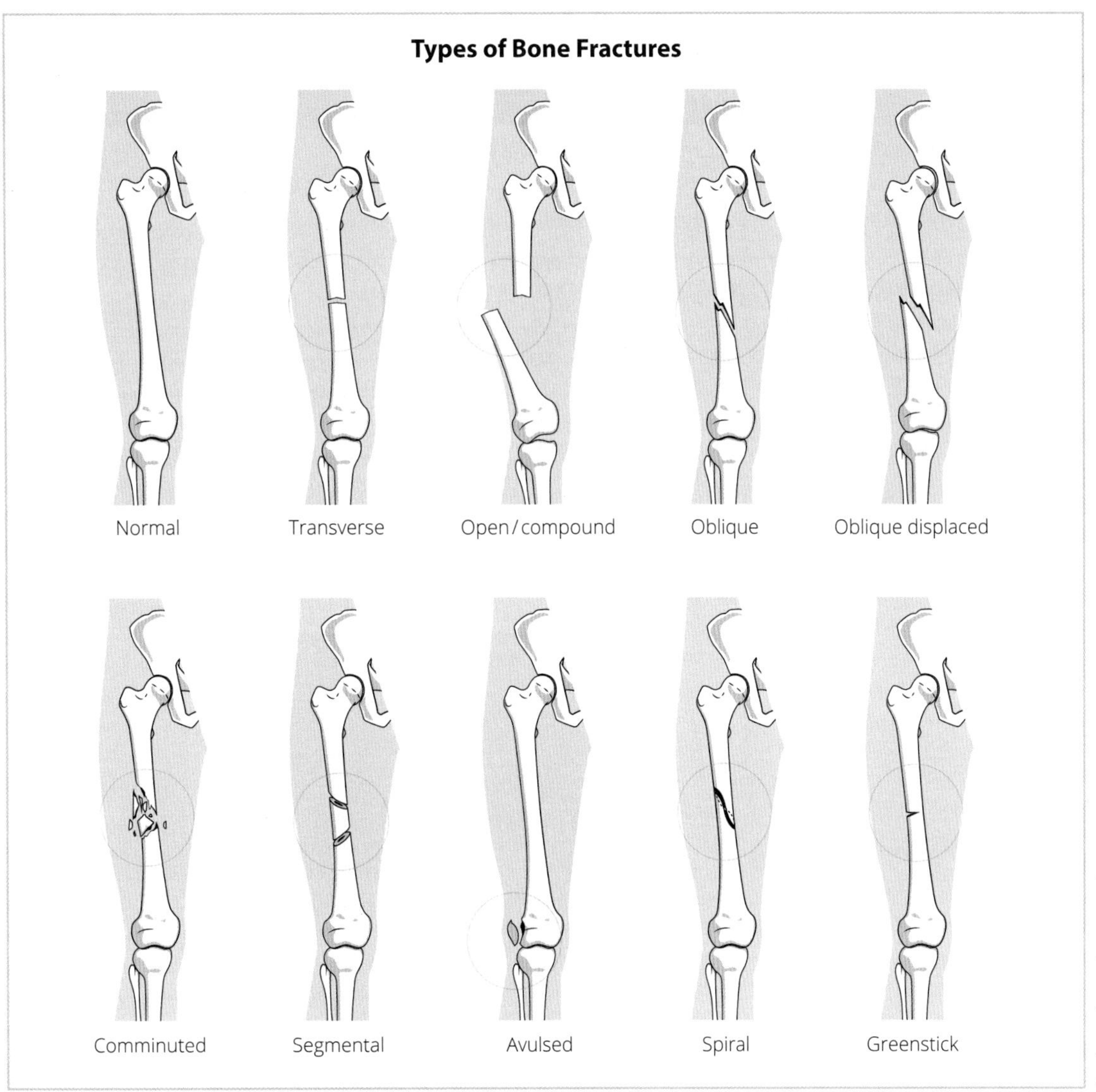

FIGURE 6-13 Commonly seen types of bone fractures.

Table 6-7 Types of fracture lines

FRACTURE	DEFINITION
Hairline fracture	Very thin fracture line that resembles a strand of hair on an X-ray.
Longitudinal fracture	Vertical cracks that goes the length of a bone.
Transverse fracture	Horizontal lines spanning across a bone at a 90-degree angle
Oblique fracture	A transverse pattern
Spiral fracture	A crack that twists around a bone
Satellite fracture	Cracks that appear in a star-like pattern

Table 6-8 Terms associated with fractures based on location

FRACTURE	DEFINITION
Intracapsular fracture	Occurs in the inside of a joint capsule
Extracapsular fracture	Occurs in the outside of a joint capsule
Intertrochanteric fracture	Occurs in the trochanter of the femur
Femoral neck fracture	Cracks in the neck of the femur
Subcapital fracture	Break in the femur at the proximal end
Colles' and Pott's fracture	At the end of the radius of a bone, typically seen in wrist and ankle injuries

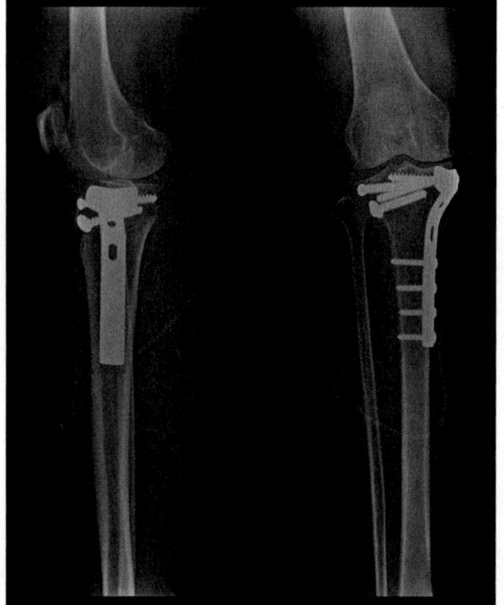

FIGURE 6-14 X-ray image taken at different angles of an open reduction internal fixation with plate and screws.

CLINICAL CONNECTION 6.1

Some patients will ask why his or her muscles are weaker or smaller after his or her cast is taken off than they were before the cast was put on. All muscles have a tone, known as tonus. Tonus occurs in the presence of resistance or stretching that causes muscles to contract partially. Since the cast was preventing the patient from using those muscles, they began to become flaccid or lose tone. Another term for this is atrophy (**a- = without, -trophy = growth.**) This tone will come back after the cast is removed, and the patient returns to normal function.

Just as with any procedure, complications can also occur with bone fractures. These include:

- Mal-union, which occurs when the bone heals in an abnormal position, possibly making it nonfunctional.
- Nonunion is when the bone does not heal back together.
- Avascular necrosis happens when there is an interruption in proper blood supply to the bone causing it to die.

6-13c Bone Repair

Bone repair is done in a series of steps that depend on the patient's age, overall health, severity of the fracture, and blood flow to the site of injury. All of these factors play a role in successfully healing and returning the bone back to as normal as possible. The steps of bone repair are presented in Table 6-9.

6-13d Osteoporosis

Osteoporosis is a bone disease that causes a gradual decrease in bone density, causing the bones to become porous with sponge-like holes (Figure 6-15). More often found in women, this slow, progressive disease is the most common bone disease seen globally. Factors that contribute to osteoporosis include:

- Age-related bone loss causes osteoporosis to occur in both men and women similarly
- Postmenopause bone loss because of:
  - Estrogen deficiency
  - Calcium deficiency

Signs and symptoms do not always readily present themselves. This condition is often silent and creeps up on the patient. However, there are signs that show that an individual has a lessened bone density. For example, an individual can become shorter in height because of compression fractures in the spine.

Table 6-9 Steps of bone repair

Step 1	Bleeding occurs at the site of injury that clots and begins to develop granulation tissue formation.
Step 2	The damaged tissue begins to proliferate, meaning that it begins to quickly produce new tissue cells that form a soft bone deposit at the site of the break.
Step 3	These new young cells become osteoblasts, which are bone cells, while other cells might become cartilage.
Step 4	Inorganic salts at the site of injury cause the new bone cells to strengthen and become hard.
Step 5	The bone is repaired to its previous shape and function.

This causes the abdomen and thoracic cavity to become smaller and restrict the amount of air the patient can get into his or her lungs, causing shortness of breath. Hip breakages show osteoporosis at a later stage.

Since other diseases, such as bone cancer, can cause bones to weaken and break, the physician has to be sure to diagnose the patient properly. This can be done through bone mineral density tests (BMD) and dual X-ray absorptiometry (DEXA), and blood and urine samples to look for any signs of bone metabolism. Another method used to diagnose is to measure the patient's bone thickness via a densitometry. If these tests are conclusive that the patient has osteoporosis, the patient can undergo treatment.

Even though osteoporosis cannot be reversed, its progression can be slowed by stopping smoking, eliminating or decreasing the amount of alcohol consumption, and decreasing caffeine intake. Another therapy, which is controversial because it increases the chances of cancer, is hormone therapy to increase estrogen levels in women. Taking vitamin D and calcium supplements also can help slow progression.

Medications used to prevent bone fractures from occurring in individuals affected by osteoporosis include Actonel, Boniva, Fosamax, and Reclast. These drugs belong to a classification called bisphosphonates. New bone is created by osteocytes to repair and replace old bone tissue removed by osteoclasts. A small amount of bone reabsorption is normal, but is balanced by bone building and bone reabsorption. While these medications can pull calcium out of the blood to help make new bone, this can lead to low calcium levels in the blood as a possible side-effect. With some bone diseases such as osteoporosis, the bone breaks down and degrades faster than it is being repaired. These drugs are used to prevent the normal reabsorption of bone so the bone building phase can win out (see Figure 6-15).

Since women are at higher risk of osteoporosis, prevention should begin by age 30. Eating a healthy diet, along with vitamin D and calcium supplements, and exercising regularly will help build strong bones and bone mass.

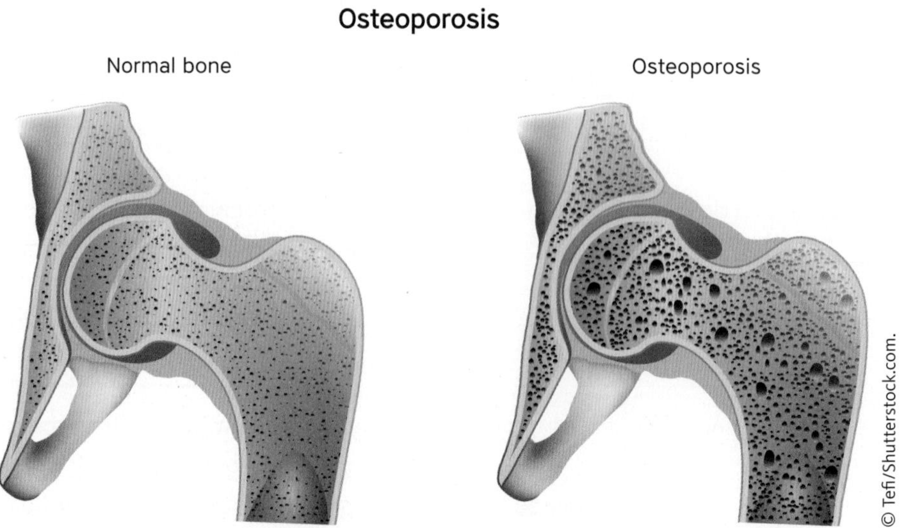

FIGURE 6-15 Image of the effects of osteoporosis on the bones.

6-13e Osteomyelitis

Osteomyelitis is an inflammation of the bone, typically in the legs and arms, which is caused by an infection by the bacteria *staphylococcus aureus*. This condition is categorized as either acute or chronic. There are many ways for this bacterium to enter the body. Staph can enter the blood by a wound on the skin or mucous membrane. After it is in the blood stream, it can infect bone since bone is vascularized.The most commonly affected patient demographic is young children, usually from a sore throat caused by a staph infection. Another way this bacteria can make its way to the bone is from a traumatic injury that would give the bacteria direct access to the bone.

This disease can have lifelong effects, such as stunting a child's bone growth plate, causing the bone to be shorter than the one on the other side of the body. Those infected exhibit a high fever from the infection, increased leukocytes or white blood cells in a response to fight infection, and bacteria in the blood known as bacteremia.

This condition can be diagnosed by obtaining specimen samples of blood, joint fluid, exudative fluid, or bone tissue and identifying the causative organism. After it is identified as a bacterial staph infection, antibiotic therapy should be started via IV. Examples of antibiotics used are Ceftriaxone, Fluoroquinolone, Ceftriaxone, and Vancomycin. If this condition is not treated promptly, it will become a chronic disease that will require medical attention throughout the rest of the patient's life.

Prevention involves performing wound care, especially to deep lacerations. Before undergoing any dentistry or surgical procedures, individuals should take antibiotics if they had a joint replaced or surgically implanted metal rods to prevent an infection from reaching bone tissue.

6-13f Osteomalacia

Osteomalacia means softening of the bones. The etiology, or reason for this disease, is that bones do not have enough vitamin D, which is vital in the absorption of key minerals, such as phosphorus and calcium. If the body does not have enough vitamin D, it will not be able to maintain strong and hard bones. This disease affects both children and adults; however, when a child has this condition, it is called rickets.

Symptoms of osteomalacia are bone pain, especially in the legs, pelvis, and spine. Weight-bearing bones often show a degree of deformity. For example, the legs and spine might appear bent in an abnormal fashion. This disease can even decrease the growth rate of bones, making them unable to function normally.

A patient will undergo a blood test to measure the level of vitamin D present for diagnosis. In addition, X-ray imaging can show cracks in the bone.

After a physician is sure the patient has osteomalacia, treatment is started with appropriate doses of vitamin D. The patient also should be encouraged to get a safe degree of sun exposure to allow the body to produce its own vitamin D. Foods high in vitamin D, including milk, cereal, eggs, and fish can be consumed to help the body reach a healthy level of vitamin D. Like any vitamin or drug, too much of a good thing also can be unhealthy; vitamin D is fat soluble and can build up to toxic levels in the body.

6-13g Spinal Deformities

Three of the more commonly found spinal deformities are **kyphosis**, **scoliosis**, and **lordosis**. Compare and contrast these conditions in Table 6-10.

Table 6-10 Types of spinal deformities

	KYPHOSIS	SCOLIOSIS	LORDOSIS
Definition	Causes a humpback curvature of the spine (see Figure 6-16)	Exaggerated posterior curvature of the spine. The spine appears to be in an "s" shape from the lateral or sideways curvature of the spine. Typically affects both genders, but females have a more severe spinal curvature.	Anteroposterior curvature of the lumbar of the spine, also called swayback.
Etiology	Can be caused by a congenital defect, cancer, or osteoporosis	Unknown	Pregnancy and obesity are most common causes.
Signs/ Symptoms	A visual exam can indicate abnormal spine curvature; however, no signs or symptoms might be present. Pain might occur as a result of spinal curvature. Shortness of breath and decrease in appetite from deformity causing a smaller sized abdominal thoracic cavity.	Appearance of a hump at the shoulder blade, as well as asymmetrical shoulder blades with one appearing lower or higher than the other, even an uneven waist can be seen. Pain might be felt as a result of this condition.	Patient's abdomen and buttocks stick out farther than normal, causing pain and discomfort.
Diagnosis	MRIs and X-rays can be used to determine if the condition is kyphosis and to determine the cause if it can be seen (i.e., tumor, infection)	Screen for deformity by having individual touch his or her toes while spine is checked for any curvature. This is done in grade school. Further imaging can be done with an X-ray or MRI.	The patient can lie on his or her back. If the person has lordosis, a larger than normal gap will be seen between the floor and the lumbar region of the spine. MRI and X-rays can be used to determine if the patient does have lordosis.
Treatment	In children, braces are used to prevent further deformity. In severe cases, a surgical procedure can be performed to place rods into the spinal column. If patient experiences pain, analgesics can be used.	Using braces to prevent further distortion of the spine has a better outcome if caught in the early stages. The braces are discontinued after bone growth stops. Surgery, in which the spine can be fused or metal rods can be installed into the spine, is a last resort. If patient experiences pain, analgesics can be used.	Braces are used in children, while severe cases might indicate a need for surgery. Patients are encouraged to lose weight if obese. If patient experiences pain, analgesics may be used.
Prevention	None	None	Maintain a healthy weight.

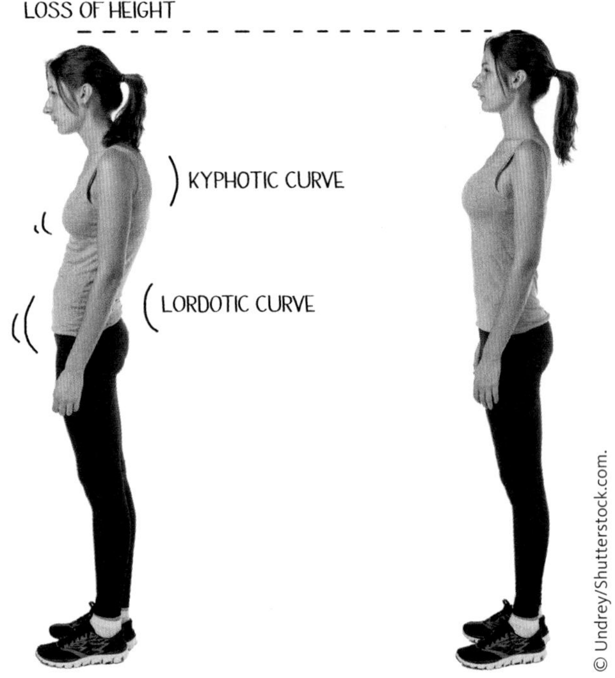

FIGURE 6-16 Visual differentiation between kyphosis and lordotic curvatures.

6-13h Summary of Diseases and Conditions of Bones

See Table 6-11 for a summary of the diseases and conditions of the bones.

Table 6-11 Summary of diseases and conditions of the bones

DISEASE/ CONDITION	ETIOLOGY	MAJOR SIGNS/ SYMPTOMS	DIAGNOSTIC TESTS	MAIN PHARMA-COLOGIC TREATMENT
Osteoporosis	Age-related bone loss, postmenopause, estrogen deficiency, calcium deficiency	Pain Decreased height Feeling of fullness	Bone mineral density tests (BDM), dual X-ray absorptiometry (DEXA), and blood and urine samples	Bisphosphonates: Actonel Boniva Fosamax Reclast
Osteomyelitis	Bacterial infection	Pain Fever	Sampling of blood, joint fluid, exudative fluid, or bone tissue X-ray, CT, and MRI imaging to check for any bone irregularities	IV antibacterial; Ceftriaxone, Fluoroquinolone, Ceftriaxone, and Vancomycin

(continued)

Table 6-11 Summary of diseases and conditions of the bones—*continued*

DISEASE/ CONDITION	ETIOLOGY	MAJOR SIGNS/ SYMPTOMS	DIAGNOSTIC TESTS	MAIN PHARMA-COLOGIC TREATMENT
Osteomalacia	Vitamin D deficiency	Pain Decrease in the growth rate of bones	Testing of blood samples X-ray	Vitamin D supplements
Kyphosis	Congenital defect, cancer, or osteoporosis	Pain	MRIs and X-rays	Analgesics
Scoliosis	Unknown	Pain	MRIs and X-rays	Analgesics
Lordosis	Pregnancy and Obesity	Pain	MRIs and X-rays	Analgesics

LEARNING OBJECTIVE 6.4 **Discuss the pathopharmacology of the joints.**

KEY TERMS

Arthritis Inflammation of a joint.

Gout Condition of build-up of uric acid in the blood causing pin like crystals to develop.

Osteoarthritis (OA) Degenerative joint disease.

Rheumatoid Arthritis (RA) Common autoimmune condition that is known to attack the lining of joints.

Systemic Lupus Erythematosus (SLE) Chronic autoimmune disease where the body mistakes tissue such as joints, kidneys, skin, and other organs as a foreign invader.

Temporomandibular Joint Dysfunction (TMJ or TMD) Inflamed disk-like joints in the jaw.

6-14 DISEASES OF THE JOINTS

We talked about joints earlier in the chapter, now we will look at some of the common diseases that can affect our joints. You might have a patient who was active until developing one of the joint conditions in this section. These conditions can take a toll on the body and make movement tough. What was once considered an easy everyday chore can become a daunting task with joint disease.

6-14a Arthritis

Arthritis is used in a few of the upcoming disease names, so let's make sure we understand what this term means. When breaking down the word, *arthro* means joint and *itis* means inflammation of. Another common name is rheumatism, which causes pain and stiffness. We will take a look into both of these terms and uses.

6-14b Osteoarthritis

Osteoarthritis (OA) is a degenerative joint disease and is associated with joints wearing out. All arthritic patients are not older people. An individual in his or her 20s can develop signs of arthritis. The exact cause of this condition is unknown, although certain factors can contribute to developing osteoarthritis. Risk factors include being a female, obese, participating in activities that cause increased wear on the joints, age, and family history.

Signs and symptoms of this disease include pain and inflammation. A person's fingers might have a crooked appearance. Other joints that are commonly affected are the knees and hips, because they are weight-bearing joints, accelerating the process in obese patients. The weight and pressure helps erodes the articular cartilage. As wear and tear continue, the cartilage eventually rubs away and eventually the actual bone will be affected. In response to the rubbing, the end of the bone becomes hardened. This bone-on-bone condition will not improve, and the joint must be completely replaced, known as total replacement surgery.

Treatment of osteoarthritis consists of medication such as anti-inflammatory agents and analgesics. If severe enough, the patient might benefit from steroid injections into the joint itself. The application of heat also can soothe the pain.

A patient history will be very helpful in diagnosing the patient. Imaging also can be done to see how advanced the condition is. It is best to avoid this situation altogether, which often can be done by exercising regularly and maintaining a healthy diet. Low-impact exercises, such as bicycling and swimming, are great choices to eliminate stress on joints.

6-14c Rheumatoid Arthritis

Affecting more women than men, **rheumatoid arthritis (RA)** is a common autoimmune condition that attacks the lining of our joints. Our joints produce synovial fluid so they can glide frictionless and without pain or discomfort. In this autoimmune disease, the body attacks the synovial fluid with antibodies, causing inflammation.

This chronic inflammatory disorder also affects other areas of the body besides just joints. For example, the heart, lungs, and other structures made of connective tissue, such as blood vessels and eyes, all can be affected. Therefore, this type of arthritis affects the entire body and the lives of younger individuals, not just senior citizens.

Symptoms of RA include swollen, tender joints, joint stiffness, weight loss, and fatigue. In the early stages, the patient's hands and feet are affected first (see Figure 6-17). Often, the joints that were attacked on one side of the body eventually will be affected on the other side. Currently, there is no cure for this condition. However, exercise and medications help to slow its debilitating progression.

Medications can be used to help the patient cope with the effects of the disease. NSAIDs are used to manage mild cases, while more severe cases require antirheumatic drugs known as disease-modifying antirheumatic drugs (DMARDs). Gold injections (that's right, gold) such as Myochrysine are given on a weekly to monthly basis and are more effective than the oral version, called

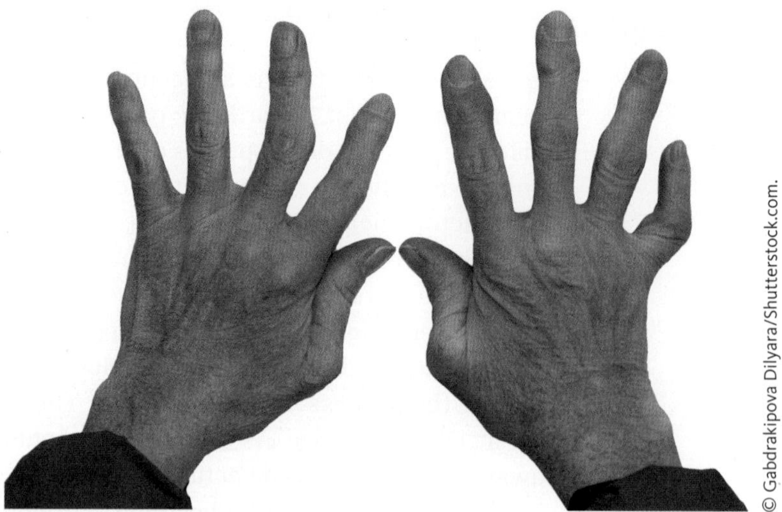

FIGURE 6-17 Hands affected by RA.

Ridaura. These drugs work by slowing the progression or even stopping the inflammatory process that damages the body's organs and joints. However, it might take a long time to notice any results from these drugs (weeks to months.) Steroids might calm exacerbations or flare-ups.

CLINICAL CONNECTION 6.2

Although gold helps decrease joint inflammation, like all drugs, there is a risk of side effects, and in this case they are very serious. This includes suppression of bone marrow, bleeding disorders, and kidney damage. Because of the high risk of serious side effects, this therapy is not widely used.

MRIs are used to track the progress of the disease over time. Blood tests can be taken to see if the body is producing excessive amounts of C-reactive protein, which would indicate that the body has an increased inflammatory process. Physical therapy helps maintain usage of joints by keeping them active.

6-14d Systemic Lupus Erythematosus

Another disease caused by the body attacking itself, particularly joints, is **systemic lupus erythematosus (SLE)**, a chronic autoimmune disease in which the body mistakes tissue such as joints, kidneys, skin, and other organs as an enemy. The body produces antibodies that try to destroy their tissue cells. This disease typically is seen in women more than in men.

While targeting people between 10 and 50 years of age, SLE can occur at any age and tends to be more prevalent in those of Asian and African-American decent. Symptoms vary, but typically, one experiences consistent episodes of exacerbation and remissions. Although this disease affects everyone differently, joint inflammation and pain are commonly found in almost all of those affected with SLE. Other symptoms include fatigue, weight loss, facial skin rashes shaped in a butterfly pattern, and even hair loss. This disease is more than just a nuisance. It is possibly a life-threatening condition. If SLE affects the kidneys, swelling, or edema, is seen in the patient's legs. When SLE attacks the kidneys, it causes inflammation of the region that filters fluids, known as the glomerulus. Eventually, the organ will waste away. If the brain is affected, there will be complaints of headaches, numb/tingly feeling, and vision or demeanor issues.

Diagnosing this disease is not easy. Many tests are used to help find a diagnosis. The most valuable test done to ensure a correct diagnosis is a positive antinuclear antibody test. Other tests are a CBC, urinalysis, CXR, and serum creatinine.

Although this disease might go into remission, it will crop up again. There is no cure, but medications can help alleviate exacerbations. NSAIDs and analgesics are used to decrease inflammation and pain symptoms, respectively. To treat a fever caused by the body's immune response, antipyretic agents can be administered. Corticosteroids are used to counteract an exacerbation that is life-threatening. No preventative measures can be taken to lessen the likelihood of developing SLE.

6-14e Gout

Gout is a form of arthritis, sometimes called gouty arthritis. It is not caused by the wear and tear of joints or autoimmune disease. Instead, it is caused by a build-up of uric acid in the blood. Usually, uric acid is removed from the body by the kidneys. However, if the kidneys are not functioning properly or if there is too much uric acid in the blood, it will all not be excreted by the kidneys. When this occurs, uric crystals develop in joints. Typically, the feet are affected, more particularly, the base of the big toe. Other joints, such as the ankles, knees, wrists, and hands also can be affected.

Gout crystals are like needles that cause tremendous pain and inflammation within the joint. A gout attack usually happens at night, causing the individual to awaken in pain. The joint feels as if it is burning and hot. Other symptoms are redness and tenderness. The afflicted toe might be so tender that even the slightest touch will cause extreme pain. Once an attack occurs, the most severe pain is felt within 4–12 hours, although discomfort in the joint can be felt for days or even weeks. To diagnose gout, a sample of fluid can be extracted from the irritated joint to check for the presence of uric crystals. The blood and urine also can be examined. Imaging such as an X-ray is also useful.

Foods such as beer and steak cause higher levels of uric acid in the blood. More men than women suffer from this condition, although women do have an increased risk of developing gout after menopause.

This condition is both treatable and preventable. First, corticosteroids will decrease inflammation of a joint and can be delivered in a pill or injection form. If injected, the steroid, such as prednisone, can be directly injected into the joint. NSAIDs such as naproxen (Aleve, Naprosyn) and ibuprofen (Motrin, Advil) are used to decrease inflammation and pain.Another drug used to treat gout is colchicine, which is a pain reliever.

Medications can prevent gout in two ways: blocking uric acid production and increasing the removal of the uric acid. Medications that prevent the production of uric acid are known as xanthine oxidase inhibitors. These drugs, which decrease the uric acid levels in the blood, include Uloric, Lopurin, Zyloprim, and Aloprim. Medications, such as Probalan, can improve the kidneys' ability to remove uric acid from the body.

6-14f Temporomandibular Joint Dysfunction

Our jaw has two joints that connect our mandible, or jaw bone, to our skull. Their disk-like joints can become inflamed for various reasons, such as grinding or clenching our teeth while sleeping or during stressful times in our life. **Temporomandibular joint dysfunction (TMJ or TMD)** can occur in both or only one joint. TMD is commonly seen in 20- to 40-year-old patients. Symptoms of TMD are jaw pain during movements, popping sounds, and locking open or closed. Other symptoms include headache, toothache, tinnitus (ringing in the ears), or pain in the shoulder, neck, or around the ear.

Imaging can be done to verify that TMJ is present. X-rays can be used to check the status of joints for inflammation. An MRI can see if the joint is in the correct position, while a CT scan will show the bone around the joint in detail. A physical examination can be used to check for popping or clicking sounds when the jaw is moving.

If the individual does have TMJ, treatment consists of NSAIDs for pain and inflammation, and muscle relaxants for a few days to relax tense jaw muscles. If the cause of gritting the teeth is stress related, the patient might benefit from anti-anxiety medication. Another drug class used to treat TMJ is tricyclic antidepressants for his or her pain relief effect by blocking neuroreceptors where the pain is triggered.

Preventative techniques are using a mouth guard while sleeping and consuming soft foods when the jaw is irritated.

Table 6-12 summarizes the pathopharmacology of joint disease.

Table 6-12 Summary of pathopharmacology of joint disease

DISEASE	ETIOLOGY	MAJOR SIGNS/ SYMPTOMS	DIAGNOSTIC TESTS	MAIN PHARMACOLOGIC TREATMENT
Osteoarthritis	Degenerative joint disease from wear and tear	Pain Inflammation Stiffness Crooked finger appearance	X-Ray MRI Physical examination	To treat this condition, anti-inflammatory agents and analgesics are used. If severe enough, the patient might benefit from steroid injections into the joint. The application of heat can also soothe pain.
Rheumatoid arthritis	Autoimmune disorder	Swollen Tenderness Stiffness Weight loss Fatigue	MRIs Blood sample	NSAIDs Antirheumatic drugs known as disease-modifying antirheumatic drugs (DMARDs) such as gold injections (Myochrysine) the oral version called (Ridaura) Corticosteroids

Table 6-12 Summary of pathopharmacology of joint disease—*continued*

DISEASE	ETIOLOGY	MAJOR SIGNS/ SYMPTOMS	DIAGNOSTIC TESTS	MAIN PHARMACOLOGIC TREATMENT
Systemic lupus erythematosus	Chronic autoimmune disease	Joint inflammation and pain Fatigue Weight loss Facial rash Hair loss Weight gain Edema Inflammation of glomerulus Headaches Numb/tingly feeling Vision Change in demeanor	Antinuclear antibody test CBC Urinalysis CXR Serum creatinine	NSAIDs Analgesics Antipyretic agents Corticosteroids
Gout	Build-up of uric acid in the blood	Pain Inflammation Redness Tenderness Warmth	Sample fluid in joint Blood testing Urinalysis X-ray	Corticosteroids NSAIDs Xantrine oxidose inhibitors
Temporomandibular joint syndrome (TMJ or TMD)	Injury Grinding or clenching the teeth	Popping sounds and locking open or closed Headache Toothache Tinnitus Pain in the shoulder, neck, or around the ear	X-rays MRI CT scan Physical examination	NSAIDs Muscle relaxants Antianxiety meds Tricyclic antidepressants

LEARNING OBJECTIVE 6.5 Explain normal neuromuscular transmission.

KEY TERMS

Acetylcholine (ACh) A chemical neurotransmitter found in both parasympathetic and sympathetic nervous system at the preganglionic sites and only the postganglionic sites of the parasympathetic nervous system.

Acetylcholinesterase (AChe) Deactivates acetylcholine.

Astrocytes Cells that keep blood vessels and neurons close together.

Autonomic system Controls functions automatically.

Axon Long fiber-like structure of a nerve cell stemming from the cell body.

Axon terminal The end of an axon.

Central nervous system Consists of the brain and spinal cord.

Dendrites Branch-like structures that receive information from other nerve cells or environments and transmits the signals to the body.

Ependymal cells Nerve support cells that act as epithelial cells by covering the surfaces of cavities.

Microglia Neural support cells that attack microbes and remove any debris.

Myelin sheath Soft, fatty, white covering for certain nerve fibers or axons.

Neuroglia Cells that support and protect structures in the nervous system.

Neurons Nerve cell that transmits impulses.

Oligodendrocytes Cells that hold nerve fibers together and also make up the fatty or lipid covering known as myelin.

Peripheral nervous system All of the nerves outside of the brain and spinal cord.

Somatic system Controls voluntary muscles.

Synapse The gap or space between the axon terminal and another cell.

6-15 COMPONENTS OF THE NERVOUS SYSTEM

Before diving into the micro components of the central nervous system, let's take a look at the primary structure of the central nervous system to understand better how it functions.

The nervous system is made up of two parts, the **central nervous system (CNS)** and the **peripheral nervous system (PNS)**. The central nervous system consists of the brain and spinal cord, while the peripheral nervous system is composed of all the nerves outside of the brain and spinal cord. The CNS will be discussed in the Nervous System chapter; we will focus on the PNS because this is where the neuromuscular connection comes into play.

The PNS has two systems, the **somatic system**, and the **autonomic system**. The somatic system controls voluntary (skeletal) muscles. We have to be consciously aware of telling these muscles to move. The autonomic system resembles another word you should be familiar with, automatic. This branch moves on its own without conscious effort. Therefore, you don't have to think about moving cardiac and smooth muscles, as well as glands.

The autonomic controls two more branches: the parasympathetic and the sympathetic systems. The parasympathetic branch maintains the daily maintenance of your body or our homeostasis (our body's normal state), which was discussed in Chapter 1. This branch controls our resting and digesting.

The sympathetic branch comes into play in times of danger or stress, controlling our fight or flight mechanism. It is the body's alert system that protects us from danger. See Figure 6-18 for a visual breakdown of this system.

6-15a Nerves

Now that we covered the main components of the nervous system, we will take a look at its tissues and see how signals are transmitted throughout our nervous system. The nerve cells or **neurons** are excitable cells that carry out all signals of the nervous system and transmit from one cell to another by an electric

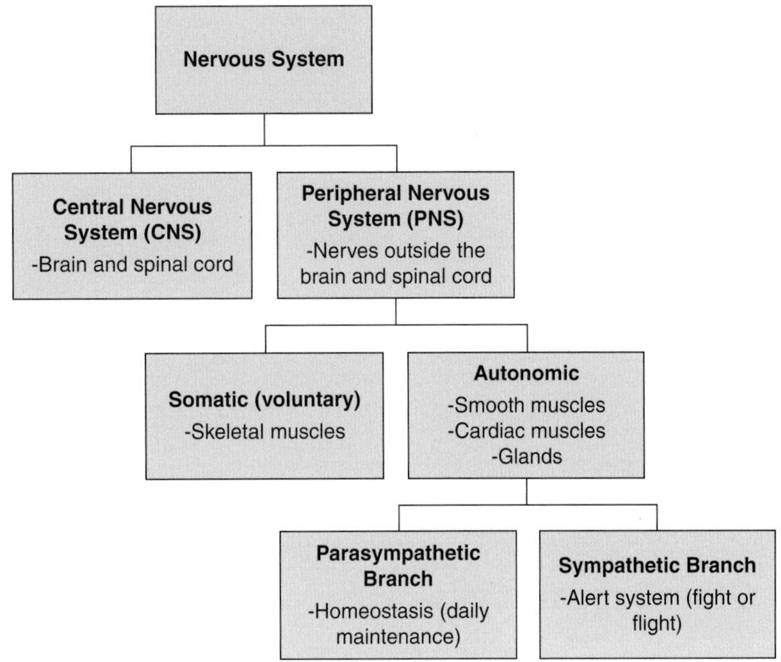

FIGURE 6-18 Main components of the CNS.

charge and a neurotransmitter chemical. The appearance of the cells is quite unusual, consisting of a head (cell body) and tail (axon) and many protruding branches (see Figure 6-19).

The cell body of the neuron maintains functionality by way of cell metabolism. Attached to the cell body are branch-like structures called **dendrites**, which receive information from other cells or environments.

Stemming from the cell body is a long fiber-like structure called an **axon**. Signals are picked up from the cell body and transmitted down the axon to the **axon terminal** (the end of the axon), which is located next to cells of other nerves or glands or even muscle. The axon terminal does not physically connect to the next junction but is in very close proximity. This microgap or space between the axon terminal and another cell is called a **synapse**. If the terminal axon is sending a signal to a muscle cell, it is called a neuromuscular synapse or neuromuscular junction, Figure 6-20.

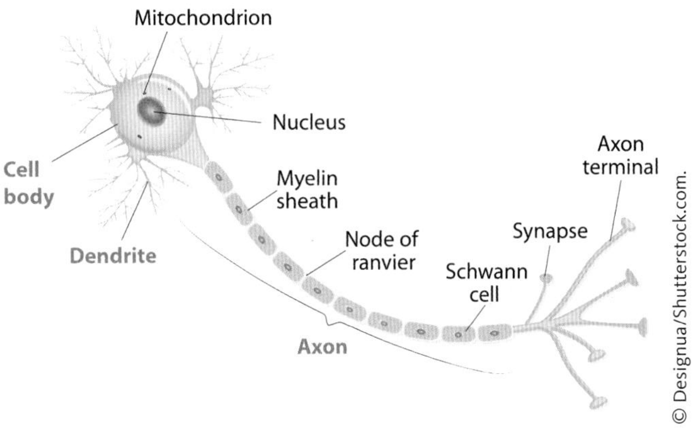

FIGURE 6-19 Anatomy of a neuron.

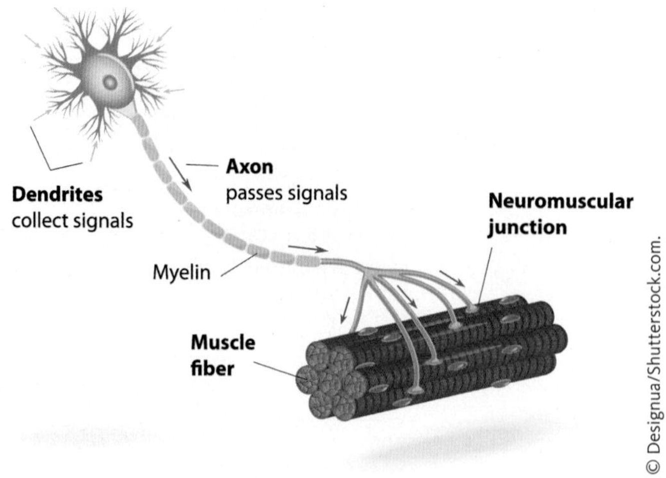

FIGURE 6-20 Neuromuscular junction.

6-15b Other Support Cells

Another component of neuron tissue is the **neuroglia**, which does not send signals, but instead supports and protects structures in the nervous system. In fact, *glia* means glue, and you can think of these support cells as the glue that holds the neural tissue together. There are four types of cells in the CNS (brain and spinal cord):

1. **Astrocytes** Cells that keep blood vessels and neurons close together. The cells comprise part of the blood–brain barrier, and provide metabolic support, energy, and function.
2. **Ependymal cells** Act as epithelial cells by covering the surfaces of cavities within the CNS.
3. **Microglia** Attack microbes and remove any debris from the CNS.
4. **Oligodendrocytes** Cells that hold nerve fibers together and also make up the fatty or lipid covering known as myelin. The myelin insulation or covering surrounds the outside of nerve fibers. This **myelin sheath** is a fatty, white covering for certain nerve fibers or axons. The myelin sheath is needed to increase the speed of impulses through the nerve fiber (axon). Think of an insulated electric wire in your home. If the insulation is torn, the wire will short out as the electricity escapes through the damaged area and does not continue through the length of the wire. You will see this mentioned in disease states shortly.

In the PNS, there are two types of glial cells:

1. Satellite or support cells.
2. Schwann cells that make myelin insulation for the PNS.

6-15c Impulse Conduction

A neuron is a special cell that transmits nerve impulses to other neurons, glands, and muscles. Special electrical and chemical functions must occur for any communication to be made. Let's say an electrical signal has traveled down an axon

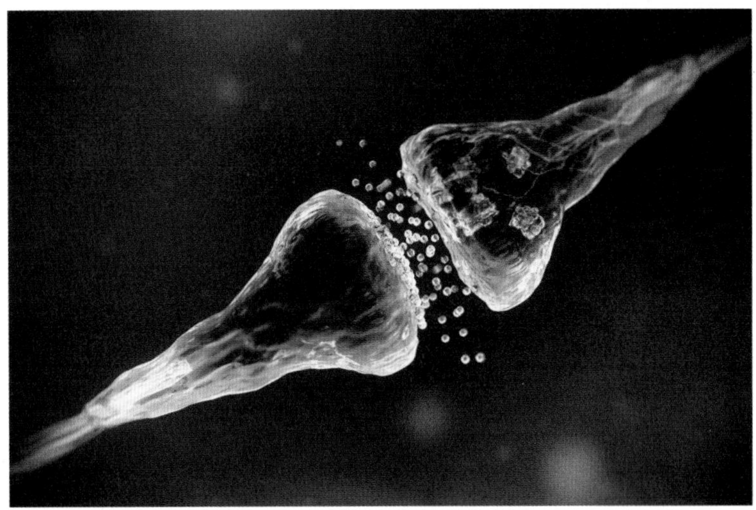

© adike/Shutterstock.com.

FIGURE 6-21 Neuron cells sending chemical signals across the synapse.

to the terminal axon. The signal cannot just make the jump to the receptor sites of the cell on the other side of the synapse (gap.) Instead, for neurotransmission to continue a neurotransmitter chemical must be released to send the signal to the next neuron, or onto the gland or muscle.

The neuron where the signal originates is called the presynaptic (before the gap) neuron. The signal now needs to travel from the presynaptic neuron to the postsynaptic (after the gap) neuron. When the electrical signal reaches the terminal end, vesicles located inside the presynaptic neuron release a neurotransmitter chemical, which travels across the gap and stimulates the receptors in the postsynaptic neuron to pass it on (see Figure 6-21). The neurotransmitter substance varies according to the area of the nervous system, but in most areas is acetylcholine (ACh).

Let's talk about the specific portion of the somatic nervous system that deals with muscular movement. A signal is sent from the CNS through a motor axon to a certain muscle to contract. The signal is received by the cell body and then sent through the motor axon via electrical transmission. At the terminal axon, vesicles release ACh to travel across the neuromuscular junction to reach receptors on the muscle and cause contraction. After all of this occurs, it is time for the neurotransmitter to be cleaned up or the muscle would remain in that state of contraction. Acetylcholine now must be broken down by an enzyme called acetylcholinesterase (AChe). You will soon see how important these chemical are in neuromuscular disease.

LEARNING OBJECTIVE 6.6 Discuss the pathopharmacology of neuromuscular diseases.

KEY-TERMS

Guillain-Barre A disease of an unknown etiology causing paralysis which progresses from the outer most extremities to the face.

Muscular Dystrophy (MD) Disease caused by a defective gene resulting in the degeneration of the affected tissue.

Myasthenia Gravis Autoimmune disorder causing muscle weakness, beginning at the patient's face to the outermost extremities.

Plasmapheresis Procedure used to remove antibodies from the patient's bloodstream.

Tetanus Also known as lockjaw; life-threatening condition caused by *Clostridium tetani* bacteria.

6-16 DISEASES OF THE NEUROMUSCULAR SYSTEM

Let's use the basic knowledge of our neuromuscular system and how our body sends signals throughout our nervous system to understand common neuromuscular disease processes. As with other bodily systems, our neuromuscular system can also fall victim to disease that range from acute and chronic.

6-16a Muscular Dystrophy

Muscular dystrophy (MD) is caused by a defective gene among the genes used to protect muscle fibers from damage, resulting in the degeneration of the affected tissue shown in Figure 6-22. It can occur at any age. There are different forms of this disease, each caused by a genetic mutation. Some people might not be affected by the illness, but might be a carrier of the mutated gene, which then might be passed on to their offspring. We will focus on Duchenne's muscular dystrophy, which affects nearly half of those affected by MD. This disease is seen in 2- to 3-year-olds, affects more boys than girls, and eventually leads to lower limb paralysis.

MD affects the somatic or voluntary muscles of the body. Typically, the legs and pelvic muscles are affected first, causing symptoms of pain, stiffness, and the appearance of large calf muscles from fat deposits. Pain is more of a secondary condition to muscle weakness caused by muscle straining.

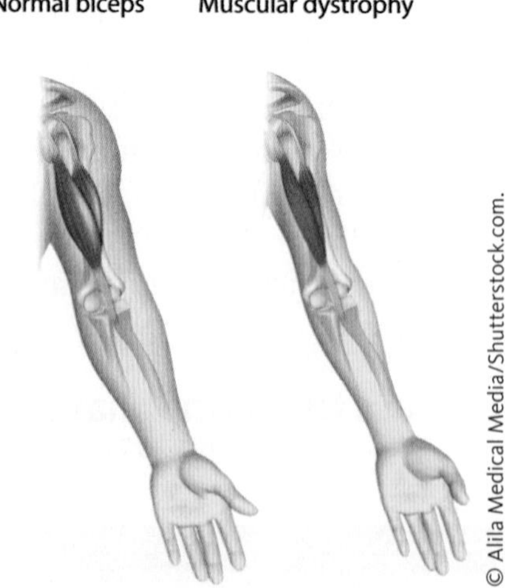

FIGURE 6-22 Normal biceps muscle contrasted to muscular dystrophy.

The patient's cognitive abilities also are affected, causing learning difficulties. The individual might appear to walk on their tip toes or waddle. Those affected are known to have difficulty standing up after lying down. Eventually, the disease leads to the child being forced to use a wheelchair by age 9 and likely dying in his or her 20s, usually because of cardiac or respiratory failure. A diagnosis is confirmed through a physical examination of the patient, muscle biopsy, and electromyography.

There is no cure for Duchenne's muscular dystrophy, but managing the disease prolongs mobility as long as possible, providing a better quality of life. Management is done through exercising and wearing braces to give the patient stability, while analgesics are given to control pain. Eventually, a wheelchair will be required. Unfortunately, there is no preventative action for this disease.

6-16b Tetanus

When you were a kid you might have been told to stay away from rusty nails or you might need a tetanus shot. It is not the rusty nail that causes the infection, but a bacteria that could be found on a rusty nail or anything else, for that matter. The bacteria is known as *Clostridium tetani* and is often found in dirt or even in the GI tract of animals. The nail is only a vehicle for spores from the bacteria to enter your body. The spores have been known to survive in the dirt and remain infectious for up to 40 years. After these spores enter an open wound, they turn into an active bacteria that produces a poisonous toxin that interferes with the signaling between the brain and spinal cord causing muscle contraction.

Tetanus, or lockjaw, is a life-threatening condition that can cause respiratory failure by paralyzing muscles needed to breathe. Symptoms include muscle spasms in the jaw, neck, back (causing aching), chest, abdominal muscles, and even the arms and legs. Other symptoms are fever, drooling, dysphasia, and tachycardia. If the individual survives, the disease will run its course within 6–8 weeks. Studies have concluded that the patient will not have any permanent disability, nor will the person have built up an immunity to another exposure.

Currently, no laboratory studies can diagnose this condition. Instead, physicians rely on a history and physical examination and bedside tests, such as the spatula test. The spatula test involves using a tool to touch the back of the throat. If the patient gags, it is a negative indication for tetanus (see Figure 6-23). However, if the patient has no gag reflex and instead bites down on the tool in response to the stimuli, then it is a positive sign for tetanus.

Supportive treatment, such as mechanical ventilation if the patient is not breathing on his or her own, is carried out until the toxins are resolved. Treatment includes cleaning out the wound and providing muscle relaxants and antibiotics. A tetanus shot is given every 10 years to prevent bacteria from progressing to the infectious stage into the body.

6-16c Myasthenia Gravis

Myasthenia Gravis is an autoimmune disorder that causes muscle weakness, beginning in the face and then down to the outermost extremities, such as the legs and feet (descending paralysis). What makes this disease so deadly

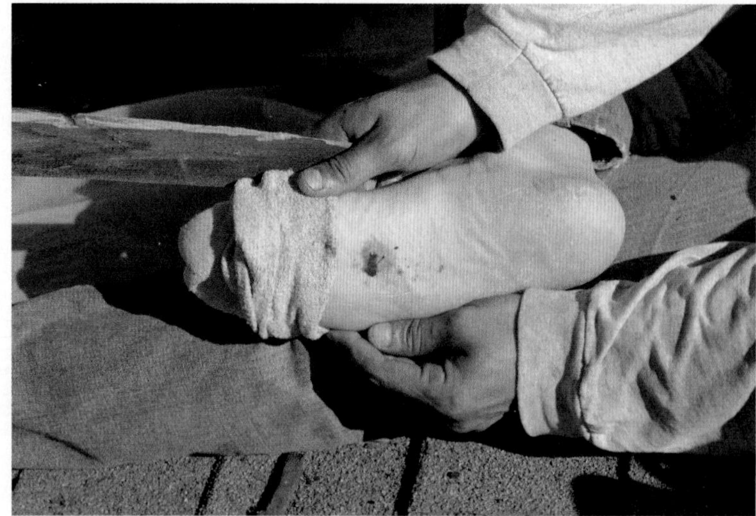

FIGURE 6-23 Puncture wound as a result of stepping on a nail at a construction site.

is the likelihood of respiratory failure. The condition interferes with the transmission of the nerve signals to the muscle at the neuromuscular junction. The muscles are unable to receive a signal from the neurotransmitter, *acetylcholine (Ach)*, because of the muscle receptors being attacked by antibodies. (see Figure 6-24).

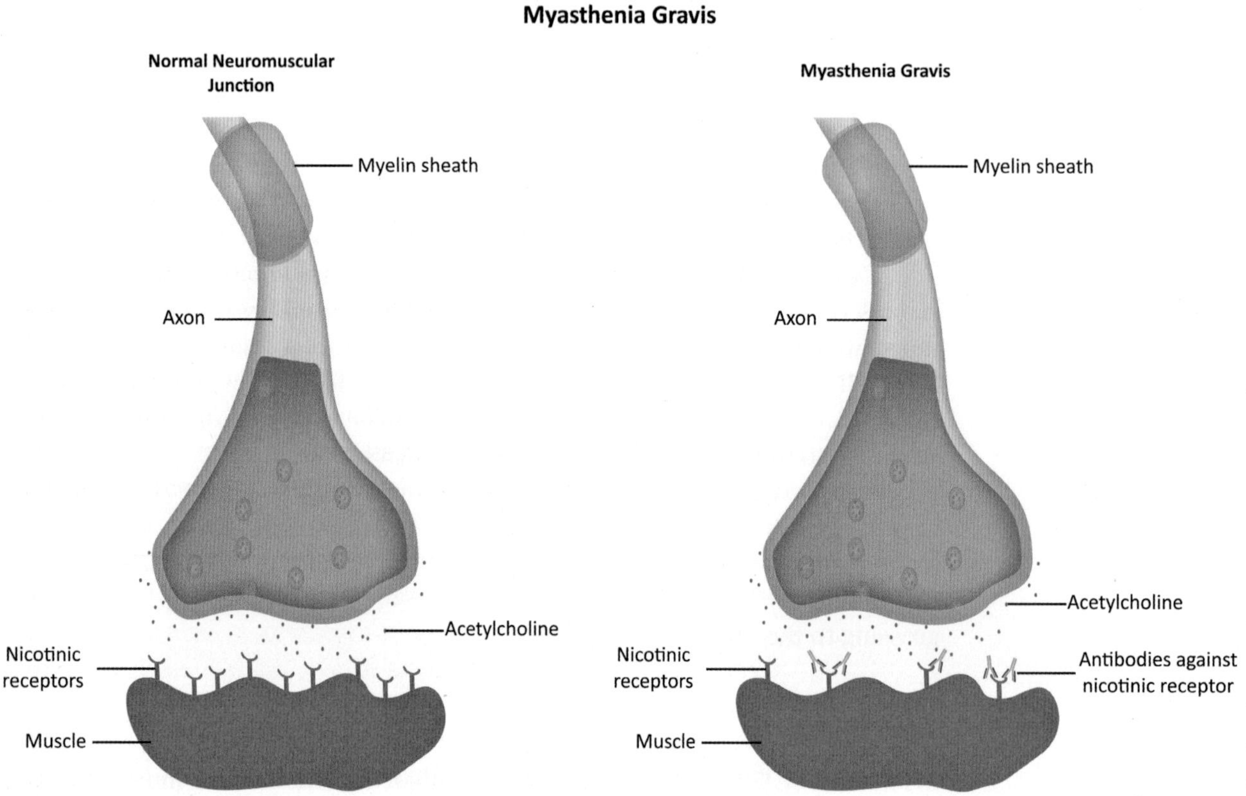

Myasthenia Gravis

Normal Neuromuscular Junction

Myelin sheath
Axon
Acetylcholine
Nicotinic receptors
Muscle

Myasthenia Gravis

Myelin sheath
Axon
Acetylcholine
Nicotinic receptors
Antibodies against nicotinic receptor
Muscle

FIGURE 6-24 An illustration showing the difference between a normal neuromuscular junction and one affected by myasthenia gravis.

This causes muscles to become weak and lessens their ability to contract. Symptoms caused by this disease have a slow onset. The first area to be affected are the facial muscles. Noticeable affects are drooping eyelids (pytosis), double vision (diplopia), difficulty swallowing (dysphagia), and problems speaking (dysphonia). Eventually, the patient will experience muscle fatigue in all voluntary muscles as the descending paralysis progresses. Those affected are also known to experience episodes of exacerbations and remissions.

A diagnosis can be reached by a physical exam and blood testing to check for antibody levels that are fighting against acetylcholine receptors.Other tests are electromyography to test muscle fatigue as well as spirometry to monitor respiratory muscle function.

Several approaches are used to prevent the breakdown of the neurotransmitter acetylcholine, with all having the goal to increase Ach at the receptor sites to allow for normal contraction and muscle tone.Cholinergic medications such as Mytelase stimulate acetylcholine production and allow it to build up in the body. Acetylcholinesterase (AChE) inhibitor medications such as Pyridostigmine allow acetylcholine to build up in the body indirectly, by stopping the substance that is breaking acetylcholine down.

Another drug class used is immunosuppressive drugs or corticosteroids to decrease the effectiveness of the patient's immune system to slow the autoimmune destructive response. Another treatment method is to remove the antibodies causing the autoimmune response from the blood. This is done by a procedure called a plasmapheresis. However, if the disease has progressed enough to paralyze respiratory muscles, mechanical ventilation will be required to sustain life until the patient can maintain their own breathing. Unfortunately, it is not possible to prevent this disease from occurring.

6-16d Guillain-Barre

Guillain-Barre is a progressive disease with a rapid onset. There are different types, based on how it affects the nervous system. Although it has an unknown origin, it is thought to be an autoimmune disease since antibodies attack support cells of the peripheral nervous system, causing demyelination, or the stripping of the insulation around cells in the nervous system, inhibiting muscle movement. This condition is known to occur within 10–21 days after a fever-producing illness, such as a respiratory infection. Symptoms associated with Guillain-Barre are fever, discomfort, nausea, paresthesia, muscle weakness, and eventual paralysis. Numbness and pain are also contributing symptoms. Usually, Guillain-Barre begins in the legs and works its way up to the upper body, making it an ascending paralysis. To remember this, think about the name *G*uillain-*B*arre and *g*round to *b*rain.

That being said, this disease can last days, even weeks, while a full recovery can take up to a year or so. What makes this disease so deadly is its effects on the respiratory system by causing paralysis of respiratory muscles, mainly the diaphragm, which is the main muscle of ventilation.

It is important to understand the methods used to diagnose Guillain-Barre. Diagnosing a patient can be done in many different ways.

- Physical examination
- Testing antibody levels

- Obtaining a blood sample
- Cerebral spinal fluid sample
- Electromyography.

Treatment for Guillain-Barre includes **plasmapheresis** to remove antibodies from the patient's bloodstream. Mechanical ventilation will be needed to ventilate the patient if the disease process has diminished the ability for the patient to breathe on their own. To control pain, analgesics can be given and rehabilitation is required to regain speech and muscle loss.

6-16e Summary of Neuromuscular Pathopharmacology

Table 6-13 summarizes conditions and diseases of the neuromuscular system.

Table 6-13 Summary of conditions and diseases of the neuromuscular system

DISEASE	ETIOLOGY	MAJOR SIGNS/ SYMPTOMS	DIAGNOSTIC TESTS	MAIN PHARMACOLOGIC TREATMENT
Muscular dystrophy	Genetic	Pain, stiffness, appearance of large calf muscles, learning difficulties, walking on tip toes, waddling, and difficulty standing up	Physical examination Muscle biopsy Electromyography	Analgesics
Tetanus	Bacteria	Fever, drooling, dysphasia, tachycardia, muscle spasms in jaw, neck, back, chest, abdominals, arms, and legs.	History, physical exam, and spatula test	Muscle relaxants, antibiotics, and tetanus vaccination
Myasthenia gravis	Autoimmune disorder	Ptosis, diplopia, dysphagia, dysphonia, and respiratory distress	Physical exam, blood samples, electromyography, and spirometry	Cholinergic drugs such as (Mytelase) are used to mimic acetylcholine and acetylcholinesterase (AChE) inhibitors (Pyridostigmine) block acetylcholinesterase from breaking down acetylcholine. Immunosuppressive agents (azathioprine) or corticosteroids might be given to decrease the body's immune response.
Guillain-Barre	Unknown, possibly autoimmune	Fever, discomfort, paresthesia, muscle weakness, numbness, pain, paralysis, and respiratory distress	History and physical exam; Blood samples, cerebral spinal fluid sample, electromyography, spirometry	Analgesics Antipyretics (for fever)

Module 7

Pathopharmacology of the Integumentary System

Module Introduction

Covering about 20.83 square feet, your skin is the major part of the **integumentary system** (from the Latin word *tegere*, meaning to cover) that covers your entire body. It is interesting to note that your skin is actually the body's largest organ, weighing about 20 pounds for an average adult. While skin is the largest component of the integumentary system, other accessory organs make up our outer covering. Other main parts of the integumentary system include:

- Hair, formed from compressed cells that arise from the hair follicle
- Nails, located on the dorsal surface of the ends of your fingers and toes
- Sweat glands, tiny coiled, tubular structures that secrete sweat through the pores on the surface of your skin
- Sebaceous glands, secrete oil (called *sebum*) into the hair follicles.

A doctor who specializes in the care, diagnosis and treatment of the skin and its related conditions is a **dermatologist**. (*Dermat/o* is one of the main word roots for skin.) This individual has spent many years studying the skin (**dermatology**) and its related structures.

Interestingly, although your skin can develop conditions related directly to a skin problem, as you will learn in this chapter, skin conditions often are a result of diseases from other parts of your body.

LEARNING OBJECTIVE 7.1 Explain the normal anatomy and physiology of the integumentary system.

KEY TERMS

Acrocyanosis Bluish hue in the outer skin because of lack of oxygen, combined with hemoglobin in the peripheral area or extremities.

Albinism Condition of lacking melanin that leads to loss of skin color resulting in very white skin and hair.

Alopecia Condition of balding.

Anhidrosis Condition of decreased or lack of ability to sweat.

Apocrine sweat glands Glands found in the groin and anal regions that become active around puberty.

Arrector pili muscles Muscles that allow the hair to stand erect for thermoregulation of our body and in times of fright.

Carotene Skin pigment that gives a normal yellowish hue to the skin.

Cyanosis Bluish hue in the outer skin because of lack of oxygen combined with hemoglobin.

Dermatologist Medical doctor who specializes in the treatment of skin conditions and diseases.

Dermatology Study of skin and its related structures.

Dermis Considered the true skin containing nerve, blood vessels, elastic fibers, hair follicles and glands; lies below the epidermis.

Eccrine glands Sweat glands located over the body to allow perspiration and cool the body by evaporation to aid in temperature regulation.

Epidermis Outermost, visible layer of skin.

Fibroblasts Cells that produce connective fiber.

Freckles Concentrated patches of melanin on the skin.

Hair shaft Visible portion of hair on the epidermal layer.

Hypodermal layer Also known as the subcutaneous layer; innermost layer of skin that is composed of elastic and fibrous connective tissue and fatty tissue.

Jaundice Skin that has a deeper yellow or orangish coloration because of the build-up of bilirubin; often found with liver disease.

Integumentary system Composed of skin and other accessory organs that make up our outer covering. Other main parts of the integumentary system are hair, nails, sweat glands, and sebaceous glands.

Keratin Protein that hardens cells and forms hair and nails.

Lipocytes Cells that produce fat needed to provide padding to protect the deeper tissues of the body and act as energy storage.

Lunula White, half-moon shaped area at the base of the nail.

Melanin Dark pigment produced by melanocytes that provides for skin color.

Melanocytes Specialized cells located deep in the epidermal layers responsible for our skin color.

Nail root Part of epidermis where specialized cells that form the nail are located.

Peripheral perfusion Amount of blood reaching the furthest extremities.

Peripheral vascular disease (PVD) Disease that affects the amount of blood reaching the extremities.

Pustule Small bump in skin filled with pus; a pimple.

Sebaceous glands Oil glands that secrete sebum to keep the skin from drying out.

Sebum Oily secretion of the sebaceous glands that keeps the skin lubricated; also acts as an anti-infective agent because of its acidic nature.

Stratum basale Deepest layer of the epidermis where new cells are formed.

Stratum corneum Outermost layer of the epidermis made up of flat, hardened dead epithelial cells.

Subcutaneous layer Also known as hypodermal layer; innermost layer of skin composed of elastic and fibrous connective tissue and fatty tissue

Sudoriferous glands Sweat glands located in the skin for cooling and release of toxins.

Wound debridement Process of removing of foreign material, dead and damaged tissue from a wound to stimulate healing.

7-1 NORMAL INTEGUMENTARY SYSTEM ANATOMY AND PHYSIOLOGY

Before getting deeper into the anatomy and physiology of the skin, let's look at its important functions. First and foremost, the skin acts as a protective barrier for our entire body. This barrier actually prevents the body from drying out and is the first line of protection against many infections. Without our skin, we could not regulate our body temperature and therefore would die. The skin also provides much-needed sensory input so we can perceive the world around us and be alerted to potential dangers. While the skin acts as a protective sunscreen, it uses the sunlight to produce the essential vitamin D. The skin is also critical in storing fatty tissue needed for energy. Now, let's take a detailed look at the anatomy of our largest organ in Figure 7-1.

Don't be intimidated by all the layers as their importance will soon be clear. For now, study the figure and focus on the three main layers; the epidermis, dermis, and subcutaneous or hypodermis.

7-2 THE EPIDERMIS

The **epidermis** is the layer of skin you can see. The underlying **dermis** is considered the true skin so it makes sense that the epidermis (***epi*** **= above**) sits above the dermis. The epidermis, as can be seen in the figure, is made up of several smaller layers with specialized cells. This layer contains no blood vessels and is therefore avascular. The outermost layer is the **stratum corneum**, which

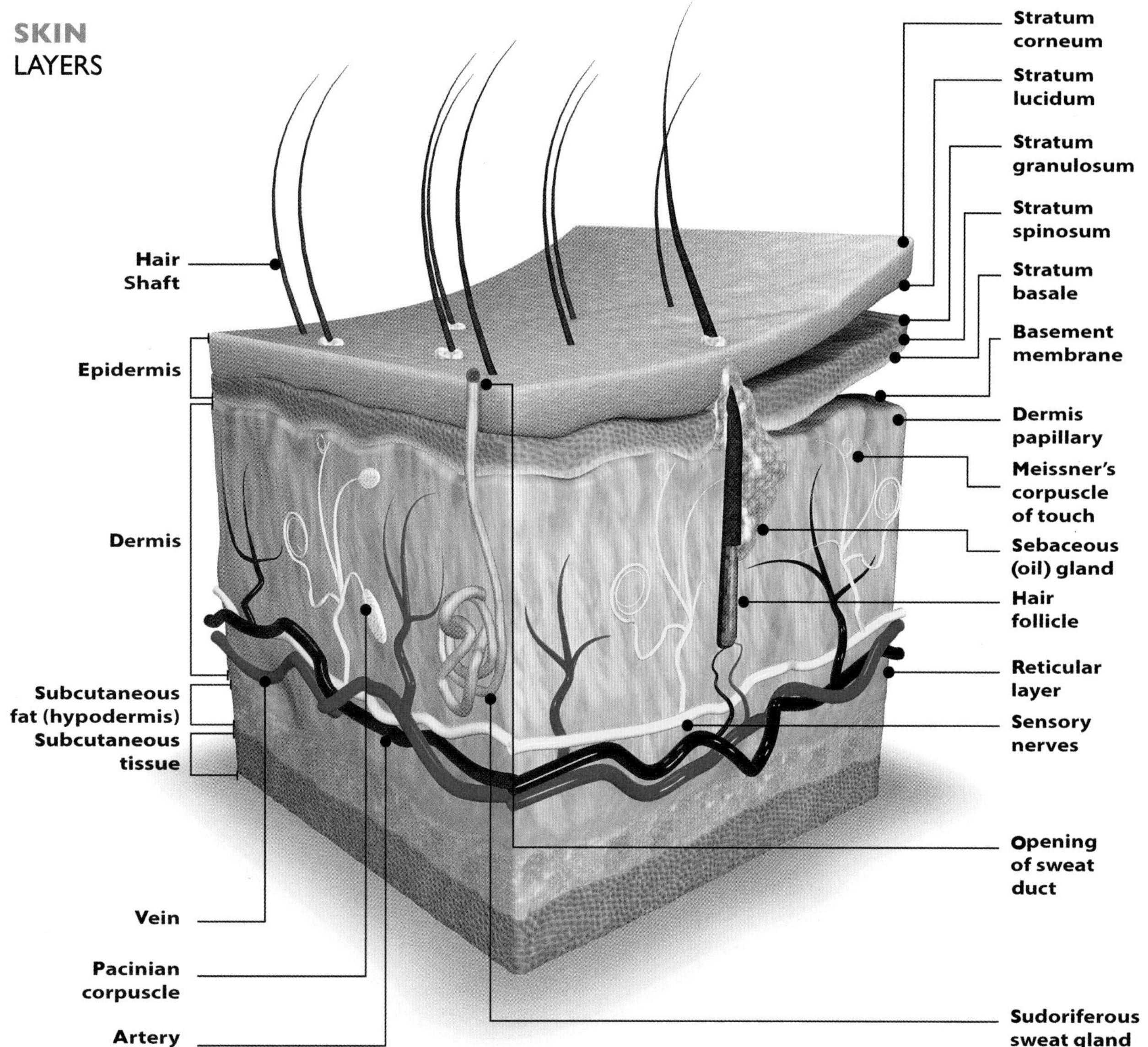

FIGURE 7-1 Labeled diagram of the skin.

is made up of flat, hardened, and dead epithelial cells. These surface cells are constantly shedding and sloughing off as we move around, dry ourselves after showering, or even while we sleep. Dandruff is actually excessive sloughing of dead skin scales because of excessively dry skin from the scalp.

We lose about 500 million dead skin cells per day, and obviously, they need constant replacements. The new cells form in the deepest layer called the **stratum basale**. They work their way up through the layers and eventually die, filling with a protein called **keratin** that hardens them when they reach the surface. This renewal is important for normal wear and tear, but it also can be kicked in high gear with tissue damage.

7-2a The Epidermis and Skin Color

Specialized cells called **melanocytes** located deep in the epidermal layers are responsible for our skin color. Melanocytes produce a dark pigment called **melanin**. All individuals contain roughly the same number of melanocytes; the variations in skin color occur mainly as a result of the amount of melanin produced by these cells. When exposed to ultraviolet (UV) rays of the sun, the melanocytes are stimulated to produce more melanin as a protective measure; that is why we tan. Unless you sun bathe in the nude, you will notice tan lines attesting to melanin being produced as needed. Regardless of the individual's skin color, all skin types respond to sun exposure. Melanin can concentrate in patches on the skin and this is commonly known as **freckles**.

Carotene (think carrot and don't confuse with keratin) is another skin pigment that gives a normal yellowish hue to the skin. However, in liver disease, an orange/yellow pigment found in bile called bilirubin builds up in the blood and can give the skin a deeper yellow or orangish coloration. This is called **jaundice**, which is a French term for yellow. See Figure 7-2. Jaundice can especially be seen in the sclera, or whites, of the eyes.

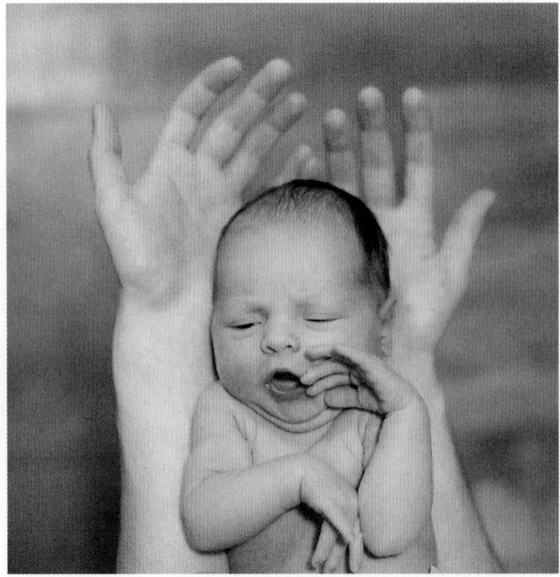

FIGURE 7-2 Infant with neonatal jaundice.

Individuals with albinism have little pigment because they produce little or no melanin. They have very white skin and hair, and even lack pigment in their eyes, which often causes vision problems.

CLINICAL CONNECTION 7.1

When oxygen combines with hemoglobin in the blood it turns a bright red color. Sometimes lack of oxygen in the blood can cause it to appear a darker red as less is combined with the hemoglobin. In the skin, this lack of oxygen or deoxygenation of blood will give a bluish hue to the outer skin called cyanosis. If the cyanosis occurs only in the peripheral area or extremities, it is known as acrocyanosis.

7-3 DERMIS

Sitting right below the epidermis is the dermis. Refer to Figure 7-3 that highlights this area. This is known as the true skin and contains the following:

- Capillaries for nourishment
- Collagenous and elastic fibers for support and integrity
- Nerve endings for sensations
- Lymph vessels to transport excess fluid from tissue back to blood
- Sudoriferous glands or sweat glands for cooling and release of toxins

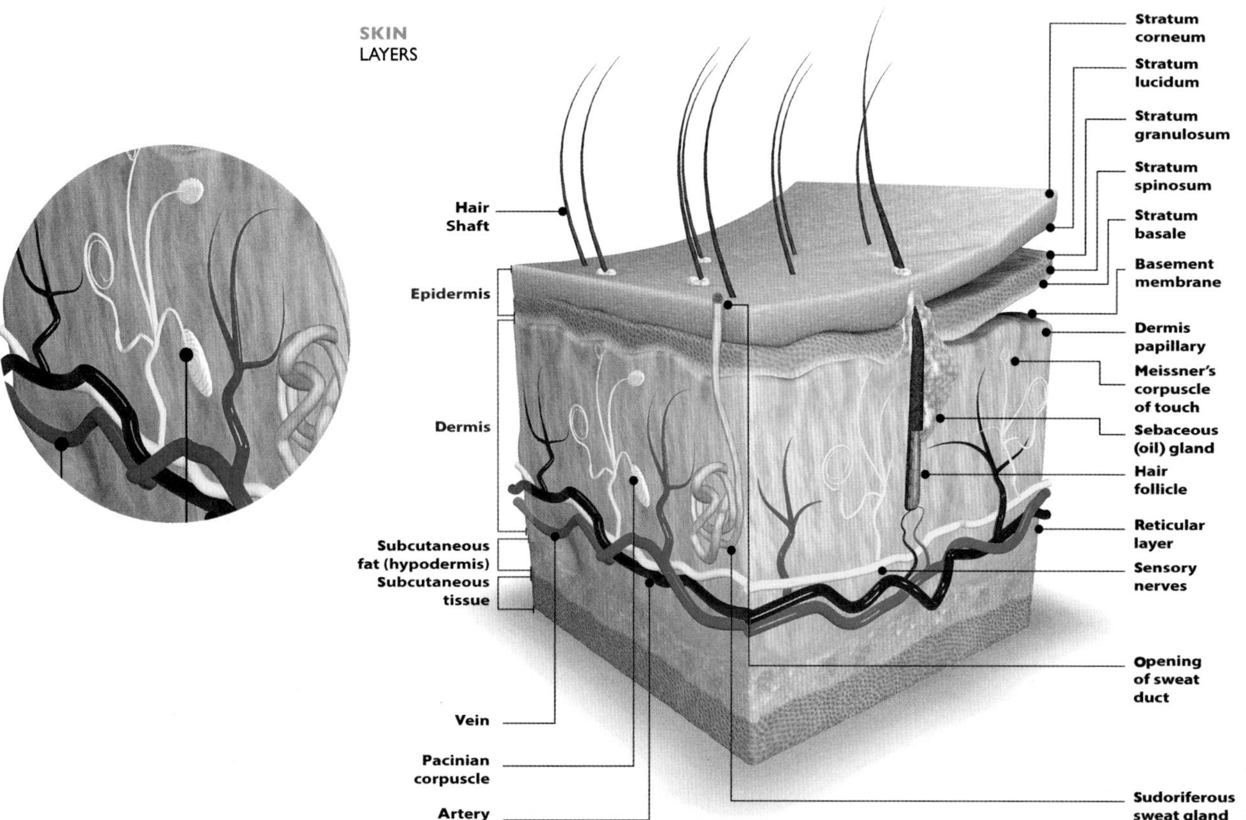

FIGURE 7-3 Layers of the skin with the dermal layer highlighted.

- **Sebaceous glands** (oil glands) to secrete sebum to keep the skin from drying out
- Hair follicles, located everywhere except for the palms of the hands and soles of the feet.

The collagenous and elastic fibers help your skin to flex or expand while moving, and then return to its original resting state or normal shape. As we age, skin loses this elastic recoil property and the skin begins to wrinkle and sag.

7-3a Sweat Glands

You actually have two types of sweat glands. **Apocrine sweat glands** are found in the groin and anal regions and become active around puberty. They are believed to have acted as sexual attractants in our early evolution. The glands with which you are probably most familiar are **eccrine glands**, located all over your body to allow you to perspire and cool your body through its evaporation to aid in temperature regulation. Your body has approximately 3 million sweat glands, and sweat itself does not have a strong odor. If left on the skin, however, bacteria degrade substances within the sweat, giving off strong body odors.

Sebaceous glands secret **sebum**, which keeps the skin lubricated and acts as an anti-infective agent because of its acidic nature. This helps to destroy pathogens on the skins surface. Sometimes sebaceous glands can become blocked or obstructed and the sebum can become stagnant, dry out and turn black, causing a *blackhead*. If the blackhead becomes infected and filled with pus, a pimple, medically known as a **pustule** will develop. When we get to the pathopharmacology section, you will learn about the different types of pustules and skin conditions that can develop.

CLINICAL CONNECTION 7.2

In Module 5, cancer was discussed. In advanced stage cancer, **anhidrosis** can be common. *An* means without and *hidro* refers to sweat, so anhidrosis is a condition of a decreased or lack of ability to sweat. This situation means air conditioners can be critical for comfort in many end-stage cancer patients.

7-4 SUBCUTANEOUS FASCIA OR HYPODERMIS

The **subcutaneous layer** or **hypodermal layer** is the innermost layer of skin and is composed of elastic and fibrous connective tissue and fatty tissue (Figure 7-4). **Lipocytes** produce the fat needed to provide padding to protect the deeper tissues of the body. The fatty layer also acts as insulation to help make temperature regulation easier. In addition, fat stores energy that can be called upon in times of need. The hypodermis is the layer of skin that actually attaches to your muscles.

CLINICAL CONNECTION 7.3

The hypodermal layer is a convenient place to administer injections because it contains no vital organs. This layer of skin gave its name to the hypodermic needle.

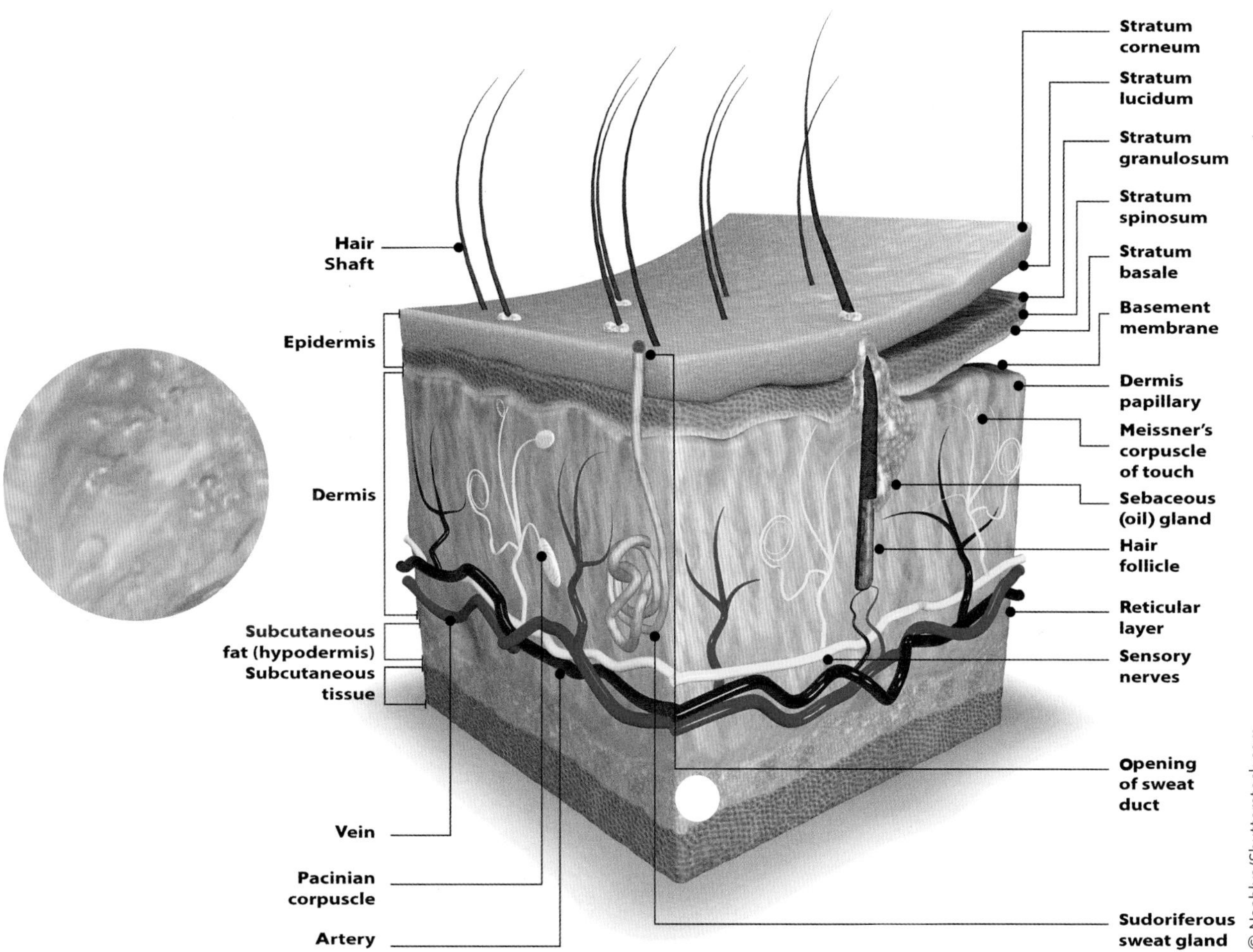

FIGURE 7-4 Layers of the skin with the hypodermal layer highlighted.

7-5 NAILS

Nails are specialized cells originating from the **nail root** (see Figure 7-5). As the cells grow out and over the nail bed, which is actually part of the epidermis, they become hardened or keratinized (there is that hard protein again) forming the hardened nail. This is a similar process as in the formation of the horns on a bull. The cuticle is the small fold of tissue covering the nail root and the portion we see is the nail body. **Lunula** means little moon, and this is the white half-moon shaped area at the base of the nail. The pinkish color of the nails comes from the blood vessels (vascularization) of the tissues under the nails.

CLINICAL CONNECTION 7.4

Peripheral perfusion or the amount of blood reaching the most distal extremities is an important indication of **peripheral vascular disease (PVD)**. To assess your peripheral perfusion, pinch one of your fingernails with the thumb and index finger of your other hand and hold for 5 seconds. Release pressure, and you will notice the nail bed should go from a blanched white appearance back to pink in a few seconds. This shows the blood rushing back to feed the tissue. If you have poor perfusion, it will remain white for a while. It normally takes less than 3 seconds to return to pink. Try it in the cold. Diabetes can cause PVD.

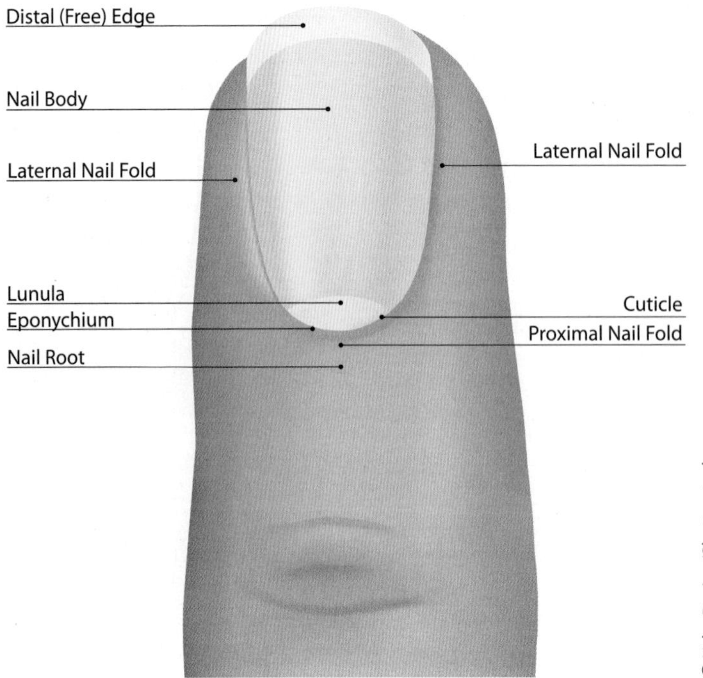

FIGURE 7-5 The nail and related structures.

7-6 HAIR

Hair is also composed of the fibrous protein keratin, just like your nails. The hair you see in the epidermis is called the **hair shaft**; and the follicle and anchored hair root are below the surface in the dermal layer. Similar to the skin layer, the cells grow and divide at the base of the follicle. Then as they are pushed up, they die and become keratinized, so the hair you see is actually dead hardened skin cells. Balding is called **alopecia**, derived from the Greek word for fox mange. Hair loss is not always part of aging; it can be caused by serious illness, hormonal disorders, chemotherapy, toxins, tissue trauma, and radiation.

7-7 SKIN AND TEMPERATURE REGULATION

The integumentary system is responsible to help maintain thermoregulation of our body. Your hair helps insulate your body to retain heat. Hairs can actually stand erect using **arrector pili muscles**, giving you goose bumps. Pockets of still air form around the standing hairs and act as insulation.

If your body is extremely hot, your sweat glands excrete and you perspire. The evaporative cooling effect of the sweat allows for heat to leave your body. In addition, vasodilation can allow more of the heat in your blood to get near the body surface and dissipate, radiating heat away from your body. Conversely when you are cold, vasoconstriction helps keep the blood closer to the body core where it is warmer, in order to maintain the body heat.

7-8 HOW SKIN HEALS

Since skin is exposed to the elements and hazards of everyday life, it will become damaged on a regular basis. We discussed the regenerative layers that continually replace skin cells. However, what if a deeper wound causes damage to the dermal layer? First, the wound fills with blood, which will begin to clot, forming a scab (nature's Band-Aid) over the wound to prevent more pathogens from entering. Now the deeper layers must heal. White blood cells attack the pathogens that have entered the wound, attempting to keep the infection from growing and spreading.

Fibroblasts (cells that produce connective fiber tissue) are then stimulated to develop at the edge of the wound to begin to pull it together. The basal layer now hyper-produces cells to repair the wound. If the wound is severe, scar tissue may develop. Scars are composed of collagen fibers and contain no nerves or blood vessels so you can't feel them.

CLINICAL CONNECTION 7.5

Scars can be minimized with stitches, adhesive strips or specialized glue to bring the edges or margins of the wound closer together and lessen the stress of healing. Ideally, the wound starts to heal from the inside working out toward the outside, which aids in preventing pathogens from being trapped in the deeper layers of skin and developing pockets of infections. This is why some wounds are purposely left open if an infection is suspected so the infection will not be encapsulated within the wound and then spread. Often foreign material, dead and damaged tissue, must be removed from the wound to stimulate healing. This process is called **wound debridement**.

LEARNING OBJECTIVE 7.2 Discuss the various types and routes for skin medications.

KEY TERMS

Antipruritics Medications used to relieve itching.

Corticosteroids (for integumentary use) Agents used to treat skin disorders from allergic reactions.

Emollients Agents used to soothe irritation and protect skin damage.

Enzymatic agents Promote removal of necrotic and fibrotic tissues (aids in debridement).

Keratolytic agents Loosens and breaks down epithelial skin scaling.

Pediculicides Agents used to treat lice infestation.

Scabicides Agents used to treat mite infestations (scabies).

Topical route Drug administration applied to local area.

Transdermal route Use of a skin patch to deliver various medications.

7-9 ROUTES OF SKIN MEDICATION

By far, the most common route used to treat skin conditions is the **topical route**, which will be the primary focus of this section. However, some serious conditions do require oral or parenteral medications. In addition, while not used to treat skin conditions, the **transdermal route** of drug administration uses the controlled absorption of a medicated patch through the skin to deliver various medications. The transdermal delivery route is advantageous because it is easy to apply, effective for long periods, so frequent dosing is not needed, and maintains a consistent blood level of the drug over long periods of time. The key to how the transdermal patch works is that the drug molecules are in a variety of shapes and sizes that allow for absorption at varying rates. One such transdermal patch contains nicotine and is used to help smokers quit by reducing or eliminating the nicotine cravings. A patch used to treat chest pain in cardiac conditions is the Nitro-Dur patch containing nitroglycerine, which dilates the coronary arteries supplying oxygen to the heart (see Figure 7-6). More about specific types of transdermal drugs will be given in their respective body system chapter, but the subject is introduced here because it does use the skin as a delivery route.

7-10 TOPICAL SKIN MEDICATIONS

We are going to briefly discuss the nine categories of topical skin medications before going into detail about the specific disease states. This will give you an overview of the types of skin medications in the drug arsenal for use on various conditions within the integumentary system. Soon you will see that some are needed in combination; for example, an antibiotic to fight the infection in conjunction with a medication to prevent itchiness (pruritus), which would lead to scratching which would lead to further irritation. The nine categories of skin preparations are:

1. **Antipruritics** to relieve itching
2. **Corticosteroids** to treat skin disorders from allergic reactions
3. **Emollients** and protectants to soothe irritation and protect skin damage
4. **Keratolytic agents** to loosen and break down epithelial scaling such as in dandruff
5. **Enzymatic agents** to promote removal of necrotic and fibrotic tissues (aids in debridement)
6. **Scabicides** and **pediculicides** to treat scabies or lice infestation

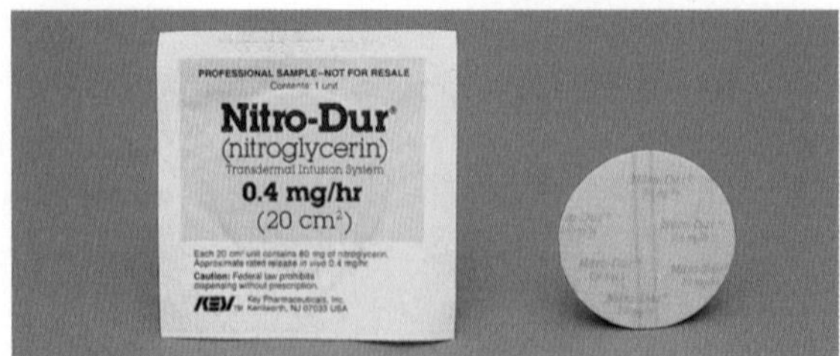

FIGURE 7-6 Nitro-Dur is a transdermal system of delivering medication used for prevention and long-term management of angina pectoris.

7. Local anti-infective agents to prevent and treat bacterial, fungal, and viral skin infections
8. Agents to treat acne
9. Burn medications.

7-10a Antipruritics and Corticosteroids

Antipruritics (***anti* = against**, ***pruritus* = itchiness**) are used to relieve the discomfort and itchiness of dermatitis (rash). Dermatitis can have several different etiologies, such as allergic reactions, hives, insect bites, poison ivy exposure, and so on. Types of antipruritics are as follows:

- Local anesthetic agents that deaden the skin sensation (benzocaine and dibucaine)
- Drying agents that reduce discomfort (calamine lotion)
- Antihistamines that reduce the release of histamine, which causes allergic reaction (Benadryl)
- Corticosteroids that prevent or decrease the allergic reaction (Cortaid and Kenalog).

Antihistamines and corticosteroids can be given both topically and systemically. If the patient is itchy but has no inflammation, use of corticosteroids should be avoided because of potential side effects. In addition, oral antihistamines should be used for only a few days in a hypersensitive reaction. First-generation antihistamines can cause sedation, so later-generation non-sedating antihistamines might be a better choice. In addition, antihistamines have been known to cause paradoxical agitation in children.

Side effects of long-term topical corticosteroid use could cause slow healing (because it reduces the immune system) and fragile skin with frequent tearing or bruising. For this reason, its use is not recommended on open wounds. Table 7-1 contrasts the medications discussed in this section.

7-10b Emollients, Keratolytics, and Enzyme Preparations

Emollients or protectants are used to soothe, soften, and protect minor dermatologic conditions. They seal out wetness and act as a protective barrier by topically creating a lipid barrier. They are used for diaper rash, skin irritation/abrasions, and minor burns. Desitin and Balmex are two common examples. Protectants also can block the harmful UV radiation from the sun.

Keratolytic agents are used to control integumentary issues involving abnormal skin scaling, such as dandruff or as occurs in seborrhea and psoriasis (see Figure 7-7A). In addition, it can be used for excessive keratinization as in hard corns, callouses, and even wart formations (see Figure 7-7B). Keratolytics use should be monitored for side effects such as skin irritation, pruritus, and stinging sensations. Clearasil for acne use and Compound W for wart removal are examples of keratolytic agents.

Table 7-1 Topical Antipruritics

GENERIC NAME	TRADE NAME	AVAILABLE TOPICAL FORM	CONSIDERATIONS
Local Anesthetics			
benzocaine	Lanacane, Orajel	Ointment, spray, gel, lotion, cream, liquid, lozenge	Can cause hypersensitivity reaction
dibucaine	Nupercainal	ointment	Can cause hypersensitivity reaction
Antihistamine			
diphenhydramine	Benadryl	Lotion, cream, gel, spray	Not as effective as when given orally (PO)
Corticosteroids			
high potency form	Diprolene, Temo-vate, others	Ointment, cream, lotion, solution, gel, foam, shampoo	Duration is maximum 2–4 weeks and do not discontinue abruptly but taper use.
low potency forms	Cortaid, Topicort, Kenalog, Synalar, others	Ointment, cream, lotion, solution, gel, foam, shampoo	Lower potency preferred for face, groin, armpits, and large treatment surface.

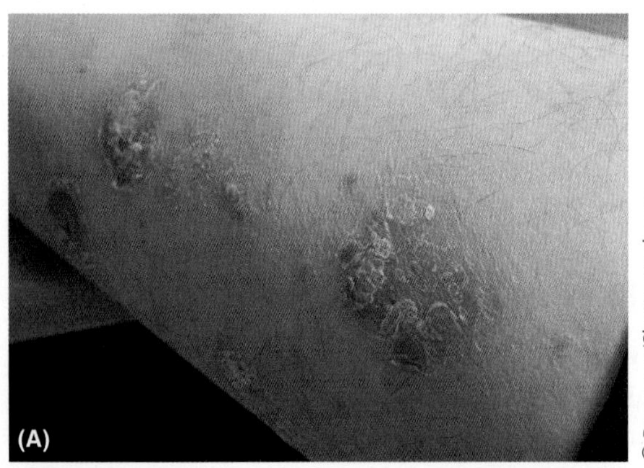

FIGURE 7-7A Psoriasis condition showing scale-like skin.

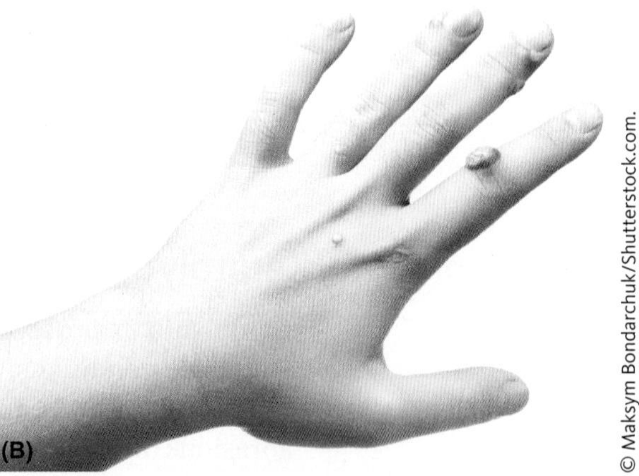

FIGURE 7-7B Common warts on hand.

Enzyme preparations are used to remove dead skin to promote regenerative skin healing. Necrotic skin can occur because of a variety of reasons, but is often seen in bedridden patients in the form of decubitus ulcers (pressure sores) and in foot ulcers in diabetic patients. Colagenase (Santyl) is a topical enzyme ointment used for topical debridement.

7-10c Summary of Emollients, Keratolytics, and Enzyme Preparations

Table 7-2 summarizes the medications in this section.

Table 7-2 Emollients, Keratolytics, and Enzyme preparations.

GENERIC NAME	TRADE NAME	AVAILABLE TOPICAL FORM	CONSIDERATIONS
Emollients			
ammonium lactae	AmLactin	Cream, lotion	Moistening agent; also used in sunscreen products
vitamins A & D	A&D Desitin	Ointment for both	Moistening agent; also used in sunscreen products; used as protective barrier for diaper rash
zinc oxide	Balmex	Cream, ointment	Moistening agent; also used in sunscreen products; used as protective barrier for diaper rash
Keratolytics			
coal tar	Neutrogena T/Gel, Polytar	Shampoo, oil, cream, lotion, ointment, soap, solution	Used for dandruff, seborrheic dermatitis, or psoriasis; stains clothing
salicylic acid	Clearasil, Fostex, Compound W	Cream, liquid, gel, patches	Indicated for dandruff, psoriasis, acne, warts, corns, and calluses
Enzyme Preparations			
collagenase	Santyl	Ointment	For use in debridement of necrotic skin

7-10d Scabicides and Pediculicides

Scabies is caused by a tiny female mite that burrows into the skin to lay her eggs. The most common signs are severe itchiness and a pimple-like rash. Pediculosis is caused by an infestation of lice in the hairy regions of the body, include the scalp, pubic area, and chest. Both conditions are highly contagious and can be transmitted by direct contact or through contact with contaminated clothing, bed linen, or towels. See Figure 7-8A and Figure 7-8B.

Effective treatment includes scabicides and pediculicides (***cide*** **= killing**) along with replacing or laundering in hot water all potentially contaminated clothing and bedding. Scabicides include permethrin 5% or lindane lotion applied, according to packet directions, and left in place for a specified time and then rinsed thoroughly. Pediculicides include permethrin 1% (Acticin) and lindane shampoo. Pyrethrins (RID) shampoo is effective for head lice only. A recently approved topical ivermectin lotion (Sklice) is safer to use on younger children and is approved for patients 6 months or older.

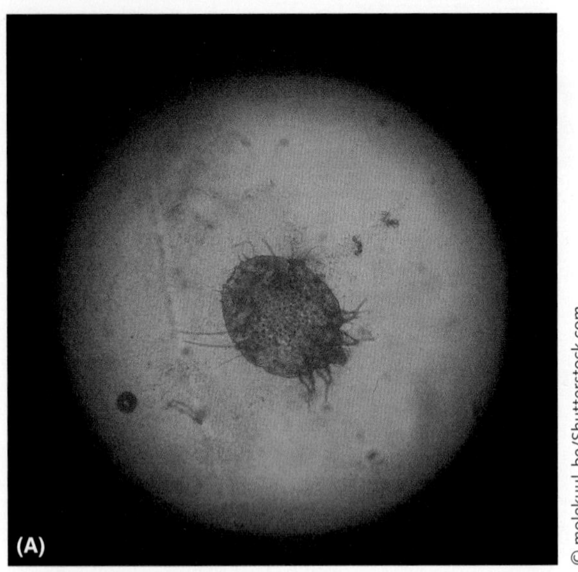

FIGURE 7-8A Light microscopy image of 7-year itch mite.

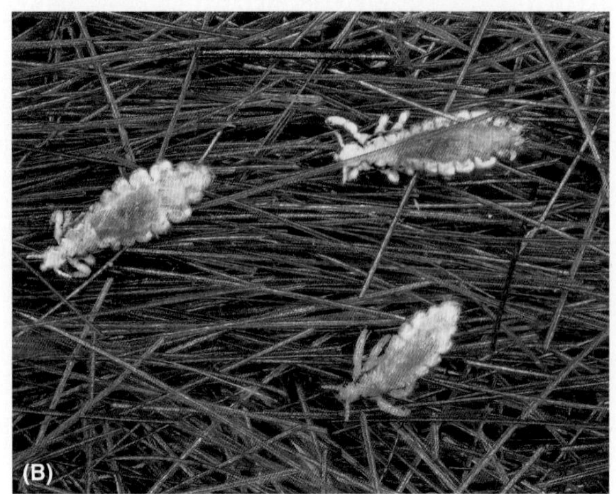

FIGURE 7-8B Head lice on human hair.

LEARNING OBJECTIVE 7.3 Discuss the pathopharmacology of infectious integumentary diseases.

KEY TERMS

Abscess Localized collection of infected material or pus.

Acne Skin condition characterized by hyperactivity of oil glands and red pimples on the face, back and chest.

Antifungal agents Medications used to treat fungal infections.

Antiseptics Chemicals that inhibit the growth of bacteria.

Candidiasis Caused by the candida yeast, it is an opportunistic infection that surfaces if normal flora is wiped out by antibiotic use or an immunosuppressant condition. Infections can occur in the mouth (thrush), vagina (vaginitis), intestines, and fingernails (onychomycosis).

Carbuncle Large grouping of furuncles.

Cellulitis Bacterial infection of the skin caused by *streptococcus* and/or *staphylococcus* bacteria.

Disinfectants Chemicals that kill bacteria on surfaces.

Erysipelas Acute skin infection that extends into the underlying fat layer; more commonly found in children caused by group A *streptococcus* bacteria.

Folliculitis Infection of the hair follicle on the skin from *staphylococcus* bacteria.

Furuncle Small abscess developed around a hair follicle.

Herpes simplex Viral infection causing clusters of fluid-filled vesicles called cold sores or fever blisters and genital herpes.

Herpes varicella Viral infection causing chickenpox.

Herpes zoster Viral infection causing shingles.

Human papilloma virus (HPV) Viral infection causing warts. Genital warts, the most commonly sexually transmitted disease, has been shown to increase risk for cervical cancer.

Impetigo Highly contagious pustule forming skin disease usually found in children and affecting the hands and face.

Lesion General term for any abnormal damage or change in tissue especially on the skin.

Lyme Disease Transmitted by the bite of an infected deer or blacklegged tick that harbors the bacterium *Borrelia burgdorferi*; often forms a bull's eye rash.

Methicillin-resistant staphylococcus aureus (MRSA) *Staphylococcus aureus* bacteria that has become pathogenic and resistant to antibiotic.

Open comedo Blockage and stagnation of the sebaceous gland; a blackhead.

Shingles Viral disease caused by herpes zoster that causes painful skin lesions that follow the course of a spinal nerve.

Tinea barbae Fungal infection affecting bearded area of neck and face; barber's itch.

Tinea capitis Fungal infection of the skull or cap of head.

Tinea corporis Fungal infection found on smooth skin of arms, legs, and body; called ringworm because of its appearance, but no worm is involved.

Tinea cruris Fungal infection of the scrotal and groin area; jock itch.

Tinea pedis Fungal infection of the feet; athlete's foot.

Tinea unguium Fungal infection of the fingernails or toenails causing white patches on the nail; difficult to treat, can destroy the entire nail.

Verrucae Medical term for warts caused by a virus (papilloma virus).

7-11 LOCAL ANTI-INFECTIVE AGENTS

Numerous skin diseases are caused by various types of microorganisms. This chapter will focus on topical agents used to treat skin disease, and other anti-infective agents will be discussed in their respective body system chapters for more systemic-wide disease. Infectious skin disease can be fungal, as in jock itch, viral, as in shingles, or bacterial, as in impetigo.

7-12 ANTIFUNGAL INTEGUMENTARY DISEASES

Tinea is the key term to remember that describes contagious fungal infections. For example, **tinea pedis** (***ped* = foot**) is a fungal infection of the feet, commonly known as athlete's foot. **Tinea capitis** affect the skull or cap of head. Fungi like warm moist areas where they can grow and feed off dead skin cells. Symptoms of fungal infections include itching and cracking or weeping of the skin that can lead to skin fissure formations. If left untreated fungal infections can lead to secondary bacterial infections. Diagnosis is made on patient history, clinical appearance of the affected region, and microscopic examination of skin scrapings showing fungi.

One other fungal infection is caused by a yeast, which is actually a specialized form of a fungus. **Candidiasis** is caused by the fungus *candida*, actually a normal flora in our body. This is an opportunistic infection that surfaces if our normal flora are wiped out by antibiotic use or an immunosuppressant condition.Infection in the mouth is called thrush, but it can occur in the vagina (vaginitis), intestines, or even in fingernails, where it is called onychomycosis (***myco* = fungi**).

Table 7-3 describes the various types of tineas.

7-12a Treatment of Fungal Diseases

Antifungal agents, such as nystatin are indicated in candidiasis-like infections, such as thrush, diaper rash, and vaginitis. Other antifungals such as clotrimazole are used to treat tinea-like infections such as ringworm, jock itch, and athlete's foot. Sometimes antifungals are combined with corticosteroids, but these products are not recommended by dermatologists. Although rare, side effects of topical antifungal agents can include contact dermatitis, itching, and burning sensations.

Table 7-3 Forms of Tinea or Fungal Infections

FUNGAL DISEASE	AREA FOUND AND COMMENTS
Tinea corporis	Found on smooth skin of arms, legs, and body. Commonly called ringworm because of its appearance, but no worm is involved, Figure 7-9A. 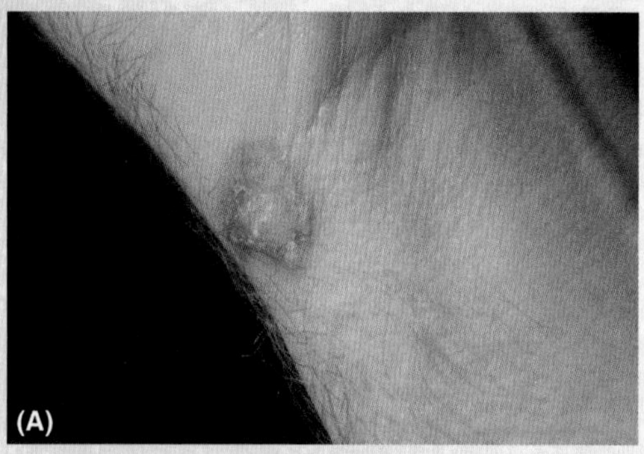 (A) © Rodrigo Bellizzi/Shutterstock.com. **FIGURE 7-9A** Ringworm.
Tinea pedis	Highly contagious athlete's foot first found between toes but can spread to entire foot, Figure 7-9B. Wearing sandals helps prevent and treat fungus. 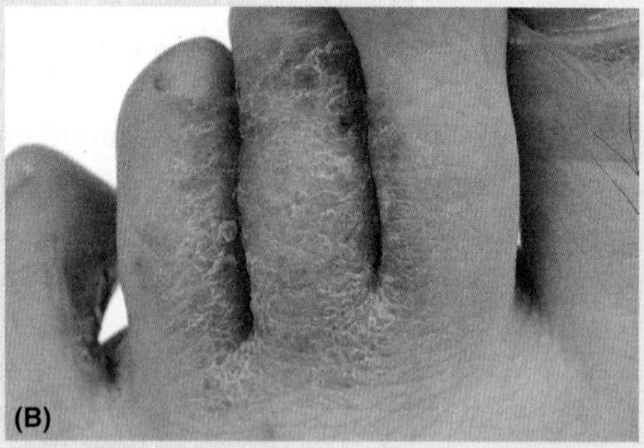 (B) © carroteater/Shutterstock.com. **FIGURE 7-9B** Athlete's foot.
Tinea cruris	Affects scrotal and groin area and lay term is called jock itch. Aggravated by sweat and tight fitting pants/underwear.
Tinea capitis	Affects the scalp and can cause hair loss. Most commonly found in children.
Tinea barbae	Affects bearded area of neck and face; commonly called barber's itch

Table 7-3 Forms of Tinea or Fungal Infections—*continued*

FUNGAL DISEASE	AREA FOUND AND COMMENTS
Tinea unguium	Affects fingernail or toenails and has white patches on the nail. Hard to treat and can destroy the entire nail causing it to thicken, overgrow and become brittle, Figure 7-9C. (C) © tugolukof/Shutterstock.com. **FIGURE 7-9C** Fungal nail infection.
Candidiasis (thrush)	Yeast infection of the skin, mouth, vagina, or intestines, Figure 7-9D. Taking antibiotics that kill the normal flora or immunosuppression can cause yeast to form this opportunistic infection. (D) © Victoria 1/Shutterstock.com. **FIGURE 7-9D** Oral candidiasis fungal infection. (Thrush)

Effective treatment requires strict adherence to the topical application directions according to the drug insert. In addition, good hygiene practices such as proper washing and drying to maintain a clean dry environment along with exposure to air whenever possible will facilitate healing.

Table 7-4 provides a summary of antifungal medications.

7-13 TOPICAL ANTIVIRAL AGENTS

The viral family of herpes causes many skin conditions. **Herpes simplex** is responsible for clusters of fluid-filled vesicles called cold sores or fever blisters, and genital herpes. **Herpes varicella** causes chickenpox and **herpes**

Table 7-4 Antifungal Medications

GENERIC NAME	TRADE NAME	AVAILABLE FORMS	COMMENTS/ CONSIDERATIONS
clotrimazole	Lotrimin	Cream, lotion, solution for oral use, vaginal cream	For oral (thrush), topical, or vaginal application
ketoconazole	Nizoral	Cream, 2% shampoo (Rx only)	Topical antifungal, shampoo for dandruff
miconazole	Monistat	Cream, gel, ointment	Also in vaginal cream and suppositories; for vaginal infections; refrain from intercourse until healed
nystatin	Mycostatin	Oral suspension, lozenges, cream, ointment, powder	Use oral suspension or lozenges pc then NPO for 1 hour
terbinafine	Lamisil	Cream, gel, spray, tablets	Tablets effective for hard to treat nail infections
tolnaftate	Tinactin	Aerosol spray, cream, powder, solution	Avoid spray or powder contact with eyes

zoster causes **shingles**. It should be noted that many viral diseases are acute and can resolve without medication, but many viral infections are lifelong and can remain dormant and re-emerge at a later time to cause an acute exacerbation. Chickenpox is a classic example of the virus remaining in your body from initial infection as a child, with the potential to re-emerge in your adult years as shingles. Shingles are painful skin lesions that follow the course of a spinal nerve. Diagnosis is made by patient history, observation and location of vesicles, and if needed, a blood test for herpes antibodies.

Acyclovir is used to treat herpes infections. Acyclovir (Zovirax) cream is used only for the treatment of cold sores. It does not cure them, but does reduce the frequency and appearance of new lesions. It can be used for first-time eruptions of genital herpes, but is not effective in later occurrences. Docosanol (Abreva) is an OTC medicated cream that shortens the healing time and duration of cold sore symptoms. It is most effective when applied as soon as first symptoms of tingling, itch or redness appear. In other words, before the vesicles form.

For effective treatment of shingles, oral systemic doses of antivirals are needed. Acyclovir (Zovirax) is available in oral form, as are derivatives of Zovirax that include valacyclovir (Valtrex) and famciclovir (Famvir). The derivatives require less frequency in dosing and therefore have better patient compliance. All oral antivirals need to be started within 72 hours of rash onset but are most effective when started within the first 48 hours. Zostavax is an FDA approved vaccine for those 50 or older to reduce the risk of getting shingles (see Figure 7-10).

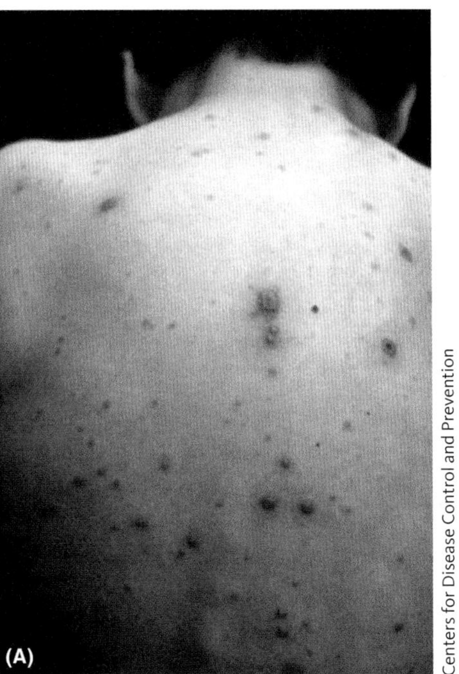
Centers for Disease Control and Prevention

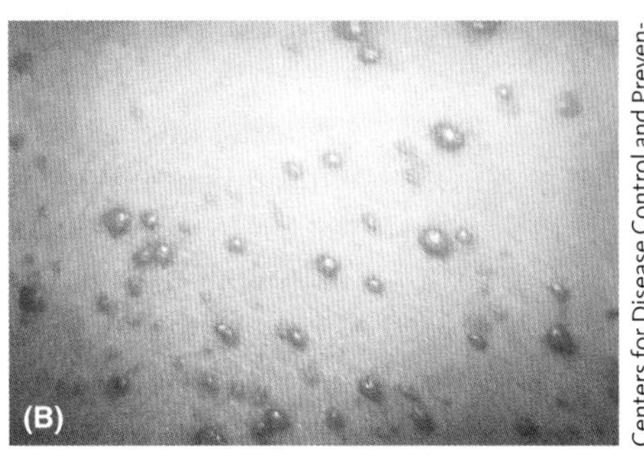
Centers for Disease Control and Prevention/Joe Miller

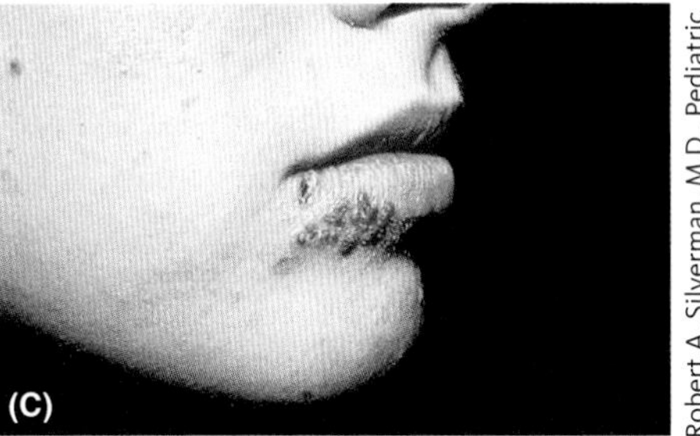
Robert A. Silverman, M.D., Pediatric Dermatology, Georgetown University

FIGURE 7-10 (A) Chickenpox caused by varicella zoster. (B) Shingles, a later eruption of the chickenpox virus as the herpes zoster virus. (C) Cold sores of the mouth caused by herpes simplex virus.

7-13a Warts

Verrucae is the medical term for warts. Warts are caused by the papilloma virus and spread by contact and scratching. While this was discussed in a previous section under keratolytics, it deserves re-mentioning because the etiology is viral in nature. Common warts, which appear on the hand and fingers of children, are painless and often disappear spontaneously. Warts on an adult should be checked for skin cancer. Plantar warts occur on the soles of the feet and do cause pain while walking; therefore, they need to be removed surgically.The topical solution containing salicylic acid, such as Compound W, can be used for common warts. Genital and plantar warts are often surgically removed (see Figure 7-11).

The **human papilloma virus (HPV)** is the most commonly transmitted sexually disease, and also has been shown to increase risk for cervical cancer. A HPV vaccine (Gardasil or Cervarix) is recommended for pre-sexually active boys and girls.

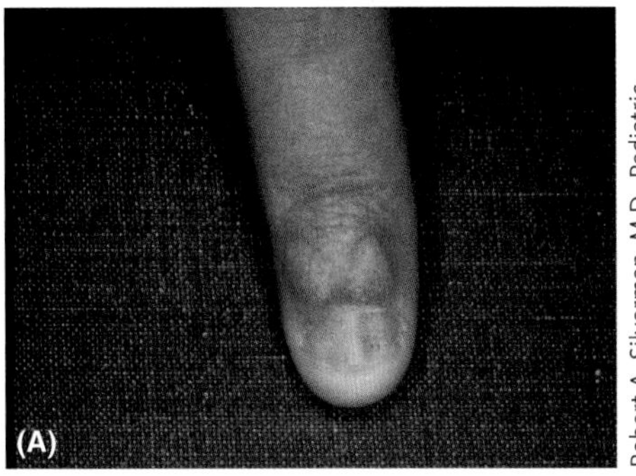
Robert A. Silverman, M.D., Pediatric Dermatology, Georgetown University

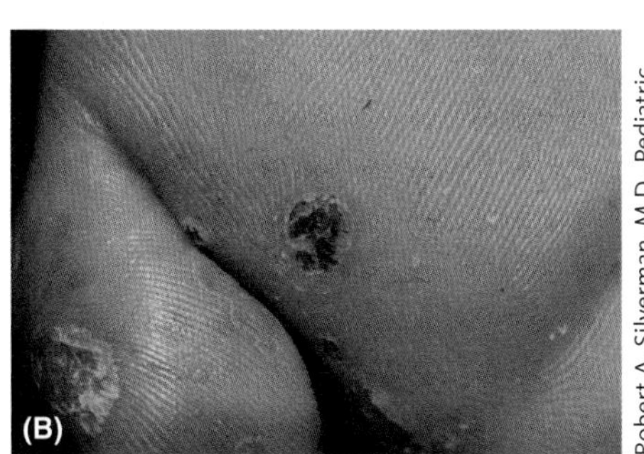
Robert A. Silverman, M.D., Pediatric Dermatology, Georgetown University

FIGURE 7-11 (A) Common wart. (B) Plantar wart.

7-14 TOPICAL ANTIBACTERIAL AGENTS

Bacterial infections can be caused by many etiologies but often affect patients who have compromised immune systems, poor hygiene, or trauma wounds. Bacterial skin diseases range from the simple pimple to the life-threatening methicillin-resistant staphylococcus aureus (MRSA) infection.

7-14a Skin Lesions

A **lesion** is a general term for any abnormal damage or change in tissue. The lesions that affect the skin seem almost legion in numbers. One of the most common bothersome lesions of growing up is the dreaded pimple. When the sebaceous gland within the skin becomes blocked, the sebum it produces becomes stagnate and dries out, forming an **open comedo**, commonly known as a blackhead. If the blackhead becomes infected, a *pustule* or pimple forms. See Figure 7-12.

7-14b Acne

Treatment of blackheads and pimples includes proper skin hygiene by washing with soap and water. If the inflammation and infections of sebaceous glands are widespread, and pimples cover large areas such as the face, neck, back, or shoulders, it is known as **acne**, Figure 7-13. Mild acne can be treated with OTC topical medications that include sulfur, salicylic acid, and benzoyl peroxide.

More severe forms need more aggressive treatment from a dermatologist that can include prescribed topical antibiotics, such as clindamycin or erythromycin, to reduce inflammation. In addition, retinoid medication, such as isotretinoin, can be given to decrease oil production of the glands. For the most severe

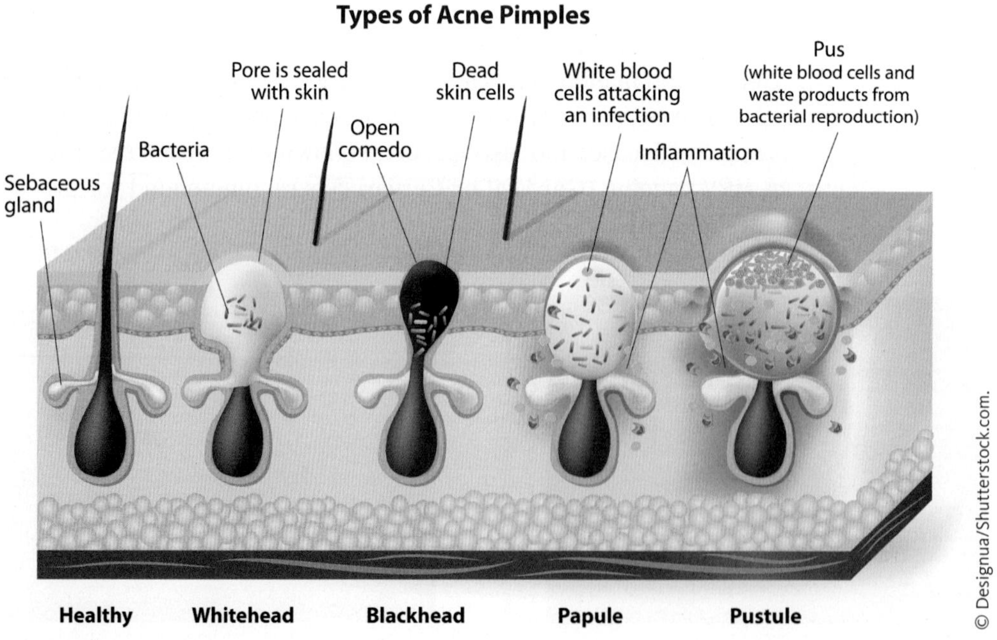

FIGURE 7-12 Types of acne pimples.

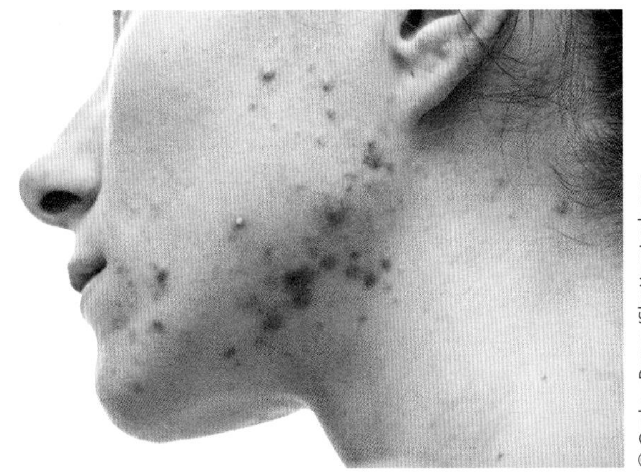

FIGURE 7-13 Acne.

forms, a course of oral antibiotics, such as tetracycline, is prescribed to produce a systemic affect, in addition to the topical medications. Table 7-5 describes some of the common acne medications.

7-14c Wounds and Abscesses

An **abscess** is a localized collection of infected material or pus that can occur in any tissue of the body, but often occurs in the skin because of wounds or trauma. A small abscess is known as a **furuncle**, commonly called a boil. See Figure 7-14.

Table 7-5 Acne Medications

GENERIC NAME	BRAND NAME	FORMS AVAILABLE	CONSIDERATIONS/ COMMENTS
benzoyl peroxide	Panoxyl	Bar, cream, foam, liquid, gel, lotion	Has antibacterial and drying activity
salicylic acid	Clearasil, Neutrogena	Cream, liquid, gel, pads	For mild acne
sulfur	In many combinations with other keratolytics	Cream, soap, lotion, gel, pads	For mild acne
tretinoin	Retin-A	Cream, gel	Increases sensitivity to sun or photosensitivity, meaning you can burn more easily
isotretinoin	Claravis	In various capsule dosages	For severe acne, but absolutely contraindicated in pregnancy
clindamycin or erythromycin		Topical antibiotic cream	For mild acne
tetracycline		Pills	For severe acne

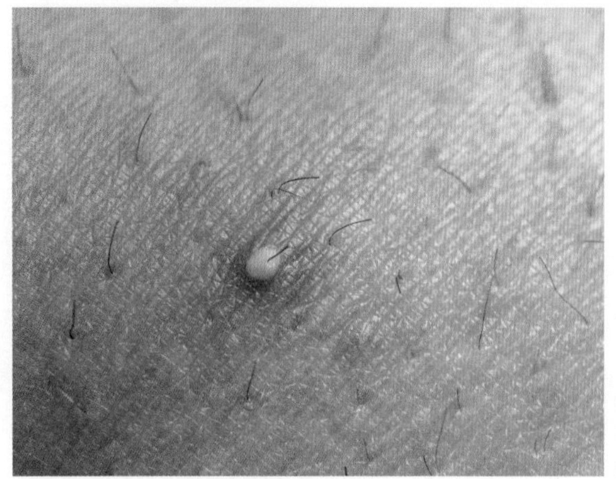

FIGURE 7-14 Furuncle showing ingrown hair.

Furuncles usually develop around a hair follicle; tip to remember: think of a "furry uncle." A large grouping of furuncles is a **carbuncle**. The treatment of both is warm moist compresses to relieve pain and promote drainage of the infected material. Topical OTC antibacterial agents such as Neosporin also can be used.

7-15 SKIN TRAUMA

Trauma or certain diseases can cause larger areas or wounds that can become infected and fill with pus. Severe wounds can actually erode or ulcerate the skin as can be seen in Figure 7-15.

Obviously, the wound must be kept clean, and antibiotics can be given topically or systemically for more severe wounds to prevent the infection from entering the blood stream, which can cause septicemia.

Often, the wound is cleaned with **antiseptics**, which are chemicals that inhibit the growth of bacteria (bacteriostatic). **Disinfectants** are chemicals that kill bacteria (bacteriocidal), and often are too strong to use on tissue. They normally are reserved for objects, such as instruments used to treat the wound. The two major antiseptics used are chlorhexidine (Hibiclens) and povidone-iodine

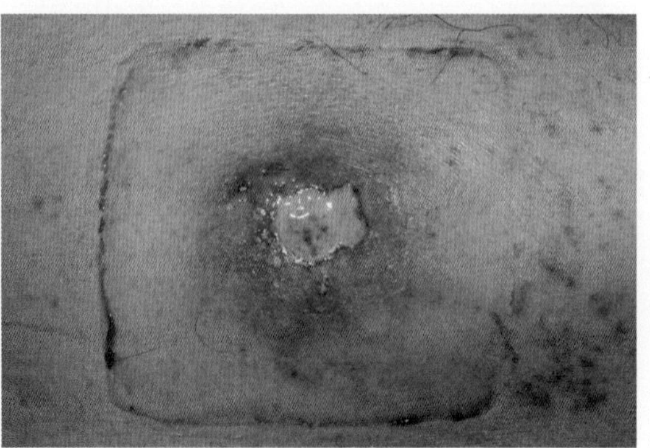

FIGURE 7-15 Ulcer.

(Betadine). These come in solution form and can be used to clean wounds or as surgical scrubs prior to surgical procedures. Hibiclens should not be used on wounds involving more than the superficial skin layers.

7-15a Impetigo

Impetigo is a highly contagious skin disease usually found in children. It often affects the hands and face, but can be found in other areas as shown in Figure 7-16. Pustules form and rupture, producing a yellowish crust over the skin lesions. Treatment includes proper washing and drying the affected area several times a day and using topical antibiotics. Mupirocin (Bactroban) is a prescribed topical ointment used to treat impetigo caused by *Staphylococcus aureus* and forms of *Streptococci*. Bactroban nasal ointment is used to reduce the risk of infection during institutional outbreaks of MRSA, which will be discussed next. Severe cases of impetigo might require oral antibiotics.

7-15b Methicillin-Resistant Staphylococcus Aureus

Staphylococcus aureus is a common normal flora of the skin and is usually harmless. Therefore, your skin is colonized with this microorganism but no illness occurs. **Methicillin-resistant staphylococcus aureus (MRSA)** comprises a group of this bacteria that has become pathogenic and resistant to antibiotics. While bacteria, like any organism driven by survival, can become resistant over time, we have speeded up the evolutionary process by the misuse and overuse of antibiotics. For example, antibiotics have been given to treat viral infections, on which they have no effect. Some individuals can harbor colonized MRSA but not have any infections. They can, however, pass it on to someone in an immunocompromised situation, such as a patient in a hospital, which is why MRSA can spread throughout a hospital.

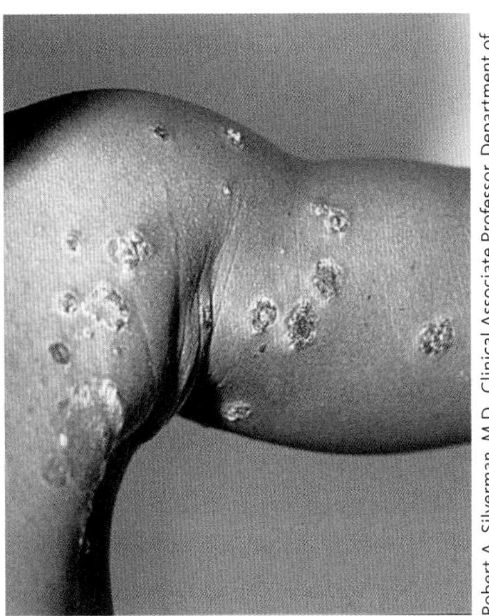

Robert A. Silverman, M.D., Clinical Associate Professor, Department of Pediatrics, Georgetown University

FIGURE 7-16 Impetigo is a highly contagious bacterial skin infection commonly found in children.

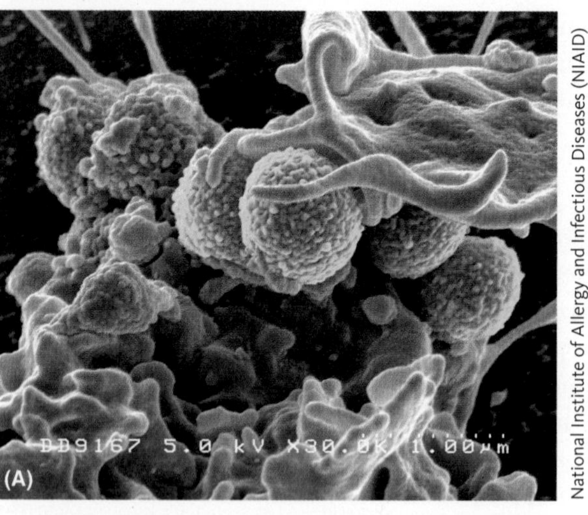

National Institute of Allergy and Infectious Diseases (NIAID)

FIGURE 7-17A Colorized electron micrograph of MRSA (green spheres) being attacked by white blood cells.

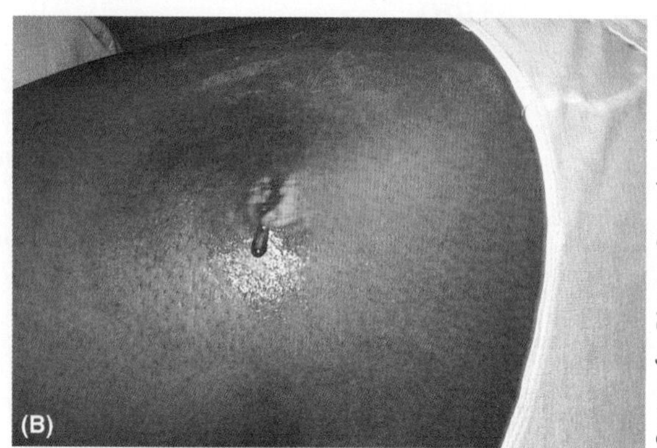

Centers for Disease Control and Prevention/ Bruno Coignard, M.D.; Jeff Hageman, M.H.S.

FIGURE 7-17B Skin abscess caused by MRSA.

Symptoms of MRSA often start with small red, pimple-like bumps on the skin. These can quickly develop into deep abscesses or travel into the bloodstream. Sepsis occurs when the infection is within the bloodstream, giving staph a route to attack organs of the body, such as heart, lungs, and bones. Sepsis symptoms include fever, chills, diffuse rash, headaches, joint pain, and shortness of breath. Diagnosis is confirmed by culture and sensitivity testing. See Figure 7-17A and Figure 7-17B.

Prevention is key in healthcare facilities and requires sanitation of all surface areas and disinfectant of all equipment, along with proper hand washing hygiene. Vancomycin is the drug currently used to treat MRSA. It often needs to be given intravenously for serious infection because it is not absorbed well orally.

7-15c Cellulitis

Cellulitis is a bacterial infection of the skin, usually caused by *streptococcus* and *staphylococcus* bacteria. It can occur after an insect bite, blister, or burn and is a diffuse inflammation of the both the skin and subcutaneous tissue. Cellulitis also appears in open areas of the skin, such as a wound or ulceration, Figure 7-18. This condition is not to be confused with cellulite, which looks like cottage cheese (lumpy dimples) on the surface of the skin and is caused by fat cells pushing against the underside of the dermis.

Symptoms include pain, redness, swelling, warmth, and tenderness in the affected area. Advanced symptoms can include headaches, fever or chills, and development of red streaks showing further spread of the disease.

Oral antibiotics are needed in mild to moderate cases, with IV antibiotics indicted in severe cases. Analgesics are used to treat the associated pain. Severe pain can indicate that necrotizing fasciitis (flesh-eating disease) is developing, which requires immediate surgical intervention. Cellulitis in the facial area is

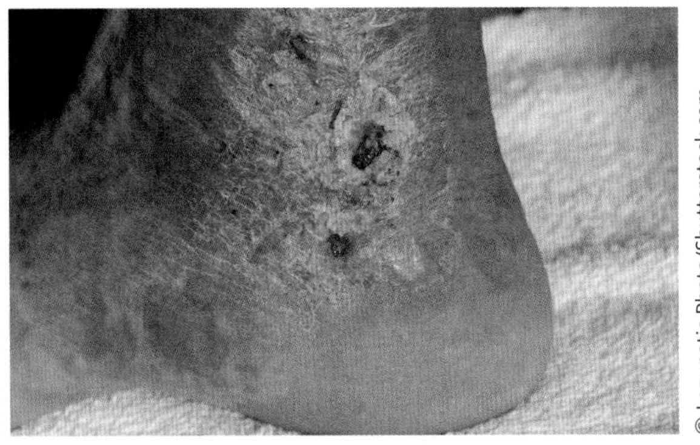

FIGURE 7-18 Cellulitis occurring after a wound.

concerning because it has the potential to spread to the sinuses and therefore into the skull. Like most skin diseases, good handwashing and proper wound care can prevent the occurrence of cellulitis.

7-15d Erysipelas

Erysipelas is an acute infection of the skin that extends into the underlying fat layer, usually in the face and legs. It is more commonly found in children. Its etiology is group A *streptococcus* bacterial infection. The diffuse rash is red, warm, hardened, and painful and has aptly been called red skin or holy fire. The skin has an orange peel-like texture, Figure 7-19.

Symptoms of erysipelas can include fatigue, fever, chills, headache, and vomiting. Ultrasound tests should be done to rule out deep vein thrombosis, which can exhibit a similar rash, as can herpes zoster and contact dermatitis.

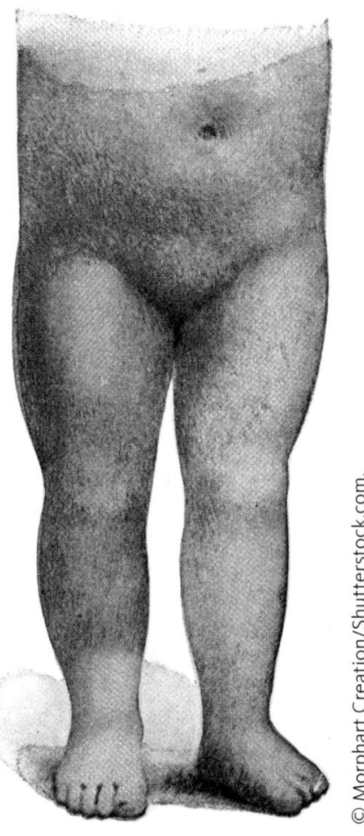

FIGURE 7-19 Erysipelas or red skin; note the orange peel-like texture.

Oral or IV antibiotics, such as penicillin and clindamycin, are indicated, depending upon severity. Care must be taken as it can spread to blood (bacteremia) and also advance to necrotizing fasciitis (flesh-eating bacteria). Prevention includes good skin hygiene, injury avoidance, and properly treating any *strep* infection such as *strep* throat commonly found in children.

7-15e Lyme Disease

Lyme disease is named after Lyme, Connecticut, the town where it was first discovered in 1975. This disease is transmitted by the bite of an infected deer or blacklegged tick that harbors the bacterium *Borrelia burgdorferi*.A bull's eye rash appearing days or weeks after the bite is a common sign as seen in Figure 7-20, although it appears only in approximately one-third of cases. Diagnosis is confirmed from history and a positive blood test showing the presence of antibodies for the disease.

In addition to the rash, other symptoms of Lyme disease include joint pain, malaise, fever, and chills, similar to flu-like symptoms. If untreated, it can lead to serious neurological, cardiovascular, and arthritic complications. Antibiotic treatment with doxycycline or amoxicillin, or even more powerful antibiotics in stubborn cases, is recommended. Most cases are treated successfully in a few weeks, but some can last longer or progress even with treatment.

Prevention is the key by avoiding being bitten by a tick. Wearing long-sleeves shirts and long pants with the bottoms tucked into socks or boots, along with insect repellant, when hiking or camping in grassy and/or wooded areas are good preventative measures. Showering and inspecting for ticks after being outdoors, especially in natural areas, is highly recommended.

7-15f Folliculitis

Folliculitis is an infection of the hair follicle anywhere on the skin. The infection usually begins with damage to the hair follicle from abrasions or shaving, where *staphylococcus* bacteria can enter the follicular area. Common symptoms are rash, itching, and formation of small pimples around the hair.

Warm, moist compresses can help ease pain and promote drainage. Daily cleansing and OTC antibiotic or antifungal creams, depending on the type of

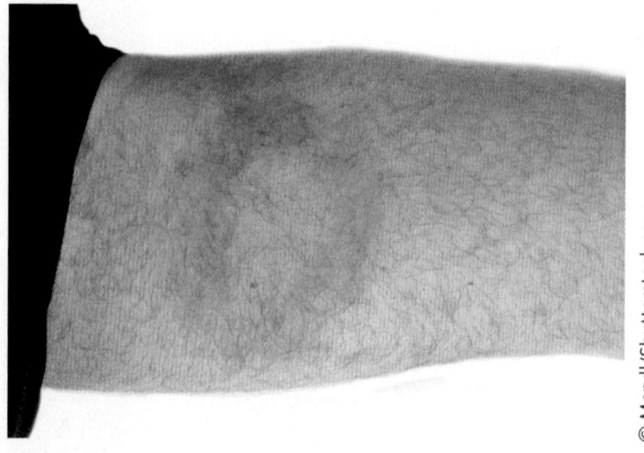

FIGURE 7-20 Bull's eye rash appearing in Lyme disease.

infection, usually resolves folliculitis in a few weeks. Severe cases might need oral antibiotics.

Reducing friction from tight clothing and clean, dry skin are excellent preventative measures. Also avoid shaving the area when infected.

LEARNING OBJECTIVE 7.4 Describe the pathopharmacology of the non-infectious integumentary conditions.

KEY TERMS

Basal cell carcinoma Most common form of skin cancer that does often not metastasize; appears as a raised nodule with depressed center or a smooth shiny tumorpinkish to whitish in color.

Contact dermatitis Inflammation of the skin because of contact with an irritating substance.

Dermatoplasty Surgical repair of the skin such as skin grafting needed to replace damaged skin with healthy grafted skin.

Eczema Genetic hypersensitivity skin reaction often found in infants.

Hemangiomas Common benign, often cherry red, childhood tumor made up of blood vessels; usually appears on the face and neck.

Keloids Raised mass of scar tissue that usually develops after trauma or surgery.

Malignant melanoma Most deadly form of skin cancer often resulting from overexposure to the sun or harmful radiation.

Psoriasis Non-contagious, chronic, idiopathic skin disease that presents as a series of red raised lesions with silvery scaling generally on the elbows, knees and scalp.

Rosacea Chronic, non-contagious, idiopathic skin condition that presents as redness and inflammation of the face, especially around the nose and cheeks.

Seborrheic keratosis Non-cancerous overgrowth of skin cells that appears as a wart-like growth; tan or black.

Squamous cell skin cancer Form of skin cancer with high cure rate that usually appears as a firm, red nodular lesion with a crusty-looking appearance; usually found on face, arms, or neck.

Sun protection factor (SPF) Value of protectiveness of sunscreen.

Urticarial Raised reddened area of skin because of allergic reaction.

Wheal Raised, reddened, swollen, and itchy area of the skin; hives

7-16 URTICARIA

Another condition of the skin that forms a raised reddened, swollen, and itchy area is known as **wheal**. This condition also is called **urticaria**, or more commonly, hives. See Figure 7-21.

This often occurs with contact of an external skin irritant such as an insect bite, plants (poison ivy, stinging nettles), dyes, jewelry, and laundry product. Therefore, because contact with the skin causes this condition, it is also known as **contact dermatitis**. An allergic reaction to certain foods and drugs also can cause hives.

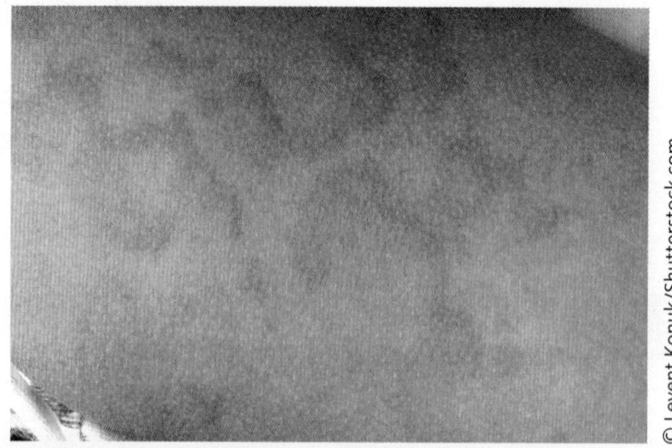

FIGURE 7-21 Example of a wheal with severe urticaria.

Identifying and avoiding the irritant or allergen is obviously the best treatment. However, when the rash develops, itching can be relieved with a topical antipruritic discussed earlier. Antihistamines, such as diphenhydramine (Benadryl), can be given orally to diminish the allergic reaction, but it also can cause drowsiness. Cool water soaks also can help alleviate the itch.

7-16a Eczema

Eczema is also known as atopic (allergic) dermatitis because it tends to run in families that have a genetic tendency toward hypersensitivity or allergic reactions. See Figure 7-22. Often it begins with infants because of food allergies, such as to milk or fruit juices. The obvious treatment for food allergy-related eczema is to identify and eliminate the offending food.In addition to heredity, other skin irritants, severe environmental conditions, and even stress can cause a flare up of the condition. In adults, the rash takes on a dry leathery appearance with pustules, scaling, and crusting.

Medications include topical cortisone creams such as hydrocortisone to reduce the inflammation caused by the allergic reaction. Antihistamines and antipruritics are often needed to relieve the itchiness. In addition, the avoidance of sunlight on the affected area is recommended. This condition is not contagious.

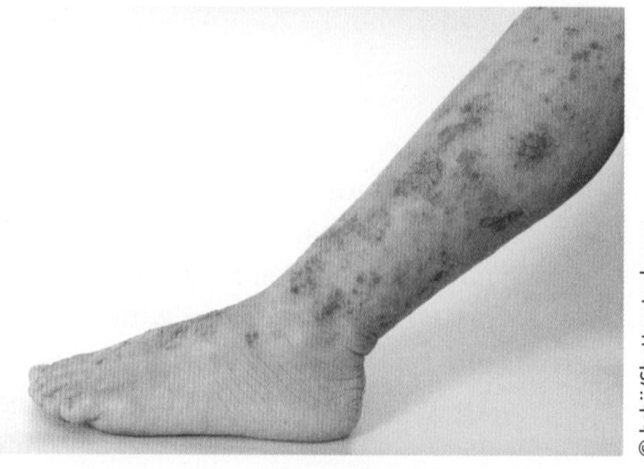

FIGURE 7-22 Eczema on the leg of a child.

7-16b Psoriasis

Psoriasis is a non-contagious chronic skin disease that has no known cause, but it is thought to have a genetic predisposition because it does tend to run in families. (A disease with no known identifiable cause is known as *idiopathic*.)

Psoriasis most often affects people between the ages of 15 and 35 and presents as a series of red, raised lesions with silvery scaling generally on the elbows, knees, and scalp, Figure 7-23. While the cause is not known, the condition does exacerbate during infections, stress, and skin trauma/irritation.

Medications include antipruritics for the associated itching along with keratolytics, such as coal tar creams and salicylic acid creams, to remove the dead scaly skin cells. In addition, topical and oral steroids can be given to reduce inflammation, along with vitamins A and D for skin health. UV light treatment have proven beneficial in some cases, and oatmeal baths have been shown to loosen the scales. Using emollients to moisten the skin can diminish the extent of the rash.

7-16c Rosacea

Rosacea is a chronic, non-contagious, idiopathic skin condition that presents as redness and inflammation of the face, especially around the nose and cheeks, Figure 7-24. While not dangerous, it can lead to self-esteem issues given the facial rash, and often affects fairer skinned woman ages 30–50. In addition to the rash, the nose can become reddened and bulbous, and spider-like blood vessels can appear in the face. A stinging or burning sensation and irritated, watery eyes also are associated with the rash.

There is no cure, but symptoms can be managed. The first step is identifying any triggers that cause the exacerbation. Triggers can include prolonged sun exposure, stress, alcohol, spicy foods, and extreme changes in temperature. Topical antibiotics can control any skin eruptions, such as pustule formations, and laser surgery can reduce the redness. Rhinoplastic procedure to reduce the size of the nose is an option in moderate to severe cases of bulbous nose formation.

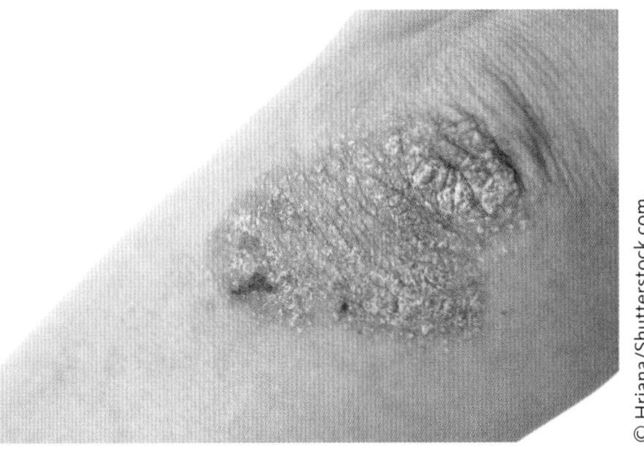

FIGURE 7-23 Psoriasis of the elbow.

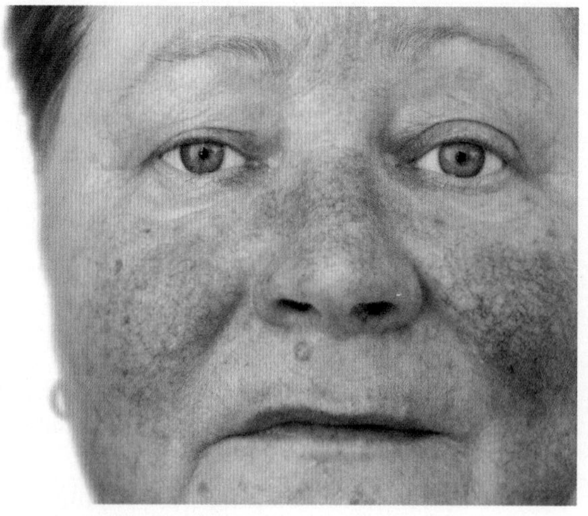

FIGURE 7-24 Rosacea.

7-17 BURNS

Burns are a special class of skin injury that can be caused by heat, radiation, or chemicals. The severity of burns of the skin can be classified by the depth of the burn and the size of the area that the burn covers. Let's look at burn classifications based on the depth of the burn.

A *first-degree burn* has damaged only the epidermis and is classified as a *partial-thickness burn* (i.e., a burn that does not affect the entire depth of the skin). A first-degree burn exhibits skin redness and pain, but no blistering. The pain usually subsides in 2 to 3 days with no scarring. The damaged layer of skin usually sloughs off in about a week or so. A sunburn is a classic example of a first-degree burn.

Second-degree burns involve the entire depth of the epidermis and a portion of the dermis. These burns are still considered partial-thickness burns because they do not go all the way through the skin. Such burns cause pain, redness, and blistering. Blisters continue to enlarge even after the initial burn. Excluding any additional complications, such as infection, these blisters usually heal within 10 to 14 days. Burns reaching deeper into the dermis require anywhere from 4 to 14 weeks to heal. Scarring in second-degree burn cases is common.

Small second-degree burns can be treated at home. The patient should run cool water over a burn without open blisters. The burn should be dried carefully, in order to avoid breaking the blisters, and a dry, sterile dressing applied to the burn. Ibuprofen can be taken to help with the pain. Larger second-degree burns or burns with open blisters might need to be treated by a doctor. The doctor might prescribe intravenous fluids to replace those lost by your body and antibiotics to fight infection. Stronger pain medicine also might be prescribed.

Third-degree burns affect all three of the skin layers and, therefore, are classified as *full-thickness burns*. The surface of the skin has a leathery feel to it and varies in color: black, brown, tan, red, or white. Initially, the victim will feel no pain at the affected site because pain receptors are destroyed by third-degree burns. Also destroyed are the sweat and sebaceous glands, hair follicles, and blood vessels. Third-degree burns can be life-threatening, but improvements in burn care have reduced the number of mortalities. A doctor might prescribe antibiotics to fight infection and intravenous fluids for rehydration. Surgical debridement is needed for severe burns to remove dead, charred tissue. A form of **dermatoplasty** called skin grafting might be necessary to replace damaged skin with healthy grafted skin that will hopefully take hold and grow. See Figure 7-25 for a contrast of types of burns.

7-17a Specific Burn Medications

Topical medications used for more serious second- and third-degree burns include sulfadiazine (Silvadene) and mafenide (Sulfamylon) creams. These are applied with a sterile glove to prevent or treat infections associated with the damaged skin layers. The affected area should be covered with the cream and a sterile dressing. Side effects can include pain and burning at the site and possible allergic reaction. These medications can stain the skin temporarily.

Varying Degrees of Burn Injuries

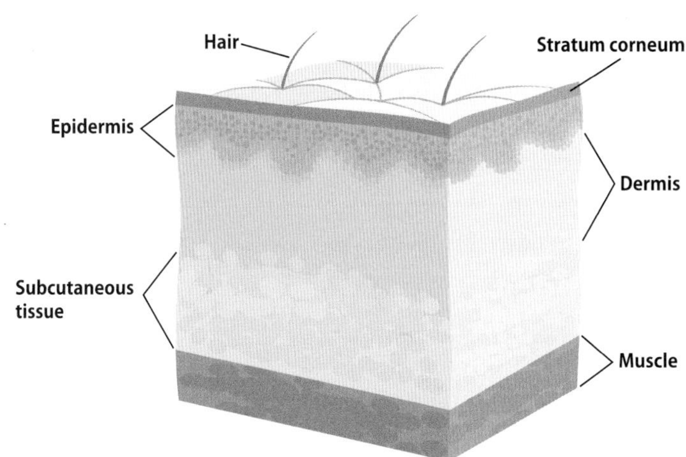

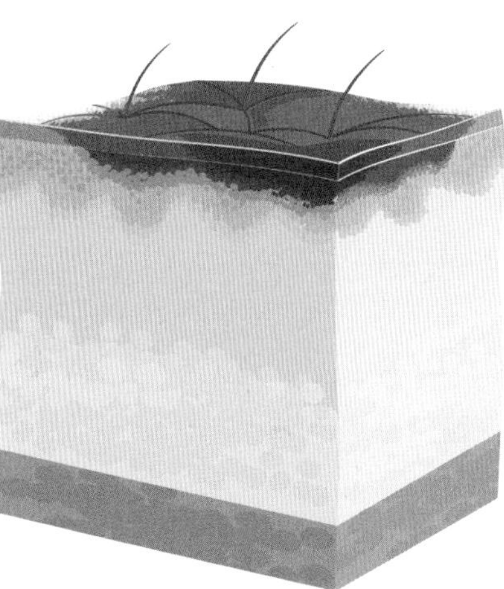
First Degree Burn Injury
Involves of skin

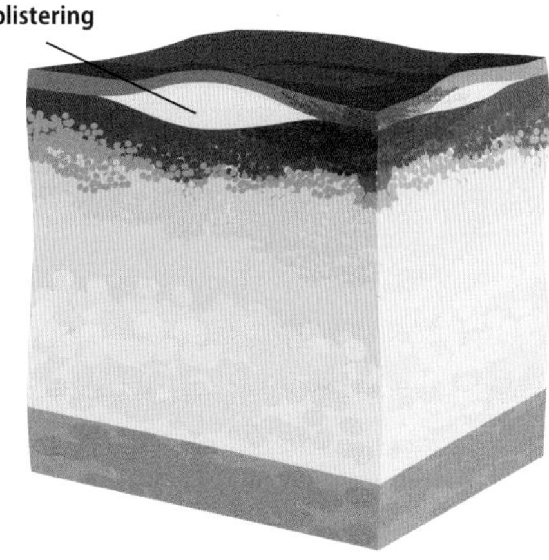
Second Degree Burn Injury
Involves top of skin and dermis
Deep blistering

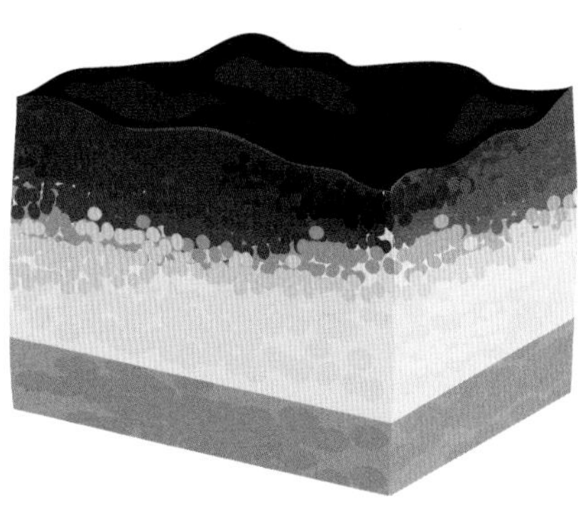
Third Degree Burn Injury
charred dermis and subcutaneous tissue

FIGURE 7-25 Burn classification system.

Of course, prevention of the most common type of first-degree burn or sunburn is accomplished with the use of sunscreens. UV radiation from the sun causes the burn; there are two types of UV radiation: UVA and UVB. Use broad-spectrum sunscreens to protect against both types.The **sun protection factor (SPF)** values should be equal to or greater than 30 SPF to reduce the risk of cancer and premature skin aging.

7-18 BENIGN TUMORS

Benign tumors of the skin are common and tend to run in families. **Seborrheic keratosis** is an overgrowth of skin cells and often occurs in older adults. It appears like a wart-like growth, whether tan, brown, or black in color. While not cancerous, it can be confused with skin cancer, and therefore should be biopsied to be sure. Treatment consists of curettage or scraping off the skin growths for cosmetic purposes; they do not have to be removed for medical reasons.

Hemangiomas are the most common childhood tumors and usually appears on the face and neck, Figure 7-26. As their name blood tumor implies, hemangiomas are made up of small blood vessels that form a reddish or pink mark. They have colorful names according to their appearance, color, and shape. A port-wine stain hemangioma leaves a dark red or purplish birthmark, usually on the face. A strawberry hemangioma is rougher and appears like a strawberry in both texture and color. A cherry hemangioma is a small, circular, deep red spot. There is usually no treatment, as they often disappear or just leave a colorful birthmark.

Keloids are scar tissue gone wild, Figure 7-27. The raised mass of scar tissue usually develops after trauma or surgery. While of cosmetic concern, keloids

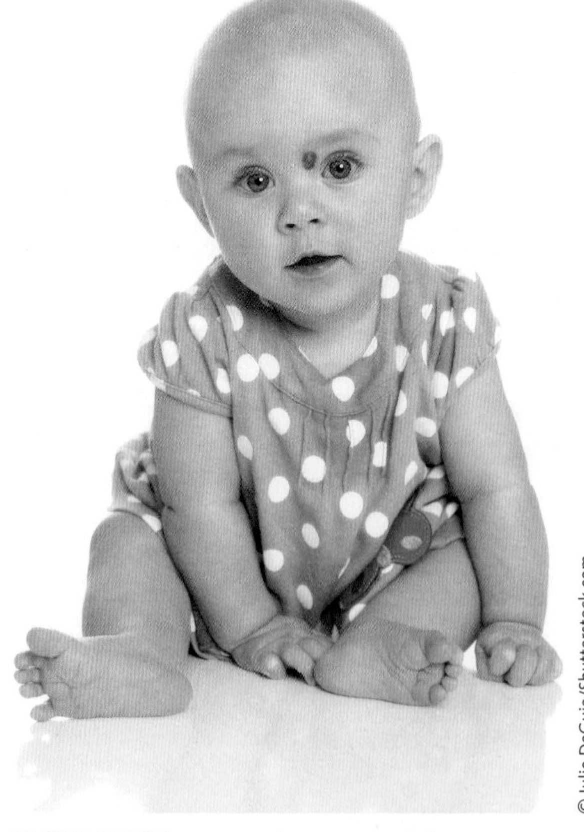

FIGURE 7-26 Hemangioma on an infant.

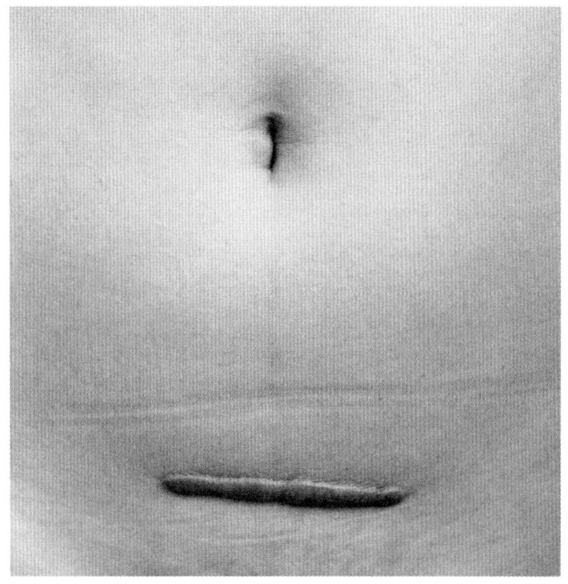
© WEERACHAT/Shutterstock.com

FIGURE 7-27 Keloid formation.

are medically harmless. Surgical removal usually does not work because it can cause additional keloid formations. Radiation and cryotherapy (freezing) can help reduce the keloid's size; steroid injections can reduce the inflammatory process that causes the over-scarring.

7-19 SKIN CANCER

The most common and most preventable type of cancer is skin cancer because most cases are because of excessive UV exposure. There are three types with **basal cell carcinoma** most common, then **squamous cell**, with **malignant melanoma** being the most deadly. The best prevention, previously discussed, is avoiding over-exposure to the sun and its harmful radiation and using sunscreen when exposed.

Basal cell is the most common form of skin cancer, is slow growing, and does not metastasize. The tumor's appearance varies but often appears as a raised nodule with depressed center or a smooth, shiny tumor pinkish to whitish in color, Figure 7-28. Diagnosis is confirmed by biopsy and microscopic

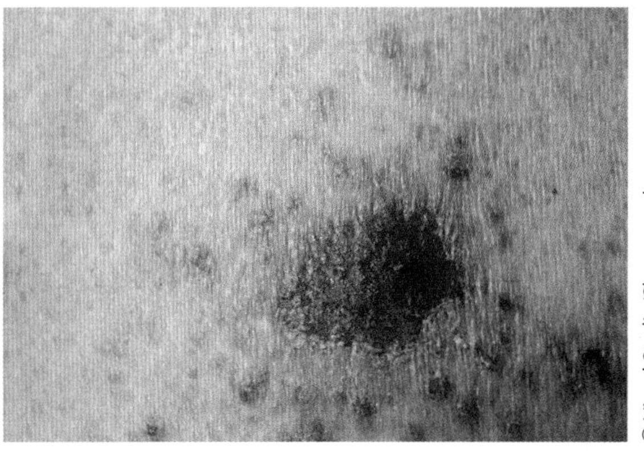
© Vizual Studio/Shutterstock.com.

FIGURE 7-28 Basal cell skin cancer.

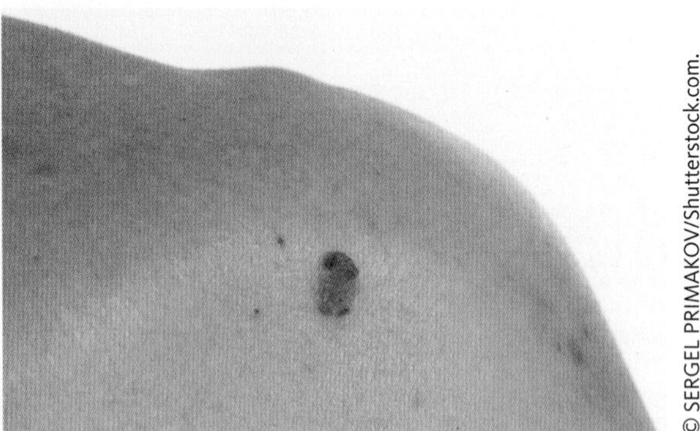

FIGURE 7-29 Squamous cell skin cancer.

examination of cell type. Treatment is primarily surgical removal. However, basal and squamous skin cancer also can be treated with fluorouracil, which is available in a topical cream called Efudex. Fluorouracil is an antimetabolic cancer drug that interferes with DNA synthesis, repair, and cellular replication and therefore can help slow or stop the proliferation of the cancerous skin cells.

Squamous cell cancer, while less common than basal cell cancer, can grow and spread more rapidly and can metastasize. This form of skin cancer usually appears as a lesion that is firm, red, nodular, and crusty looking, and usually found on face, arms, or neck, Figure 7-29. Confirmed by biopsy and microscopic examination, this form of skin cancer has a high cure rate if found early and is treated with surgical removal and radiation treatments.

Malignant melanoma is the most serious form of skin cancer and is found more commonly in men. It results from the uncontrolled growth of the pigment-forming melanocytes. The tumor is dark in appearance and can arise from a mole that changes its shape or color, Figure 7-30. This form is deadly because it metastasizes rapidly through the lymphatic system. Treatment depends on spread and can include surgical removal, radiation, and chemotherapeutic drugs. Prevention is key, but early detection can increase survivability. Therefore, frequent skin examinations for suspicious growths, changes in moles, or suspicious bleeding should be investigated immediately.

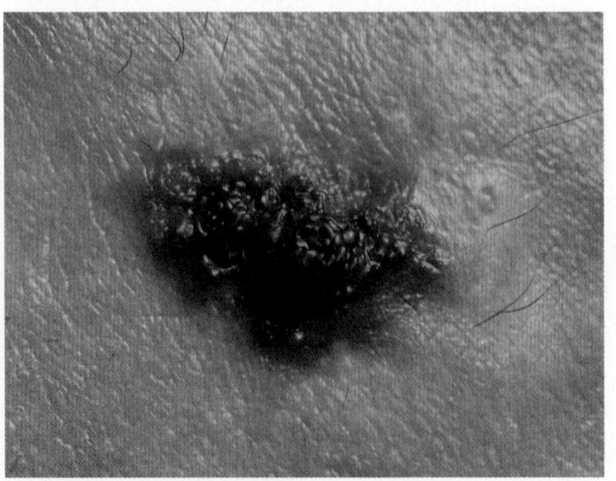

FIGURE 7-30 Malignant melanoma.

Module 8

Gastrointestinal Diseases and Medications

Module Introduction

The gastrointestinal system has other names with which you might be familiar: GI tract, alimentary tract, and alimentary canal. This network is made up of multiple organs that add up to be about 30 feet long. This system is, in basic terms, a large muscular tube that begins at the mouth and ends at the anus, with many other organs and structures in between.

This system, like others, is vital for homeostasis. It turns food and drink into fuel for the body to function properly every day and rids the body of waste products. Earlier chapters discussed how drugs are broken down and absorbed and then eventually eliminated by our GI tract, and accessory organs, such as the liver and kidneys. This chapter focuses on the basic anatomy and physiology of this system and discusses ailments and treatments.

LEARNING OBJECTIVE 8.1 Explain the normal anatomy and physiology of the upper gastrointestinal system.

KEY TERMS

Bicuspid A tooth with two cuspids, also referred to as a premolar tooth.

Body Largest portion of the stomach.

Canines Long, pointed teeth used to hold onto food.

Cardiac sphincter A circular or ring-shaped muscle leading to the stomach.

Cardiac (stomach) Portion of the stomach located around the lower esophageal sphincter.

Cementum Surface of the tooth root that is a bone-like connective tissue adhering teeth to the jaw bone.

Chyme Puree of acidic fluid containing partially digested food moving from the stomach to the small intestine.

Crown Upper visible portion of a tooth usually consisting of enamel.

Dentin Hard layer of the tooth found directly under the enamel.

Duodenum First part of the small intestine between the stomach and the jejunum.

Enamel Hard, white outer layer of a tooth providing durability and protection against everyday wear and tear.

Esophagus Flexible, yet muscular tube that connects the pharynx with the stomach allowing food to pass through.

Fundus Midportion and most superior part of the stomach.

Ileocecal valve Valve attaching the ileum to the large intestine.

Ileum Last portion of the small intestine after the jejunum that is connected to the large intestine.

Incisors Teeth located in the front of the mouth, used for cutting.

Jejunum Second part of the small intestine located between the duodenum and ileum.

Lower esophageal sphincter (LES) a ring-like muscle that leads to the stomach

Molars Last teeth in the back of the mouth used to grind and crush food.

Oral cavity Beginning of the GI tract where food and drink are mechanically broken down by chewing.

Parotid salivary glands Glands that assist with chewing and swallowing of food by lubricating with saliva.

Peristalsis Unconscious, wave-like motion or contraction of the smooth muscle in the intestinal walls necessary to move contents through the GI tract.

Pharyngoesophageal sphincter Muscular ring located at the beginning of the esophagus.

Pharynx Passageway more commonly referred to as the throat allowing for food and air to pass.

Premolars Flat teeth located behind the canine teeth used to crush food.

Pulp Connective tissue inside the tooth beneath the dentin layer supplying it with nerves and blood.

Pyloric sphincter Muscular ring that prevents stomach contents from prematurely moving into the duodenum.

Pylorus Funnel-shaped, terminal end of the stomach.

Small intestine Nearly 20-foot-long, hollow organ consisting of three parts, the duodenum, jejunum and ileum that is located between the stomach and large intestine.

Stomach Pear-shaped organ located between the esophagus and small intestine.

Sublingual salivary glands Salivary glands located between the tongue and mandible on each side of the mouth, which also happen to be the smallest of the three salivary glands.

Submandibular salivary glands Salivary glands located under the jaw.

Vagus nerve Tenth cranial nerve, responsible for motor and sensory input in the digestive tract organs.

8-1 ORAL CAVITY

In this section you will journey through the upper GI tract from the mouth to the small intestines. The mouth is where food is mechanically broken down by chewing. Also known as the **oral cavity**, it has a mucosal lining, like other parts of this tract, Figure 8-1. The labia or lips act as a door to allow for the intake of food, and their movement articulates speech. The top of the oral cavity consists of the soft and hard palates; the tongue is located on the bottom. The small dangling piece of tissue that resembles a punching bag is called the uvula. The oral chamber is separated from the throat or pharynx by the uvula and where the tongue is attached. The uvula assists in swallowing and prevents substances from coming out of the oral cavity and into the nasal cavity or nose. Also found in the back of this cavity are lingual tonsils, which are part of the lymphatic system and serve as a guardian to this importance entrance to help fight infection.

8-1a Oral Cavity Glands

The tongue provides the body with the ability to taste and sense hot or cold. The tongue also aids in chewing by moving food around and assists with swallowing and speaking. As a kid, have you ever held your tongue in place with your fingers and tried to talk? It does not sound the same as when your tongue is free to move about on its own.

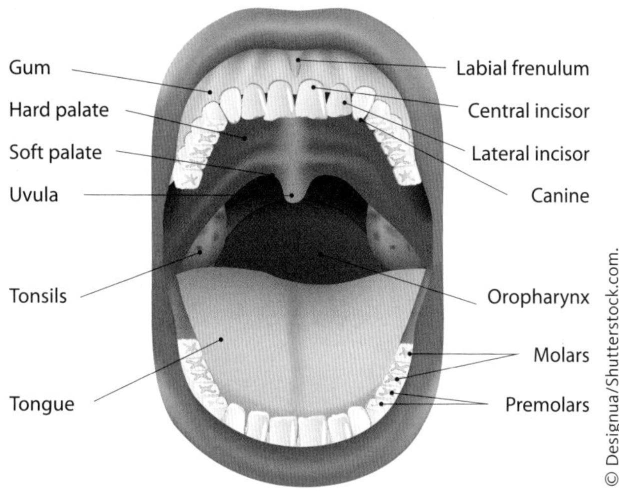

FIGURE 8-1 Basic anatomy of the oral cavity.

Another important feature found in the mouth are three salivary glands controlled by the autonomic system, so they operate on their own, without conscious effort. These glands produce enzymes to help increase the speed of the digestive process. The **submandibular salivary glands** are found inside of both sides of the mandible. The **sublingual salivary glands** are the smallest of the three glands and are found in a small space under the tongue. The **parotid salivary glands** are the largest of the three glands and are found in front of and just below both ears. See Figure 8-2.

8-1b Teeth

Another important feature in the mouth is the teeth, which come in many different types as shown in Table 8-1. Teeth mechanically break down food into manageable pieces, allowing us to swallow and to assist in the digestive process.

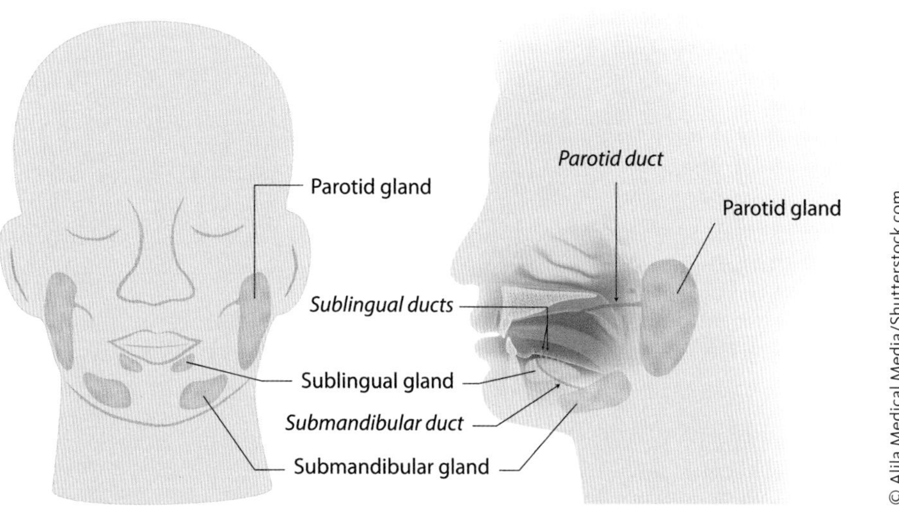

FIGURE 8-2 The salivary glands.

Table 8-1 Types of Teeth

TYPE	DEFINITION
Incisors	Blade-shaped teeth used to cut food; located in the front of the mouth.
Canines (Eye teeth or cuspids)	Used to cut, tear, and hold food.
Premolars or **bicuspids**	Transitional teeth used to grind food; four of these are found on each side of the mouth, two on top and two on bottom.
Molars	Used to grind and crush food; have flat tops.

We only get two sets of teeth in our lifetime. The first teeth are known as our primary or deciduous teeth, more commonly known as baby teeth, which appear from 6 months of age to 2½ years. A way to remember that baby teeth are called deciduous teeth is to think of a deciduous forest, which consists of trees that lose their leaves, just as we lose our baby teeth.

After we lose our primary teeth, 21 permanent teeth take their place around the ages of 6–12. The exception to this is our wisdom teeth, which make their appearance when we are about 21 years old and hopefully a lot wiser.

CLINICAL CONNECTION 8.1

IDENTIFYING TEETH

We have many teeth in our mouth, or at least we should. So, how do dental workers label teeth to keep accurate records when charting or communicating with other clinicians? As an adult, you may have heard the dentist call one of your teeth 9 or 7. This is because adult teeth are labeled numerically. Baby teeth, however, are identified alphabetically.

Although our teeth are not the same in shape, they have a similar interior. Every healthy tooth has a root, neck, and crown. In short, the crown is the part of the tooth that we see. The neck is the portion between the crown and the root. The root is anchored into the gum, where it is connected to nerves and a blood supply.

Our teeth are made up of different layers, Figure 8-3. The outer layer of the **crown** has a very hard covering called **enamel**, which is the hardest material produced by our body. The next layer, found below the enamel, is **dentin**, which is a bone-like substance. Underneath the dentin layer is connective tissue called **pulp**, which is found within the pulp cavity. It is inside this pulp cavity that the nerves and blood vessels are located, by way of the root canal. The gums help keep our teeth in place by making a tight seal around our teeth to prevent foreign debris and bacteria from contacting the **cementum**, which is the thin bony tissue layer covering the root.

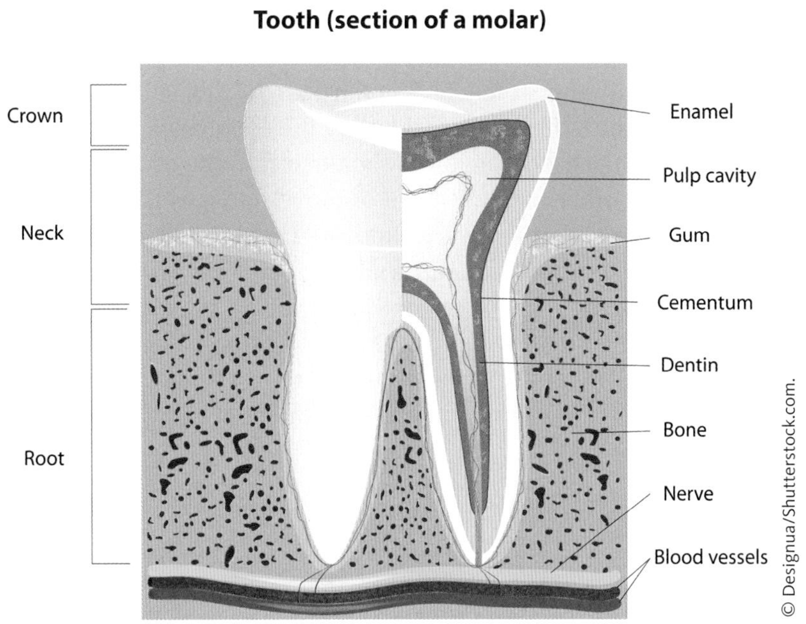

Tooth (section of a molar)

Crown
Neck
Root
Enamel
Pulp cavity
Gum
Cementum
Dentin
Bone
Nerve
Blood vessels

FIGURE 8-3 Anatomy of a tooth.

8-2 PHARYNX

After food leaves the oral area, it must travel through the **pharynx**, a hollow muscular passageway commonly called the throat. The pharynx has three parts: the nasopharynx, oropharynx, and laryngopharynx. Breathing, eating, and drinking are all be accomplished within these passageways. In the respiratory chapter, we will discuss the nasopharynx in relationship to breathing, while food and beverages must travel within the oropharynx.

What directs air into the lungs and food and liquid into the esophagus for digestions? When you swallow, the passageways to the respiratory tract are protected by the epiglottis, which covers the airway during swallowing, while the soft palate blocks the nasopharynx to prevent food from going up your nose.

8-3 ESOPHAGUS

The act of swallowing closes off the epiglottis, thus shutting the door to the opening of the trachea, which leads into the lungs. The food is now forced through the only other open tube or passageway, which is the esophagus. The **esophagus** is a muscular tube about 10 inches long, reaching from the pharynx through the thoracic cavity to the peritoneal cavity, where it meets the stomach. The esophagus, unlike the trachea, does not have cartilaginous rings, so it remains collapsed until food passes through. As the food moves through the esophagus, the content reaches a muscular ringed structure called the **pharyngoesophageal sphincter**. When swallowed contents reach this sphincter, it relaxes. allowing food into the esophagus.

The esophagus consists of muscles: a longitudinal layer and circular muscle layer. To move food through the esophagus and reach the stomach, the muscles of the esophagus contract, making a wave-like motion called **peristalsis**.

After the contents make their way through the esophagus, the **cardiac sphincter** or **lower esophageal sphincter (LES)** relaxes to allow food to move into the stomach. The purpose of this sphincter is to keep gastric acids within the stomach from entering the esophagus. We will discuss the issues that arise when gastric acid does make it into the esophagus later in this chapter.

Another handy feature of our esophagus that helps transport food to our stomach is that it is very slippery. This lubrication is caused by the esophagus excreting mucus from its walls. A sip of hot liquid burns your tongue, but you don't feel any heat after it is swallowed because of the thick cellular mucus layer that makes up the esophageal walls. This lining of stratified squamous epithelium makes the esophagus resistant to extreme temperature, irritation from chemicals, and even abrasions. Figure 8-4 shows the relationship of these structures.

8-4 STOMACH

From the esophagus, the food or liquid enters the **stomach**, which is located below our diaphragm in the left central region of our abdominal cavity. The length of most people's stomachs is about 10 inches, however, the diameter varies, depending on how much a person can eat. Our stomach has the ability to increase and decrease its size, thanks to a feature called rugae. Rugae are folds covered in mucus that give the stomach the ability to change its size, similar to the action of an accordion.

The stomach secretes enzymes and gastric juices to assist digestion, and it also absorbs small amounts of water to form a small ball of food, called **chyme**, which then leaves the stomach by way of the **pyloric sphincter** and enters the duodenum (the first part of the small intestine). It can take as long as 4 hours

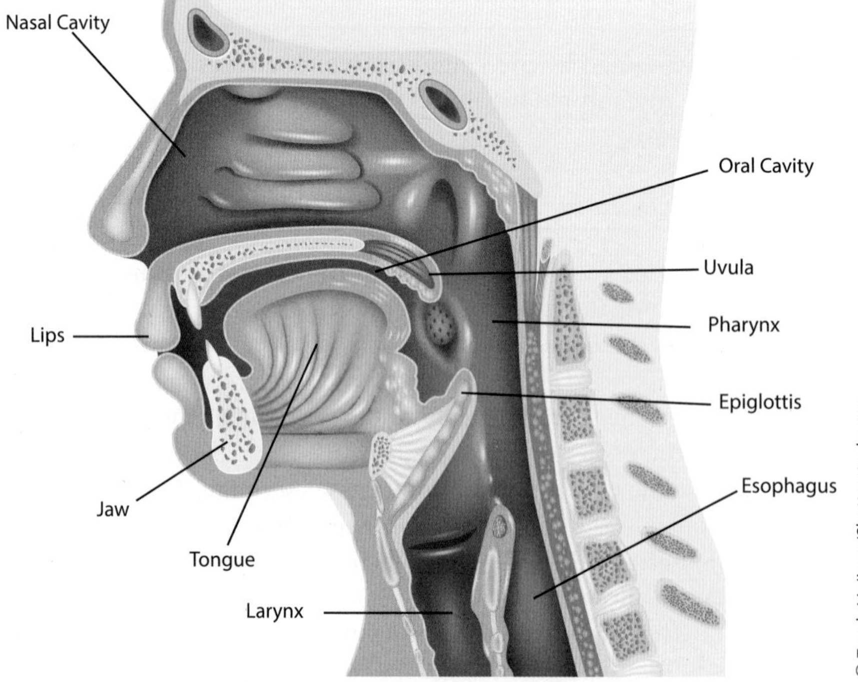

FIGURE 8-4 Image of the oral portion of the digestive tract.

Table 8-2 Four Sections of the Stomach

REGION	DEFINITION/LOCATION
Cardiac	Encompasses the lower esophageal sphincter (LES) or cardiac sphincter; this area gives the term heartburn its name.
Fundus	Food contents are briefly held here before they enter the stomach; located laterally and superiorly of the cardiac region.
Body	The largest part of the stomach and the middle portion.
Pylorus	End of the stomach; resembles a funnel.

for food to pass through the stomach; fluids pass faster than solid contents. Contents high in protein can take a little longer than 4 hours to pass, while fats take the longest, up to 6 hours.

Although it contains gastric juices that can cause irritation to the esophagus, the stomach does not usually become irritated or injure itself. The stomach actually has a barrier of protection set up by mucous cells, which produce a thick secretion of mucus that lines the organ. This ability is tied into the autonomic system's parasympathetic branch, which provides homeostasis and daily maintenance. The **vagus nerve** is what integrates the stomach secretion ability into the nervous system. In essence, when the stomach moves around due to having food or liquid within, the signal is sent to produce more protective mucus secretion.

The stomach itself is divided into four sections as described in Table 8-2 and shown in Figure 8-5.

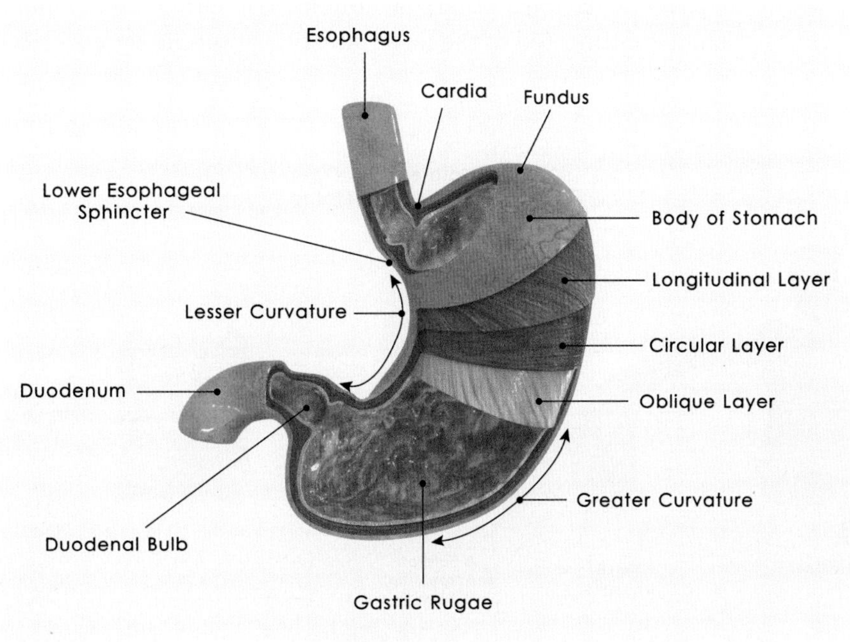

FIGURE 8-5 Anatomy of the stomach.

CLINICAL CONNECTION 8.2

IN THE STOMACH

Our stomach cells produce hydrochloric acid secreted from parietal cells and pepsinogen from chief cells. When these two secretions come together, they create pepsin, which breaks down proteins in meat that we consume.

8-5 SMALL INTESTINE

The **small intestine** is the bridge between the stomach and the large intestine, and is where nutrient absorption takes place. This organ is about 20 feet long and is 1–1½ inches in diameter. Located in the central and lower regions of the abdominal cavity, the small intestine is where most of the contents we consume are digested.

The walls of the small intestine emit digestive enzymes, and up to 80% of nutrient absorption occurs as the chyme substance contacts the intestinal wall. Contents absorbed into the bloodstream are water, vitamins, amino acids, sugars, fatty acids, and ions.

This long organ has three parts: the duodenum, jejunum, and ileum.

The first section, the **duodenum**, is where contents enter after being received from the stomach. The stomach does not push all of its contents out at one time. The pyloric valve allows for small amounts of chyme to enter the small intestine. The duodenum is about 10–12 inches long. Interestingly enough, this section gets its name from its length. *Duo* means two and *denum* means 10, and their sum is 12, which is the number of finger widths that add up to 10 inches.

Located in the mid-section of the small intestine, between the duodenum and the ileum, is the **jejunum**, which is 8 feet long.

The third and last section of the small intestine is the **ileum**, which is 6–12 feet long, longer than the combined length of duodenum and jejunum. The ileum is connected to the large intestine at the **ileocecal valve**. See Figure 8-6.

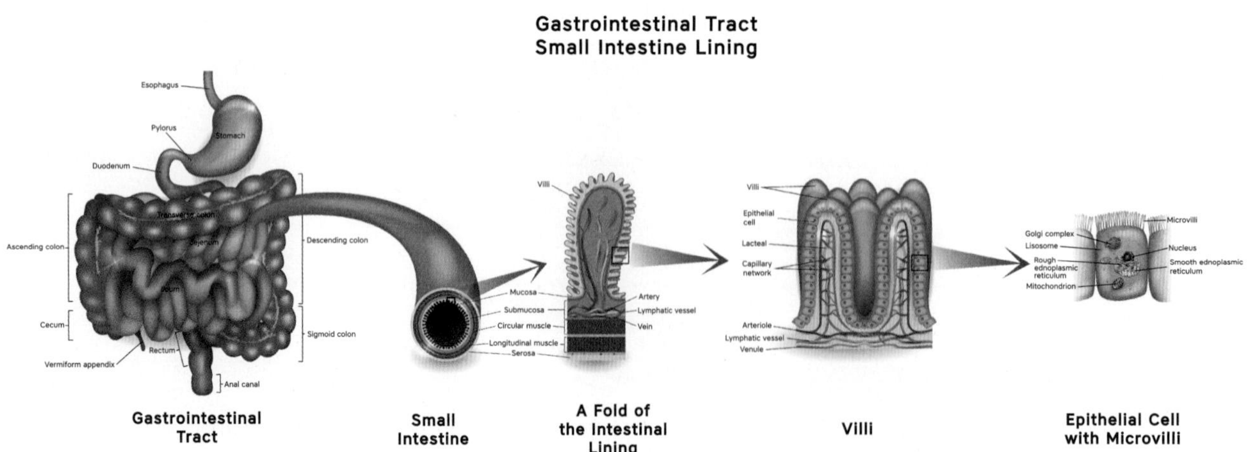

FIGURE 8-6 Anatomy of intestinal lining showing its vascular nature at a micro level.

LEARNING OBJECTIVE 8.2 **Describe the pathopharmacology of the upper gastrointestinal tract.**

KEY TERMS

Achlorhydria Absence of hydrochloric acid in stomach acid.

Antacids Medication taken to neutralize stomach acid.

Barrett's esophagus Damage caused by chronic acid reflux causing the cells to change from its normal squamous cells to a specialized intestinal metaplasia cell found in the small intestine.

Beta blockers Drugs causing decreased heart rate.

Cavities Small holes that can develop in teeth.

Crohn's disease Common, chronic inflammatory bowel disease causing inflammation in the lining of the digestive system.

Duodenal ulcer Peptic ulcer located in the duodenum.

Endoscopic mucosal resection Removal of abnormal lesions with a scope instrument.

Esophageal varices Dilated (varicose) veins in the lower portion of the esophagus.

Esophagogastroduodenoscopy (EGD) Upper GI endoscopy used to diagnose and treat.

Gastric cancer Cancer of the stomach.

Gastritis Inflammation of the lining of the stomach.

Gastroenteritis Inflammation of the gastrointestinal tract.

Gastroesophageal reflux disease (GERD) Flow of gastric juices from the stomach into the esophagus.

Gastrointestinal stromal tumors (GIST) Tumors that develop from the walls of the GI tract from cells in the autonomic system responsible for regulating the body's digestion.

H-2 blockers Medication used to block the production of stomach acid.

Helicobacter pylori Gram-negative bacterium that can cause stomach ulcers.

Hiatal hernia Portion of the stomach pushes through the diaphragm.

Inguinal hernia Intestinal tissue pushes through a weakened area of the abdomen wall.

Malabsorption syndrome Condition preventing the absorption of nutrients in the small intestine.

Oral cancer Mouth cancer.

Peptic ulcers Crater-like lesions that may occur in the esophagus, stomach, or duodenum.

Periodontal disease Destructive gum disease.

Pharyngitis Inflammation of the pharynx.

Proton pump inhibitors Medication used to reduce the amount of acid produced.

Sclerosing Irritates tissue causing an inflammatory response to initiate fibrosis or scarring.

Squamous cell carcinoma Cancer developing from an abnormal growth of squamous cells.

Subtotal gastrectomy Removal of part of the stomach, usually the lower portion.

Total gastrectomy Removal of the stomach in its entirety.

8-6 DISEASES OF THE MOUTH

When thinking about diseases of the mouth, most people think of a cavity or someone with bad breath. However, mouth diseases often develop over time and can be quite serious. Bacteria harbored in the mouth over time can actually cause heart disease. That is why poor oral hygiene can be a risk factor for developing cardiac disease. Other serious diseases, such as cancer, can also affect this cavity.

8-6a Mouth Cancer

As with other regions of the body, the mouth, too, can be affected by cancer. Statistically speaking, one person dies every hour each and every day from mouth cancer. Those affected with this type of cancer have a bleak survival rate of only 57 %, according to the Oral Cancer Foundation.

Oral cancer is typically found in men in the lower lip region, although it also can be located in the tongue, gums, cheek, or palate. One of the most common types of oral cancer found on the lips is **squamous cell carcinoma**.

Oral cancers can be attributed mainly to tobacco usage, including both smoke and smokeless varieties; sun exposure is also a known cause. See Figure 8-7. When a patient encounters this disease, symptoms include a small whitish bump on the affected oral tissue that is often painless.

When cancer is suspected, testing must be done to ensure a correct diagnosis. This is done by taking a tissue biopsy of the tissue lump. After confirmed cancerous, treating with regimens of chemotherapy and radiation can begin in an effort to decrease the likelihood of metastasis before it is surgically removed.

The primary method used to treat oral cancer is chemotherapy such as cisplatin. This anticancer drug also goes by the brand names Platinol-AQ and Platinol. There is no pill form; it must be given intravenously.

To prevent this disease from occurring, sunscreen and limited sun exposure are recommended, as well as the wearing of protective gear, such as hats, to shade the face from the sun's harmful rays. Another critical measure in preventing mouth cancer is to stay away from any tobacco usage.

8-6b Periodontal Disease

The word periodontal means around the teeth, which describes the gums. **Periodontal disease** primarily affects adults and those older in age. This disease causes structural problems in the mouth by damaging the gums, which help keep your teeth anchored in place. (See Figure 8-8.) The main cause of periodontal disease is poor oral hygiene and diet. There is a saying: "You don't have to floss all of your teeth, just the ones you want to keep." People who lack proper teeth cleaning have a much greater risk of developing periodontal disease.

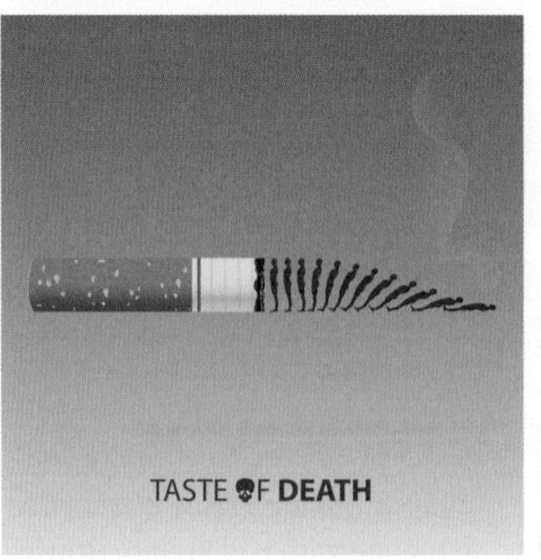

FIGURE 8-7 Greatly decrease the odds of oral cancer by not using tobacco products.

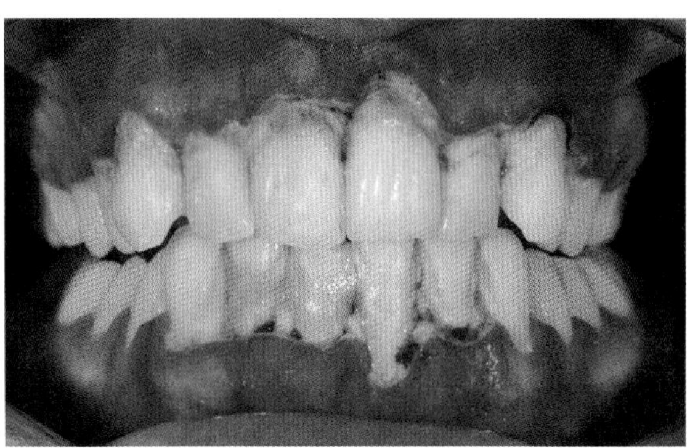

FIGURE 8-8 Periodontal disease.

Symptoms of this condition include red and inflamed gums to the point where they bleed and become painful. To diagnose, the dentist will do a visual inspection of the oral cavity and use a small ruler called a probe to measure the depth of the pocket in which the tooth sits. If the gums are healthy, the pocket should measure between 1 and 3 millimeters.

Treatment of periodontal disease requires cleaning plaque off the teeth and treating inflammation. Drugs used to treat gum disease come in many different forms. Oral antibiotics can be taken to manage infected gums; they are used only on a short-term basis to treat an acute infection. Another form of antibiotic is used to decrease the periodontal pockets and keep bacterial growth in check. An antibiotic called minocycline, which is in the form of tiny spherical particles, is placed into the pockets by a periodontist and then releases over a period of time.

Another type of antibiotic that is directly placed into the gum pocket is doxycycline, which is a gel and basically works the same as minocycline. An antimicrobial implant called a PerioChip (chlorhexidine gluconate) is a gelatin implant placed directly into the dental pockets to be released over time. Finally, the last form of medication we will discuss is an antimicrobial mouth rinse. The drug found in this type of mouth wash is called chlorhexidine.

The best way to manage periodontal disease is to prevent it from occurring. This means brushing and flossing regularly and routine dental appointments to clean your teeth and prevent plaque build-up and gingivitis.

8-6c Cavities (Dental Caries)

When it comes to cavities, poor dental hygiene again comes to mind. Inside the mouth, microorganisms routinely assault the teeth and gums. This bacterium is found in plaque, the same substance that is found on the surface of our enamel and tends to sit in the tough-to-reach cracks of our teeth, near the gum line.

Coffee, tea, and citrus fruit cause damage to teeth because of their acidic content. Plaque is an acidic substance that sticks in crevasses of our teeth. The bacteria in the plaque cause the acid to wear away at the enamel, eventually making a hole or cavity in the tooth and potentially causing pain, Figure 8-9.

A dental hygienist or dentist can spot cavities on the visible regions of our teeth, but an X-ray is required to check difficult to see areas, such as between the teeth.

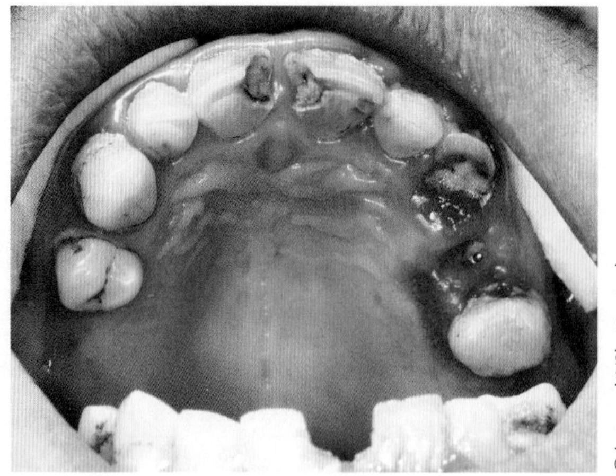

© botazsolti/Shutterstock.com.

FIGURE 8-9 Pictured is a diseased mouth complete with caries (cavities).

If decay is not too bad, the cavity can be filled. The dentist will inject the gum near and around the affected tooth with a local anesthetic such as Novocain (procaine) to numb the tooth's nerves before drilling out the damaged portion of tooth and inserting a filling. Sometimes, a crown or root canal might be required. If the decay is too severe and the tooth cannot be salvaged, it might need to be extracted.

Cavities can be prevented by routine oral cleaning and dental cleanings. Using mouth rinse and toothpaste with fluoride, along with water supplemented with fluoride, will decrease the chances of having a cavity. Another way is to decrease the amount of sugar (carbohydrates) ingested.

8-6d Summary of Diseases of the Mouth

See Table 8-3 for a summary of diseases of the mouth.

Table 8-3 Diseases of the Mouth

DISEASE/ CONDITION	ETIOLOGY	MAJOR SIGNS/ SYMPTOMS	DIAGNOSTIC TESTS	MAIN PHARMACOLOGIC TREATMENT
Mouth cancer	Tobacco Sun exposure	Small lump White coloration	Tissue biopsy	Anticancer: Platinol-AQ and Platinol Chemotherapy: Cisplatin
Periodontal disease	Poor oral hygiene Old age	Swollen Painful bloody gums	Inserting a probe to measure tooth pocket	Oral antibiotics: Minocycline Doxycycline Antimicrobial implant: PerioChip (chlorhexidine gluconate) Antimicrobial mouth rinse: Chlorhexidine
Dental caries	Poor dental hygiene Poor diet	Pain	Oral exam X-ray	Analgesic Local anesthetic: Novocain (procaine)

8-7 DISEASES OF THE PHARYNX AND ESOPHAGUS

Leaving the mouth, we will discuss the ailments that can affect the pharynx and esophagus.

8-7a Pharyngitis

A painful, scratchy, and inflamed throat is called **pharyngitis**, which can be caused by viral or bacterial microorganisms. Tonsillitis, a common type of pharyngitis, is caused by microorganisms. An acute form of pharyngitis is strep throat, which is caused by *Streptococcus* bacteria (Figure 8-10). This type of infection can be more than just a nuisance; it can be dangerous if it gets into the patient's bloodstream, where it can cause serious complications, such as endocarditis or glomerulonephritis.

A throat culture is performed to determine whether a patient's sore throat is caused by *streptococci*. The physician uses what appears to be a large cotton swab to rub the back of the throat to obtain secretions. The swab is then sent to a lab where it can be examined for strep. Another and much faster way to test for strep is by using a rapid antigen test, which can identify the presence of antigens in the throat. This takes only minutes to perform.

If the sore throat is identified as strep, it must be treated using antibiotics such as amoxicillin, cephalexin, and penicillin. To help alleviate symptoms such as pain, inflammation, and fever, over-the-counter agents, such as acetaminophen and ibuprofen, can be used.

Use proper hand washing techniques and avoid individuals who are sick to prevent this condition. Also, after you have overcome this illness, throw away your old toothbrush because it can harbor infectious organisms and cause you to become re-infected.

8-7b Gastroesophageal Reflux Disease

The cardiac sphincter, located in the lower end of the esophagus, usually prevents stomach acids from backing up into the esophagus. However, when gastric juices overcome this mechanism and make their way past the cardiac sphincter, the individual experiences what is commonly known as heartburn. This reflux or movement of acid from the stomach to the esophagus is known as **gastroesophageal reflux disease (GERD)**, Figure 8-11.

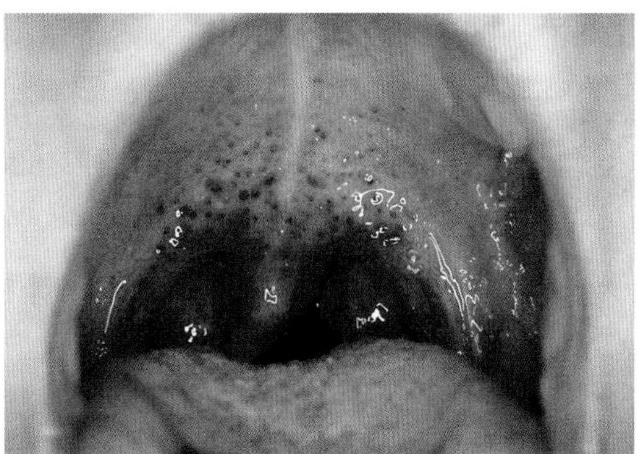

Centers for Disease Control and Prevention/Heinz F. Eichenwald, MD

FIGURE 8-10 Strep throat.

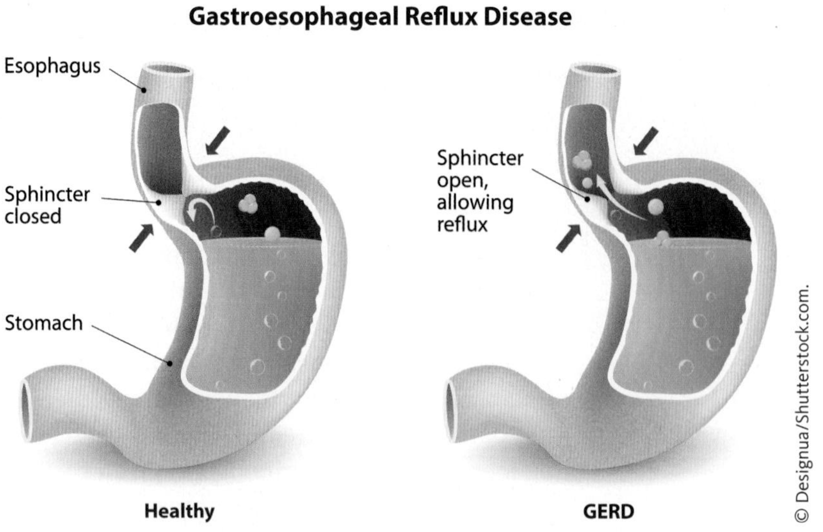

Gastroesophageal Reflux Disease

Esophagus
Sphincter closed
Stomach
Sphincter open, allowing reflux
Healthy
GERD

© Designua/Shutterstock.com.

FIGURE 8-11 Image shows how a slightly opened cardiac sphincter can allow stomach acid to enter into the esophagus, causing GERD.

Symptoms of GERD include heartburn and a burning sensation in the epigastric region. Other symptoms include a sour taste in your mouth, chest pain, hoarseness, dry cough, difficulty swallowing, or feeling like there is a lump in the throat. This acidic reflux action can be damaging if it is a chronic occurrence, eventually causing ulcers, bleeding, and even scarring. This scarring will cause the individual to have difficulty with swallowing. Occasional heartburn is no cause for alarm, but a person who experiences episodes twice a week or more should seek medical attention. The acidic contents will cause esophagitis and eventually lead to a precancerous condition known as **Barrett's esophagus**.

GERD can be diagnosed by using many different tests. Endoscopy involves a flexible tube, equipped with a camera, guided down the throat and into the esophagus to look for signs of erosion and to collect tissue samples for examination. Another method is a barium swallow. The patient is instructed to drink a liquid that coats the lining of the esophagus. This allows the physician to get a better view of the esophagus, stomach, and duodenum on an X-ray film.

The last method we will mention is an esophageal pH test. A probe is inserted via a catheter placed through the patient's nose. After it is in the esophagus, the probe monitors the acid level by connecting it to a small, portable computer worn by the patient for 24 hours.

Treatment of GERD can be as simple as changing the patient's diet (limiting caffeine and spicy foods). If a change in diet is not enough, medications, including stool softeners, laxatives, and antacids, can be used to treat GERD successfully. To prevent GERD from occurring, the patient is urged to maintain a healthy diet and exercise regimen.

Table 8-4 lists medications used to treat acid reflux, and can be referred to for other acidic stomach conditions that will be discussed in this module.

Another approach to correcting acid reflux is to reduce or block acid production to give the esophageal tissue time to heal. This action can be

Table 8-4 Medications Used to Treat Acid Reflux

Proton pump inhibitors INHIBIT RELEASE OF ACID	H-2 blockers BLOCK RECEPTORS THAT PRODUCE ACID	Antacids HELP TO NEUTRALIZE ACID ALREADY PRESENT
Prilosec (omeprazole)	Zantac (ranitidine)	Rolaids
Protonix (pantoprazole)	Pepcid (famotidine)	Maalox
Nexium (esomeprazole)	Axid (nizatidine)	Mylanta
Prevacid (lansoprazole)	Tagamet (cimetidine)	Tums

accomplished by proton pump inhibitors that reduce acid production, such as Prilosec OTC (omeprazole) and Prevacid 24 HR (lansoprazole).

The third method used to stop symptoms of heartburn is by blocking the amount of acid produced by using acid blocking medicine such as Pepcid AC (famotidine) or Zantac 75 (ranitidine).

If these medications still don't stop the symptoms, a stronger form may be prescribed. Preventative therapy such as avoiding alcohol, smoking, spicy foods, and caffeine can be helpful in reducing episodes of acid reflux.

8-7c Hiatal Hernia

In our diaphragm is a hole called a hiatus, through which the esophagus goes to reach the stomach. Unfortunately, it is possible for part of the stomach to push through this hole because of a weakened diaphragmatic muscle as shown in Figure 8-12. This might be caused by heavy lifting, coughing, vomiting, or injury to that area. When this condition occurs, the patient might be asymptomatic or might complain of GERD.

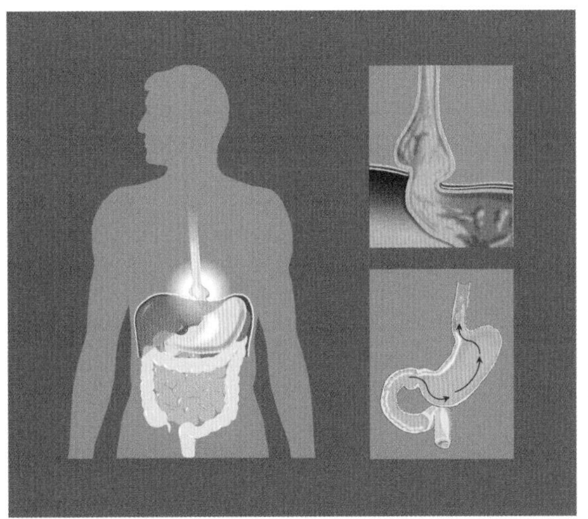

FIGURE 8-12 This image shows how stomach acid can reach the esophagus because of a hiatal hernia.

Confirmation of a **hiatal hernia** can be done by an upper GI X-ray (barium swallow), or an endoscopy examination or manometry, which is performed by inserting a pressure-sensitive catheter through the patient's nose, through the esophagus, and into the stomach. The catheter then measures pressure levels in the esophagus.

An operation likely will not be needed to manage this condition, unless it is an emergency. Medications prescribed are typically the same as those used for heartburn to control acid reflux. OTC antacids such as Rolaids, Tums, Mylanta, or Maalox can provide fast relief to heartburn symptoms by neutralizing stomach acid.

8-7d Esophageal Varices

From medical terminology, you learned that *varix* (plural: *varices*) means varicose veins. Esophageal varices are varicose veins in the esophagus, even though you might have thought they affect only the legs (see Figure 8-13).

Esophageal varices are caused by high pressure within the veins. Any condition that causes venous congestion in the liver, including a liver obstruction, can cause enlargement of the esophageal veins.

This condition can be life-threatening; treatment is aimed at preventing bleeding from a burst vein. Symptoms of this condition are black stool from blood passing through the GI tract, or vomiting blood.

To diagnose, an endoscopic exam can be done to look for dilated veins in the esophagus. This condition also can be suspected if there are signs of chronic liver disease. To confirm the diagnosis, an **esophagogastroduodenoscopy (EGD)** is done.

Portal vein bypass surgery can be performed to decrease venous pressure in the portal vein of the liver, and some medications can reduce liver congestion. For example, beta blockers decrease blood pressure in the portal vein to lessen pressure in the esophageal veins. Examples of **beta blockers** are Inderal (propranolol) and Corgard (nadolol).

If a vein looks as though it will burst, an elastic band can be used to tie off blood flow through that particular vessel (band litigation).

Esophageal Varices

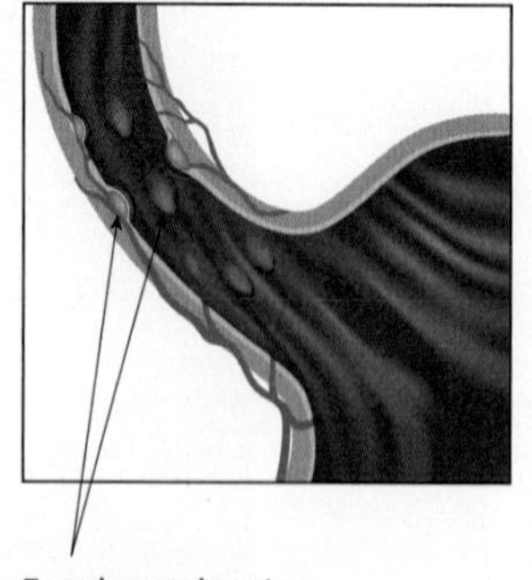

FIGURE 8-13 Varicose veins in the esophagus.

Another way to treat bleeding is by using a **sclerosing** agent, which hardens the vessels and destroys them to prevent blood flow. This technique is used for chronic bleeding. If the bleed is acute, pressure can be applied to the site by nasogastric tube or lavaging the site with cold saline to constrict the vessels.

8-7e Summary of Diseases of the Pharynx and Esophagus

Table 8-5 will summarize the conditions and medications discussed thus far.

Table 8-5 Summary of Pathopharmacology of Diseases of the Pharynx and Esophagus

DISEASE/ CONDITION	ETIOLOGY	MAJOR SIGNS/ SYMPTOMS	DIAGNOSTIC TESTS	MAIN PHARMACOLOGIC TREATMENT
Pharyngitis	Viral or bacterial microorganism	Pain Inflammation Fever	Throat culture	Antibiotics: Amoxicillin Cephalexin Penicillin Pain relievers: Acetaminophen Ibuprofen
GERD	Gastric juices going past the cardiac sphincter Poor diet	Heartburn Sour taste Chest pain Hoarseness Dry cough Difficulty swallowing Lump-like feeling in the throat Ulcers Bleeding Scarring	Endoscopy Barium swallow Esophageal pH test	Stool softeners Laxatives Antacids
Hiatal hernia	Heavy lifting Pregnancy Coughing Vomiting Injury	Acid reflux	Barium swallow Endoscopy Manometry	OTC antacids Proton pump inhibitors H-2 blockers
Esophageal varices	Increased pressure from liver disease or blockage	Black stool Vomiting blood	Endoscopy Esophago-gastroduo-denoscopy	Beta blockers: Inderal (propranolol) and Corgard (nadolol) Sclerosing agents

8-8 STOMACH DISEASES

Our stomach, shown in Figure 8-14, plays a major role in our digestive system. This chamber acts much like a cement mixer as it churns food and drink with gastric juices to further break down ingested contents. This stretchable, pear-shaped organ is located in the upper left side of the abdomen and is found in-between the esophagus and the small intestine. This section will focus on many diseases that are chronic in nature and have the possibility of becoming life-threatening if not properly managed.

8-8a Gastritis

Gastritis is not a certain type of disease, but rather, it describes many different conditions that cause inflammation of the stomach lining. Gastritis can be acute or chronic, and is commonly caused by overuse of NSAIDs (aspirin and ibuprofen). Other contributing factors are drinking alcohol and smoking, as well as certain types of bacteria known to cause gastritis, called ***Helicobacter pylori***. People especially affected with chronic gastritis might be linked to this bacterium, because it is known to weaken the mucous lining of the stomach, allowing the walls to become exposed to stomach acids and bacteria.

Gastritis also can be caused by a lack of stomach acid, which kills the bacteria that have been ingested. The amount of stomach acid also decreases with age, leading to a condition called **achlorhydria**, meaning no hydrochloric acid. Another cause can be from an autoimmune disease that allows the body to attack cells of the stomach lining.

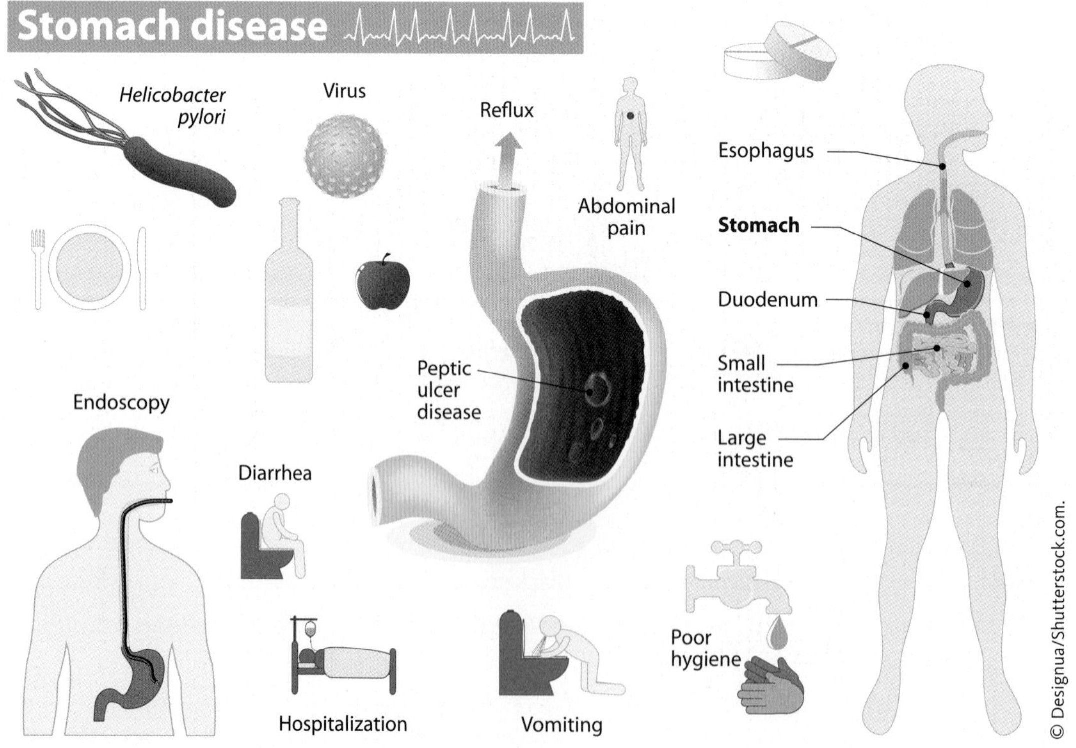

FIGURE 8-14 Infographic about stomach disease.

Those affected by gastritis often exert symptoms of nausea, indigestion, abdominal pain, vomiting, and belching. However, not everyone shows signs or symptoms.

An upper GI endoscopy helps diagnose the patient by letting the physician see what is going on in the stomach. A barium swallow also can be performed, and a stool sample can be checked for blood and the presence of *H. pylori* bacterium. A blood sample might be taken to check for anemia. A patient interview might provide clues, as well, such as if symptoms increase after taking certain pain relievers.

Medications are given to decrease stomach acid production over a period of time to allow the tissue to heal. If a bacterium was the cause, an antibiotic will be required; changing the patient's lifestyle also can be helpful. For example, avoiding certain foods or avoiding alcohol consumption should decrease the odds of a flare-up. Lists of drugs used to treat gastritis are as follows:

Antibiotics to treat *H. pylori*:

- Biaxin (clarithromycin)
- Flagyl (metronidazole)
- Moxatag (amoxicillin)

Proton pump inhibitors are used to stop acid production and allow healing to occur. Examples of the kinds of medications used are:

- Prilosec (omeprazole)
- Protonix (pantoprazole)
- Nexium (esomeprazole)
- Prevacid (lansoprazole)

Agents called H-2 blockers or H2 receptor antagonists are used to decrease the production of acid (known as histamine). These examples include:

- Zantac (ranitidine)
- Pepcid (famotidine)
- Axid (nizatidine)
- Tagamet (cimetidine)

Finally, antacids are used to neutralize stomach acid and quickly give relief to symptoms such as pain and indigestion. Examples include Rolaids, Maalox, Mylanta, and Tums.

8-8b Peptic Ulcer

Peptic ulcers are not caused by a poor diet or high stress levels, contrary to what many believe. These crater-like ulcers are linked to certain medications and *H. pylori* bacterium. In addition, overproduction of pepsin also can cause these ulcers to develop. Pepsin is produced by the stomach to break down proteins. Peptic ulcers include esophageal, gastric, and duodenal ulcers. See Figure 8-15.

The main symptom associated with this condition is abdominal pain. Pain can be worse on an empty stomach. Bleeding can occur, causing vomiting a substance that might be red or black in color.

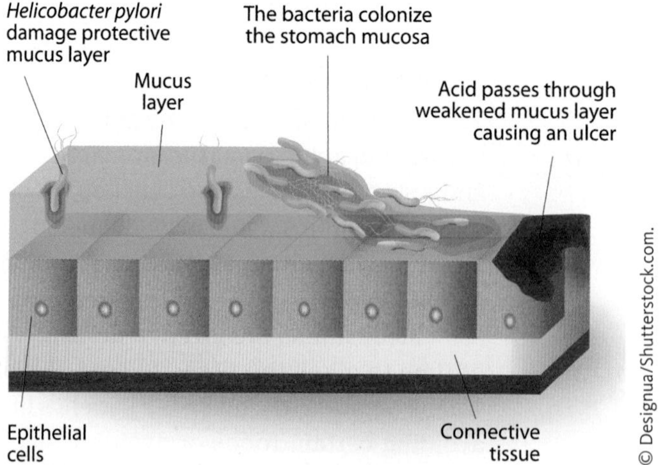

FIGURE 8-15 This image shows how *H. pylori* bacterium can cause an ulcer.

To ensure a correct diagnosis, tests such as a barium swallow are completed. The liquid used in this procedure coats the GI structures, allowing for the ulcers to be seen on film.

The patient also can undergo an endoscopy and stool test for *H. pylori*.

Medications used to treat peptic ulcers are the same as discussed for gastritis to reduce stomach acid and allow time for the damaged tissue to heal. If *H. pylori* is confirmed present, then antibiotics are used.

8-8c Stomach Cancer (Gastric Cancer)

Although not commonly found in the United States, **gastric cancer** often goes undetected until it metastasizes to other regions of the body. The cancer spreads from stomach to other organs nearby, including the esophagus, intestine, and pancreas. If the cancer cells enter the bloodstream and lymphatic system, it can spread throughout the body.

Often diagnosed after age 50, stomach cancer occurs more than twice as often in men than in women. Our diets can increase the risk of developing stomach cancer. Foods high in salt, smoked meats, pickled foods, and other highly processed foods greatly increase the risk for this condition. Smoking, obesity, and *H. pylori* are other causes and risk factors.

Common symptoms of stomach cancer include a loss of appetite, abdominal pain, a feeling of fullness, heartburn, and vomiting.

Testing for gastric cancer include a barium swallow, CT scan, PET scan, and an endoscopy with a biopsy of questionable tissue. The biopsied tissue sample can be sent to a lab for a definite diagnosis.

Treatment of stomach cancer depends on the patient's overall health and cancer stage. Surgery is done to remove all of the cancer while leaving as much of the healthy gastric tissue as possible. Table 8-6 lists and briefly describes the various forms of surgical procedures.

Radiation uses X-ray beams of energy to kill cancer cells, making it a localized therapy. Before undergoing surgery, radiation can shrink stomach cancer tumors to allow for easier removal. This can also be done after the surgery to kill any cancer cells that might still be in that region.

Table 8-6 Surgical Procedures to Remove Stomach Cancer

Endoscopic mucosal resection	Removing gastric cancer from stomach lining
Subtotal gastrectomy	Removing the part of the stomach affected by cancer
Total gastrectomy	Removing the entire stomach and connecting the esophagus to the duodenum

Another cancer treatment is by using chemotherapy, which uses chemicals to kill cancer cells, and similar to radiation, it can be used pre- or post-surgery.

Chemotherapy drugs used to slow or stop cancer cells in the stomach include:

- Taxotere Intravenous (docetaxel)
- Adrucil (fluorouracil)
- Platinol-AQ (cisplatin)

Other drugs are used to treat **gastrointestinal stromal tumors (GIST)**. These tumors can be either malignant or benign. Stromal tumors can be found elsewhere in the body, but one of the most common sites is in the walls of the gastrointestinal system. Stomach cells support organ function and are made of connective tissue cells. Drugs used to target cancer cells are:

- Sutent (sunitinib)
- Stivarga (regorafenib)
- Gleevec (imatinib)

8-9 SMALL INTESTINE DISEASES

Many diseases affect the small intestine, making it even more important to thoroughly investigate the history and signs and symptoms present along with appropriate diagnostic tests.

8-9a Duodenal Ulcer

A **duodenal ulcer** is another type of peptic ulcer, Figure 8-16. Ulcers are crater-like, open sores, but instead of being external, they are found internally in the GI tract. Duodenal ulcers can be caused by certain OTC pain relievers such as aspirin, while other possible causes are from our own stomach acids and bacteria such as *H. pylori*. Refer to Section 8.8b, the peptic ulcer section in stomach diseases, for more information such as symptoms, diagnostics, and treatments.

8-9b Gastroenteritis

Gastroenteritis, shown in Figure 8-17, is a condition consisting of inflammation of the stomach *and* intestine. The occurrence can be caused by three

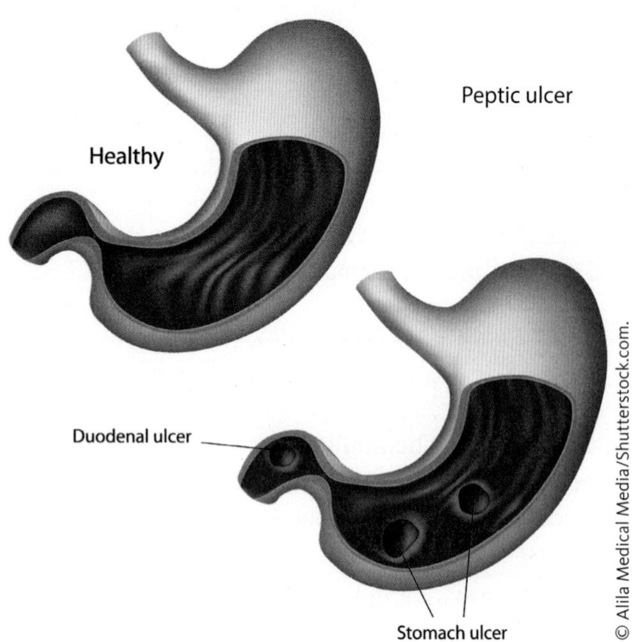

FIGURE 8-16 A duodenal ulcer is the same as a peptic ulcer, but it is located in the duodenum.

Gastroenteritis

Health

Inflammation

© Designua/Shutterstock.com.

FIGURE 8-17 Comparison between the inflammation of the stomach and intestinal tissue and its normal state.

different microorganism sources: bacteria, virus, and parasite. This illness is quite common and can spread by way of food and drink, or even just by coming into contact with someone who is infected. The most common cause is a virus, such as the rotavirus or norovirus that from time to time pops up on cruise ships.

The symptoms of gastroenteritis include nausea, abdominal pain, headache, fever, chills, vomiting, and diarrhea, and can range from mild to severe.

To diagnose the patient, a stool sample might be required to discover the origin (bacterial, viral, or parasite).

This illness usually does not require any treatment; however, antibiotics or antivirals can be given, depending on the cause. Antidiarrheal and antinausea medications also might be used (see Table 8-7). The best way to prevent this illness is maintaining proper hand hygiene.

Table 8-7 Common Types of Antidiarrheal and Antinausea Medications

ANTIDIARRHEAL AGENTS	ANTINAUSEA AGENTS
Lomotil, atropine/diphenoxylate	Anzemet, dolasetron
Imodium, loperamide	Benadryl, diphenhydramine
Kaopectate, bismuth subsalicylate	Emend, aprepitant
Motofen, atropine/difenoxin	Kytril, granisetron
Lonox, atropine/diphenoxylate	Zofran, ondansetron

8-9c Malabsorption Syndrome

Malabsorption syndrome is a term used to describe a wide array of disorders that cause the small intestine not to properly absorb nutrients from digested contents into the bloodstream. Possible causes are insufficient pancreatic function, lactose intolerance, poor bile production, celiac disease, cystic fibrosis, diabetes mellitus, and bacterial growth. The level of severity varies; one patient might have abdominal cramps or an upset stomach while another experiences ulcerative conditions.

Because the varied conditions causing malabsorption syndrome affect the ways fats, sugars, vitamins, proteins, and minerals are absorbed, many different symptoms can be seen. Possible symptoms are:

- Weight loss
- Diarrhea
- Steatorrhea (excess fat discharge in stool)
- Foul smelling, sticky, greasy, and light-colored stool
- Abdominal pain
- Muscle cramping
- Poor growth in children
- Heart arrhythmias
- Anemia
- Blood clotting disorder
- Edema
- Fatigue/weakness
- Decreased bone density.

Many diagnostic exams are required to pinpoint the exact cause, but often begins with a test of the patient's stool. The stool can tell the physician a lot about digestive issues, including whether it contains blood, fat, and parasites. Stool samples are collected over a 3-day period; a measurement of 7 grams of fat is indicative of an absorption disorder. Other tests include imaging via a CT scan, barium swallow, MRI, ultrasound, and an endoscopy. A GI culture can also be done to see if an overgrowth of bacteria is present.

Treatment depends on the cause of the disorder. For example, if the syndrome is caused by the overgrowth of bacteria, then antibiotics are used. To treat inflammation, anti-inflammatory and corticosteroids might be used. Because the body is not getting the nutrition it requires to properly function, vitamins and mineral supplements are taken.

The causes of this syndrome are often hereditary, so it cannot be prevented. However, those caused by dietary elements, such as celiac disease, require the individual to avoid foods containing gluten.

8-9d Regional Enteritis (Crohn's Disease)

Crohn's disease is a type of inflammatory bowel disease with an unknown cause. This disease causes chronic inflammation in the tissue make-up of the walls of the intestines. This condition can occur in both the small and large intestines; however, it is most commonly found in the ileum of the small intestine. This disease causes the patient to experience many recurring exacerbations followed by periods of remissions.

Symptoms of Crohn's disease can happen suddenly, without warning. This makes it that much more difficult for those affected. Common symptoms include abdominal pain and cramping resulting from ulceration and inflammation affecting the movement of contents through the GI tract and possible low-grade fever.

An inconvenient and common symptom is urgent diarrhea, which might require an antidiarrheal agent such as Imodium (loperamide). Bleeding can develop as a result of the ulcerations, leading to blood being found in the patient's stool. The patient also might experience weight loss, a decrease in appetite, flatulence, and even constipation.

A physical and history will help uncover the patient's symptoms. A colonoscopy can be performed to visually inspect the inside of the large intestine with a long flexible scope. A barium swallow is used to check the upper GI tract, while other methods include endoscopy, an MRI, and CT imaging. A patient's stool sample can be tested for blood.

This disease is currently incurable, so treatment focuses on managing symptoms and decreasing inflammation. Drugs used to manage Crohn's include antibiotics such as Cipro (ciprofloxacin) and Flagyl (metronidazole) to help decrease the presence of bacteria causing inflammation and to treat any abscesses present. To reduce inflammation and prevent damage, corticosteroids such as prednisone can be given. Surgery might be required if the patient experiences an obstruction or perforation of the intestine.

8-9e Inguinal Hernia

An **inguinal hernia** can develop from a weakened abdomen or from a birth defect caused by the dissension of the testes from the abdomen to the scrotum. Either way, this condition is more commonly seen in men than women (see Figure 8-18).

This condition can cause problems in the digestive tract and can be life-threatening because part of the small intestine and stomach cavity lining (peritoneum) can protrude into the groin. The affected region can become twisted, preventing blood flow to that portion of the organ. If this is the case, it is called a strangulated hernia.

Those affected experience pain that occurs with lifting and bending. The patient might have a bulge in the groin region. A patient who has episodes of vomiting and nausea likely has a strangulated hernia.

After a physical exam of the groin, a CT and ultrasound can be done to confirm the diagnosis of an inguinal hernia. Surgical intervention is done to correct the problem, while analgesics might be used to control pain if needed.

Table 8-8 summarizes the upper GI conditions and medications discussed thus far.

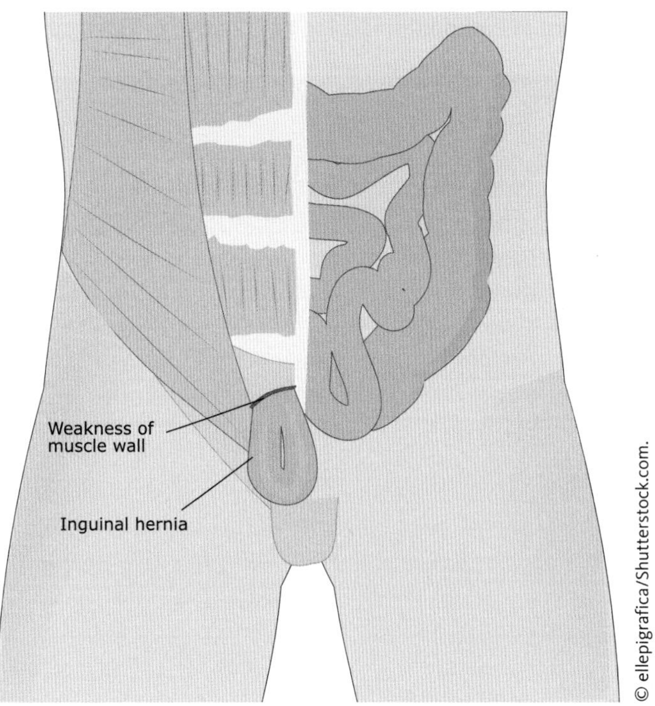

FIGURE 8-18 Pictured is an inguinal hernia because of muscle weakness of the abdominal wall.

Table 8-8 Summary of Pathopharmacology of the Upper Gastrointestinal Tract

DISEASE/ CONDITION	ETIOLOGY	MAJOR SIGNS/ SYMPTOMS	DIAGNOSTIC TESTS	MAIN PHARMACOLOGIC TREATMENT
Gastritis	Pain relievers *H. pylori* Achlorhydria	Nausea Indigestion Abdominal pain Vomiting Belching	Endoscopy Barium swallow Stool sample Blood sample	Antibiotics Proton pump inhibitors H-2 blockers Antacids
Peptic ulcer	Medications *H. pylori* Pepsin	Abdominal pain Bleeding Vomiting	Endoscopy Barium swallow Stool sample	Agents to decrease stomach acid Antibiotics
Stomach cancer	Smoking Obesity *H. pylori* Poor diet	Loss of appetite Abdominal pain Feeling of fullness Heartburn Vomiting	Barium swallow CT scan PET scan Endoscopy with a biopsy	Chemotherapy drugs: Taxotere intravenous (docetaxel) Adrucil (fluorouracil) Platinol-AQ (cisplatin) Sutent (sunitinib) Stivarga (regorafenib) Gleevec (imatinib)

(*continued*)

Table 8-8 Summary of Pathopharmacology of the Upper Gastrointestinal Tract—*continued*

DISEASE/ CONDITION	ETIOLOGY	MAJOR SIGNS/ SYMPTOMS	DIAGNOSTIC TESTS	MAIN PHARMA-COLOGIC TREATMENT
Duodenal ulcer	(See **peptic ulcer**)	(See **peptic ulcer**)	(See **peptic ulcer**)	(See **peptic ulcer**)
Gastroenteritis	Bacteria Virus Parasites	Nausea Abdominal pain Headache Fever Chills Vomiting Diarrhea	Stool sample	Antibiotics Antivirals Antidiarrheal Antinausea
Malabsorption syndrome	Hereditary insufficient pancreatic function, lactose intolerance, poor bile production, celiac disease, cystic fibrosis, diabetes mellitus, and bacterial growth	Weight loss Diarrhea Steatorrhea Foul smelling, sticky, greasy, and light-colored stool Abdominal pain Muscle cramping Poor growth in children Heart arrhythmias Anemia Blood clotting disorder Edema Fatigue/weakness Decreased bone density	Stool sample GI culture CT scan Barium swallow MRI Ultrasound Endoscopy	Anti-inflammatory Corticosteroids Vitamins Mineral supplements
Crohn's disease	unknown	Abdominal pain Cramping Ulceration Inflammation Low-grade fever Diarrhea	Physical exam Colonoscopy Barium swallow Endoscopy, MRI, and CT imaging Stool sample	Antibiotics: Cipro (ciprofloxacin) and Flagyl (metronidazole) Corticosteroids: Prednisone Antidiarrheal agent: Imodium (loperamide)
Inguinal hernia	Weakened abdomen Birth defect	Pain experienced with lifting and bending A bulge in the groin region Vomiting Nausea	CT Ultrasound	Analgesics

LEARNING OBJECTIVE 8.3 **Explain the normal anatomy and physiology of the lower GI tract.**

KEY TERMS

Appendix A long, thin pouch on the outside wall of the cecum.

Ascending colon The first of four segments of the colon that extends in an upright direction.

Cecum A short pouch-like structure that connects the small intestine to the large intestine.

Colon The large intestine.

Colonoscopy A procedure that uses a scope to visually inspect the colon.

Descending colon A section of the colon that moves in a downward direction and meets the sigmoid colon.

Large intestine Located between the small intestine and the anal opening that plays a major role in absorption.

Rectum A short, tube-like structure located between the sigmoid colon and outside of the body.

Sigmoid colon The portion of the large intestine that is in an "S" shape leading to the rectum.

Transverse colon The section of the large intestine that goes across the abdomen below the stomach and liver.

Vermiform A slender, hollow, blind-ended tube connected to the cecum.

8-10 THE LOWER GI TRACT

The lower portion of the GI tract begins at the large intestine and ends at the rectum. Now that needed nutrients have been absorbed in the small intestines, the rest of the trip will consist mainly of reabsorbing some more water and concentrating the fecal matter for expulsion.

8-11 LARGE INTESTINE

The **large intestine**, shown in Figure 8-19, is about 5 feet long and 2.5 inches in diameter. This organ is connected to the small intestine at the ileocecal orifice and extends to the anus. This organ is divided into three parts: the **cecum**, the **colon**, and the **rectum**. Keep in mind, the large intestine is not longer than the small intestine, but it is greater in diameter. The large intestine has important duties such as water and vitamin absorption as well as compacting waste products to prepare for excretion.

The cecum is a pouch-like structure that passes on undigested food and water from the ileum (part of the small intestine) to the first portion of the large intestine. The cecum does absorb a small amount of water to help the body maintain a proper fluid balance. Attached to the cecum is the appendix, which is about 3 inches in length, has a worm-like appearance, and is a hollow tube that is closed on one end. Often called the **vermiform** appendix because of its worm shape, the appendix is lined with lymphatic tissue. In the past it was thought that the **appendix** had no purpose, and it was termed a vestigial organ, meaning evolution had rendered it useless. That is no longer the belief, however. Instead, it is thought that this small worm-like structure serves as a reservoir for

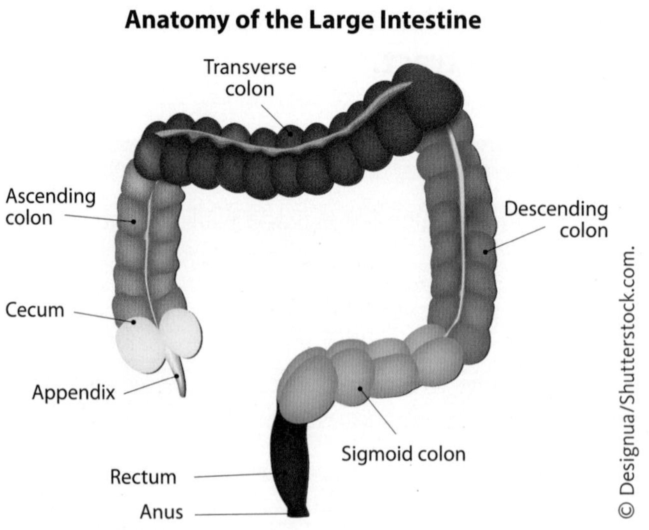

Anatomy of the Large Intestine

Transverse colon
Ascending colon
Descending colon
Cecum
Appendix
Sigmoid colon
Rectum
Anus

FIGURE 8-19 The large intestine.

good bacteria that can replenish the large intestine if need be. Also, because it contains lymphatic tissue, it is thought to help fight infection.

Now let's continue on our way along the large intestine to the colon. The colon consists of four parts: the **ascending**, **transverse**, **descending**, and **sigmoid colon**. The ascending colon goes in an upward direction on the right side of the body, leveling off at the liver. In Figure 8-19, the ascending colon is on your left, but it is the patient's right. The transverse colon travels across the abdomen just below the stomach and liver. The descending colon moves down the left side of the body, where it becomes the sigmoid colon, which connects to the rectum.

The unconscious movement of the large intestine, like the small intestine, is called peristalsis (intermittent waves), but the action is slower in the large intestine. The slower movement gives the large intestine time to remove water from the solid waste, so the watery waste product has time to become a semisolid product. If not enough water is removed, it results in diarrhea; if too much water is absorbed, rock-hard stool and constipation will occur.

Bacteria located in the large intestine (*E. coli*) help break down ingested contents and produce vitamins K and B complex. It is from these bacteria that we produce gas or flatulence. If the good bacterium gets out of its normal area, it can cause a life-threatening bacterial infection.

8-11a Diagnostic Testing of Lower GI

Before moving onto diseases of the large intestine, let's take a look at a valuable test that will be mentioned frequently throughout this chapter: a colonoscopy. (See Figure 8-20.) A **colonoscopy** itself is relatively fast, but the preparation for it takes time, as the patient must drink a large amount of prep solution the day before. An 8-ounce glass should be consumed every 10 minutes until contents from the bowel run clear, or the 2-liter jug of electrolyte solution is finished. This solution does not taste good, and many patients say it is best to drink it cold and fast. This solution cleanses the colon of all waste so the physician can get a clean view. All that cleansing liquid means you will be spending a lot of time in the bathroom, so plan ahead by stocking up on good reading material.

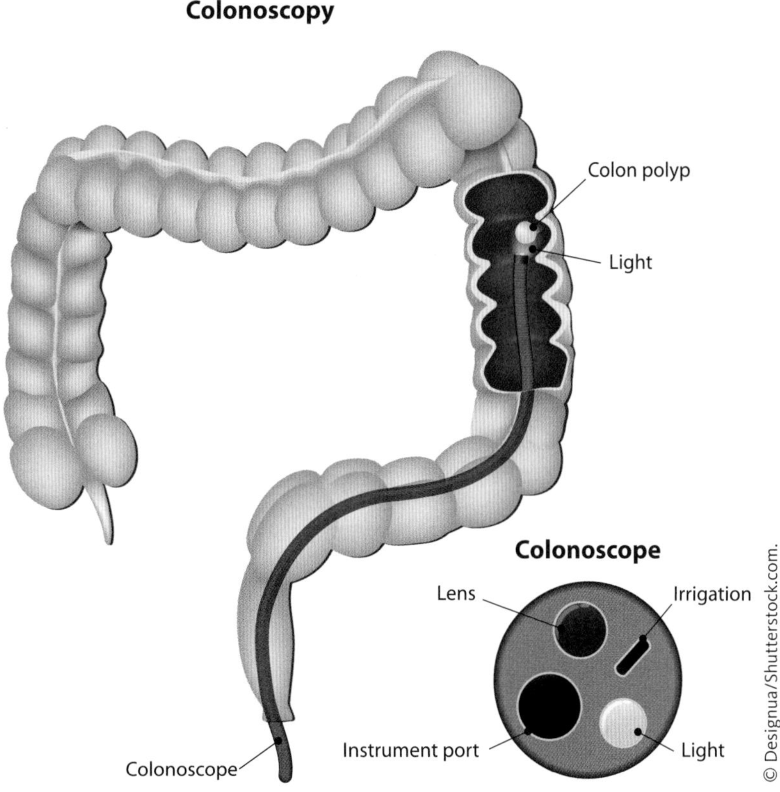

FIGURE 8-20 A colonoscope inside the large intestine.

8-12 RECTUM

Connected to the sigmoid colon, the rectum opens to the anal canal. When waste reaches the rectum and fills it with feces, it stimulates stretch receptors and the rectal muscles start to contract. Then the anal sphincters relax to allow the feces to pass through and thus eliminate the waste products of digestion.

LEARNING OBJECTIVE 8.4 Describe the pathopharmacology of the lower GI tract.

KEY TERMS

Adenomatous polyps Gland-like growths that develop in the large intestines on the mucous membrane.

Anoscope Tube-like instrument that is inserted into the anus to examine the walls of the lower rectum and anal region.

Appendicitis Inflammation of the appendix.

Colon polyps Growths developed from a cluster of cells on the intestinal wall that may become cancerous.

Colorectal cancer Cancer of the colon or rectum.

Diverticula Outward sac that develops in the wall of the large intestine.

Diverticulitis Condition developing from the inflammation of diverticula.

Dysentery Bacterial infection of the intestines causing severe, infectious diarrhea.

Fecal impaction Hardened stool causing a blockage.

Hemorrhoids Inflamed veins of the anus and rectum.

Ileus Inability of the intestines to move contents by way of peristalsis.

Inflammatory bowel disease Conditions causing inflammation to the intestinal tract.

Inflammatory polyps Type of polyp that usually occur in individuals who suffer from an inflammatory condition of the bowel.

Intestinal obstruction Blockage of the intestines.

Intussusception Condition occurring when part of the intestine folds into itself.

Irritable bowel syndrome Chronic condition affecting the large intestine causing pain, cramping constipation or diarrhea.

Proctoscope Slightly larger instrument than the anoscope used to examine the anus and rectum.

Sclerotherapy Procedure usually involving the direct injection of a salt solution into a vessel causing inflammation and the vessel to stick together.

Serrated polyps Flattened saw-toothed appearing growths.

Sigmoidoscopy Procedure utilizing a scope to examine the sigmoid colon.

Ulcerative colitis Inflammatory bowel disease causing ulcer-like lesions in the large intestine.

Volvulus Condition where the intestine becomes twisted.

8-13 DISEASES OF THE LARGE INTESTINE

The large intestine, also called the colon, can be affected by disease at all ages; however, colon disease is primarily seen in middle-aged adults to senior citizens, with some exceptions. These conditions range in severity from acute to chronic.

8-13a Appendicitis

This condition can occur at any age, but is most common in people between the ages of 10 and 30. **Appendicitis** is inflammation of the appendix, shown in Figure 8-21. It is commonly caused by the appendix becoming blocked, resulting in an infection. As the bacterium multiplies, the appendix swells and fills with pus. The swollen appendix can rupture and be life-threatening. Symptoms include abdominal pain that moves to the lower right side of the abdomen, vomiting, nausea, loss of appetite, bloating, even diarrhea or constipation.

To diagnose, the physician can apply pressure to this site, which causes pain. A blood sample shows high white blood cell count. A urinalysis can be ordered to rule out a urinary tract infection or kidney stone, which can have similar symptoms. Imaging such as an abdominal X-ray, abdominal CT scan, or an ultrasound can best confirm the correct diagnosis.

Treatment consists of surgical removal of the appendix. To prevent spread of infection, the patient may be given antibiotics, while analgesics may be prescribed to help the patient manage post-surgery abdominal incision pain.

8-13b Intestinal Obstruction

An **intestinal obstruction** is a blockage preventing GI contents (solids and liquids) from moving through the small or large intestine. Obstructions can be caused by:

- Hernias
- Tumors, cancerous and benign

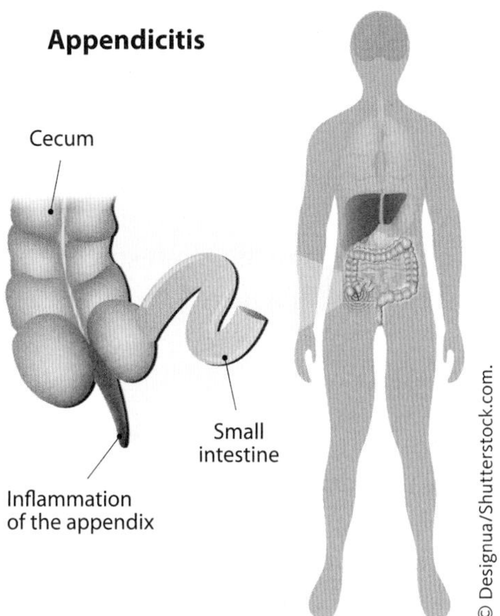

FIGURE 8-21 Inflammation of the appendix.

- Adhesions, which can occur after abdominal surgery where fibrous strands of tissue stick together
- Inflammatory bowel disease, such as Crohn's disease
- Diverticulitis
- Cancer
- **Fecal impaction** (dry mass of solid stool causing blockage)
- **Ileus**, the lack of peristalsis movement in the intestines
- **Volvulus**, a twist in the intestines
- **Intussusception**, part of the intestine folds into itself like a collapsing telescope

Whatever the cause, the obstruction must be remedied as soon as possible; otherwise, it can be life-threatening. Blood supply can be cut off, causing tissue death (necrosis), and infections can develop from a perforation (tear) in the intestine, and then enter the bloodstream and become a systemic infection.

Symptoms depend on the severity and type of blockage, but can include abdominal distention (swelling), inability to expel gas or feces (constipation), vomiting, decreased appetite, abdominal cramping, and pain.

During a history and physical examination, the physician might suspect an abdominal obstruction of the patient who presents with an abdominal lump, distention, or tenderness. The physician might notice a lack of bowel sounds upon auscultating regions of the abdomen with a stethoscope. The physician might order a CT scan, X-ray, or ultrasound to help locate and determine the type of blockage. A barium enema or air enema, in which liquid barium or air are inserted into the rectum, can help provide a better image of the colon.

Treatment can be accomplished in different ways, depending on the condition. For example, a hospitalized patient can be relieved of gas and fluid that is causing the abdominal distention by inserting a nasogastric tube to allow the gas and fluid to escape and thus release the extra pressure. An IV is often started to give the patient proper hydration. The patient will undergo surgery for severe blockages.

To prevent the occurrence of an obstruction, a patient might be directed to take laxatives or stool softeners to allow bowel contents to keep moving. An off-label use of acetylcysteine (one for which the drug was not intended) is used in newborns with an intestinal obstruction because the drug has the ability to loosen and thin mucus.

8-13c Ulcerative Colitis

Ulcerative colitis is a condition in which ulcers develop in the rectum and/or colon because of repeated inflammatory exacerbations as shown in Figure 8-22. This disease is chronic in nature and is a type of inflammatory bowel disease. There is no cure and those affected experience periodic exacerbations. While ulcerative colitis can occur in anyone at any age, those at higher risk for the disease are Caucasian men and women younger than 30 years of age. Unfortunately, they are also at a greater risk of developing colon cancer. Different types of ulcerative colitis are based on how much of the colon and rectum are affected.

Although the cause is unknown, flare-ups or exacerbations seem to be more likely during times of stress. While the origin is still a mystery, it is thought to be possibly linked to autoimmune, hereditary, or dietary issues.

Symptoms experienced develop over time and can vary depending on the severity. Symptoms include abdominal pain and cramping, fever, rectal pain, bloody diarrhea, anemia, fatigue, weight loss, and a sensation of needing to have a bowel movement, only to be unable to do so.

A diagnosis of ulcerative colitis starts with a blood sample, which can provide information about signs of infection (high white blood cell count) and anemia (low red blood cell count), which can occur from prolonged bleeding. A stool sample is required to check for the presence of blood. The presence of bacteria, viruses, and parasites—all of which would cause an infection—can also be detected. A colonoscopy is performed, and in most cases of ulcerative colitis, the ulcers will be clearly seen. A biopsy can be done on any suspicious tissue.

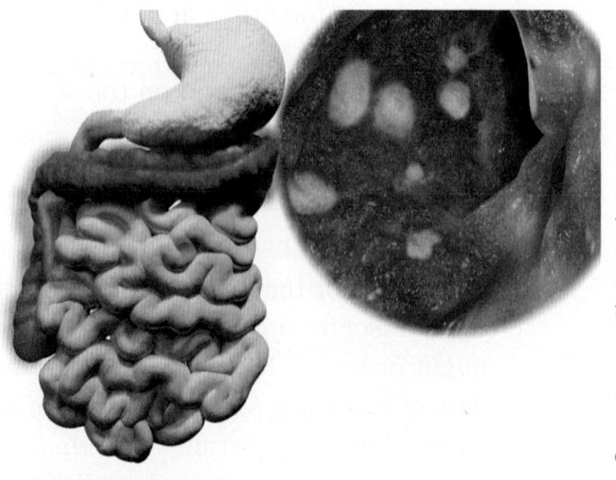

FIGURE 8-22 Ulcers in the large intestine as a result of ulcerative colitis.

Other procedures that can be done are X-rays and CT scans. The X-ray can determine if a perforation or hole is present, while a CT scan can be used to determine where the ulcers are located and how much inflammation is present.

Pharmaceuticals can help manage this chronic condition. The first class of drugs used to manage ulcerative colitis are anti-inflammatory drugs, such as corticosteroids (prednisone). These drugs can be delivered orally, intravenously, or rectally (via suppository or enema), depending on where the ulcers are located.

Aminosalicylates are used to treat not only ulcerative colitis but also exacerbations. While it's not completely understood what causes this medication to work, it is thought to change the way the lining of the gut releases chemicals, which otherwise irritate the bowel. This class of drugs can be given long term, if needed. A list of these drugs includes:

- Dipentum (olsalazine)
- Colazal (balsalazide)
- Asacol, Canasa, Lialda, others (mesalamine)

Another class of anti-inflammatory medication is corticosteroid. This is used to treat more moderate to severe cases that do not respond favorably or at all to other treatments. Because of the severity of potential side effects, it is not given on a long-term basis. For severe cases, IV corticosteroids can be given, while mild forms can be treated with tablets. If the condition is affecting the lower portion of the large intestine, an enema can be used to administer medication; if the rectum is the site of inflammation, then suppositories are used.

Examples of corticosteroids are:

- Entocort (budesonide)
- Baycadron (dexamethasone)
- Cortef, Cortenema, and Proctofoam (hydrocortisone)
- Medrol (methylprednisolone)
- Orapred (prednisolone)
- Predsol (prednisone)

Another drug class that can be used to treat ulcerative colitis is immunosuppressant drugs. These work by decreasing the body's immune system, thus preventing the inflammatory response. These can be given with corticosteroids to maintain control and prevent another relapse. Examples of commonly used immunosuppressant drugs are:

- Purinethol and Purixan (mercaptopurine)
- Imuran and Azasan (azathioprine)

If the condition persists and medications are not effective, surgery might be performed to put in a colostomy, in which a healthy portion of the large intestine is brought through the abdominal wall, where it is sutured into place to bypass the affected site.

8-13d Irritable Bowel Syndrome IBS (Spastic Colon)

Spastic colon is another name for irritable bowel syndrome. Note that **irritable bowel syndrome** (IBS) and **inflammatory bowel disease** (IBD) are not the same. IBD is used to describe chronic enteritis conditions with ulcers, while IBS is also a chronic issue but without any inflammation or ulcers. While the exact cause is unknown, patients with IBS—often young adults—have episodes of flare-ups that tend to be triggered by stress. Symptoms include flatulence, bloating, abdominal pain, constipation, and diarrhea. You might wonder why both constipation and diarrhea are listed as symptoms, as they are two opposite extremes. Some people experience constipation, others diarrhea, and some might have a mixture, meaning that the patient might have constipation (hardened stool) during one bowel movement and diarrhea (loose stool) during another.

Those living with IBS have to closely monitor what kind of foods and drinks they consume. For example, beverages with caffeine and alcohol and spicy foods can cause an exacerbation.

To determine whether the patient has IBS, a series of tests can be done, including a blood test, endoscopy, colonoscopy, and imaging such as an X-ray. The best way to manage this disease is to avoid triggers; however, medications can help the patient cope with this condition (antidiarrheals, gut antispasmodics, antibiotics, and laxatives). Table 8-9 lists medications commonly used to treat IBS.

CLINICAL CONNECTION 8.3

PROBIOTICS

Have you ever heard of probiotics? Maybe you have but you are not sure what exactly they are or how it can benefit you. Probiotics are good bacteria that we need to have a healthy gut. They are actually live bacteria and yeast that help your gut with the digestive process and can be taken to replenish the good bacteria that might have been wiped out by drugs or disease.

Table 8-9 Common Drugs Used to Treat IBS

DRUG CLASS	PURPOSE	COMMON EXAMPLES
Antidiarrheal	To decrease urgency and frequency of bowel movements.	• Imodium (loperamide) • Pepto-Bismol, Select, and Kaopectate (bismuth subsalicylate) • Lomotil (atropine/diphenoxylate)
Antibiotics	Used to kill bacteria and treat IBS by working only in the intestines and not absorbed into the bloodstream.	• Xifaxan (rifaximin)
Gut antispasmodic	Slows the movement of GI contents in the intestines by decreasing the ability for muscles to contract.	• HyoMax-SL, Levsin and Oscimin (hyoscyamine) • Bentyl (dicyclomine)
Laxative	Used to treat constipation and increase bowel movements.	• Amitiza (lubiprostone) • Dulcolax and Fleet (bisacodyl)

8-13e Dysentery

Dysentery is also known as infectious diarrhea. This condition causes intestinal inflammation and is spread by way of contaminated food or water. Most often dysentery is caused by *Shigella* bacterium, but it also can be caused by an ameba-type microorganism.

Symptoms encountered by the patient include fever, discomfort, abdominal pain and cramping, flatulence, vomiting, dehydration, and weight loss, with bloody diarrhea being the classic hallmark.

A stool sample is tested for the presence of blood and pathogenic microorganisms. Treatment can help clear up the cause of the dysentery infection. If caused by *Shigella* bacterium, a commonly used antibiotic called Bactrim (sulfamethoxazole and trimethoprim) is effective. If caused by an ameba, however, an antiprotozoal agent such as Diaquinol or Yodoxin (diodoquinol) is required.

This condition can be avoided by maintaining proper hygiene, such as hand washing. When traveling abroad, avoid drinking untreated water (including ice cubes) and eating fresh produce.

8-13f Diverticulosis/Diverticulitis

Little pouches called **diverticula** develop in the colon wall. These pockets bulge outward through weak spots in the colon wall resulting in a condition called diverticulosis. These pouches are commonly seen in people older than 40 and rarely cause any issues. Inflammation occurs when feces fills these pouches, although a patient might be asymptomatic until irritation occurs. When the sacs get blocked, they become inflamed; that condition is called **diverticulitis**. (See Figure 8-23.)

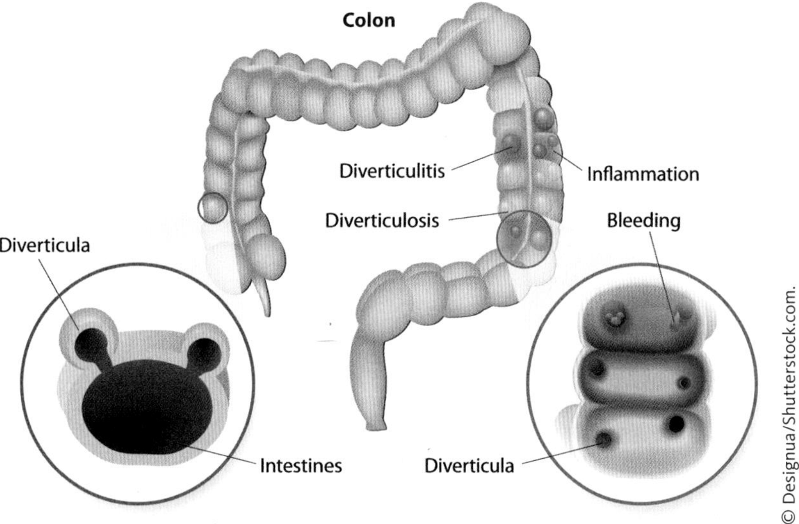

FIGURE 8-23 Pictured are the conditions known as diverticulosis and diverticulitis. Diverticula are pockets that develop in colon wall. These small pouches bulge outward through weak spots in the colon wall resulting in a condition called diverticulosis. When these sacs in the intestinal wall get blocked, they become inflamed causing diverticulitis.

Common symptoms experienced by affected individuals include lower abdominal cramping and pain, fever, vomiting, and abdominal tenderness. Also, because of the inflammation, bleeding and even a perforation of the colon can happen. Inflammation and swelling of the pouches cause the lumen of the intestine to become smaller or narrower, making it difficult for GI contents to pass, and can even cause total obstruction.

A diagnosis can be done by visually inspecting the colon by a colonoscopy. Other testing includes a CT scan, blood, stool and urine (to rule out infections), and liver function tests (to rule out other causes of abdominal pain). Treatment consists of the patient adding more fiber to his or her diet to allow stool to remain softer and pass easier. Antibiotics are used in the presence of an infection, while basic pain relievers such as Tylenol (acetaminophen) are used to treat associated pain. If the condition is severe, IV antibiotics might be required.

8-13g Colon Polyps

While the cause is largely unknown, **colon polyps**, shown in Figure 8-24, can develop. These polyps are cellular clusters found on the lining of the intestine that protrude into the lumen. Anyone can develop polyps at any age; however, it is most common for people to develop polyps in their 50s or older, those who are obese, and smokers. Polyps are harmless the majority of the time, but they can become cancerous and be deadly if not caught early. There are three types of polyps as shown in Table 8-10.

Many symptoms can develop as a result of colon polyps, including rectal bleeding. If the bleeding occurs chronically, it can cause anemia from blood loss. The patient also might experience abdominal pain and discomfort such as cramps, nausea, vomiting, and diarrhea. Most often, however, the patient is asymptomatic.

To diagnose the patient, a colonoscopy or **sigmoidoscopy** can be done to visually examine the colon. A biopsy can be performed through the scope to check for malignancy. It is also likely that the physician will remove all of the polyps found at this time.

No medications are used to treat colon polyps themselves, but supportive care such as stool softeners might be ordered.

8-13h Colon Cancer

Cancer found in the colon is called **colorectal cancer**, which is shown in Figure 8-25. Cancer developing in the rectum is called rectal cancer.

Most cases of colorectal cancer begin as a small benign growths, such as adenomatous polyps. Because these polyps might not cause any symptoms, and patients 50 years and older should be screened regularly with a colonoscopy. While the exact cause is unknown, ulcerative colitis and polyps are known predisposing factors. Rectal abnormalities can be found with a digital rectal exam.

Symptoms vary depending on the region of the cancer. Individuals might experience bowel habit changes, such as constipation or diarrhea. The stool appearance can be thin and narrow, with the possibility of blood. Other symptoms are rectal bleeding, flatulence, anemia, abdominal pain and cramping, and fatigue.

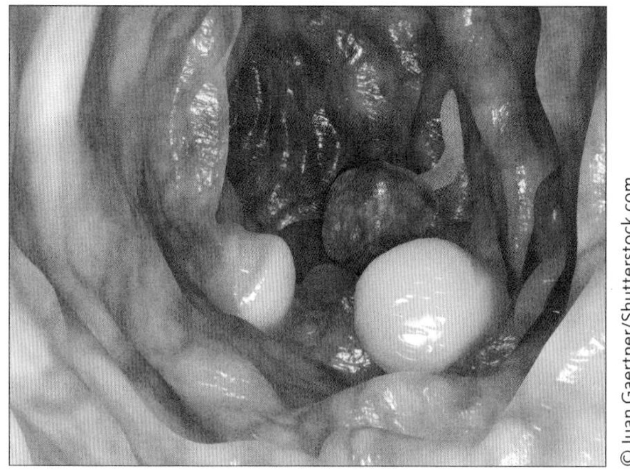

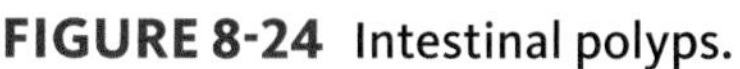

FIGURE 8-24 Intestinal polyps.

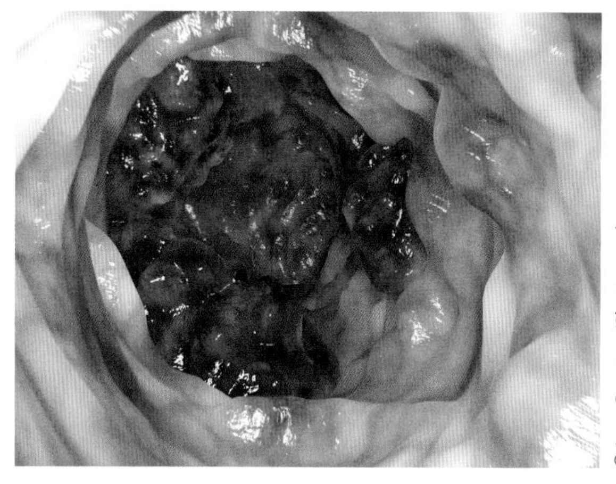

FIGURE 8-25 Colon cancer.

Table 8-10 Types of Colon Polyps

Inflammatory polyps	Occur after the body responds to an inflammatory condition such as Crohn's disease or other ulcerative condition.
Adenomatous polyps	Comprise the majority of polyps encountered; not likely to be cancerous.
Serrated polyps	Found in different regions of the colon; can be difficult to find because they can lie flat. Smaller serrated polyps do not typically result in cancer, but larger ones are likely to be a precancerous condition.

Treating colorectal cancer depends on the size and region of the condition. The patient might undergo surgical procedures such as removing part or even all of the colon, known as a colectomy. To kill the cancer cells, chemotherapy drugs are used. Chemotherapeutic drugs used to treat colorectal cancers include bevacizumab, cetuximab, oxaliplatin, capecitabine, and fluorouracil. Cancer treatment can make a patient feel nauseated, so antinausea medication might be given for relief.

Avastin (bevacizumab) is used not only to treat colorectal cancer, but other cancers such as breast and kidney cancers. Injected once every 14 days, the drug works by attaching to a protein called vascular endothelial growth factor (VEGF). This factor is used by cells to grow new blood vessels (angiogenesis). Cancer cells, because of their uncontrolled rapid growth, demand more blood flow to feed the hyperreproduction and rely on angiogenesis to thrive. Avastin blocks angiogenesis and therefore slows or stops the cancerous growth.

Erbitux (cetuximab) is another drug used to treat colorectal cancer. This drug also can be used with another cancer drug to help to treat cancer that has metastasized from the colon or rectum.

Xeloda (capecitabine), although primarily used to treat breast cancer, also is used to treat colorectal cancer. It is used when the cancer has metastasized and after surgery to decease the likelihood of metastasis.

Adrucil (fluorouracil) comes in two forms: an injection (Adrucil) and a topical agent called Efudex. The injection form is used to treat colorectal cancer. This drug stops cancer growth by mimicking the nutrient cells in the body cancer uses to grow. The cancer cells consume the drug, which stops the cancer's growth. This makes this drug part of the drug class called an antimetabolite because it interferes with the cancer cell's needed metabolic processes.

8-14 DISEASES OF THE RECTUM

Finally, we will end our journey of the alimentary tract by discussing the rectum, the end of the digestive tract.

8-14a Hemorrhoids

Hemorrhoids are varicose veins that can develop both inside and outside of the rectum. External hemorrhoids can be seen at the lower opening of the anus, while internal hemorrhoids are found on the rectal wall and can be seen with an instrument called an **anoscope** (or **proctoscope**), allowing the physician to look inside the anus. Hemorrhoids can be caused by any activity that causes an increase in pressure at the anus, including pregnancy and strenuous bowel movements from constipation. (See Figure 8-26.)

The most common symptoms of hemorrhoids are rectal pain, bleeding, and itching. It can be difficult for the patient to sit, stand, or lay down. To treat hemorrhoids, the patient can undergo **sclerotherapy**, which can be used to shrink the size of the hemorrhoid. This is done by directly injecting the hemorrhoid

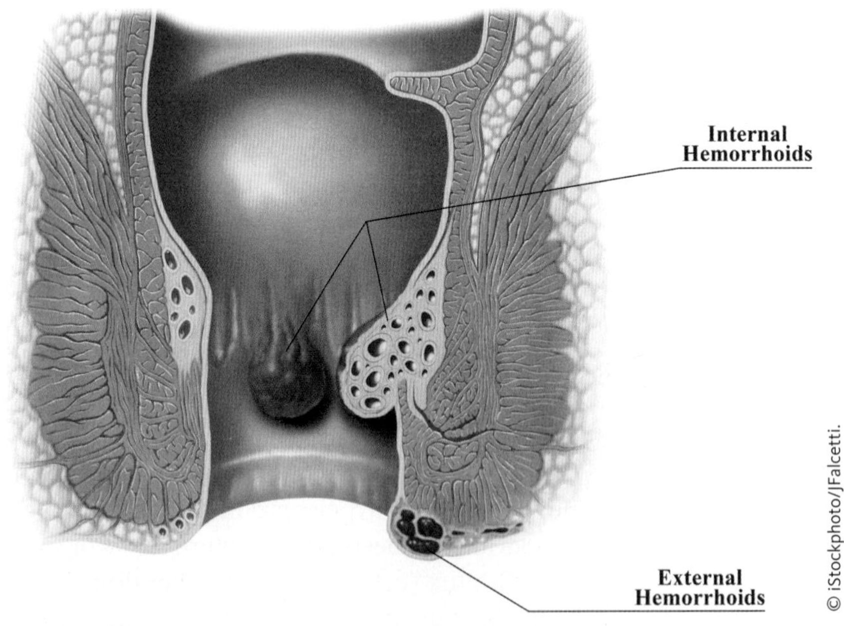

FIGURE 8-26 This illustration shows the differences between internal and external hemorrhoids.

with a chemical causing coagulation to harden and dry up the hemorrhoid. Another minimally invasive procedure is rubber band litigation, which entails placing rubber bands at the base of the hemorrhoid to cut off its blood supply. Finally, a surgical removal or hemorrhoidectomy can be done to remove a severe case of hemorrhoids.

Medications used to treat hemorrhoids come in topical over-the-counter ointments, suppositories, and medicated wipes. Popular OTC drugs include Preparation H with hydrocortisone, Anucort, and hydrocortisone suppositories. These medications help decrease inflammation and itching, while analgesics such as Tylenol and NSAIDs such as ibuprofen can be used to treat pain.

8-15 SUMMARY OF PATHOPHARMACOLOGY OF THE LOWER GI TRACT

Review Summary Table 8-11 for a recap of the causes, symptoms, diagnostic tests, and main pharmacology treatment for disease of the lower GI tract.

Table 8-11 Lower GI Pathopharmacology

DISEASE/ CONDITION	ETIOLOGY	MAJOR SIGNS/ SYMPTOMS	DIAGNOSTIC TESTS	MAIN PHARMACOLOGIC TREATMENT
Appendicitis	Appendix obstruction	Abdominal pain Vomiting Nausea Loss of appetite Bloating Diarrhea Constipation	Blood sample Urinalysis X-ray CT scan	Antibiotics Analgesics
Intestinal obstruction	Hernias Tumors Adhesion Inflammatory bowel disease Diverticulitis Cancer Fecal impaction Ileus Volvulus Intussusception	Abdominal distention Constipation Vomiting Decreased appetite Abdominal cramping Pain	Auscultation CT scan X-ray Ultrasound Barium enema Air enema	Acetylcysteine

(continued)

Table 8-11 Lower GI Pathopharmacology—*continued*

DISEASE/ CONDITION	ETIOLOGY	MAJOR SIGNS/ SYMPTOMS	DIAGNOSTIC TESTS	MAIN PHARMACOLOGIC TREATMENT
Ulcerative colitis	Unknown	Pain Cramping Rectal pain Bloody diarrhea Anemia Fatigue Weight loss Urgency sensation to have a bowel movement Fever	Blood sample Stool sample Colonoscopy Sigmoidoscopy X-rays CT scans	Aminosalicylates: Dipentum (olsalazine) Colazal (balsalazide) Asacol, Canasa, Lialda, and others (mesalamine) Corticosteroids: Entocort (budesonide) Baycadron (dexamethasone) Cortef, Cortenema, and Proctofoam (hydrocortisone) Medrol (methylprednisolone) Orapred (prednisolone) Predsol (prednisone) Immunosuppressant drugs: Purinethol and Purixan (mercaptopurine) Imuran and Azasan (azathioprine)
Irritable bowel syndrome (spastic colon)	Unknown	Constipation Diarrhea	Blood test Endoscopy Colonoscopy X-ray	Antidiarrheal: Imodium (loperamide) Pepto-Bismol, Select, and Kaopectate (bismuth subsalicylate) Lomotil (atropine/ diphenoxylate) Antibiotics: Xifaxan (rifaximin) Gut antispasmodic: HyoMax-SL, Levsin, and Oscimin (hyoscyamine) Bentyl (dicyclomine) Laxatives: Amitiza (lubiprostone) Dulcolax and Fleet (bisacodyl)

Table 8-11 Lower GI Pathopharmacology—*continued*

DISEASE/ CONDITION	ETIOLOGY	MAJOR SIGNS/ SYMPTOMS	DIAGNOSTIC TESTS	MAIN PHARMACOLOGIC TREATMENT
Dysentery	*Shigella* bacterium Ameba	Fever Discomfort Abdominal pain Cramping Flatulence Vomiting Dehydration Weight loss Bloody diarrhea	Stool sample	Antibiotic: Bactrim (sulfamethoxa-zole and trimethoprim) Antiprotozoal agent: Diaquinol and Yodoxin (diodoquinol)
Diverticulosis/ diverticulitis	Feces fill diverticula	Lower abdominal cramping pain Fever Vomiting Abdominal tender-ness Inflammation Bleeding Perfora-tion Obstruction Inflammation Narrow lumen of the intestine narrower	Colonoscopy CT scan, blood, stool, and urine tests (to rule out infections) and liver function tests (to rule out other causes of abdomi-nal pain).	Antibiotics Pain relievers such as Tylenol (acetaminophen)
Colon polyps	Unknown	Rectal bleeding Anemia Abdominal pain Discomfort Cramps Nausea Vomiting Diarrhea Asymptomatic	Colonoscopy Sigmoidoscopy Tissue biopsy	Stool softener
Colon cancer	Unknown	Bowel habit changes (constipation and diarrhea) Stool appearance can be thin and narrow (possibly with blood) Rectal bleeding Flatulence Anemia Abdominal pain Cramping Fatigue	Colonoscopy Digital rectal exam (DRE)	Chemotherapy drugs: Avastin (bevacizumab) Erbitux (cetuximab) Xeloda (capecitabine) Adrucil (fluorouracil) Eloxatin (oxaliplatin)

(*continued*)

Table 8-11 Lower GI Pathopharmacology—*continued*

DISEASE/ CONDITION	ETIOLOGY	MAJOR SIGNS/ SYMPTOMS	DIAGNOSTIC TESTS	MAIN PHARMACOLOGIC TREATMENT
Hemorrhoids	Any activity causing increased pressure around the anus	Rectal Pain Bleeding Itching	Visual inspection Anoscope Proctoscope	Corticosteroids: Preparation H with hydrocortisone Anucort and other hydrocortisone suppositories Analgesics: Tylenol NSAIDs: ibuprofen Sclerotherapy

LEARNING OBJECTIVE 8.5 Explain the normal anatomy and physiology of accessory organs and their associated pathopharmacology.

KEY TERMS

Cholecystectomy Surgical removal of the gallbladder.

Cholecystokinin (CCK) Hormone that is released to assist in the digestion of protein and fat.

Gallbladder Sac-like organ which stores bile from the liver before releasing the bile to the small intestine.

Gallstones Hardened deposits of bile that forms in the gallbladder.

Hepatitis Inflammation of the liver.

Hepatitis A (HAV) Infectious liver disease caused by contaminated food or water.

Hepatitis B (HBV) Chronic viral liver infection caused by the Hep B virus.

Hepatitis C (HCV) Chronic inflammatory liver disease caused by the Hep C virus.

Liver Large organ located below the right side of the abdomen with important digestive and metabolic roles.

Magnetic resonance elastography (MRE) An MRI with the ability to show the stiffness of body tissue.

Pancreas Located behind the liver, this gland secretes digestive enzymes into the duodenum.

Pancreatitis Inflammation of the pancreas.

8-16 LIVER

Found inferior to the diaphragm in the upper right quadrant, the liver, weighing 3.3 pounds, is the body's largest glandular organ, and, in fact, the largest organ located within the abdominopelvic cavity. Playing a major role in our survival, the liver receives 1.5 quarts of blood every minute from the hepatic portal vein, blood that is loaded with byproducts of digestion.

The liver stores vitamins, produces cholesterol, and helps regulate blood sugar, to name only a few of its metabolic functions. As for digestion, the liver produces bile, which breaks up fats to aid in making digestion. Bile causes the fats to be broken down, allowing more surface area for enzymes to work on and digest fat. Bile can absorb certain substances such as bilirubin and excess cholesterol, to then allow them to be eliminated from the body.

Bile does not stay in the liver. Instead, it leaves the liver by way of the hepatic duct, makes its way through the cystic duct, until reaching the gallbladder, where it will remain until the small intestines need it.

Hepatitis is inflammation of the liver, which is usually caused by a pathogenic viral microorganism. Hepatitis can be broken down into three distinct types. **Hepatitis A (HAV)** is spread by consuming food or water contaminated with infected fecal matter. This disease occurs suddenly and requires rest. It is not chronic and, therefore, is not going to last a lifetime.

Hepatitis B (HBV) causes more severe symptoms than HAV. This type of hepatitis causes an acute illness that can become a chronic condition. If this happens, the liver might be permanently damaged. This form of hepatitis is acquired by sharing needles, sexual intercourse, and blood transfusions.

Hepatitis C (HCV) is usually transmitted through contaminated blood and can cause serious damage to the liver. Many people have no idea they are infected because not everyone who acquires the disease has symptoms. In fact, it might be decades before it flares up. Baby boomers are five times more likely to develop Hepatitis C than people born outside of this era.

Symptoms of hepatitis include ascites (fluid accumulation in abdominal region), jaundice (yellowing of skin and whites of the eyes), fatigue, leg edema, and weight loss. When chronic, this condition can cause scarring of the liver known as cirrhosis. A blood sample can determine whether the patient is affected. Other tests are used to check if liver scarring is present. Transient elastography can estimate liver thickness by using ultrasound to measure the speed of the vibrations moving through the liver and how fast the waves disperse. A stiff, thick liver means there is scarring from chronic hepatitis.

Another non-invasive test of liver thickness is **magnetic resonance elastography (MRE)**. This method combines magnetic resonance imaging with sound waves used to bounce off the liver to build a visual image of the organ. Another way to diagnose hepatitis is through an invasive biopsy procedure. This entails the insertion of a needle into the liver by going through the abdominal wall. The tissue sample can then be sent to a laboratory where a conclusive diagnosis can be made.

Antiviral medications are used to treat Hepatitis C. The patient should not have the virus in his or her system 2 weeks after the treatment is completed. Common antiviral drugs used to treat HCV include Ribasphere, Copegus, ribavirin, Pegasys (peginterferon alfa-2a), and Harvoni (ledipasvir and sofosbuvir). See Figure 8-27.

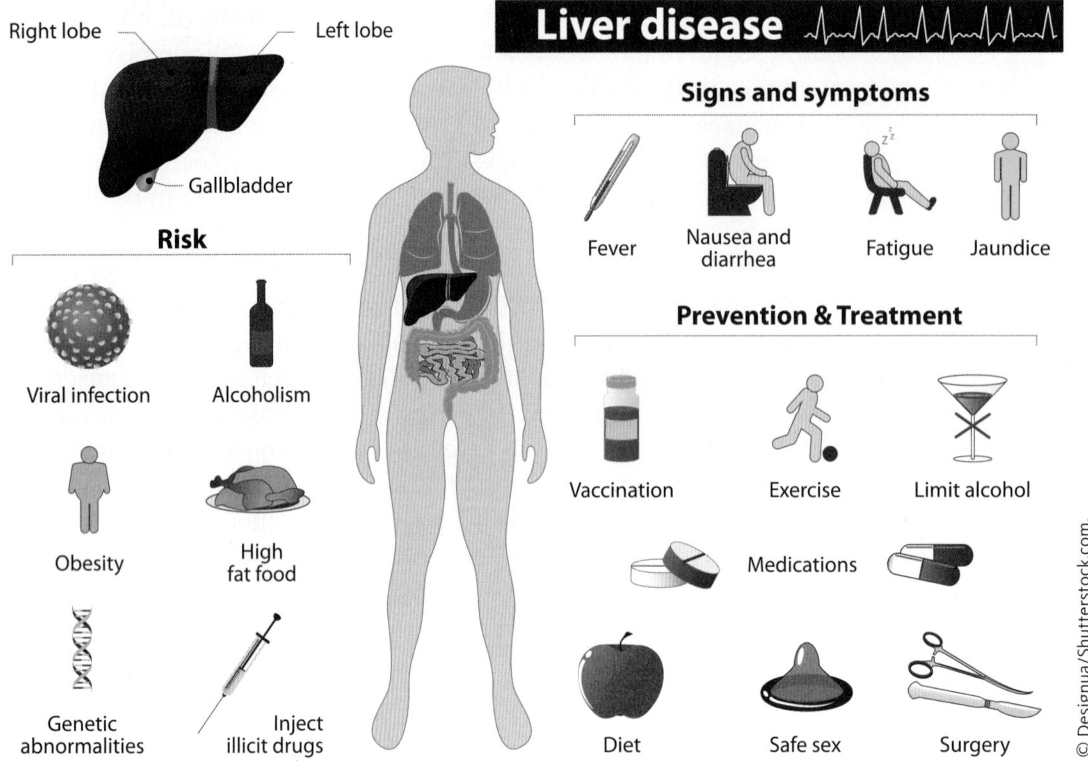

FIGURE 8-27 Liver disease infographic.

8-17 GALLBLADDER

The **gallbladder**, shown in Figure 8-28, is a green sac-like organ about 4 inches long, located below the right lobe of the liver. Bile produced by the liver is stored by the gallbladder and concentrated 6–10 times by reabsorbing water

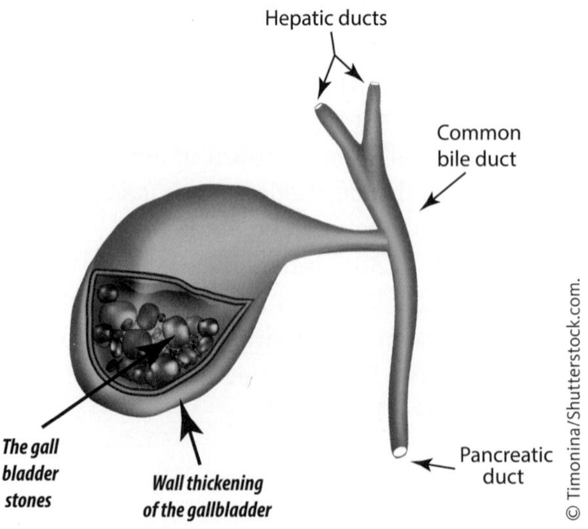

FIGURE 8-28 Cholecystitis.

from it. Gallstones can be formed by bile salts if too much fluid is removed, making it important to have the right consistency of bile. Bile is released into the duodenum when fatty foods enter. Bile release causes a hormone called **cholecystokinin (CCK)** to be released. When this hormone is released, the smooth muscle of the gallbladder contracts, allowing more bile to enter the cystic duct, the common bile duct, and duodenum to aid in the digestion of proteins and fats.

While waiting to be released into the small intestine, bile is stored in the gallbladder, where it is possible for gallstones to develop. **Gallstones**, more formally known as *cholelithiasis*, are formed from too much cholesterol. These hardened deposits vary in size and can range anywhere from a grain of sand to larger than a marble. If the stone becomes lodged, the patient will experience tremendous pain that often radiates into the right shoulder between the shoulder blades, and acute pain within the center of the abdominal cavity. Serious signs and symptoms requiring prompt medical treatment include high fever and chills and jaundice.

Procedures done to diagnose gallstones include ultrasound, CT scan, blood samples (to rule out other conditions), or using a special dye to better show the patient's bile ducts during a hepatobiliary iminodiacetic acid (HIDA) scan, a type of nuclear medicine scan that is used to create visual images of the liver, biliary duct, and small intestine.

If gallstones are present, the entire organ can be removed by a procedure called a **cholecystectomy**. Surgery can be avoided, however, if the stones can be dissolved by either lithotripsy or medication. Lithotripsy uses ultrasound waves to break up gallstones, a procedure typically used only for patients who are unable to undergo a cholecystectomy. Dissolving a stone with medication is a lengthy process, taking months, even up to 2 years. Examples of medications used to dissolve gallstones include Actigall and Ursa (ursodiol).

8-18 PANCREAS

Located behind the stomach and spanning across laterally from the duodenum to the spleen, the **pancreas** is shown in Figure 8-29. The pancreas plays an important role in the digestive system, buffering the acidity of the chyme in

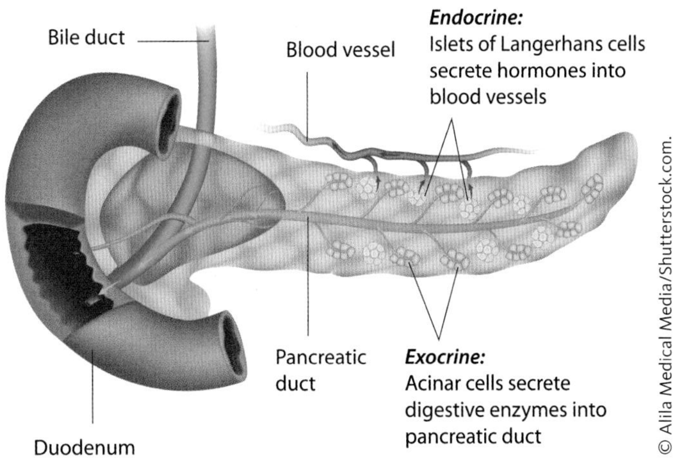

FIGURE 8-29 The pancreas showing its role in digestion.

Table 8-12 Pancreatic Enzymes

ENZYME	PURPOSE
Carbohydrases	Break down sugars and starches
Lipases	Break down fats
Proteinases	Break down proteins
Nucleases	Break down nucleic acids

the small intestine to prevent damage. The duodenum causes the pancreas to release its substances to neutralize the chyme pH to about 7.5–8.8. To learn more about enzymes used to breakdown different types of food substances, see Table 8-12.

Inflammation of the pancreas can occur when there is a blockage in a bile duct, which can push bile back into the pancreas. The enzymes in the bile start to inflame and destroy the pancreas causing **pancreatitis**. There are other causes for pancreatitis, and this condition can be an acute or chronic condition.

Symptoms can include nausea, vomiting, upper abdominal pain and tenderness, weight loss, and greasy, foul smelling stool. Examinations include but are not limited to blood samples, stool tests, MRI, and CT scan.

Often dehydration occurs and IV fluids are indicated. Pain relievers are given to control the abdominal pain, which can be severe. Surgery might be required not only to drain accumulated fluid in the pancreas, but to also to remove a portion of the diseased organ.

Module 9

Pathopharmacology of the Endocrine System

Module Introduction

Working alongside the nervous system, the **endocrine system** regulates the body's physiological function, controlling all of the body's organs. The nervous system receives and sends out signals with tremendous speed; the endocrine system also sends and receives signals, but at a much slower pace.

Another difference between the two systems is the duration of the signals. Those from the nervous system last for only a short time and immediately take control. The endocrine system, on the other hand, sends out signals that last a long time and control the body until another signal is sent to change the body's response.

An example of the nervous system and endocrine system working together is the fight or flight response when a person senses danger. Immediately, the body prepares for the event by increasing heart rate, breathing, and undergoing several other physiologic changes. The nervous system immediately senses the dangers and sends signals throughout the body. The adrenal glands release adrenaline into the bloodstream to reach receptors all over the body and gets ready to fight or flee. Even when the danger is over, and the nervous system no longer needs to send signals, it takes some time for the body to come down from the adrenaline rush, as it cleared from the bloodstream.

LEARNING OBJECTIVE 9.1 Explain the normal anatomy and physiology of the endocrine system.

KEY TERMS

Adrenal glands Glands located on top of each kidney.

Adrenal medulla gland Inner section of the adrenal gland.

Anterior pituitary gland Frontal portion of the pituitary gland.

Endocrine system System that produces and secretes hormones to control everyday bodily functions.

Gonads Testes in men and ovaries in women.

Hormones Chemical signal that is secreted into the bloodstream to control bodily functions.

Negative feedback loop Physiological process used to bring the body back to its normal point.

Pancreas Produces and secretes insulin.

Parathyroid glands Four pea-sized regions in the posterior side of the thyroid.

Pineal gland A small gland located in the brain responsible for maintaining our circadian rhythm.

Positive feedback loop Physiological process that takes the body farther way from its normal point and will continue to do so until the cycle is broken.

Posterior pituitary Rear portion of the pituitary gland.

Thymus gland A gland found in the chest behind the breastbone that plays a role in our immune system.

Thyroid gland Important structure located in the middle section of the neck that secretes thyroid hormones.

9-1 HORMONES

We know that the nervous system sends electrical signals that cause a chemical neurotransmitter to pass the signal on to another nerve or muscle. The endocrine system sends commands through chemical signals called **hormones**, which are secreted from various glands and organs throughout the body with the main purpose of keeping the body's organs working in a state of homeostasis.

These endocrine glands and organs secrete their hormones into the bloodstream on an as-needed basis. This function is actually spelled in its name, *endo-* meaning into and *-crine* meaning to secrete. We do have other types of glands in our body, such as exocrine or sweat glands, but they secrete outside (*exo*) of the body.

The endocrine system is made up of both glands and organs. Organs are made up of more than one type of specialized cell, which has the ability to secrete a substance and also perform other functions. For example, the pancreas is an organ that produces the hormone insulin to regulate blood sugar levels, but it also performs digestive functions. A gland is made up of just one type of cell and it secretes substances only inside the body (see Figure 9-1).

9-1a Hormone Function

Hormones are released into our bloodstream, which transports them all throughout the body. Hormones function can last for various periods of time, ranging from several minutes to multiple days.

To perform their duty, hormones must do more than just float around in our blood. Instead, they must seek out and bind to receptor cells. These receptors can be found both inside and outside of a cell. When a hormone binds to a target cell or receptor cell, it can change the cell's activity by causing the cell

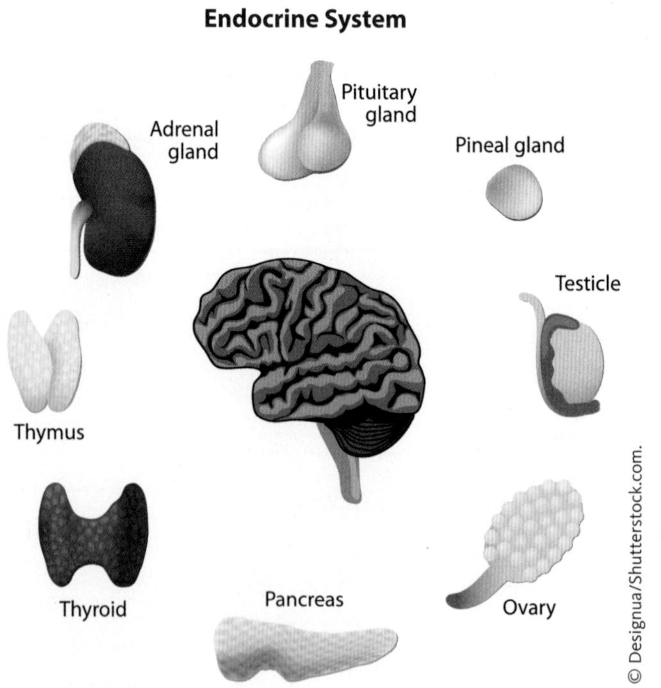

FIGURE 9-1 Parts of the endocrine system.

to make more protein, decrease the amount of protein production, or even stop the production of protein entirely.

Two very powerful types of hormones are steroids and thyroid hormones, which have the ability to bind to receptors inside the body's cells. This means these two hormone types can enter a cell and cross over into the cell's DNA, where they can make changes to the cell. Steroids are released by the adrenal glands, while the thyroid gland releases thyroid hormones. Another difference from nervous system control is that endocrine glands secrete hormones on a continual basis. This means our endocrine glands are always at work to maintain our hormone levels at a proper level and to keep our bodies at a homeostatic state.

Let's show how the two control systems work in a common situation, such as being in a cold environment well below the body's homeostatic body temperature of 98.6 degrees Fahrenheit. When the nervous system senses the body temperature dropping, the hypothalamus will be triggered by sensory neurons to produce body heat by shivering (neuromuscular control) and the hypothalamus stimulates the thyroid to release hormones to increase metabolism, which also generates more body heat.

9-2 FEEDBACK LOOPS

Our bodies have two different types of feedback processes that keep our bodies working at its proper levels.

The majority of our homeostatic regulation is accomplished by a **negative feedback loop**. Negative feedback occurs when your body is trying to get itself back to its correct level of function, such as body temperature, by working in opposition to the out-of-range value. Keeping with the temperature theme, an example of negative feedback is the thermostat found in your home, shown in Figure 9-2. Let's say you like to keep your house at 68 degrees Fahrenheit. If you get ill, you might turn the thermostat up to a new set point of 72 degrees. Because the house was colder than the new set point, the heating system will have to run until the temperature of the house reaches the new setting of 72 degrees. The too-cold sensation caused the opposite effect of adding heat, demonstrating a negative feedback system to bring the temperature back to the desired set point.

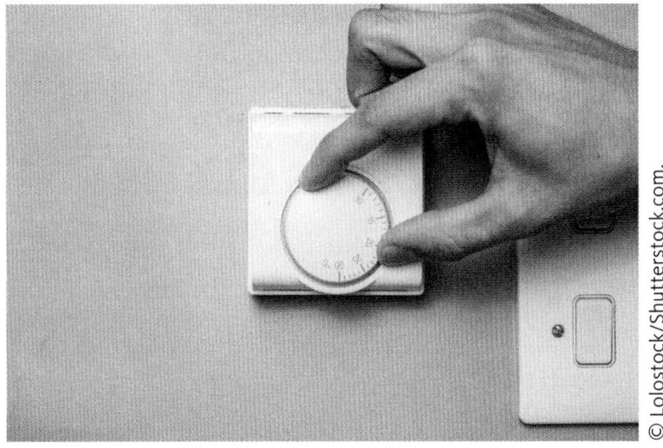

FIGURE 9-2 A home thermostat is an example of negative feedback.

Other examples of bodily functions controlled by negative feedback include blood pressure and blood sugar control.

The second type of feedback is the **positive feedback loop**. Instead of maintaining homeostasis like the negative feedback does by bringing the change back toward normal, this feedback mechanism causes an increase in the change within the body. In most cases, positive feedback is a vicious cycle that can be harmful as it moves farther and farther away from normal. A good example, however, is uterine contractions during childbirth. The hypothalamus sends a signal releasing oxytocin, which causes contractions to begin. As the uterus contracts, the baby moves down the birth canal, which increases signals to the hypothalamus, causing even more oxytocin to be released, which increases the uterine contractions. This cycle continues to increase in intensity until the baby is born, thus relieving the pressure and signaling the hypothalamus to stop calling for more oxytocin.

9-3 HORMONE LEVEL CONTROLS

Our hormone levels are controlled by three different sources, all of which play a very important role in hormone regulation. First is *neural control*, which is done through the nervous system. Reacting to danger, the nervous system initiates the fight or flight response. It increases the heart rate, dilates pupils, and increases the diameter of the airways so the body can bring in more oxygen by triggering the release of two hormones from the adrenal glands, which sit upon the kidneys. The two hormones, epinephrine and norepinephrine, cause the effects of the sympathetic nervous system, also known as the alert system.

The second type of control comes from *hormonal control*, which follows a hierarchy chain of command. A hormone is released from a gland, which is controlled by the release from another gland, higher on the chain of command. This is like a relay race in which runners cannot take off until they are given the baton. This chain of command is a form of negative feedback, so that whenever the value returns to normal the stimulus to secrete more hormone is inhibited.

The final type of hormone level control is *humoral control*. Humoral means fluid, and one of the most important body fluids is blood. Some endocrine organs have the ability to monitor body fluids, such as blood, and then use the negative feedback mechanism to make any changes. For example, humoral control is used to keep our blood sugar levels properly balanced. If the body's blood sugar is too high, the pancreas will secrete the hormone insulin to decrease the elevated blood sugar. Insulin causes the sugar or glucose to be absorbed by tissues to decrease the total blood glucose level back toward normal.

9-4 TYPES OF ENDOCRINE GLANDS

Many different types of endocrine glands and organs are found throughout the body, and are needed for the body to maintain a healthy balance.

9-4a Adrenal Glands

The **adrenal glands** are located on top of each kidney. This gland is responsible for releasing three types of hormones: aldosterone, androgen, and cortisol. Each hormone has a specific role: Aldosterone maintains a balance of potassium and

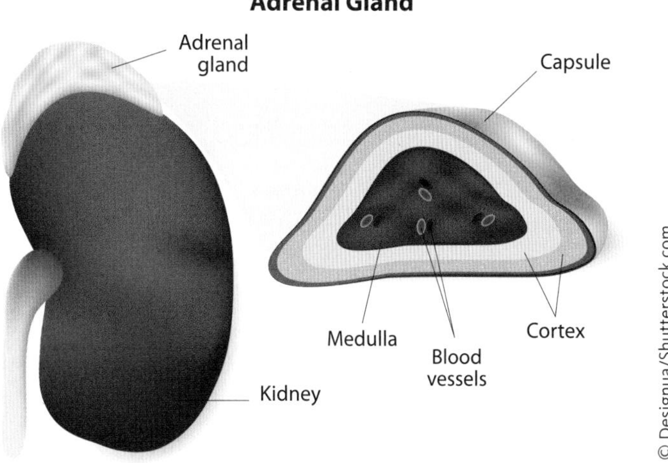

FIGURE 9-3 This image shows the location of the medulla within the adrenal gland.

sodium levels in the blood; androgen hormone produces male sex traits, such as deepening of voice and body hair; and cortisol releases glucose to the brain. The **adrenal medulla gland** is found in the inner region of the adrenal gland, which is encased by the adrenal cortex (outer core), shown in Figure 9-3. Two hormones secreted by the adrenal medulla are epinephrine and norepinephrine, which are released by the sympathetic system in response to high stress or danger.

9-4b Pancreas

The **pancreas** is found behind the stomach and spans from the right side of the body where the duodenum is attached via the pancreatic duct to the left side of the abdomen. Shown in the Figure 9-4, the pancreas secretes glucagon from alpha cells of the islets of Langerhans and insulin is secreted from beta cells. The glucagon hormone is responsible for increasing the blood glucose level to produce energy for the body, while insulin is required to decrease blood sugar levels by enhancing cellular uptake.

9-4c Thyroid Gland

The **thyroid gland**, shown in Figure 9-5, is found in the anterior region of the neck. This gland releases three hormones that play very important roles in our body's function. These are:

- Calcitonin, a hormone that helps to regulate proper levels of calcium and potassium in the blood. The parathyroid glands also play a role in regulating the calcium and potassium.
- Triiodothyronine (T3) has an effect on our body temperature, heart rate, and growth.
- Thyroxine (T4) helps to maintain appropriate metabolic processes.

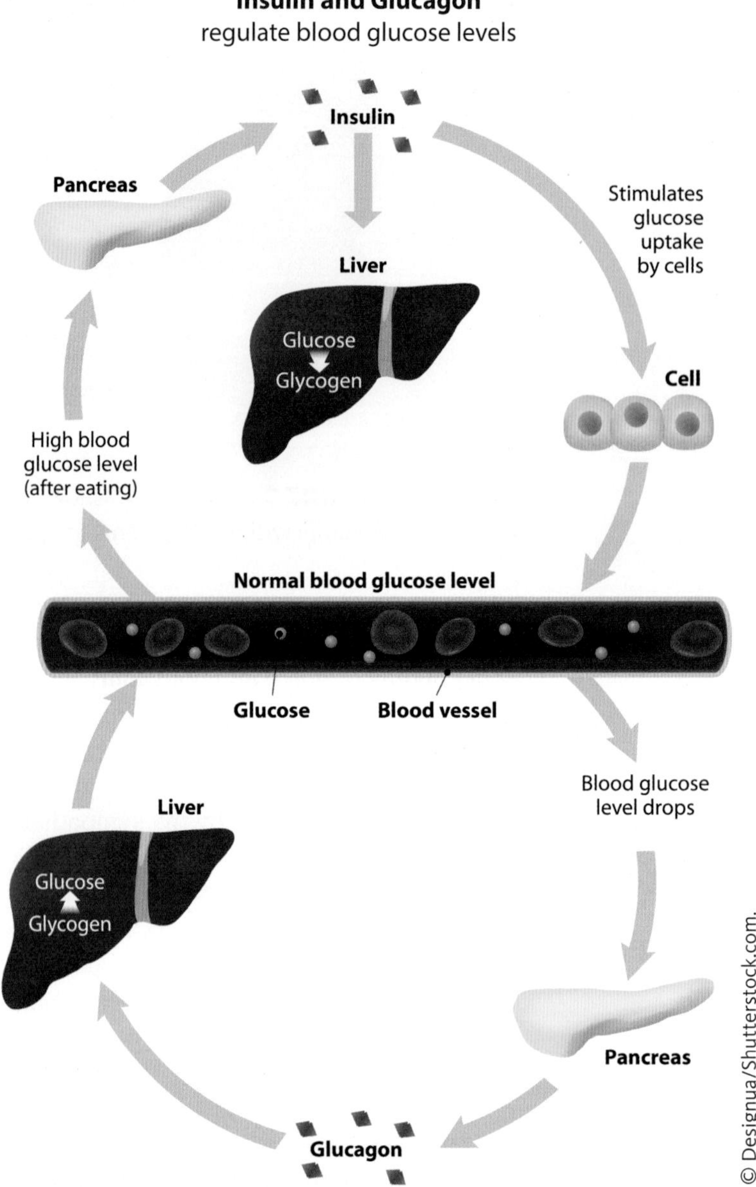

FIGURE 9-4 The roles of insulin and glucagon, which are both products of the pancreas.

9-4d Parathyroid Glands

The **parathyroid glands**, shown in Figure 9-6 are located on the posterior side of the thyroid. These four pea-sized glands on the posterior side of the thyroid secrete a hormone called parathyroid hormone. This hormone is important in regulating the levels of calcium and phosphates in the bloodstream. These minerals are needed for proper functioning of areas of the body such as the kidneys, bones, and small intestines.

9-4e Pituitary Gland

The pituitary gland is an amazing feature of our body. It is small, yet complex in how it controls many of our bodily functions.

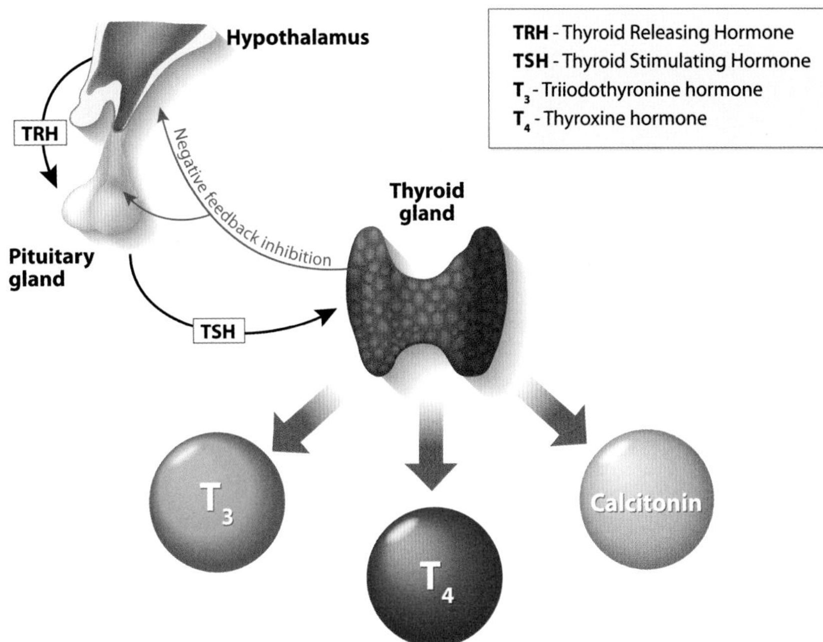

FIGURE 9-5 The release of thyroid hormones, while the negative feedback inhibition keeps these hormones at proper levels.

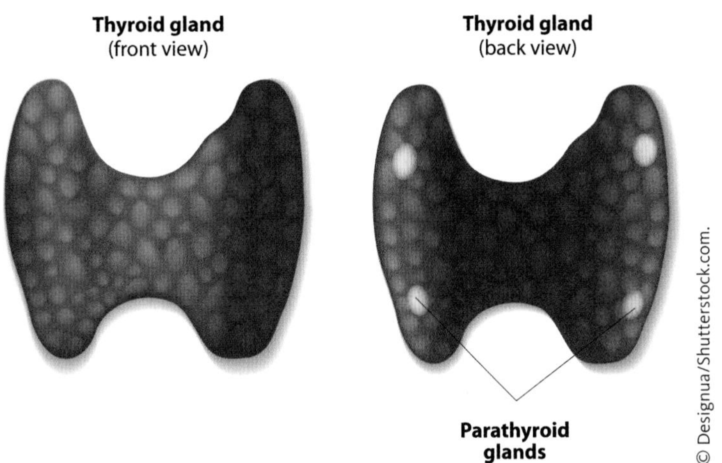

FIGURE 9-6 Image showing the difference between the thyroid and parathyroid.

The **anterior pituitary gland**, also called adenohypophysis, is located in the front portion of the pituitary gland. This gland is incredibly small, and yet is responsible for so much, which is why it is called the master gland. The anterior pituitary gland releases the following hormones:

- Adrenocorticotropic hormone (ACTH) regulates levels of cortisol, a steroid released by the cortex (the outer layer) of the adrenal gland. Cortisol is released when the body has low blood sugar, is used to regulate blood pressure, decrease inflammation, and monitor metabolism. When too much cortisol is in the body, whether caused by a tumor or drug, Cushing's syndrome can develop, while too little cortisol can cause Addison's disease. These two conditions will be discussed later in this chapter.

- Follicle-stimulating hormone (FSH) is used to produce eggs in the ovaries and plays a role in controlling the menstrual cycle. In men, it is used to produce sperm.
- Growth hormone (GH) directly affects cellular growth and reproduction.
- Luteinizing hormone (LH) is used along with FSH to control the female menstrual cycle. This hormone's level varies depending on the phase of the woman's cycle, as does FSH.
- Prolactin causes lactation stimulation.
- Thyroid-stimulating hormone (TSH) is released to control the thyroid in the body.

The **posterior pituitary**, or neurohypophysis gland, is responsible for releasing two hormones, oxytocin and antidiuretic (ADH) hormone. Oxytocin helps with lactation and uterine contractions. Antidiuretic hormone controls how much fluid the kidneys reabsorb, and therefore, the body's fluid balance. A diuretic causes fluid loss; an antidiuretic retains fluid within the body. This hormone is produced by the hypothalamus and is stored in the pituitary gland. When not enough antidiuretic hormone is secreted, it results in diabetes insipidus which will be discussed later in the chapter (see Figure 9-7).

9-4f Gonads

Next among our primary endocrine system glands are the **gonads**. Female gonads are located in the pelvic cavity and produce three types of hormones. Estrogen is produced in the ovaries and is the main sex hormone in women. The little bit of estrogen men have in their bodies comes about because the hormone is also made in the adrenal glands and even in fat tissue. While it can help maintain healthy bones in both sexes, it plays a major role in female development and pregnancy. There are actually three different types of estrogen:

1. Estradiol is the dominant form of estrogen found in women of childbearing age.
2. Estriol is the main type of estrogen found in pregnant women.
3. Estrone is the only form of estrogen found in women after they have gone through menopause.

The second type of hormone produced in ovaries is inhibin, which decreases FSH. The third hormone is progesterone, which also plays a major role in menstruation and pregnancy. In a pregnant woman, this hormone causes the endometrium to release proteins to prepare the body to nourish the fertilized egg.

Male gonads are made up of two testes, which are found in the scrotum. Two hormones are produced by the testes: testosterone and inhibin. Testosterone generates male sex characteristics and helps with sperm maturation, while inhibin is used to increase sperm count when needed.

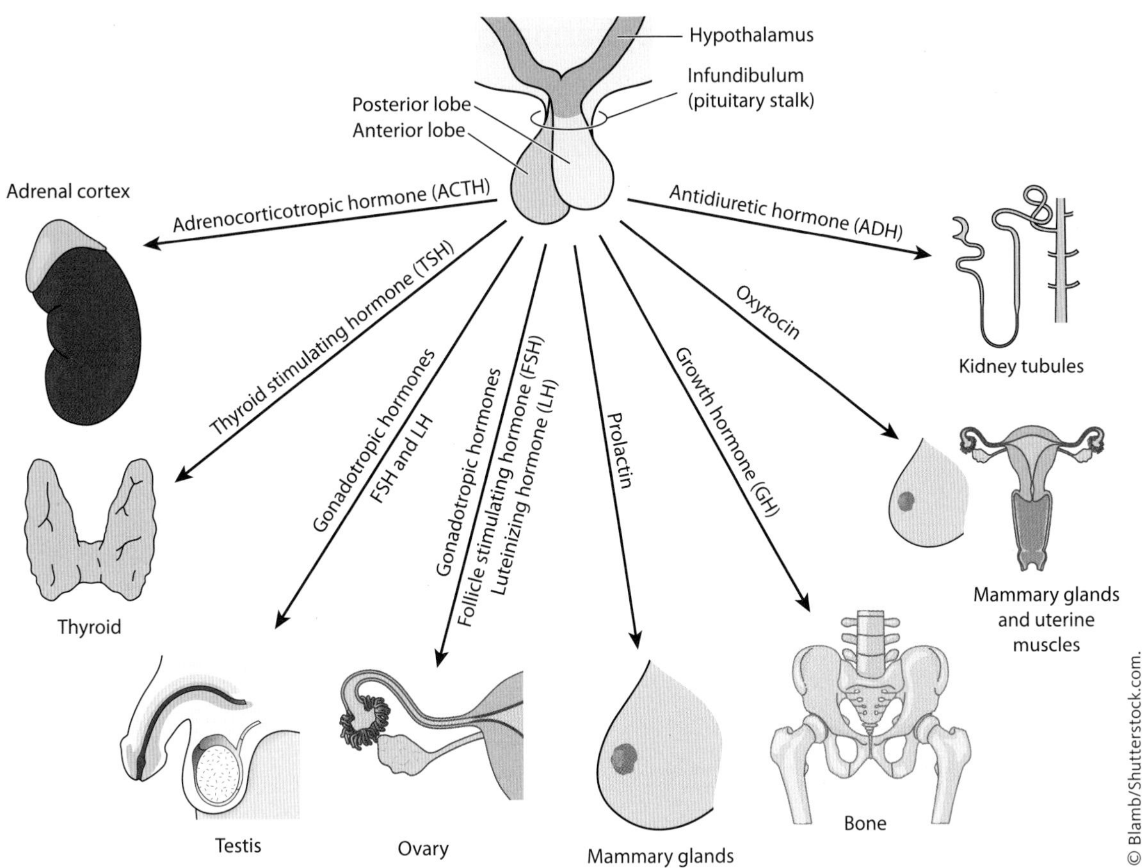

FIGURE 9-7 The functions of the anterior and posterior pituitary glands.

9-4g Thymus Gland

Located behind the sternum or breast bone is a gland called the thymus gland, which is bilobed (two lobes that are identical). T-cells are lymphocytes that are produced by the thymus gland and play a role in the body's immune system.

9-4h Pineal Gland

The pineal gland is located between the two cerebral hemispheres of the brain and is attached to the thalamus. The hormones produced by this gland are melatonin and serotonin. Melatonin helps to regulate the body's sleep cycles or circadian rhythm. The pineal gland produces melatonin based on the light in the retina as sensed by photoreceptors. For example, if it is dark outside (night time), it will be dark in the retina causing the gland to produce melatonin. When it is day time, light will be sensed in the retina by photoreceptors causing a decrease in melatonin production. The hormone serotonin functions like a neurotransmitter and vasoconstrictor. Serotonin can cause the constriction of smooth muscles and the inhibition of gastric secretions.

LEARNING OBJECTIVE 9.2 Describe the pathopharmacology of diabetes.

KEY TERMS

Antidiabetic drugs Drugs used to control Type 2 diabetes.

Atherosclerosis Hardening of blood vessels.

Central diabetes insipidus Caused by the lack of antidiuretic hormone.

Diabetes insipidus A condition caused by a lack of antidiuretic hormone, causing frequent urination and thirst.

Diabetes mellitus A group of diseases caused by too much sugar in the blood.

Diabetic coma Unconscious state caused by high blood sugar.

Diabetic gangrene Dead tissue resulting from a loss of blood flow, peripheral artery disease caused by diabetes mellitus.

Diabetic retinopathy Blindness caused by high blood sugar.

Diabetic shock Life-threatening condition caused by too much insulin in the body.

Gestational diabetes Diabetes that develops because of pregnancy.

Hyperglycemia High blood sugar.

Hypoglycemia Condition of low blood sugar.

Insulin Hormone required to control blood sugar.

Ketoacidosis Buildup of ketones (acid) in the blood when the body breaks down fat for energy.

Nephrogenic diabetes insipidus Form of diabetes insipidus caused by kidney disease.

Peripheral Vascular Disease (PVD) Disease of the blood vessels outside of the heart often resulting in partial or complete blockages of blood flow.

Prediabetes Condition of slightly higher than normal blood sugar that is not high enough to be considered diabetes.

Type 1 diabetes Also called juvenile diabetes, caused by the pancreas' inability to produce insulin.

Type 2 diabetes A chronic, lifelong condition of high blood sugar.

9-5 DIABETES INTRODUCTION

One of the most common disorders of the endocrine system is diabetes. Some people even call diabetes an epidemic, although there is much confusion because of the various types of diabetes. The most familiar type is **diabetes mellitus**, which is a chronic condition that involves insulin and blood sugar. The less familiar form is called **diabetes insipidus**, and we will begin our discussion there.

9-6 DIABETES INSIPIDUS

Diabetes insipidus causes an increase in the body's production of urine because of the kidneys inability to retain fluid. It can be caused by different situations, and each has a different name. Diabetes insipidus tends to affect men more than women and is likely to occur early in a person's life.

The hormone involved in this condition is vasopressin, also known as antidiuretic hormone (ADH), which regulates the amount of urine released by the kidneys. For example, if vasopressin levels are increased, the kidneys will increase fluid reabsorption into the body and thus output less urine. On the other hand, if the vasopressin levels are decreased there will be less antidiuretic effect and the kidneys will eliminate large amounts of urine, a condition known as diabetes insipidus.

The different variations of diabetes insipidus are as follows:

- **Nephrogenic diabetes insipidus** is caused when the kidneys do not respond to the vasopressin hormone. This can be an inherited condition or caused by kidney dysfunction.
- **Central diabetes insipidus** develops as a result of not enough vasopressin being secreted by the pituitary gland. This form can develop as a result of a head injury or brain tumor.

Patients with diabetes insipidus experience excessive thirst and urination. While normal urine output is roughly two liters in 24 hours, those with diabetes insipidus will excrete up to 16 liters per day. This amount of urine output causes extreme thirst, a signal that the body needs to replenish the fluid volume being lost. The person, however, cannot keep up with the fluid levels required to remain properly hydrated, and usually becomes dehydrated and has dry skin.

Because the patient is usually drinking and urinating a lot, a urinalysis will show low levels of dissolved waste products in the urine, as well as the urine appearing very light in color.

Central diabetes insipidus conditions are treated with replacement hormones such as Pitressin, Vasostrict (vasopressin), and Dyapid (lypressin). Another agent, desmopressin, is a synthetic analogue of antidiuretic hormone that comes in various forms, including oral, intravenous, intranasal, and subcutaneous. This medication can be given up to three times per day to help the patient's body maintain proper fluid requirements.

9-7 DIABETES MELLITUS

The sugar-regulating diabetic condition, diabetes mellitus, is a chronic condition caused by an insufficient production of **insulin**, the hormone that regulates blood sugar, or from the body becoming insensitive to insulin. This condition causes an abnormally high blood sugar (glucose) level in the blood called **hyperglycemia**. It should be noted that diabetes and hyperglycemia are not the same. If a patient's diabetes is not controlled properly, their blood sugar can rise causing hyperglycemia. Hyperglycemia can be caused by other factors such as stress and medications, not just as a complication of diabetes mellitus.

Insulin, which is secreted by the pancreas, moves sugar from the bloodstream out into the tissues, where it is used to fuel the body and causes the blood sugar level to decrease. With a lack of insulin, the sugar remains in the bloodstream, causing an increase in blood sugar. In addition, because the sugar is not able to get out into the tissues to be used as fuel, the body will break down its own muscle and fat cells to produce energy. This causes a byproduct called ketones to build up in the body, leading to a condition called **Ketoacidosis**.

Glucose comes from two main sources: the food we eat and our liver. People who need help controlling his or her diabetes must adhere to a strict diet to prevent too much glucose from entering his or her blood resulting in high blood sugar. Our liver also makes and stores glucose in the form of glucagon, which can be converted to glucose when needed, acting as a reserve store of energy.

For example, if we go a long time between meals, our body still must keep our blood sugar in check to maintain vital cellular processes. The liver will

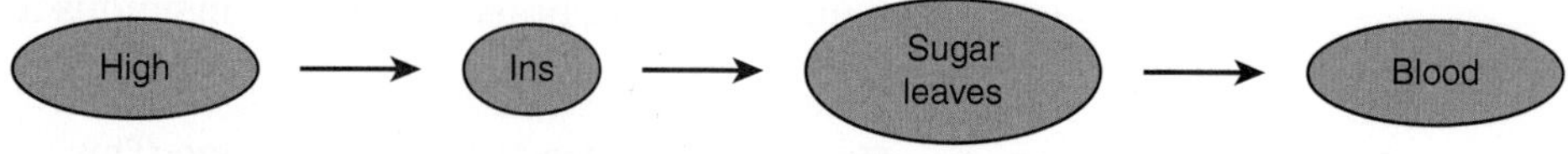

FIGURE 9-8A How high blood sugar is lowered.

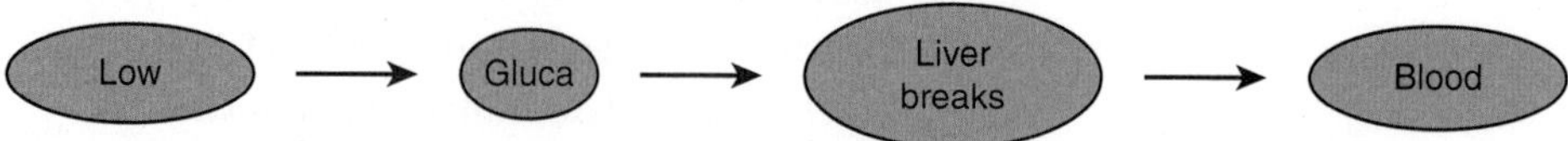

FIGURE 9-8B How low blood sugar is increased.

break down glucagon and turn it into glucose to pick up the slack. This glucose is then released into the bloodstream to increase our blood glucose levels. This increased blood sugar can then be pulled out of the bloodstream by insulin and be used by our body's cells for fuel (see Figures 9-8A and 9-8B).

9-8 NORMAL BLOOD SUGAR VALUES

Normal blood sugar levels should be less than 100 mg/dL after fasting for eight hours. Diabetes can be diagnosed by a fasting plasma glucose test higher than 126 mg/dL. Another method called an oral glucose tolerance test is done by having a patient drink a sugary drink after fasting for eight hours. A reading of 200 mg/dL or higher is positive for diabetes.

CLINICAL CONNECTION 9.1

PREDIABETES

Prediabetes has gained much focus in recent years because of the rising prevalence of diabetes. Prediabetes occurs when a patient's blood sugar is not in the diabetic range, but it is higher than normal. For example, normal blood sugar is less than 100, and the diabetic range is higher than 126. Prediabetes blood sugar levels range from 100 to 125. It is a signal that the patient should change their lifestyle—lose weight, eat healthier, and get more exercise—or they will end up with diabetes. Prediabetes causes the body to not work properly and it might not produce or respond to insulin as it should. If the condition is caught early and proper lifestyle changes are made, the person can stop the pathway to diabetes.

9-8a Type 1 Diabetes

Diabetes mellitus can be broken down further into Type 1 and Type 2 diabetes. **Type 1 diabetes**, or juvenile diabetes, usually develops before the age of 30. As shown in Figure 9-9, Type 1 diabetes is caused by the body's inability to produce enough insulin, which can be caused by an autoimmune disease that attacks the pancreas and inhibits its ability to produce insulin.

In the pancreas, insulin is produced by special beta cells in the islets of Langerhans. If not enough insulin is present, glucose will remain in the blood, and the body is unable to make energy to fuel its cells. The body then will attempt to use other substances such as proteins and fats to make energy. This

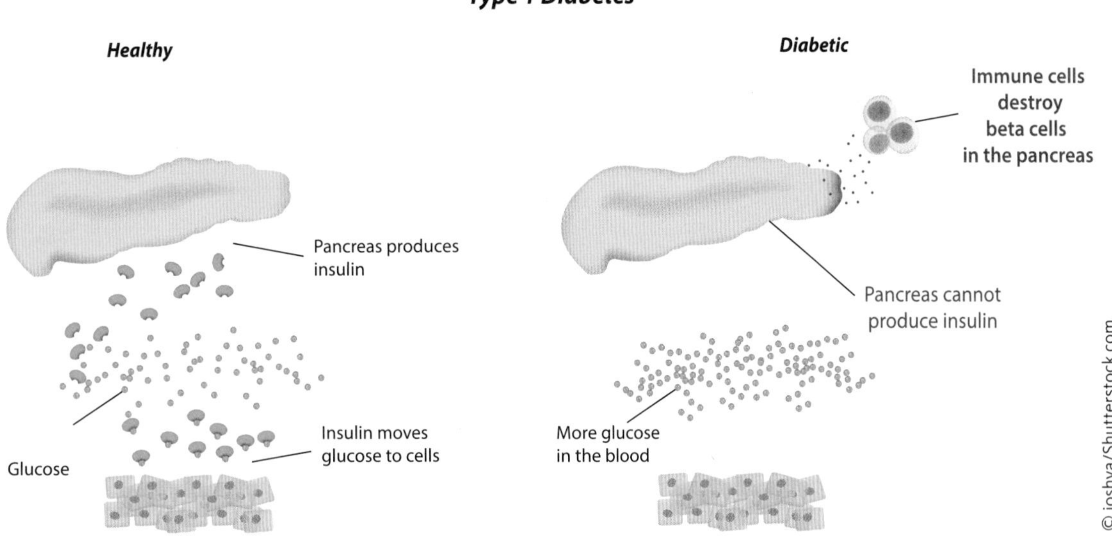

FIGURE 9-9 Type 1 diabetes.

will cause the body to store high levels of ketones in the bloodstream, creating a condition known as diabetic ketoacidosis. Both hyperglycemia and diabetic ketoacidosis cause life-threatening symptoms.

9-8b Diabetic Symptoms

The degree of symptoms experienced by a patient depends on how much glucose is in the bloodstream and the type of diabetes present. With Type 1 diabetes the symptoms are more severe and have a faster (acute) onset. That being said, Type 1 and Type 2 (to be discussed soon) share some of the same symptoms. These symptoms include increased urination, thirst, hunger, blurred vision, fatigue, irritability, and recurring infections affecting the skin, vagina, and even the gums. Often people experience sweet-smelling urine caused by an increase in ketones in the urine. Also seen with this condition is impaired wound healing, causing a much slower healing time that often requires medical attention for even minor wounds.

9-8c Monitoring Diabetes

Type 1 diabetes requires insulin injections to make up for the lack of insulin production, a situation that needs to be monitored to maintain the proper levels of blood glucose. The American Diabetes Association recommends a blood test to measure the level of glycated hemoglobin. The test is called hemoglobin A1c or HbA1c. This test gives medical providers an average of how well their patient has controlled his or her blood sugar over the past two to three months.

Glycated hemoglobin forms when the hemoglobin in the blood is exposed to high blood sugar levels. This glycated change lasts throughout the duration of the hemoglobin's life span of two to three months. The higher the blood glucose level, the higher the level of HbA1c.

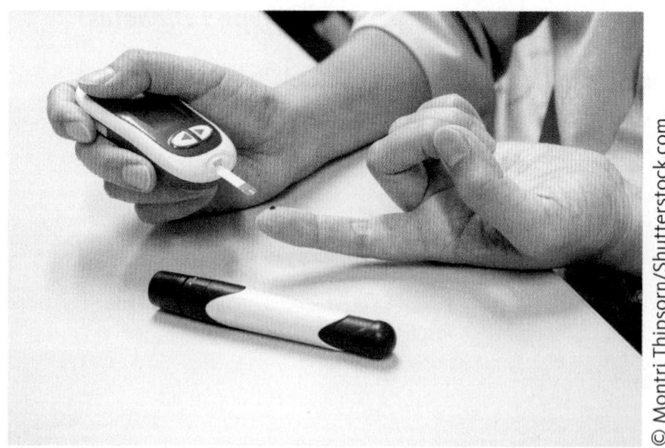

FIGURE 9-10 Checking blood sugar level with a glucose meter.

For individuals that are not diabetic, HbA1c levels of 4% to 5.9% are considered normal, while those with diabetes who poorly manage their condition will have levels above 7%. Those able to decrease their HbA1c levels actually can decrease the likelihood of developing complications of diabetes.

Type 1 diabetes is a serious medical condition and treatment will be required for the rest of the patient's life. Insulin injections are required to be given daily to control blood sugar levels. Insulin cannot be taken orally because it would be rendered ineffective by the stomach. To ensure blood sugar levels are normal, it can be checked both quickly and painlessly with a blood glucose monitoring device, Figure 9-10.

9-8d Types of Insulin

There is more than one type of insulin and each has its own specific purpose, but all are administered with an insulin syringe. Some types of insulin depend on their rate of action: rapid or fast-acting insulin, long-acting insulin, and intermediate-acting insulin. Insulin also can be natural or synthetic. A list of synthetic insulin injection preparations follows.

- Novolin N, Humulin N, others (insulin isophane) is an intermediate-acting form that takes 2–4 hours to begin to work. It peaks at 4–12 hours, and can last 12–18 hours.
- Apidra (insulin glulisine) is a short-acting insulin that does not last long in the body. It begins to work 15 minutes after injection, peaks after a 1 hour, and has a 2- to 4-hour duration.
- NovoLog (insulin aspart) is a fast-acting insulin that also begins to work 15 minutes after injection, peaks at 1 hour, and has a 2- to 4-hour duration.
- Humalog (insulin lispro) is a fast-acting insulin that works 15 minutes after injected, peaks at 1 hour, and has a 2- to 4-hour duration.
- Lantus (insulin glargine) is a long-acting insulin that begins to work hours after the injection and continues to work for 24 hours.

- Levemir (detemir) is a long-acting insulin that begins to work hours after the injection and continues to work for 24 hours.
- Humulin 70/30, Novolin 70/30, others are mixtures of different types of insulin (70% human insulin isophane suspension and 30% human insulin injection). This is a mixture of intermediate-acting insulin with fast-acting insulin. Regular insulin also known as regular human refers to human forms of insulin.

9-8e Insulin Pumps

Insulin pumps are another alternative to managing diabetes, Figure 9-11. Instead of using insulin injections to control blood sugar levels, an insulin pump can administer rapid-acting insulin 24 hours a day. This device can deliver three different dosage types under the skin via a catheter.

Basal rate dosages are given at all times to keep the blood sugar level at proper levels (maintain a baseline) between meals and at night while you sleep. A bolus dose can be given by pushing a button on the pump to deliver an extra dose when you eat or any time you check your blood sugar level and the reading is too high.

9-8f Type 2 Diabetes

Type 2 diabetes is a non-insulin dependent form of diabetes because although some insulin is being produced, it is either an insufficient amount or ineffective in pushing the glucose out of the blood and into the cells. This is the most common type of diabetes mellitus and has been increasing in the population because of poor diets, obesity, and a lack of exercise. While it usually affects those older than 40 years of age, with the rise of childhood obesity, it is becoming more common in younger age groups.

One reason the islets of Langerhans in the pancreas stop producing enough insulin or produce ineffective insulin is thought to be that the cells in the pancreas wear out from all of the carbohydrates (sugars) being consumed in mass quantities over a period of time. This causes a heavy burden on the gland to produce insulin to the point where it weakens or wears out as shown in Figure 9-12.

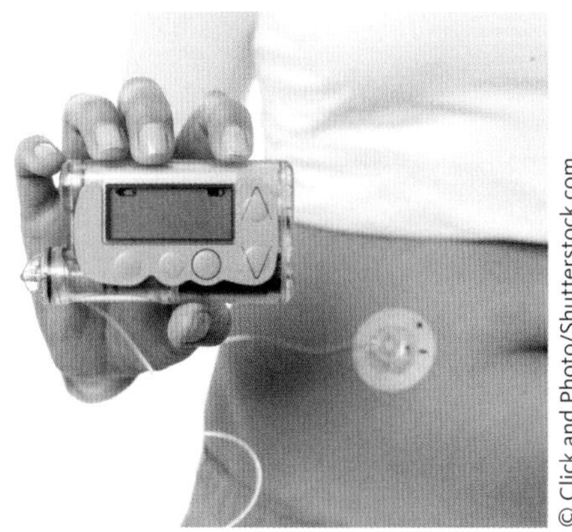

FIGURE 9-11 Insulin pump.

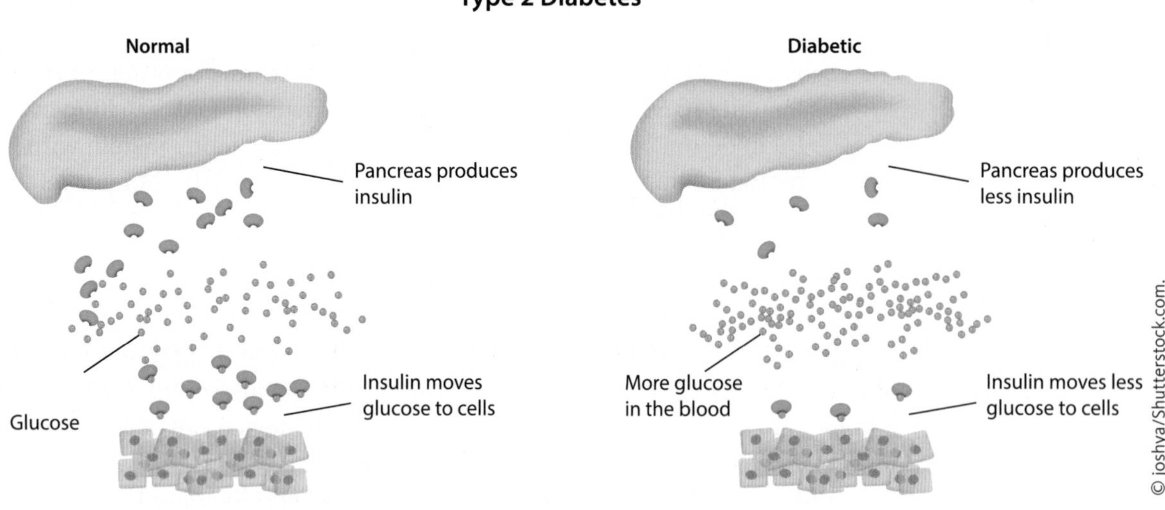

FIGURE 9-12 Type 2 diabetes.

9-8g Treatment of Type 2 Diabetes

Unlike Type 1 diabetes, Type 2 *usually* does not require injections of insulin. Instead, this condition can be controlled with a healthy diet and exercise. If this lifestyle change isn't enough, the patient also can be given antidiabetic medication that will stimulate insulin secretion.

Table 9-1 lists **antidiabetic drugs** commonly used to treat Type 2 diabetes along with a healthy diet, and exercise.

Table 9-1 Commonly used Type 2 antidiabetic agents

BRAND NAME/GENERIC NAME	ACTION
DiaBeta (glyburide) oral	Stimulates beta cells in the pancreas to release insulin.
Glucotrol (glipizide) oral	This drug assists the pancreas in the production of insulin to decrease blood sugar.
Januvia (sitagliptin phosphate) oral	Releases incretins, which increase insulin released after meals and also decrease the amount of glucose produced by the liver.
Glucophage (metformin) oral	This drug decreases the amount of glucose absorbed by the stomach and intestines.
Janumet (sitagliptin phosphate/metformin) oral	This is a combination drug that works to control blood sugar levels by releasing incretins, which increase insulin released after meals and decrease the amount of glucose produced by the liver from the drug sitagliptin. The other drug, metformin, decreases the amount of glucose absorbed by the stomach and intestines.
Actos (pioglitazone) oral	Decreases blood sugar by getting the body to respond more efficiently to insulin.

9-9 COMPLICATIONS OF DIABETES MELLITUS

Complications of diabetes mellitus can occur rapidly or over a long period of time. Some people even lose their limbs or go blind because of untreated diabetes. One complication that occurs suddenly and progresses rapidly is **diabetic shock**. This perfect storm occurs when an individual does not get enough food, exercises too much, or takes too much insulin (removing too much sugar from the blood). This severely decreased blood sugar level (**hypoglycemia**) causes the person to shake, sweat, become light-headed, and eventually confused. This condition requires immediate emergency attention as it progress quickly.

Diabetic coma is another complication that arises when a person administers too little or too much insulin or if someone consumes too many carbohydrates, spiking their blood sugar levels. Those affected experience symptoms of excessive thirst, lethargy, and excessive urination, which result in dehydration. Also present is ketoacidosis, which can produce a noticeably sweet-smelling breath. This condition progresses slowly, but will eventually lead to coma. If this condition occurs, medical attention is needed to receive proper amounts of insulin and fluids.

Atherosclerosis is a condition that causes fatty or waxy-like deposits on the walls of the arteries, causing them to thicken and harden. This condition is caused by lipids or fat cells going into the bloodstream to be used as energy instead of blood sugar. When a patient develops atherosclerosis, they are at greater risk of a myocardial infarction (heart attack), cerebral vascular accident (stroke), and peripheral vascular disease.

Peripheral vascular disease (PVD) occurs because of poor peripheral circulation. This is the culprit behind difficult wound healing and extremity loss from **diabetic gangrene** in the legs and feet, Figure 9-13. Some people develop complications from peripheral vascular disease in their eyes and kidneys. In fact, some diabetic patients go blind from the disease when the blood vessels

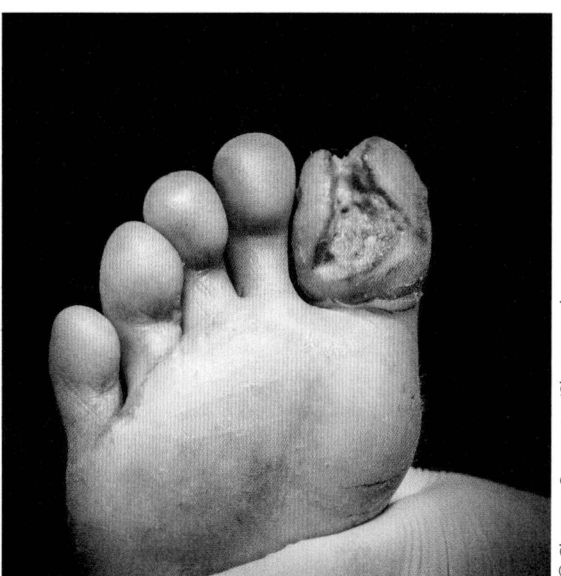

FIGURE 9-13 Diabetic gangrene because of peripheral vascular disease caused by atherosclerosis.

in their retinas are destroyed by a conditional called diabetic retinopathy. In the kidneys, renal vessels can be destroyed, causing kidney failure and death.

Because diabetes mellitus is incurable, the key to avoiding such problems is to closely monitor blood sugar levels and keep up with proper medication, diet, and exercise regimens.

CLINICAL CONNECTION 9.2

GESTATIONAL DIABETES

Some women are affected by gestational diabetes. The reason for this is linked to the hormones estrogen and progesterone. These hormones are required to maintain pregnancy, and the levels increase as the placenta grows and the pregnancy continues. Estrogen and progesterone make the body insulin-resistant, which forces the pancreas to work harder to produce more insulin. When the pancreas reaches the limit where it cannot keep up with the body's demand, the blood sugar level rises because not enough insulin is available to pull it out of the bloodstream and into the cells of the body. Gestational diabetes is treated like diabetes mellitus. This condition can cause larger baby sizes at birth and will usually disappear after the mother has delivered her baby.

LEARNING OBJECTIVE 9.3 Summarize pathopharmacology of additional endocrine disorders.

KEY TERMS

24-Hour urine-free cortisol test A diagnostic procedure used to measure the cortisol levels in urine over a 24-hour period.

Addison's disease A condition caused by the lack of cortisol produced by the adrenal glands.

Addisonian crisis A severe complication of Addison's disease.

Antithyroid Drug that stops the thyroid from producing T3 and T4 hormones.

Cushing's syndrome A condition caused by too much cortisol in the body.

Exophthalmos Abnormal protrusion of the eyes.

Hyperthyroidism Overproduction of thyroid hormones.

Hypothyroidism Underproduction of thyroid hormones.

Late-night salivary cortisol level test Salivary test done at night to measure cortisol levels.

Myxedema Condition associated with hypothyroidism.

Thyroid storm Life-threatening complication of hyperthyroidism.

9-10 THYROID DISORDERS

While diabetes is the most common endocrine disorder, other common disorders affect the thyroid gland. Our body depends heavily on our thyroid to ensure proper functioning. For example, it secretes hormones such as thyroxine (T4), which helps us maintain our metabolism, body temperature, and even assists our GI system in digesting food by stimulating gastric juice secretion and peristalsis. We will focus on both hyperthyroidism and hypothyroidism in this section.

9-11 HYPERTHYROIDISM

There are many known causes of **hyperthyroidism**, also known as thyrotoxicosis, while some causes still remain unknown. Hyperthyroidism is a condition where the thyroid gland secretes T4 in excess. To produce hormones like T4, our body requires iodine, which can be found in table salt. Some causes of hyperthyroidism include hereditary, tumors, a diet high in iodine, and taking too much thyroid hormone medication. An autoimmune disease such as Graves' disease causes hyperthyroidism because antibodies stimulate the thyroid, causing the gland to become enlarged and overproduce hormones.

Regardless of the cause, the thyroid becomes enlarged appearing as a lump called a goiter in the anterior region of the neck. The excessive production of T4 causes an increase in the body's metabolism rate, causing an increased appetite but no gain in weight because of the hypermetabolic state. Instead, the patient becomes very thin. Peristalsis is also stimulated by T4, and too much T4 increases peristalsis action, causing the bowel contents to move through the intestine at a faster pace than normal. This situation does not allow for proper fluid absorption and therefore causes diarrhea.

The increased metabolism also causes an increase in body temperature, causing the patient to sweat excessively. Both diarrhea and increased sweating will cause an increase in fluid loss, leading to dehydration. Other symptoms are a high heart rate, hyperactivity, excessive excitability, weakness, and nervousness.

A life-threatening condition called a **thyroid storm** is an acute or sudden exacerbation of hyperthyroidism, which can happen to those with severe hyperthyroidism or after the thyroid has been removed (thyroidectomy). Symptoms include excessive tachycardia (possibly reaching a heart rate of 200 bpm), tachypnea, and a rapid onset of a high body temperature.

Other patients can develop an eye-opening symptom, literally. A condition called **exophthalmos** causes the eyeballs to protrude outward in a wide-eyed appearance because of swelling of the vessels behind the patient's eyes. Exophthalmos can be so severe that the patient cannot close his or her eyelids. Even after the patient gets his or her hyperthyroidism under control, the exophthalmos might not completely resolve (see Figure 9-14).

9-11a Treating Hyperthyroidism

The main treatments for hyperthyroidism include medication, radiation, and a thyroidectomy. **Antithyroid** agents, also called thionamides, are used to bring thyroid levels back to normal. These drugs do not alter the thyroid gland as radiation would, and they also work faster than radiation therapy. Antithyroid medications decrease iodine levels in the body and thus decrease thyroid hormone production. Antithyroid hormones work best when treating mild cases of hyperthyroidism; however, this class also helps decrease the odds of experiencing worsening effects of hyperthyroidism.

Commonly used antithyroid medications include Tapazole (methimazole) and Propacil (propylthiouracil). Tapazole is taken every eight hours, with or without food, and, if used in children, the dose will vary depending on their weight. Propacil is taken every eight hours with or without food and is not recommended for children. Pregnant women and those who are breastfeeding should take special precaution in taking these drugs.

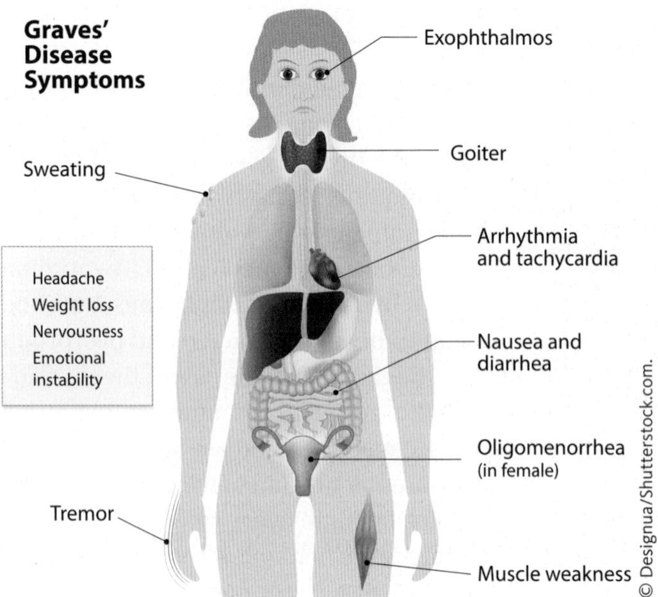

FIGURE 9-14 Graves' disease symptoms.

Propylthiouracil has fewer side effects than methimazole. Symptoms will not stop overnight. Instead, these drugs will take anywhere from one to eight weeks for symptoms to show improvements, and it may take up to six months to get the hormones back to normal levels. Common side effects of antithyroid drugs are nausea, achy joints, and a noticeable change in taste.

Another drug called ThyroSafe (potassium iodide solution) can be used to block radiation therapy treatments from causing too much damage to thyroid tissue. Radiation iodide therapy is used by nuclear medicine to destroy thyroid tissue because patients who have benign thyroid nodules produce too much thyroid hormone.

9-12 HYPOTHYROIDISM

Hypothyroidism is caused by an underactive thyroid, which decreases the body's normal production of T4. **Myxedema** is an advanced form of hypothyroidism that usually occurs in middle-aged women. Congenital hypothyroidism, also called cretinism, occurs in newborns that do not have a properly developed thyroid. This condition causes both mental and growth development problems.

Hypothyroidism is most often caused by an autoimmune disease called Hashimoto's disease. It occurs more commonly in women than men and is thought to be caused by the destruction of the body's lymphocytes, resulting in less tissue to produce proper levels of thyroid hormones. Hypothyroidism also can be caused by over-treating hyperthyroidism, in which too much thyroid tissue was damaged, preventing the thyroid from producing enough hormones to maintain proper levels.

Radiation therapy can also cause extensive tissue damage and result in decreased hormone levels, as can a thyroidectomy that removes most, if not all, of a patient's thyroid tissue. This condition requires hormone replacement therapy. Some medications, such as lithium, are known to decrease thyroid hormone levels. Lithium is used to treat patients with psychiatric disorders.

Symptoms of hypothyroidism do not usually occur suddenly. Instead, the patient will experience symptoms gradually and might even blame them on something else, such as old age. The severity of symptoms a patient experiences depends on how low the thyroid hormone levels drop. The list of possible signs and symptoms are:

- Increased weight gain
- Fatigue
- Weakness
- Hoarseness
- Constipation
- Muscle weakness
- Muscle aches and stiffness
- Joint pain
- Increased cholesterol
- Decreased fertility
- Depression
- Sensitivity to cold temperatures
- Slow heart rate
- Brittle nails
- Thinning hair
- Decreased memory

The patient also might develop a goiter because of the continuous stimulation of the thyroid gland to create more hormones (see Figure 9-15).

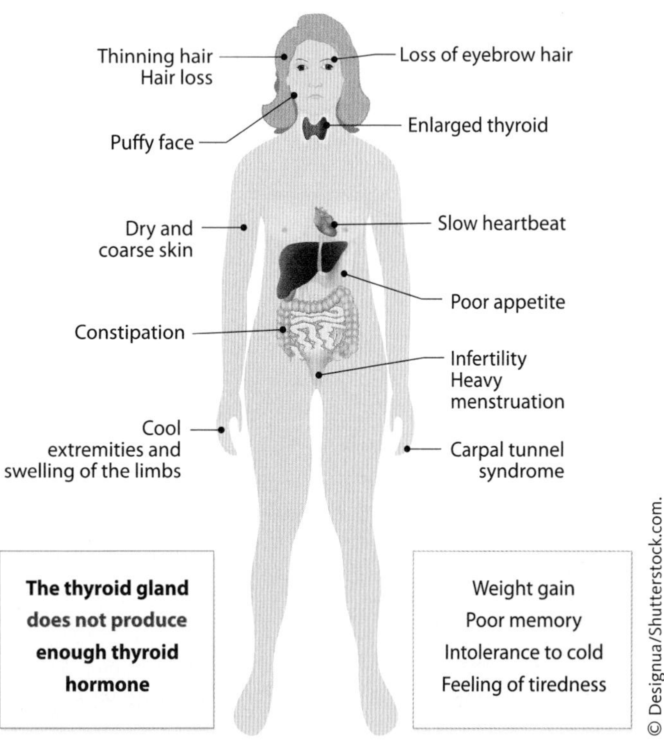

FIGURE 9-15 Symptoms of hypothyroidism.

Table 9-2 Common agents used to regulate thyroid hormones and treat hypothyroidism

Agent
Levothroid, Levoxyl, Synthroid, Tirosint, Unithroid (levothyroxine)
Cytomel (liothyronine)
Thyrolar (liotrix)

Because the thyroid gland plays a significant role in the body's metabolism and growth rate, children with hypothyroidism experience dwarfism, as well as unusual facial characteristics such as puffy eyelids, widened nose, and small eyes. Sexual organs and the muscular system do not fully develop, which might cause the patient to not be able to walk or even stand.

Hypothyroidism can be diagnosed with a thyroid stimulating hormone (TSH) blood test, which can detect this condition in its earliest stages. This is the best test at screening patients for this condition; it can even diagnose subclinical hypothyroidism meaning that it has no signs or symptoms yet.

Table 9-2 lists thyroid agents, thyroid hormone replacements, used to treat hypothyroidism.

9-13 CORTISOL ISSUES

Our body's cortisol levels also must be kept at an acceptable level to function properly. Addison's disease is caused by the body having too little cortisol; Cushing's syndrome develops from too much cortisol production.

9-14 ADDISON'S DISEASE

Addison's disease, a relatively uncommon disease of the adrenal glands, is caused by the adrenal cortex not secreting enough cortisol and aldosterone. Addison's disease, also known as hypoadrenalism or adrenal insufficiency, can be life-threatening and can occur in patients of either gender at any age. A pituitary tumor, adrenal gland infection, cancer of the adrenal gland, tuberculosis, and steroid hormone therapy all are potential causes of Addison's disease. The most common cause, however, is autoimmune disease resulting in the inability of the adrenal glands to produce adrenocortical hormones.

Symptoms of Addison's disease can range from mild to life-threatening, and can take several months to fully emerge. The symptoms of Addison's disease include:

- Vomiting
- Diarrhea
- Dehydration
- Salt cravings
- Hypoglycemia
- Darkening of skin (yellow to brown)

- Depression
- Irritability
- Joint and muscle pain
- Weight loss
- Decreased appetite.

See Figure 9-16.

Patients experiencing an **Addisonian crisis**, a life-threatening complication of Addison's disease, have decreased blood sugar and blood pressure and increased potassium levels. This is a medical emergency and requires prompt medical treatment.

9-14a Diagnosing and Treating Addison's Disease

Addison's disease can be diagnosed with blood samples. Blood tests can be used to measure the levels of adrenocorticotropic hormone and cortisol, as well as sodium and potassium. The physician also could measure the levels of antibodies that might be present causing the disease state. A test to see if the adrenal glands are producing cortisol properly is done by injecting the patient with a synthetic ATCH, which should prompt the body to increase cortisol levels. If there is adrenal insufficiency, cortisol levels will remain decreased or still not produce any at all. A CT scan can be performed to get a visual image of the adrenal glands to study for any anomalies.

Addison's disease is treated with hormone replacement therapy to increase the patient's low hormones levels. This is accomplished by taking oral or injectable corticosteroids such as Cortef oral (hydrocortisone) and Solu-Medrol injection (methylprednisolone).

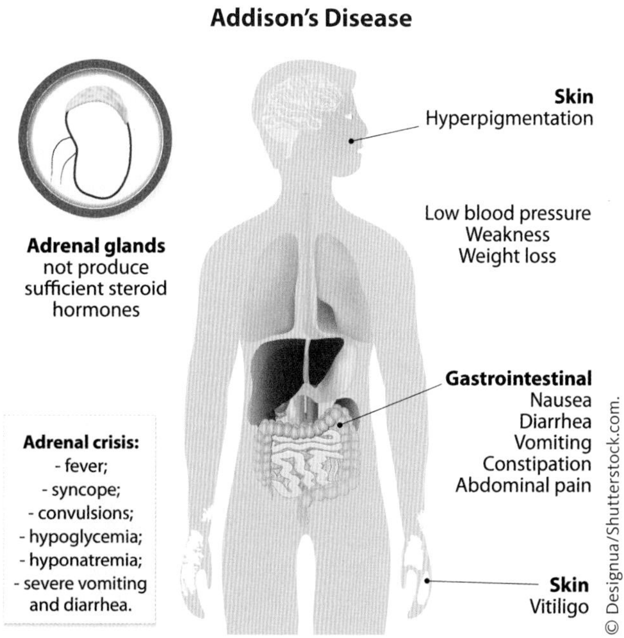

FIGURE 9-16 Additional signs and symptoms of Addison's disease.

9-15 CUSHING'S SYNDROME

Cushing's syndrome is the result of the adrenal glands pumping too much cortisol hormone in the body for too long. Cushing's syndrome is caused by a variety of different conditions.

An excessive amount of cortisol might be produced if a tumor positions itself on the adrenal glands, pituitary gland, pancreas, lungs, thyroid or thymus. In a healthy system, the pituitary gland releases adrenocorticotropic hormone (ACTH) to stimulate the adrenal glands to release more cortisol in the blood when needed. Tumors can increase the production of ACTH, signaling the adrenal glands to produce more cortisol. Tumors on the adrenal gland increase the levels of cortisol already being produced by directly causing the gland to secrete more cortisol. Cushing's syndrome most commonly is caused through prolong administration of steroid medications, the most common of which is prednisone.

Cushing's syndrome sufferers experience two classic symptoms: a round, moon-shaped face, and a buffalo hump on the upper portion of his or her back. Other symptoms are fatigue, weakness, a large abdomen with thin arms and legs, high blood pressure, stretch marks, easy bruising, poor wound healing, osteoporosis, high blood sugar, and anxiety/depression. Symptoms that are specific to women are excess facial hair and irregular menstrual cycles; for men, symptoms include decreased fertility and sex drive (see Figure 9-17).

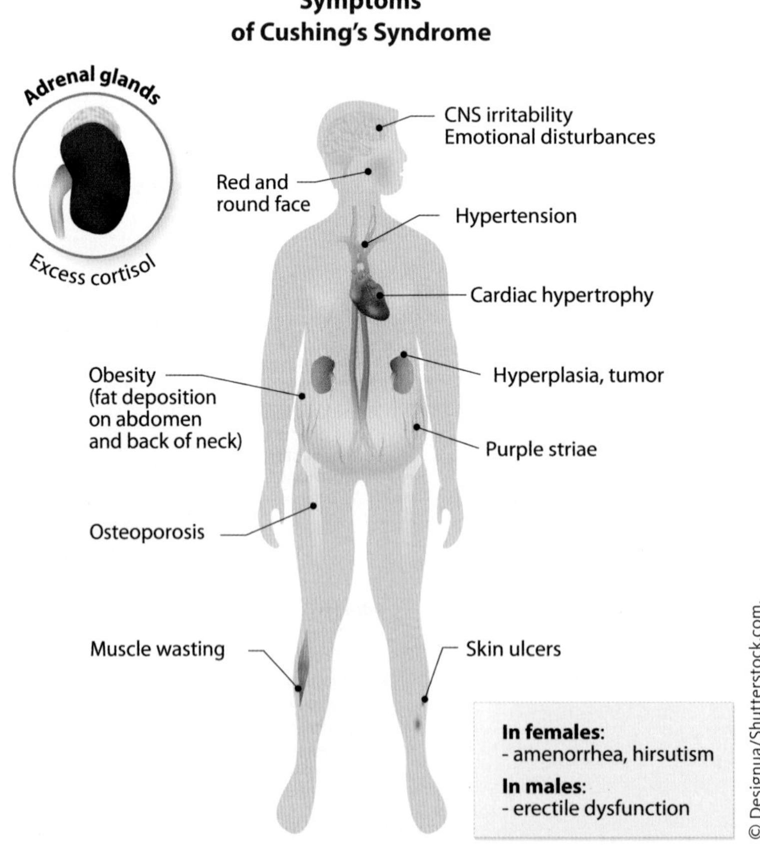

FIGURE 9-17 Symptoms associated with Cushing's syndrome.

9-15a Diagnosis and Treatment of Cushing's Syndrome

Cushing's syndrome is diagnosed if high cortisol levels exist within the blood. A dexamethasone test is a specific blood test used to measure levels of cortisol present in the body. The patient takes a low-dose steroid tablet at 11 p.m., and a blood sample is be taken in the morning to see how much cortisol the patient's body has produced. If high levels of cortisol are discovered, Cushing's syndrome is a possibility. Another test is a **24-hour urine-free cortisol test**. This is done by collecting the patient's urine over a 24-hour span to measure how much cortisol is present. The patient's saliva can also be tested at night to check for the body's cortisol levels, via a **late-night salivary cortisol level test**. Finally, to check whether a tumor is the cause of raised cortisol levels, an MRI can evaluate the adrenal and/or pituitary gland.

When treating Cushing's syndrome, the cause of cortisol over-production needs to first be identified. Depending on the situation, the patient might have to undergo surgery to remove a tumor. If that is the case, hormone therapy will be required for the rest of the patient's life. If the cause is related to steroid medication, the treatment is to decrease the dose or wean off the drug as much as possible.

Module 10

Pathopharmacology of the Urinary System

Module Introduction

The kidney can be hard to understand given all its different processes, such as filtration, absorption, secretion, and elimination, all occurring in various urinary system structures.

LEARNING OBJECTIVE 10.1 Explain the anatomy and physiology of the urinary system.

KEY TERMS

Autoregulation Protection mechanism in our body used to protect fragile filters in the kidneys from pressure fluctuations that occur throughout the day.

Bladder Expandable sac acting as a holding chamber for urine that has drained from the kidneys.

Calyces (singular: calyx) Funnel- or cup-like structure that collects urine from the renal pyramids.

Glomerular capsule or Bowman's capsule Double-layered membrane that encompasses the glomerulus, which is found inside the nephron of the kidney.

Glomerular filtrate Material filtered by the glomerulus.

Glomerulus Network of capillaries surrounded by the glomerular capsule.

Loop of Henle U-shaped loop that develops a concentration gradient in the kidney's medulla, used in the reabsorption process of sodium and water.

Nephrologist Physician that specializes in the conditions and treatment of the kidneys.

Nephron Microscopic tubules that make up the actual functioning unit of the kidney.

Renal capsule Outer covering of the kidney made of fibrous connective tissue.

Renal columns Columns of cortical tissue extensions that separate renal pyramids.

Renal cortex Outer portion of the kidney.

Renal hilum Indented area of the kidney where the renal artery, vein, and ureter connect, giving the kidney a bean-shaped appearance.

Renal medulla Middle portion of the kidney.

Renal pelvis Innermost region of the kidney that is shaped like a funnel and collects urine.

Renal pyramids Triangle-shaped structures in the medulla that are made up of tubules that collect urine.

Ureters Two hollow tubes, one from each kidney that drains urine from the kidney to the bladder.

Urethra Hollow tube used to drain urine from the bladder to the outside of the body.

Urologist Physician that specializes in the conditions and treatment of the urinary system.

10-1 URINARY SYSTEM OVERVIEW

Before delving into the urinary system, let's first do a quick overview of this system to get a basic idea about how it works, Figure 10-1. The kidneys are two bean-shaped organs that filter wastes from the blood. These wastes then are eliminated as urine, and the kidneys reabsorb the needed substances back into the body's circulation. The filtration process is done through intricate structures found in each kidney. As the kidney produces urine, it flows to the bladder through the ureters, which are tubes attached to the posterior side of the bladder. The ureters are equipped with one-way valves to prevent the backflow of urine to the kidney. Another tube attached to the bladder is the urethra, which allows urine to flow out of the body. When problems with the kidneys develop, the patient is referred to a kidney specialist or **nephrologist**. A **urologist** is a specialist who treats the remainder of the urinary tract.

10-2 KIDNEY OVERVIEW

The two kidneys are located at the superior dorsal abdominal cavity between the peritoneal cavity and back muscles (retroperitoneal). The primary job of the kidneys is to filter the blood and to maintain our body's homeostasis. Eliminating waste products is accomplished by producing urine, which is accomplished in three steps:

- Filtering the blood to produce a filtrate
- Reabsorbing any needed substances from the filtrate
- Excreting the remaining filtrate that hasn't been reabsorbed.

Urine is the result of wastes filtered from our body's blood that is not reabsorbed and is instead collected by a funnel-like structures called calyces (which will be explained later) that are directed to the passageway leading out of the body. Waste products include nitrogenous wastes and excessive nonwaste

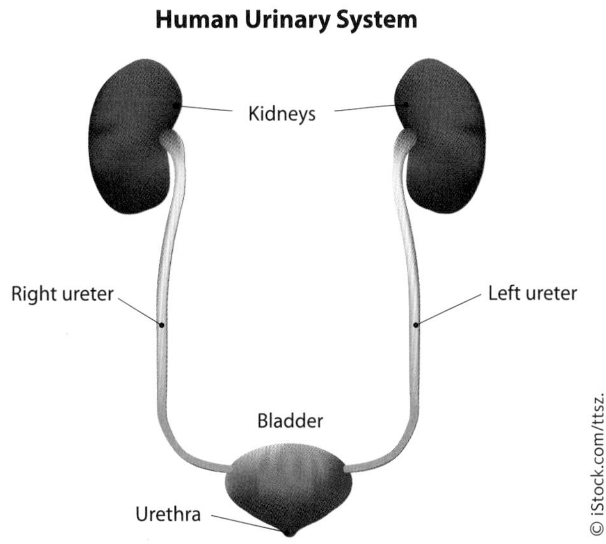

FIGURE 10-1 The urinary system.

substances such as various ions, amino acids, and proteins and other excess nutrients. The kidneys also maintain fluid and electrolyte balance; therefore, they play a major role in metabolism and blood pressure regulation.

10-3 OUTER ANATOMY OF KIDNEY

The kidney is encapsulated by a layer of fibrous connective tissue called the **renal capsule**. It has an indented area, called the **renal hilum**, which gives its bean-like appearance. Hilum means root, and the renal hilum is where the renal artery brings blood to the kidney to undergo filtration. The renal vein carries blood containing the reabsorbed substances back into circulation. Also stemming from the hilum is the ureter, which carries urine away from the kidney and to the bladder. See Figure 10-2.

10-4 INTERNAL ANATOMY OF KIDNEY

The internal anatomy of the kidney, Figure 10-3, has three layers. The outermost portion of the kidney is the **renal cortex** (cortex meaning rind, like on a melon). It is here where millions of filters remove waste from the blood. Moving toward the center of the kidney is the **renal medulla** (medulla meaning middle), which has many triangle-shaped striations called **renal pyramids**. These pyramids, separated by structures known as **renal columns**, contain tubules that are responsible for collecting urine. The third and innermost layer of the kidney is the **renal pelvis**, which acts as a funnel. It can be divided into two or three tubes called major calyces, which then are divided into minor calyces. The **calyces** channel urine from the pyramids into the ureter, and then into the bladder.

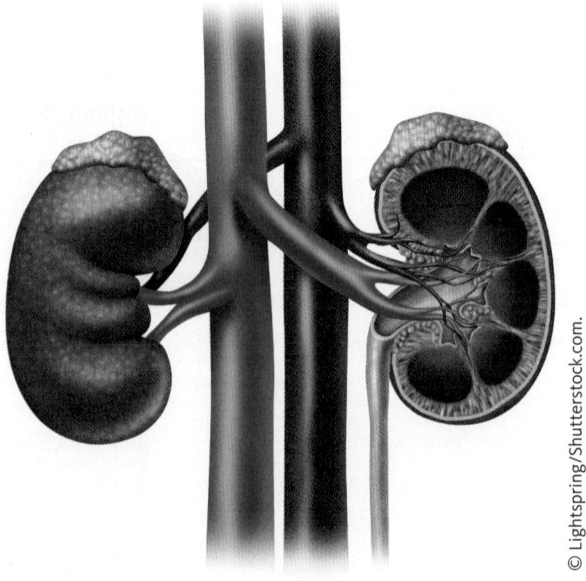

FIGURE 10-2 Outer anatomy of kidney showing the renal vein and artery and ureter stem.

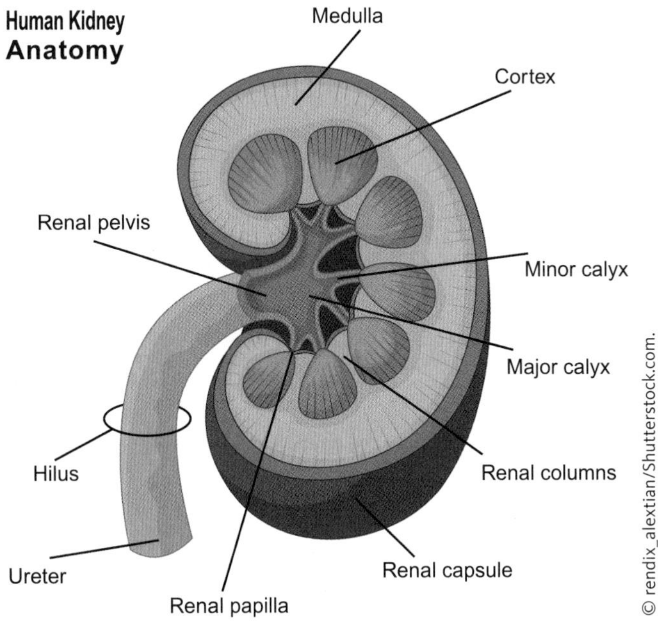

FIGURE 10-3 Anatomy of the kidney.

10-5 URETER, BLADDER, AND URETHRA

The **ureters**, tubes that connect each kidney to the bladder, are made of smooth muscle and are lined with a mucous membrane. They use peristalsis to drain fluid into the **bladder**, a stretchy sac that can expand to a much greater size when filled with urine. Connected to the outflow portion of the bladder is the **urethra**, which contains a sphincter muscle to prevent urine from leaking outside the body without conscious effort.

10-6 NEPHRON

The actual functional unit of the kidney is called a **nephron**. Each kidney has millions of nephrons, which are microscopic funnels and tubules, which provide a large surface area available to filter blood. Nephrons have two parts, the *renal corpuscle* and the *renal tubule*. The renal corpuscle acts as a filter that screens the blood coming from a ball-like network of capillaries known as the **glomerulus**.

The glomerulus receives blood from the afferent arterioles (afferent meaning toward), which are smaller branches of the renal artery. The glomerulus is surrounded by a double-layered membrane called the **glomerular capsule or Bowman's capsule**. Fluid and waste products can pass through tiny capillaries if they are small enough because these vessels are fenestrated epithelial cells. In other words, they have holes that allow ions (potassium, sodium, chloride, etc.), amino acids, and glucose to pass through. The material filtered from the blood is known as **glomerular filtrate**. Large proteins such as red blood cells and white blood cells are too large to pass through the fenestrations in healthy kidneys.

Long *tubular cells* are attached to the Bowman's capsule and glomerulus with foot-like projections called *podocytes* ("podo" meaning foot). Podocytes and specialized simple squamous epithelium form the wall of the glomerulus capillaries to

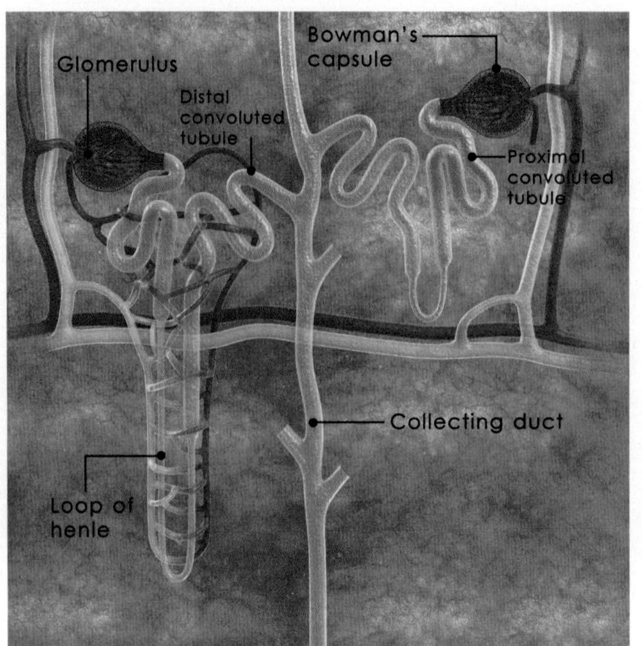

FIGURE 10-4 Anatomy of a nephron.

make a very efficient filter. After particles pass through the glomerular membrane, the filtrate leaves the Bowman's capsule and goes into the *proximal tubule*. This tube is part of a network of tubing like a city's water and sewer system. Wastes are kept in these tubules (pipes) to be sent out of the body, while fluid such as water is reabsorbed back into the body through *peritubular capillaries* (capillaries wrapped "around" the tubes to allow reabsorbing of needed substances back into circulation). See Figure 10-4.

10-6a Fluid Reabsorption

The glomerular filtrate flows into the proximal tubule or first part of the renal tubule. This tubule flows into the nephron loop, also known as the **loop of Henle**. The loop of Henle has two parts, a descending loop and an ascending loop. After the filtrate has made its way through the loop, it flows into the distal tubule.

Only water is reabsorbed in the descending loop, while no ions can leave. The ascending loop is the opposite, allowing ions to leave and be reabsorbed, while water is kept inside.

The ascending tubule leads to the *distal convoluted tubule* (distal tubule), which allows the body to reabsorb more ions that our body needs to function so they are not eliminated in the urine. From the distal tubule, the glomerular filtrate enters the collecting tubules to be sent to the bladder for storage.

10-7 CONTROL OF FILTRATION

The filters in the kidneys are selective. Think of a screen door or window screen at your house. The screens keep out bugs and other debris that are larger than the holes in the screen. However, smaller particles such as dust can still pass through if they are smaller than the holes in the screen (filter). In essence, the kidneys' filters block large particles while letting small particles pass through.

Podocytes and specialized epithelial cells that make up the capillary walls of the renal corpsule comprise the screen that filters blood. In a healthy kidney, large particles such as platelets, proteins, and red and white blood cells will not pass through the filter, while plasma (fluid portion of blood) and other smaller particles are filtered from the blood.

Therefore, if a patient has protein or red blood cells in the urine, it means the kidneys might be damaged. Very high blood pressure can force even large particles such as red blood cells through the screen.

10-8 RATE OF FILTRATION

The filtration rate is controlled by the difference in pressure across the filter (glomerular capillaries). For example, less pressure in the glomerulus will cause a decrease in filtration; an increase in pressure causes an increase in filtration.

To keep our microscopic structures protected from high and low blood pressures, our body has a mechanism called **autoregulation**. As we go about our normal daily activities, our blood pressure rises and falls, but autoregulation prevents injury to our delicate vessels from slight blood pressure changes. For example, arterioles going toward the glomerulus (afferent arterioles) will constrict in response to an increase in systemic blood pressure. This causes a decrease in the blood flow going toward the glomerulus, preventing an increase in blood pressure within the kidneys that might rupture those delicate filters.

If there is a drop in blood pressure or fluid volume, our body can override autoregulation. For instance, if a patient has lost a large amount of blood, the sympathetic system will be activated. This will release epinephrine and norepinephrine hormones from the adrenal medulla (a gland perched on top of each kidney) causing a decrease in glomerular filtration to prevent more fluid loss in the form of urine.

LEARNING OBJECTIVE 10.2 Describe the diagnostics and pathopharmacology of common infectious urinary system diseases.

KEY TERMS

Acute glomerulonephritis Sudden infection of the glomerulus.

Blood urea nitrogen (BUN) test Blood test used to check the function of the kidney.

Chronic glomerulonephritis Ongoing or recurring infection of the glomerulus.

Clean catch method Method used to collect urine to prevent contamination of the sample.

Creatinine clearance test Blood test used to see how well the kidneys are functioning.

Cystitis Inflammation of the bladder.

Cystogram Picture of the bladder.

Cystoscopy Procedure done to inspect the inside of the bladder.

Diuretics Class of medication used to eliminate excess water from the body to help control hypertension and edema.

Glomerulonephritis Group of diseases that results from an injury to the glomerulus.

In and out catheterization Temporary catheter used to drain urine and then be removed.

Indwelling catheter Catheter that remains in the patient over a period of time.

Intravenous pyelogram (IVP) Radiological technique that uses dye to obtain a better visualization of the urinary system.

Kidney-Ureter-Bladder (KUB) X-ray used to visualize the kidney, ureter, and bladder.

Loop diuretics Group of drugs used to block the reabsorption of water in the loop of Henle and the proximal and distal tubules.

Potassium-sparing diuretics Group of drugs that work in the distal tubule to eliminate water and salt while saving potassium.

Pyelitis Inflammation of the lining of the renal pelvis.

Pyelonephritis Inflammation of the structures inside the kidney.

Renal biopsy Performed to remove tissue for study.

Sterile technique Catheterizing an individual for a sample of urine.

Suprapubic catheter Type of catheter that is placed through the pelvic wall to avoid the urethra.

Thiazide diuretics Group of drugs that work in the distal tubule to prevent the reabsorption of water and salt.

Uremia Urine in the blood.

Urethritis Inflammation of the urethra.

Urinalysis Analysis of urine.

Urinary tract infection (UTI) Term used to describe an infection in any region of the urinary system.

Urine culture and sensitivity test (C&S) Study performed on urine to identify the pathogen responsible for the infection and so determine what drug can be used to treat it.

10-9 DIAGNOSTIC PROCEDURES

Some of the common diagnostic tests to assess renal functions include:

- urine sampling and analyses
- blood analysis
- imaging studies.

Catheterization is a common clinical procedure used to assist the renal system function. Let's take a more in-depth look at these assessments and procedures.

10-9a Urine Sampling

Infections are common in the urinary system and need to be identified and treated quickly. A procedure used to examine urine for bacteria or white blood cells as a result of an infection is a **urine culture and sensitivity test (C&S)**. For example, more than 100,000 bacteria per ml of urine is an indicator that a moderate urinary tract infection is present. If lower amounts are found, it shows that the patient has a mild urinary infection.

The laboratory also can use the specimen to find out what kind of bacteria is present (culture) so it can be treated appropriately with antibiotics (sensitivity). However, the way the sample is collected is critical for proper

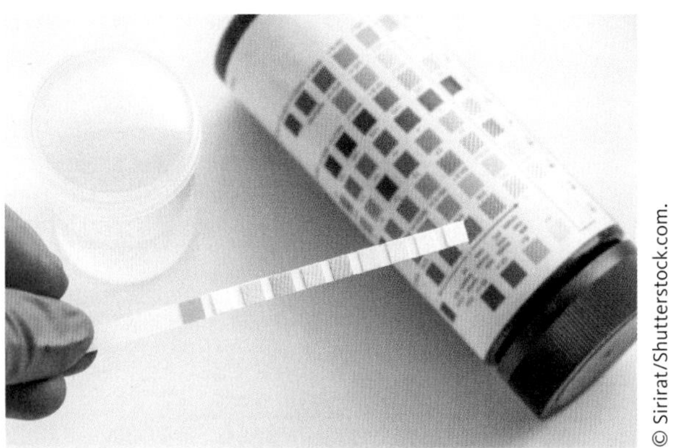

FIGURE 10-5 Urinalysis.

diagnosis and treatment. If the sample is contaminated, it might not allow a correct diagnosis and choice of treatment. A small quantity of bacteria found in the urine likely have been caused by contamination. To ensure this does not happen, a **clean catch method** or a **sterile technique** can be used. A clean catch method entails cleaning the urethral meatus to prevent any bacteria from contaminating the urine sample, and the urine is caught and sampled midstream. The sterile technique entails inserting a sterile urinary catheter through the patient's urethra and into the bladder to retrieve a sample of urine.

Another diagnostic test is a **urinalysis**, Figure 10-5. This common test is used to study the urine for any signs of glucose or larger proteins, such as red blood cells, which, if found, would indicate a problem in the patient's urinary system. Also studied from this test are the pH and specific gravity.

10-9b Blood Sample Testing

Besides checking a patient's urine, other body fluids can be used to determine whether the kidneys are functioning properly. Two common tests that measure the level of nitrogenous waste in the blood can determine how well the glomerulus is performing and whether waste products are being adequately filtered from the blood. If waste products such as creatinine and urea are building up in the blood, they are not being properly filtered within the kidneys.

A **creatinine clearance test** is used to check how well the glomerulus filtered out creatinine, while a **blood urea nitrogen (BUN) test** is used to measure the level of urea nitrogen in the blood, Figure 10-6. When too many toxins are found in the blood, it is a condition known as **uremia**, meaning urine in the blood.

10-9c Radiologic Techniques

A radiologic exam of the urinary system also can be used to diagnose diseases of the urinary system. A **kidney-ureter-bladder (KUB)** image is an X-ray used to view the structures of the urinary system. An **intravenous pyelogram (IVP)**, in which a dye is injected into the patient's blood, is used to get a better view of

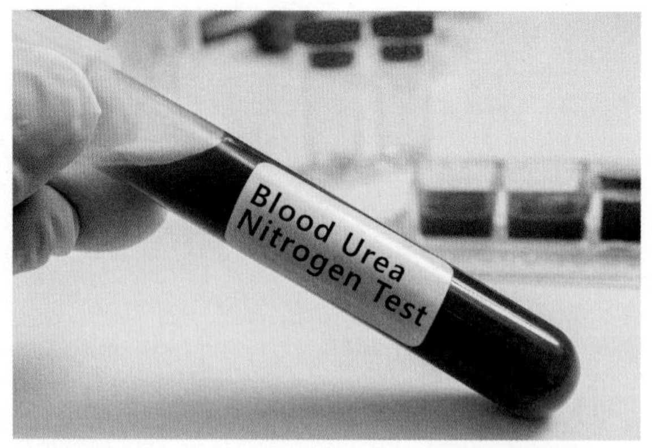

© vchal/Shutterstock.com.

FIGURE 10-6 Blood samples also can be used to check for kidney failure.

the urinary structures. The dye travels to the patient's urinary system allowing for a better visualization and diagnosing.

Another technique using dye is a **cystogram** (cysto = bladder and gram = picture). This is done by instilling a dye into the bladder to give clinicians an idea about the bladder's condition. A procedure used to visually inspect the urethra and bladder is called a **cystoscopy**, which uses a long flexible scope equipped with a light on the distal tip. This device also can harvest tissue samples from growths such as tumors, which are then sent to a laboratory for further analysis. If a biopsy is needed to extract tissue from within the kidney, however, a **renal biopsy** is performed. This entails inserting a needle into the kidney. To ensure that the needle is inserted in the correct location, the physician uses a visual aid, such as an X-ray, to guide the needle insertion.

10-9d Catheterization

Catheterization, in which a tube is inserted through the urethra into the bladder, is a commonly used practice in medicine. This is done to empty urine from the bladder or to instill medications. Care must be taken when performing this procedure to prevent urinary tract infections.

There are different types of urinary catheters and catheterization procedures. Television commercials for urinary catheters promise discrete packaging with pre-lubricated catheters. These catheters drain urine into the toilet instead of a collection bag. Lubrication is needed to prevent trauma to the inner walls of the urethra and decrease the likelihood of bleeding and scarring, which can lead to a stricture (restricted urine flow through the urethra). If the catheter is removed as soon as urine is extracted, it is called an **in and out catheterization**.

If the catheter will have to remain inside the patient for a while, however, a different catheter is used. This catheter, called an **indwelling catheter**, has a balloon toward the distal tip to keep the catheter in place and is hooked up to a collection bag.

Another way to catheterize a patient, especially those who have undergone a urinary tract surgery, is by using a **suprapubic catheter**, meaning the patient has a catheter surgically inserted through the pelvic wall.

10-10 URINARY TRACT INFECTION

The term **urinary tract infection (UTI)** is a broad term used to describe a number of infections in the urinary tract affecting the kidneys, ureter, bladder, and urethra. UTIs are more commonly found in the lower urinary tract, meaning the urethra and bladder, as opposed to the ureter and kidneys. It is also more common for women to have a UTI than men, in large part because a woman's urethra is closer to the anus, and infection can spread because of this proximity. Women also have a shorter urethra for pathogens to ascend than men. In men, the prostate gland emits secretions that act as an antibacterial agent to prevent infections.

As for the etiology, UTIs can be caused by both viruses and bacteria, although bacteria are the most common pathogens. Bacteria can cause a UTI by direct contact with the urethra as in sexually transmitted diseases. Bacteria in the bloodstream that travel to the urinary system can cause a hematogenous infection. This is a secondary infection of the urinary tract since the primary infection occurred somewhere else in the body before entering the bloodstream and spreading to the urinary tract.

There are numerous causes of UTIs, and some common examples include:

- Catheterizations or other urinary procedures
- Sexual intercourse
- Urinary blockages
- Suppressed immune system.

10-10a UTI Treatment

Some patients with UTIs are asymptomatic, but when symptoms do present, they can include:

- a strong urge to urinate often
- difficulty urinating
- burning sensation
- strong urine odor
- blood in the urine (pinkish to cola coloration)
- sudden confusion in the elderly
- pain in the lower back and flank region.

A positive test for a UTI is a bacterial count of 100,000 or more per mL of urine. Since UTIs are commonly caused by bacteria, they usually are treated using antibiotics. See Table 10-1 for antibiotics commonly used treat uncomplicated urinary tract infections. A severe infection requires an intravenous antibiotic.

10-10b Additional Antimicrobials to Treat UTIs

Other classes of antimicrobials, specifically the class called sulfonamides, are also successful in treating UTIs. Sulfonamides are useful for treating infections caused by Gram-negative bacteria such as *Escherichia coli*. This group of drugs

Table 10-1 General Antibiotics Used to Treat Uncomplicated UTIs

BRAND NAME(S)	GENERIC NAME
Zithromax, Zmax	azithromycin
Rocephin	ceftriaxone
Keflex	cephalexin
Cipro	ciprofloxacin
Monodox, Vibramycin, others	doxycycline
Monurol	fosfomycin
Levaquin	levofloxacin
Macrodantin, Macrobid	nitrofurantoin
Bactrim, Septra, others	trimethoprim/sulfamethoxazole

is separated into three groups based on how long they stay in the body: short-acting, intermediate-acting, and long-acting. Typically, short-acting sulfonamides are used in treating UTIs as they are absorbed quickly. These drugs are not to be taken by anyone breastfeeding or if younger than 2 months of age. Table 10-2 presents a list of sulfonamides used to treat UTIs.

Antiseptics also are used to combat urinary tract infections. Urinary antiseptic agents work to stop the growth of bacteria. Antibiotics and sulfonamides are used before any antiseptic drugs, but if the patient's condition does not respond or if the patient is unable to tolerate treatment antimicrobials, then antiseptic agents are administered. An example of antiseptic agents used for UTIs is NegGram (nalidixic acid) and Hiprex (methenamine hippurate).

Table 10-2 Common Sulfonamides Used to Treat UTIs

BRAND NAME(S)	GENERIC NAME
Bactrim and Septra	sulfamethoxazole/trimethoprim
Microsulfon	sulfadiazine
Truxazole and Gantrisin Pediatric	sulfisoxazole

10-10c Urethritis

The term **urethritis** means inflammation of the urethra. This type of UTI is usually accompanied by cystitis (inflammation of the bladder), which we will also discuss in this module. While injury to this region can cause inflammation, bacterial infection is the most common cause. These include the opportunistic bacteria (*E. coli*) from the GI tract, the pathogens of the sexually transmitted diseases such as *Chlamydia trachomatis* (chlamydia), *Neisseria gonorrhoeae*, or gonococcal bacteria responsible for gonorrhea, as well as the herpes simplex virus.

Signs and symptoms for urethritis include:

- Difficulty urinating
- Frequent urges to urinate
- Urethral discharge
- Pain
- Burning sensation during urination.

To diagnose, the physician will note the patient's symptoms and order urine cultures to determine the bacteria at fault. If the patient has urethral discharge, that too can be sent to the laboratory for analysis. Blood tests, although less likely to be used, also can show what bacteria are present in the patient's body.

To treat nonsexually transmitted conditions, antibiotics used to treat UTIs, as shown in Tables 10-1 and 10-2, also are used to kill the bacteria causing urethritis. However, if the etiology is from sexual transmission, then antibiotics specific to these bacteria will be chosen. Because gonorrhea and chlamydia often are seen together, concurrent dual therapy is given. Table 10-3 provides more information about the drugs used to treat sexually transmitted infections (STIs).

10-10d Cystitis

Cystitis is a term used to describe inflammation of the bladder. Similar to urethritis, this type of UTI is usually caused by a bacterial infection. Other causes are associated with spermicidal jellies, certain hygiene sprays, and soaps through chemical irritation. Also, certain medications used during chemotherapy and radiation therapy can cause cystitis.

Signs and symptoms are as follows:

- Burning sensation during urination
- Frequent urge to urinate
- Blood in urine (hematuria)
- Urine that has a strong odor
- Slight fever
- Pain and discomfort in the pelvic region.

Urinalysis can help diagnose this condition. Other diagnostic methods include a cystoscope to see the inside of the bladder or an ultrasound to check

Table 10-3 Commonly Used Antibiotics to Treat Sexually Transmitted Infections Causing Urethritis

DISEASE	BRAND NAME	GENERIC NAME
Chlamydia	• Vibramycin	• doxycycline
	• Zithromax	• azithromycin
	• Amox	• amoxicillin
Gonorrhea	• Suprax	• cefixime
	• Rocephin	• intramuscular ceftriaxone
Herpes Simplex Virus	• Zovirax	• acyclovir
	• Famvir	• famciclovir
	• Valtrex	• valacyclovir

the area around the bladder for any tumors or anything else that might cause inflammation.

Antibiotics are the primary drugs used to clear up the infection.

An antispasmodic agent called Pyridium can help alleviate some of the patient's discomfort, such as the frequent need to urinate, but it will give the urine a reddish-orange color that can stain clothing.

10-10e Pyelitis versus Pyelonephritis

Another form of UTI is **pyelitis**, or inflammation of the lining of the renal pelvis, the portion of the kidney where the ureter connects to the calyces. This is not to be confused with the inflammation of the structures inside the kidney known as **pyelonephritis**. Commonly pyelitis is the result of bacteria ascending the urinary tract; however, it also can spread to this region from a hematogenous or blood infection. Pyelonephritis is inflammation of the structures within the kidney. Both of these conditions are serious, even life-threatening infections that can cause septicemia and permanent kidney damage and therefore require prompt treatment.

The signs and symptoms of these conditions include hematuria (blood in urine), cloudy and foul-smelling urine, burning sensation, frequent urge to urinate, fever, and groin, lumbar, and abdominal pain. Tests to diagnose the patient include a urine culture, blood culture, and an ultrasound. After a diagnosis is made, the physician can treat it with oral antibiotics. If the patient has a severe infection, intravenous antibiotics will be required. The patient should see improvement over the next few days and should take the entire course prescribed to prevent the infection from returning.

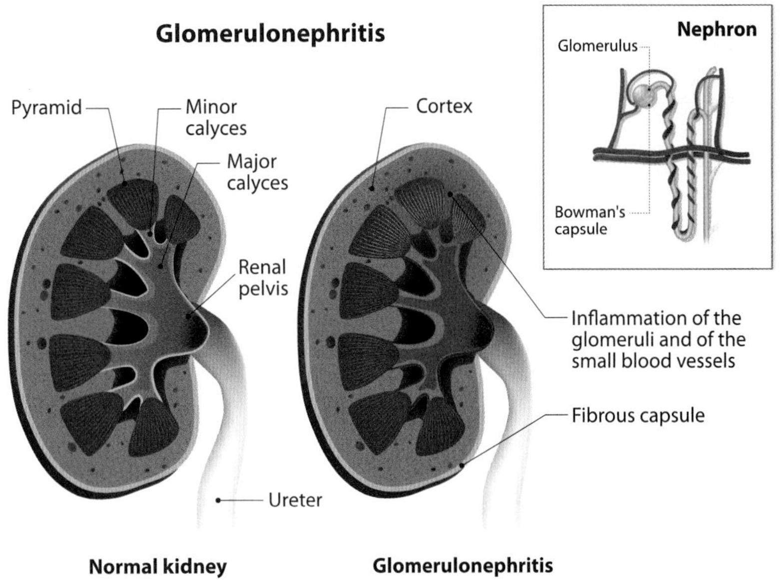

FIGURE 10-7 Glomerulonephritis.

10-11 GLOMERULONEPHRITIS (ACUTE VERSUS CHRONIC)

Glomerulonephritis is a condition that results from an injured and inflamed glomerulus, Figure 10-7. Remember, this is where the actual filtration of the blood takes place.

10-11a Acute Glomerulonephritis

Acute glomerulonephritis is caused by an infection that occurs suddenly. Those primarily affected are young adults and children who had a streptococcus infection, such as strep throat, within the previous four weeks. A case that develops as a result of a strep infection is known as post-streptococcal glomerulonephritis, but the condition also can be caused by other forms of bacteria as well as viruses and parasites.

This condition also can be caused by a malfunctioning immune system. When the immune system fights off a pathogen, it creates antibodies, which adhere to the antigen to destroy the "bug." While the antigen and antibody are bound together, they are still traveling around the circulatory system and can get stuck in the capillaries of the glomerulus and clog the filter if enough are present. This blockage can cause an increase in pressure that can damage the delicate filter. Eventually, the damaged glomerulus can become permeable to red and white blood cells and other proteins found in the blood plasma.

Signs and symptoms include:

- Pain in flank area
- Oliguria (low urine output)
- High fever
- Hematuria (blood in the urine)

- Malaise
- Feet and eye edema
- Loss of appetite
- Casts (molds of kidney tubules found in urine)
- Proteinuria (protein in urine).

A urinalysis is performed to uncover what is causing the patient's condition. Positive indicators for acute glomerulonephritis urine findings include:

- White blood cells (because of infection)
- Red blood cells (because of glomerulus damage)
- Excessive proteins (because of nephron damage).

Blood samples are also a very valuable resource. If glomerulonephritis is present, the patient's blood work will show an increased urea and creatinine level because of filter damage. Another blood test used is an erythrocyte sedimentation rate (ESR). For this test, blood is placed in a cylinder, and the erythrocytes (red blood cells) settle to the bottom of the cylinder. If inflammation is present in the body, the red blood cells will clump together. A combination of this and other test results would indicate that there is inflammation occurring in the kidney. Treatment involves controlling the patient's blood pressure to prevent further damage and treating the cause of the infection. Diuretics, which will soon be discussed, are often given to reduce the pressure.

10-11b Chronic Glomerulonephritis

Unlike the acute condition, **chronic glomerulonephritis** occurs when there is a slow, prolonged destruction of the kidney's glomeruli, which can develop into renal failure and chronic high blood pressure.

After many recurring episodes of acute glomerulonephritis, the kidney is not able to function properly and recover from the damage caused by repeated inflammation. Furthermore, a decrease in urine production and urine output will occur, and the retained fluid will cause edema in the patient's feet and, in some cases, the eyes.

The signs and symptoms are the same as those listed for acute glomerulonephritis; however, with chronic glomerulonephritis, uremia (urine in the blood), which is seen in end-stage kidney failure, and high blood pressure (hypertension) are also added.

- Pain in flank area
- Oliguria
- High fever
- Hematuria
- Malaise
- Feet and eye edema
- Loss of appetite
- Casts
- Proteinuria.

Tests to be given include:

- Urinalysis (looking for white and red blood cells, protein, infection, and casts)
- Blood analysis (looking for high blood urea nitrogen (BUN), creatinine, and elevated white blood cell count)
- Ultrasound and CT imaging to assess damage
- Tissue biopsy.

Treatment is geared toward controlling the signs and symptoms, especially hypertension. This can be done through various drugs that are covered in the cardiovascular chapter, but here we will primarily focus on diuretics as they relate to reducing blood pressure by their effects on the kidney.

10-12 DIURETICS

Diuretics help remove sodium chloride (salt) and water from the body. Whenever salt goes, water usually follows, which is why the lay term for diuretics is water pills. Diuretics decrease the reabsorption of sodium chloride in the kidneys, by keeping salt and water in the tubules to be removed via urination, thus reducing fluid retention and edema.

If the kidneys do not excrete this extra fluid, it will result in an increased blood pressure.

There are several different classes of diuretics, and which one is prescribed depends on where in the renal tubular system they have their effect. Figure 10-8 illustrates where these diuretic agents take effect.

Table 10-4 contrasts the various types of diuretics.

10-12a Side Effects of Diuretics

Diuretics are commonly prescribed and come in several categories. See Table 10-5 for a description of their specific uses and side effects for each category.

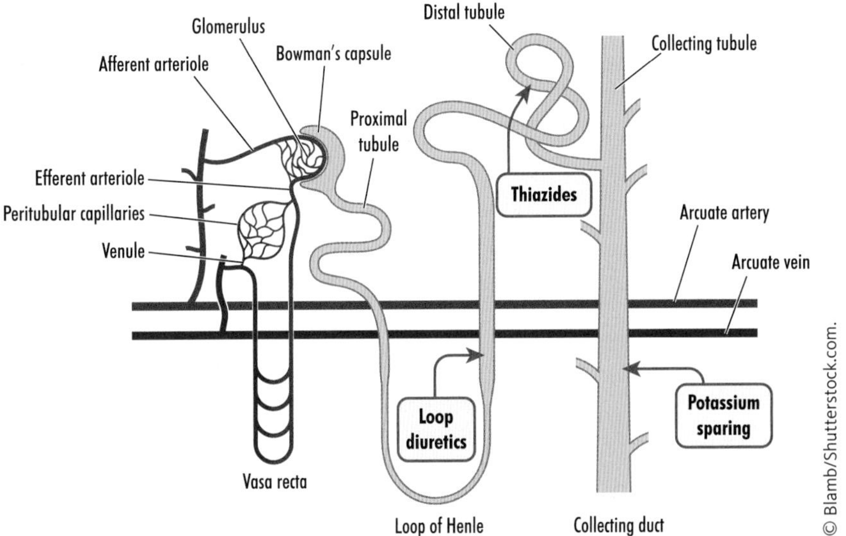

FIGURE 10-8 A visual reference showing where each diuretic takes effect.

Table 10-4 Types of Diuretics

DIURETIC CLASS	METHOD OF ACTION	COMMON BRAND AND GENERIC NAMES
Loop diuretics	These agents block the reabsorption of sodium chloride in the ascending limb of loop of Henle.	Bumex (buetanide) Demadex (torsemide) Edecrin (ethacrynic acid) Lasix (furosemide)
Potassium-sparing diuretics	While taking effect in the collecting tubule, these agents promote sodium and water loss while preventing the loss of potassium.	Aldactone (spironolactone) Dyrenium (triamterene) Inspira (eplerenone) Midamor (amiloride)
Thiazide diuretics	This class works in the distal tubule and prevents the reabsorption of sodium chloride in the body. However, potassium loss occurs in this process.	Diuril (chlorothiazide) Microzide (hydrochlorothiazide) Thalitone (chlorthalidone) Lozol (indapamide)

Note: Carbonic anhydrase inhibitors have a diuretic effect that decreases intraocular pressure in the eyes. They will be discussed more in the eye and ear module.

Table 10-5 Uses and Side Effects of Various Diuretic Agents

LOOP DIURETICS

Used to treat:

- Hypertension, used if thiazide diuretics do not work, often paired with antihypertensive agents if a patient is suffering from renal failure
- Pulmonary edema, caused from fluid backing up in the lungs from heart failure
- Edema from renal insufficiency
- Ascites, buildup of fluid in the abdomen

Side Effects and Precautions:

- Hypokalemia, low potassium in the blood, can cause muscle spasms and arrhythmias
- Hypocalcemia, low calcium in the blood
- Hypotension, must monitor patient's blood pressure often
- Hyperglycemia, caution use for diabetic patients
- Increases levels of uric acid, caution use in patients with gout

POTASSIUM-SPARING DIURETICS

Used to treat:

- Not often used alone and is likely to be given with thiazide diuretics to decrease hyperkalemia
- Counteracts the increase in blood sugar and uric acid seen with thiazides
- Used in patients suffering from hepatic insufficiency; seen in cirrhosis patients
- Decreases deaths associated with severe heart failure

Table 10-5 Uses and Side Effects of Various Diuretic Agents—*continued*

Side Effects and Precautions:

- Monitor closely for hyperkalemia
- Can cause hypotension
- Men might experience enlarged breasts (gynecomastia)

THIAZIDES

Used to treat:

- Edema
- Hypertension
- Prevent renal calculi (stone formation)

Side Effects and Precautions:

- Hypercalcemia, high calcium in the blood
- Hyponatremia, low sodium in the blood
- Hypokalemia, low potassium in the blood, can cause muscle spasms and arrhythmias
- Hyperglycemia, might be contraindicated in patients with diabetes
- Orthostatic hypotension, caused by a sudden decrease in blood pressure when standing up; often called a head rush
- Increases levels of uric acid, caution use for patients with gout

LEARNING OBJECTIVE 10.3 Describe the diagnostics and pathopharmacology of non-infectious urinary system diseases.

KEY TERMS

Alpha blockers Group of drugs used to relax the muscles of the bladder neck and prostate to allow for improved urine flow.

Antiandrogens Drugs used to decrease an enlarged prostate to decrease urine obstruction.

Anticholinergics Group of drugs used to prevent bladder constrictions to prevent the frequent urge to urinate.

Hemodialysis Method used to cleanse the blood of waste when the kidneys are unable to do so by placing a direct catheter line into the bloodstream.

Hydronephrosis Condition in which fluid (urine) is obstructed from leaving the kidney causing renal distention.

Peritoneal dialysis Method used to remove wastes from the blood by using the patient's peritoneal membrane as a filter.

Polycystic kidney disease (PKD) Inherited disease that slowly destroys the kidneys.

Renal calculi Formation of hardened crystals in the kidney.

Renal cell carcinoma Most common type of kidney cancer.

Renal failure Inability of the renal system to function and cleanse the blood of toxins.

Transitional cell carcinoma of the bladder Cancer that develops in the lining of the bladder.

Urinary incontinence Inability to control the bladder.

Urodynamic testing Testing used to study the anatomic structure and function of the bladder and urethra.

10-13 NON-INFECTIOUS KIDNEY DISEASES

While the most common type of kidney disease is of the infectious type, kidney disease also can occur with non-infectious etiologies. Two aspects stand out when we think about the anatomy and physiology of the system. First, a good flow through the system is needed for optimal functioning; therefore, anything that obstructs the flow will cause issues. Second, because the urinary system is composed of delicate filters and relatively narrow tubing, pressures that get too high will cause functional damage.

10-13a Hydronephrosis

If urine is prohibited from leaving the kidney by an obstruction, it backs up and causes an increase in pressure. This buildup will result in the renal pelvis becoming distended, a condition called **hydronephrosis**. Possible causes of an obstruction include:

- Congenital birth defects
- Tumors
- Enlarged prostrate
- UTI (because of inflammation and swelling)
- Kidney stones.

Symptoms depend on several factors, such as where the obstruction is located, if one or both kidneys are affected, and whether the patient has an acute or chronic blockage. If only a portion of one kidney is blocked, the patient might not even realize there is an obstruction. If both kidneys are backed up, then the patient will have urine in their blood (uremia) or might not be able to pass any urine at all. When the urine backs up and causes distension, the patient will have pain around the flank, lumbar, and groin areas. Some distended kidneys can be palpated or felt during a routine physical examination.

Besides a physical examination, other methods used to determine whether the patient has this condition are an intravenous pyelogram (IVP), as well as an electrolyte panel, blood urea nitrogen (BUN), and creatinine test.

This condition requires the kidneys to be drained immediately via surgery to prevent further damage. This is often a painful condition, so analgesics might be prescribed.

10-13b Renal Calculi (Kidney Stones)

Renal calculi, shown in Figures 10-9A and 10-9B, are also called nephroliths and occur more often in Caucasian men than women and typically affect those between 30 and 50 years of age. Kidney stones are hardened deposits, which make them difficult and often very painful to pass through the urinary system. Although the causes are unknown, kidney stones, which vary in size, are made up of salts and minerals that have stuck together. The risk for kidney stones increases when the patient's urine is concentrated, meaning it has less water and higher concentrations of dissolved materials.

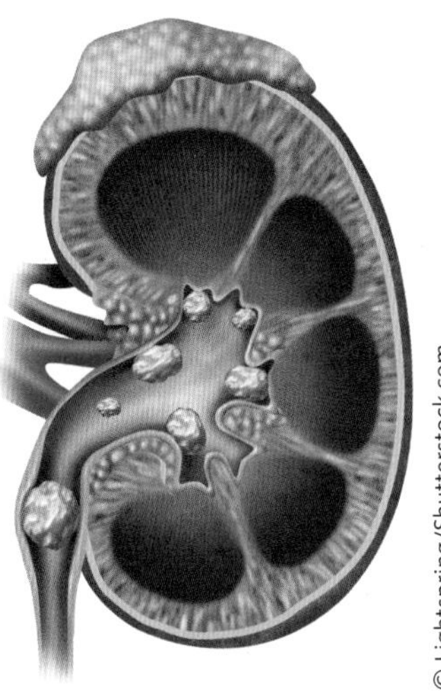

FIGURE 10-9A Renal calculi in the kidney.

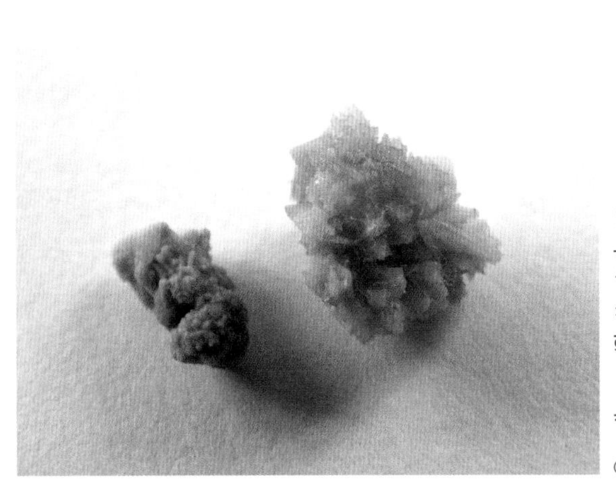

FIGURE 10-9B Actual kidney stones.

10-13c Types of Kidney Stones

Just as various stone types are found in nature, so too are kidney stones of different types, depending on what the deposit is made from. See Table 10-6 for more information.

Some situations increase the likelihood of developing kidney stones, such as:

- Gout, causing uric crystals to form
- Prolonged immobility, causing calcium to leave bones
- UTIs
- Dehydration
- Certain medications (calcium antacids)
- Diets high in sugar, protein, and sodium.

Table 10-6 Types of Kidney Stones

KIDNEY STONE TYPE	DESCRIPTION
Calcium	Most common; can result from diet
Cystine	Very uncommon; caused by genetic disorder
Struvite	Caused by infection; typically more often in women with UTIs, causing a kidney infection. Large size can cause an obstruction easily.
Uric acid	Can occur from a diet of animal protein, causing increased uric acid levels. Found more often in men than women, and those with gout or undergoing chemotherapy.

Signs and symptoms associated with renal calculi are hematuria (blood in the urine) and pain in the flank region. Some people who have experienced kidney stones say it was one of the most painful experiences in their life. This pain is referred to as urinary colic, which is the pain and spasms from the contraction of the blocked ureters.

10-13d Diagnosing and Treating Kidney Stones

Tests that can help diagnose kidney stones are:

- Intravenous pyelogram (IVP)
- Ultrasound
- Kidneys, ureter, and bladder (KUB) radiograph.

All of these imaging studies can help locate the kidney stone and obstruction to determine its severity.

Treatment depends on the type of stone and the cause. Small kidney stones can be passed on their own without any treatment. However, the patient might take medication for pain, including analgesics such as Tylenol (acetaminophen) and NSAIDs such as Aleve (naproxen), and Advil or Motrin (ibuprofen).

To help the stone to pass through the ureter faster with less pain, the patient might be given a medication known as an alpha-blocker, which dialates the ureters. Alpha blockers relax the ureter and prevent it from constricting because of the irritation from the stone. Other therapies used to remove a stone, particularly a large stone that cannot be passed, include Extracorporeal Shock Wave Lithotripsy (ESWL), which is shown in Figure 10-10. This procedure involves actually breaking up the kidney stone (litho = stone, tripsy = breaking) into smaller pieces, which are easier to pass through urination. The patient is placed in a tub of water for up to an hour, and vibrations, or shock waves, are emitted into the direction of the stone. The shock waves break up the stone into many smaller pieces.

This procedure can cause moderate pain and discomfort, so the patient might be sedated. The patient might notice blood in their urine or even bruises on their skin where the shock waves were directed.

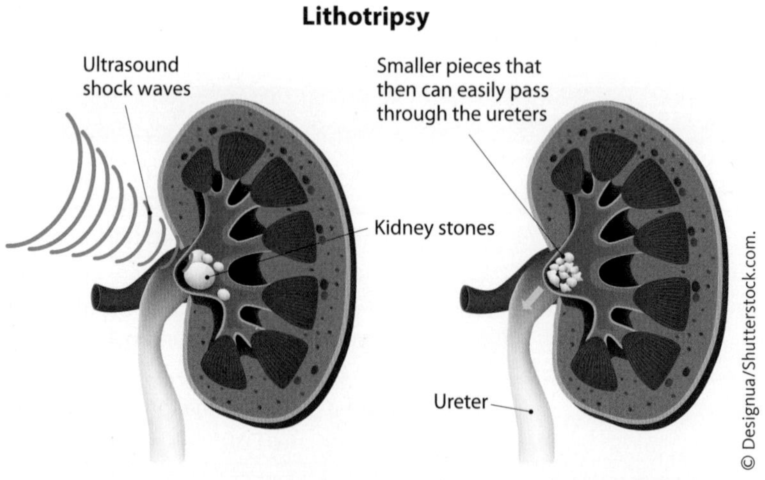

FIGURE 10-10 Extracorporeal Shock Wave Lithotripsy (ESWL).

Another treatment involves retrieving kidney stones via a urethroscope, a hollow tube that is inserted through the urethra and moves through the urinary tract up into the kidneys. The scope then breaks the stone into pieces that are small enough to fit through this hollow scope.

A surgical procedure called a percutaneous nephrolithotomy is used to remove very large renal calculi through the patient's back.

10-13e Polycystic Disease

Polycystic kidney disease (PKD) is a very serious, slowly progressing, inherited disease that affects both kidneys, Figure 10-11. With PKD, large cysts develop throughout the kidneys causing them to become significantly deformed. Symptoms include frequent UTIs, hematuria, and lower back pain. The kidneys begin to fail as the disease progresses, ultimately destroying kidney function. The patient also will experience hypertension as the failure begins.

Since this disease is inherited, a family medical history is helpful in making a diagnosis. The patient also can be injected with a dye to help visualize the kidneys during a CT scan and get a picture of the extent of damage. Medications to help treat this disease include angiotensin-converting enzyme (ACE) inhibitors, which treat hypertension by blocking an enzyme that increases blood pressure; antibiotics to treat infections; and analgesics such as Tylenol (acetaminophen) to control pain. However, when renal failure occurs, dialysis and/or a kidney transplant is required.

10-13f Renal Failure

Properly functioning kidneys are needed to rid the blood of waste products and maintain proper fluid and electrolyte balance. When renal disease stops or limits this vital function, toxins will build up in the bloodstream, and serious fluid and electrolyte imbalances can occur. Therefore, when the kidneys stop functioning (kidney or **renal failure**), the results can be serious, even deadly.

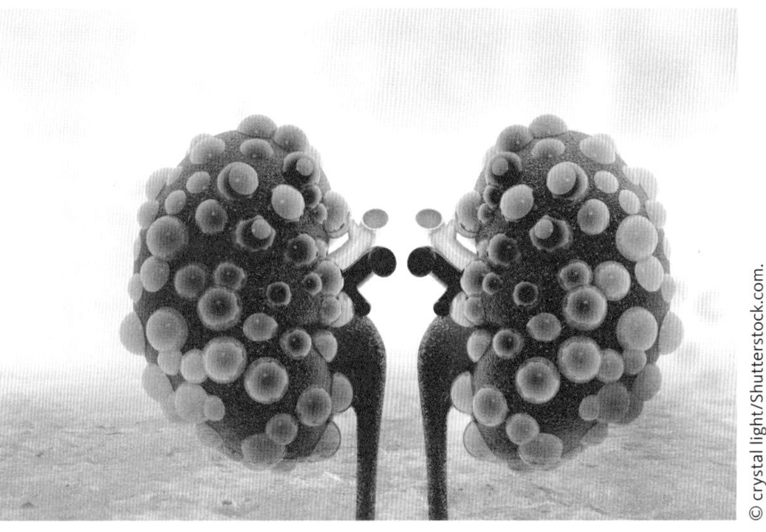

FIGURE 10-11 Two kidneys affected by polycystic kidney disease.

There are two types of renal failure, acute and chronic. Acute renal failure occurs suddenly and can be caused by a sudden blockage or decrease in blood flow. Blockages can result from tumors, calculi, scar tissue, enlarged prostate (males), or anything stopping the flow of urine from the body. Decreased blood flow also can be caused by an embolism (blood clot), dehydration, blood loss, or congestive heart failure (CHF). Either acute blockage or flow disruption will cause a buildup of waste, such as the urea produced in the liver as a byproduct of metabolism. The patient must undergo dialysis temporarily to remove waste from the blood until the cause of the kidney failure has been treated and the kidneys can filter the blood properly again.

Patients might not realize they have kidney problems until enough damage is caused for symptoms to arise. Signs and symptoms of acute renal failure include, but are not limited to, edema (retained fluid), shortness of breath (SOB), decreased urine output, nausea, chest pain, malaise, confusion, and coma. Although similar to acute renal failure, chronic signs and symptoms include edema, confusion, cramping, chest pain, shortness of breath, hypertension, weakness, and nausea.

Chronic renal failure occurs over time and at a much slower pace. Diseases such as polycystic kidney disease (PKD), renal hypertension, and other chronic kidney diseases eventually can end in chronic renal failure. Poor lifestyle choices also can cause chronic renal failure. For example, a poor diet can cause diabetes, which can damage the kidneys over time. A patient who has a history of drug and alcohol abuse also risks kidney damage.

10-13g Stages of Chronic Renal Failure

Chronic kidney disease has five stages as shown in Table 10-7. If caught early, treatment can help slow the progression of the disease. To help determine the stage of the disease, the patient's kidney function needs to be determined. To help measure the function of the kidney, the glomerular filtration rate (GFR) is calculated. First, a blood test is taken to determine the patient's creatinine level. Creatinine is a byproduct of muscle activity that is removed by the kidneys. Creatinine levels increase when the kidneys lose their ability to function properly. Other factors taken into consideration are the patient's age, race, weight, blood urea nitrogen (BUN) level, and serum albumin. Taken altogether, these factors are used in a mathematical formula to determine the patient's GFR level. Once this is determined, the patient's kidney disease can be staged accordingly.

10-13h Diagnosing and Treating Renal Failure

Diagnostic procedures used to help diagnose renal failure can be done by sampling blood to check for increased BUN and creatinine levels. High values, coupled with patient history and physical exam findings, could indicate that renal failure is present. Other methods to assess renal failure include a urinalysis, ultrasound, and biopsy of the kidney tissue.

A urinalysis is valuable in diagnosing kidney failure. After the urine is collected in a sterile specimen cut, testing can begin. A urinalysis can be done in three steps. First, the urine is examined for color and clarity, because changes can indicate problems with the kidneys. The odor of the specimen also can indicate a potential problem.

Table 10-7 Stages of Renal Failure (Kidney Disease)

Stage 1	Patient has kidney disease and a GFR that is normal or higher, ranging from 90 mL per minute or higher. Those with Stage 1 might not have any symptoms.
Stage 2	A patient with Stage 2 failure has a slight or mild case of kidney damage. The GFR score is lower than Stage 1, between 60 and 89 mL per minute. The patient still might not have any symptoms at this point.
Stage 3 (3A and 3B)	Stage 3 is divided up into two categories. A moderate case of decreased kidney function is present. The GFR of Stage 3A is between 45 and 59 mL per minute, while Stage 3B is between 30 and 44 mL per minute. Signs and symptoms include: • Changes in urine output • Kidney pain • Muscle cramping • Fluid retention causing edema • Electrolyte imbalances • Weight loss • Fatigue • Foamy urine • Urine color might become darker (Ex: tea- or cola-colored, dark orange, or reddish)
Stage 4	At this stage, the patient's GFR ranges between 15 and 29 mL per minute. Signs and symptoms worsen and other bodily systems can be affected. Patients tend to experience: • Nausea • Vomiting • Weight loss • Loss of appetite • Kidney pain • Tingling/numbness of fingers and toes • Anemia from bone disease • High blood pressure from fluid retention that puts strain on the cardiovascular system • Lethargy • Confusion • Urine might be foamy • Urine color may become darker (Ex: tea- or cola-colored, dark orange, or reddish)

(continued)

Table 10-7 Stages of Renal Failure (Kidney Disease)—*continued*

Stage 5	The patient's kidneys are not functioning and are not producing urine. The signs and symptoms are: • Weight loss • Muscle cramps • No or very little urine output • Itchy skin • Decreased alertness • Headache • Fatigue • Numbness/tingling of hands and feet • Weakness • Vomiting • Nausea • Excessive fluid accumulation causing high blood pressure, chest pain and/or edema, and shortness of breath

The second step is the dipstick test, in which a strip containing certain chemicals that will react by changing color is inserted into the urine. One value the test measures is the amount of acid in the urine, or its pH. A value outside of the normal range indicates a potential problem with the kidneys. The dipstick also measures the protein content in the urine. Because protein should not be filtered from the blood via the kidneys, when protein is found, it signifies that the kidneys are not filtering properly, indicating that kidney disease is present. If blood is found, further evaluation is needed to determine the cause.

The third step of a urinalysis is a microscopic examination, which provides information about the possible cells present in the fluid. White blood cells might indicate that an infection is present, while red blood cells might indicate a disease that affects filtration. Other possible items found in the urine sample are crystals, which might be associated with kidney stones, and casts, which are made up of various cells and protein accumulating in the small tubes in the kidneys.

Several categories of drugs can be used to treat acute renal failure. Diuretics are used to decrease edema and pressure on the kidneys resulting from retained fluid. They also can help treat the associated hypertension by reducing fluid volume. Because our kidneys help regulate electrolytes such as potassium, calcium, and sodium, if proper levels of potassium are not being excreted, for example, it can build up in the blood and cause hyperkalemia. Potassium is used for muscle contraction and too much makes the heart very irritable, and can lead to dangerous heart arrhythmias. If proper levels of potassium are not being removed from the blood, then kionex or kayexalate is given to prevent a toxic buildup of potassium in the blood.

CLINICAL CONNECTION 10.1

DIALYSIS

In addition to medications, another way to control electrolyte levels and artificially replace the kidneys' work is by transplantation or dialysis. A kidney transplant requires the donor and recipient to be compatible. Dialysis can be performed in either a medical facility or the patient's home. There are two types of dialysis, **hemodialysis** and **peritoneal dialysis**.

10-13i Hemodialysis

Hemodialysis works as an artificial kidney to remove waste products directly from the blood via a semipermeable membrane. It also maintains proper balance of electrolytes, particularly sodium, potassium, and calcium, Figure 10-12. A patient can be hooked up to the machine in different ways, but they all share routing the blood. The blood leaves the patient and goes into the machine, where filtration and ion exchange take place, and then the filtered blood is returned to the patient's bloodstream.

10-13j Peritoneal Dialysis

Peritoneal dialysis involves inserting a catheter into the patient's abdomen and instilling the dialyzing solution, Figure 10-13. The peritoneal cavity is lined with a membrane called the peritoneal membrane, which acts as a filter.

Because the fluid is allowed to sit in the cavity and acts as an exchange medium for wastes, this procedure is called an exchange. The patient might have to perform exchanges about six times per day, but this procedure can be done at home, even at night while asleep.

The solution sits in the abdomen for varying amounts of time, called a dwell time. During this time, the waste products travel across the peritoneal capillaries and are collected by the instilled solution. Then after a couple of hours, the fluid is drained, removing the waste from the body.

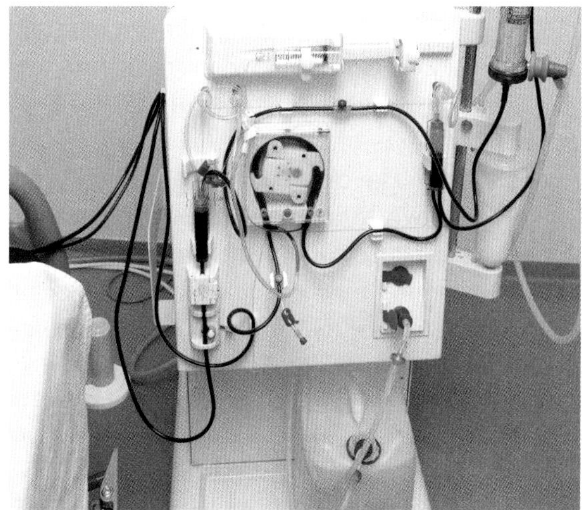

FIGURE 10-12 Hemodialysis machine.

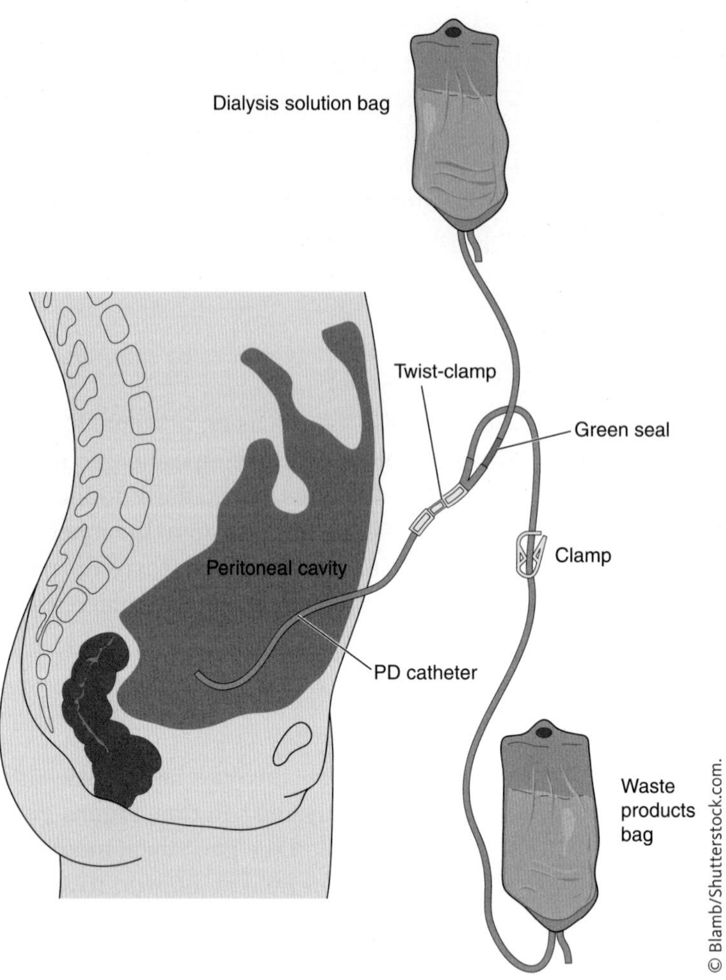

FIGURE 10-13 Peritoneal dialysis.

10-13k Kidney Cancer (Renal Cancer)

There are many different types of kidney cancer, but the most common form is **renal cell carcinoma**, which is also known as renal cell adenocarcinoma. What makes renal cell adenocarcinoma so dangerous is that it often metastasizes or spreads to the patient's bones, brain, or liver before symptoms ever occur.

While in the top 10 most common cancers affecting both men and women, kidney carcinoma tends to occur more in men than women. This form of cancer is less common in people 45 years old or younger, with the average age being 64 years old.

The exact causes of kidney cancer are not yet known, but some links are known to increase the likelihood of developing it. These risk factors include exposure to certain chemicals, obesity, which can change certain hormones thereby increasing the risk for developing renal cancer, and heredity, because inherited DNA mutations make the cells more predisposed to carcinoma.

When signs and symptoms do arise, the patient first might experience hematuria and then pain in the flank and lumbar region as the condition progresses. Other signs and symptoms are as follows:

- Loss of appetite
- Unexplained weight loss

- Fever that will not break
- Fatigue
- Mass located in the region of the kidney.

A urinalysis can detect blood (RBCs) and cancer in the patient's urine. A complete blood count (CBC) might find that there are fewer than normal RBCs, potentially indicating the patient is anemic from blood loss. The opposite can occur, however, with some patients having too many RBCs in the CBC. If this is the case, the cancer cells are making too much erythropoietin, a hormone that causes bone marrow to increase the production of red blood cells.

Other tests such as a CT scan, IVP, and KUB are used to visually inspect the kidneys for cancer. If a tumor is located, a tissue biopsy is taken to confirm the diagnosis.

Chemotherapy, surgery, and radiation can be used to treat cancer, as well as the drugs in Table 10-8.

10-14 BLADDER DISEASE

Urinary incontinence is the loss of bladder control, Figure 10-14, which is not only a nuisance but also an embarrassing problem. Both sexes are affected by this condition, though it is more likely to happen to women, and it usually occurs in those 60 years and older. For women, the odds are increased with pregnancy, childbirth, menopause, and those who have had a hysterectomy. Incontinence in men can be caused by an enlarged prostate gland. The severity of the condition can vary, from experiencing a small dribble to such a sudden urgency to urinate that the patient loses control. The incontinence can happen at any time, day or at night.

Table 10-8 Drugs Used to Treat Kidney Cancer

DRUG NAME	METHOD OF DELIVERY	METHOD OF ACTION
Avastin (bevacizumab)	Injection	Stops blood supply to tumors to slow/stop the growth
Torisel (temsirolimus)	Injection	Blocks the enzymes that signal cells to multiply (grow)
Afinator, Zortress (everolimus)	Tablet	Blocks the enzymes that signal cells to multiply (grow)
Nexavar (sorafenib)	Tablet	Blocks the enzymes that signal cells to multiply (grow)
Sutent (sunitinib)	Tablet	Blocks the enzymes that signal cells to multiply (grow)

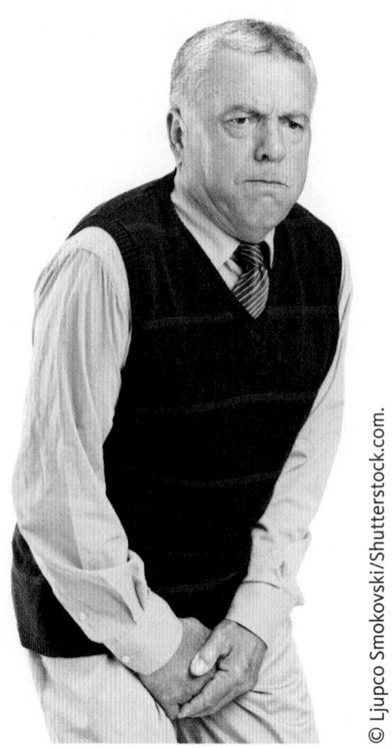
© Ljupco Smokovski/Shutterstock.com.

FIGURE 10-14 Senior citizen experiencing bladder control difficulty.

10-14a Types of Incontinence

There are several different types of urinary incontinence. *Stress incontinence* occurs when the person coughs, laughs, sneezes, lifts heavy objects, or exercises. All of these actions put extra pressure on the bladder. Normally, the bladder can handle the extra pressure with no problems, but leakage will result with stress incontinence.

Overflow incontinence results when the bladder does not empty completely, causing the individual to experience dribbling. *Urge incontinence* causes the person to urinate involuntarily following a sudden severe urgency. *Functional incontinence* is when a person cannot get to a restroom in time because of some sort of physical or mental disability. If a person has two or more of these types of incontinence, then they are diagnosed as having *mixed incontinence*.

Urinary incontinence is a symptom, and not a disease. It can be the result of the patient's diet (alcohol or coffee), medications (blood pressure or muscle relaxants), or infections (UTIs).

10-14b Diagnosing and Treating Incontinence

A diagnosis can be made after the physician takes the patient's history and physical information and looks at the patient's bladder diary, a log of urination habits and fluid input and output. Procedures such as a CBC and urinalysis are used to rule out infection while **urodynamic testing** is performed to study the anatomic structure and function of the urethra and bladder. This is done by inserting a special catheter to insert fluid and then measure the pressure in the bladder to determine the patient's sphincter and bladder endurance. Also, a cystoscopy and cystogram might be used to actually visualize possible causes, such as a tumor or other anomaly.

Treatment depends on the type of incontinence. For example, Kegel or pelvic floor exercises can be used to strengthen the pelvic or sphincter muscles. To perform this exercise, the patient flexes or tightens his or her pelvic muscles as if he or she is trying to hold in urine. These exercises are great for controlling stress incontinence.

Besides exercises, medications such as **alpha blockers**, **anticholinergics**, and **antiandrogens** are used to help control urinary incontinence.

Alpha blockers are used to help empty the bladder by blocking alpha 1 receptor sites. This allows the muscles around the bladder neck and prostate to relax and the bladder to evacuate urine. Common drugs include:

- Flomax (tamsulosin)
- Rapaflo (silodosin)
- Uroxatral (alfuzosin)
- Cardura (doxazosin)
- Hytrin (terazosin).

The bladder contraction and emptying is stimulated by the parasympathetic system. Anticholinergic agents block the nerve impulses of the parasympathetic system, which decreases the bladder tone, allowing it to fill up with more urine while also decreasing bladder contractions and stopping the patient's urgency to go. Examples are:

- Detrol (tolterodine)
- Enablex (darifenacin)
- Ditropan XL (oxytynin)
- Toviaz (fesoterodine).

Antiandrogens decrease the size of the prostate gland, which if enlarged can block the flow of urine, Figure 10-15. The patient still experiences the urgency or need to urinate but has poor urine flow. Drugs used to treat benign prostatic hyperplasia (BPH) are:

- Proscar (finasteride)
- Avodart (dutasteride).

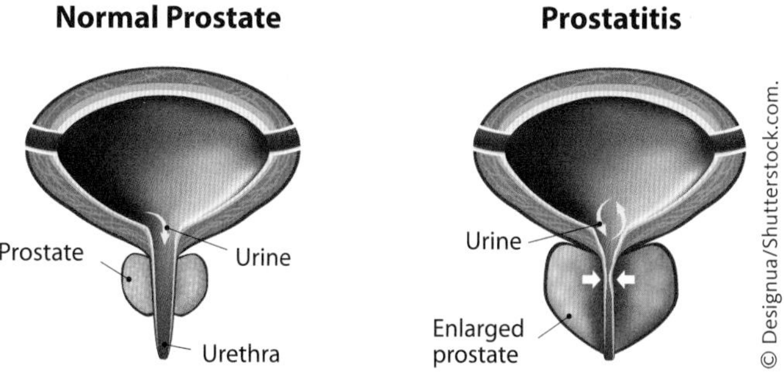

FIGURE 10-15 Inflamed prostate gland is obstructing urine flow.

10-14c Bladder Cancer (Transitional Cell Carcinoma of the Bladder)

Bladder cancer is the most common cancer of the urinary system. **Transitional cell carcinoma of the bladder** develops in the lining of the bladder, occurring mainly in people older than 60 years old. Typically, men are up to three times more likely than women to develop bladder cancer. Bladder carcinoma is more likely to spread (metastasize), usually to the bones, before symptoms arise. The exact cause is unknown; however, risk factors include smoking, chronic cystitis, and exposure to chemical agents.

While not presenting until later in the disease process, patients usually encounter:

- Hematuria
- Dysuria
- Nocturia
- Abdominal pain
- Bone pain
- Tiredness.

Confirmation of bladder cancer can be done by using a cystoscopy and biopsy procedure. As soon as the results come back positive, it should be staged to see how advanced the disease process has become. Treating bladder cancer can be done by various surgical procedures depending on the area affected.

Medications used to treat bladder cancer are:

- Tecentriq (atezolizumab), which is an immunotherapy used to reactivate a patient's immune system, specifically the T cells, which the cancer might have been stopped or slowed down.
- Pantinol, Platinol-AQ (cisplantin), stops the cancer cells from being able to divide, causing the tumor to stop growing and die.
- Thioplex (thiotepa) disrupts the cancer cells' DNA.
- Doxil (doxorubicin hydrochloride liposome) stops the cancer cells ability to divide, stopping cell growth.

Module 11

Pathopharmacology of the Respiratory System

Module Introduction

What is the purpose of the respiratory system? The obvious answer is to allow us to breathe. However, there is much more to the story. The main purpose of breathing is to bring in fresh air from the oxygen rich atmosphere, so that it can be delivered to every cell in your body for normal function and survival. However, what is often forgotten is that exhalation allows your body to remove carbon dioxide, which is a waste product of the activities conducted by all of your cells. If this gaseous waste by-product of metabolism were allowed to accumulate in the blood, it would make it very acidic, and could potentially cause damage. We will soon see how important the exchange of gas, where oxygen is taken into the blood and carbon dioxide removed, is vital for life. The respiratory system in medicine is often referred to as the *pulmonary system*, and the specialist who treats pathologies of this system is the **pulmonologist**.

The following animation shows an overview of the anatomy and physiology of the respiratory system. Don't worry if it is not all clear at this point, as we will be going over it all very soon, but it will be nice to "see the big picture" before we get into the nitty-gritty details.

LEARNING OBJECTIVE 11.1 Explain the normal anatomy and physiology concepts associated with the upper airway of the respiratory system.

KEY TERMS

Aspiration Food or liquid entering the airway, which can cause serious obstruction and damage.

Epiglottis Leaf-like fibrocartilage that, when you swallow, closes over the opening to the trachea, thus, directing food or liquid down the esophagus to prevent aspiration.

Gag reflex Protective airway reflex to prevent aspiration.

Larynx Voice box.

Lower airways Extend from the vocal cords down to the alveoli, where inspired air is transported to the alveolar region for gas exchange.

Nasal cavity Beginning of the upper airway within the nose.

Olfactory Area in nasal cavity for your sense of smell.

Palate The roof of your mouth.

Paranasal sinuses Air-filled chambers located *around* the nasal cavity.

Pathogens Disease-producing organisms.

Pharynx A hollow muscular tube for passage of food, water, and air—the throat.

Phonation The process of speech.

Tonsils Masses of lymphoid tissue that fight infection.

Turbinates Shelf-like structures called *conchae* within the nasal cavity that heats and humidifies inspired air.

Upper airway Anatomically extends from the nose to the vocal cords, where inspired air is conditioned through heating or cooling and humidification.

Vocal cords V-like structure found in the larynx that vibrates to give sound (phonation).

OVERVIEW OF THE PULMONARY SYSTEM

Air normally enters through your nose where it is warmed and moistened, making it more comfortable to breathe. The air then passes through the back of your throat and down through ever branching air passageways called *bronchial tubes*, or *bronchi*, that decrease in diameter. Once the air passes through your upper airway, it travels into the right and left lung. These tubes continue to branch and get smaller and smaller, becoming *bronchioles*. The bronchioles continue to branch in an organized manner until they end in the blind sacs, or *alveoli*, where actual gas exchange takes place. At this point, oxygen can move through the walls of the alveoli into your blood system via capillaries, allowing it to travel to the cells of your body so that they can continue to function. Carbon dioxide, the waste product, can move out of your blood vessels through the alveoli, and then into your airways to be exhaled with your next breath, thus ridding your body of carbon dioxide.

Ventilation is the term used to describe the movement of air in and out of your lungs, and consists of two main phases. *Inhalation* is the movement of air into your lungs, and *exhalation* is the movement out of your lungs. This distinction is important because you will soon see that some respiratory diseases primarily affect either inhalation or exhalation. In addition, a term that is sometimes confused with ventilation is **respiration**. Respiration is the process of gas exchange that takes place deep within the lungs at the end points, or alveolar region. Again, this distinction is important; as you will see, some diseases affect the airways (bronchi) that ventilate or bring in oxygen, and other respiratory diseases affect the peripheral regions of the lung (alveoli) where the actual gas exchange takes place.

For purposes of matching the pathology with the pharmacology, and not overwhelming you with the entire system at once, we will focus on the following three distinct regions:

- The upper airway
- The lower airway
- The lungs and chest cavity, aka the thoracic cavity

For each of these areas, we will start with what is normal, and then discuss what can go wrong, or the pathology. Finally, we will then discuss the pharmacologic treatment for the given pathology. Let's begin with the upper airway.

11-1 THE UPPER AIRWAY

Now that you have seen the big picture, let's begin a journey through the respiratory system to fill in the details. The respiratory system can be thought of as possessing three distinct regions. First is the **upper airway**, extending from the nose to the vocal cords, which conditions the inspired air through warming and humidification. The **lower airways** then transport the conditioned air to the lungs where it eventually reaches the alveolar region for gas exchange. The final region is the lung and chest cavity, which support our ability to breathe properly. We'll focus on the upper airway for now, as shown in Figure 11-1.

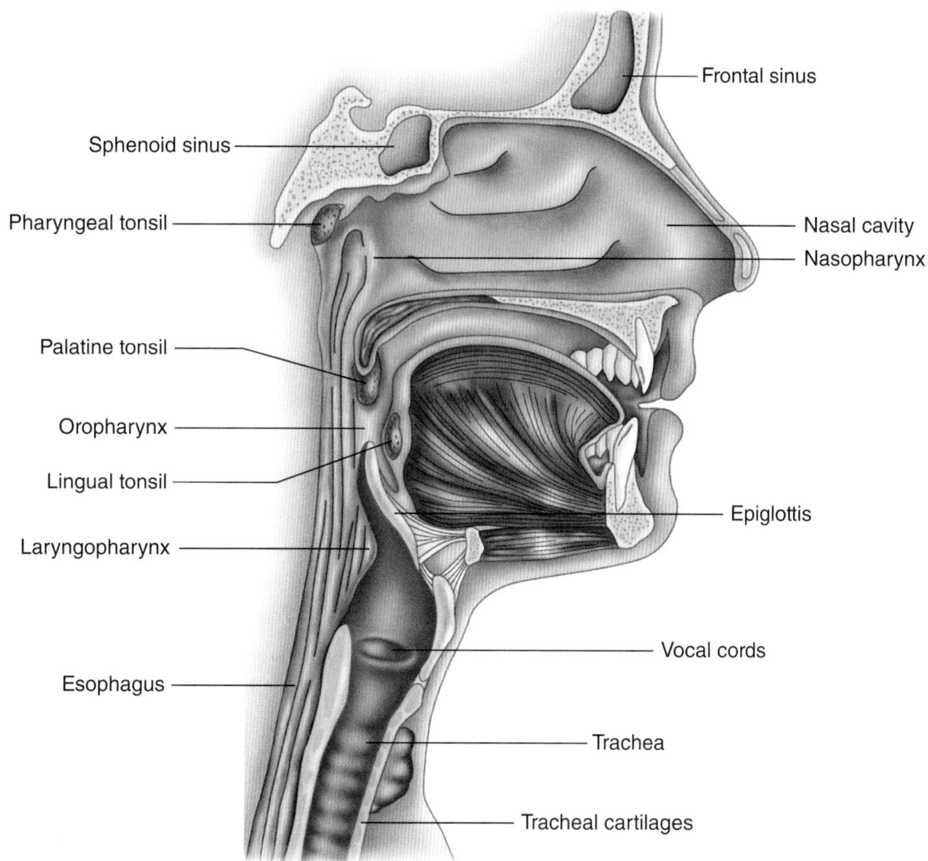

FIGURE 11-1 Structures of the upper airway.

11-1a Functions of the Upper Airway—The Nasal Region

The upper airway's main purpose is to condition the air to make it non irritating to the respiratory system. This means the following:

- Filtering out any large particles that could obstruct the airways
- Heating or cooling the inspired air to body temperature
- Adding moisture (humidification) so that the air is 100% saturated
- Keeping the upper passageways clean of debris and infection

The **nasal cavity** marks the beginning of the upper airway, and the nose begins the filtration of large particles with coarse sticky nasal hairs. These hairs will trap any large particles before they get any further into your respiratory system, which could cause blockages to the flow. Moving further into the nasal cavity, shelf-like structures called **turbinates**, or *conchae*, are lined with mucous membranes that add humidity, and heat the inspired air. They also secrete mucus that can trap dust, smaller particles, and **pathogens**. This, again, keeps these particles/pathogens from reaching deeper into the lungs, thus, preventing obstructions and infections. A very large number of blood-filled capillaries is located throughout this area. This is why a nosebleed produces a lot of blood.

Located on the roof of the nasal cavity is the **olfactory** region for your sense of smell. This is also why, when an infection causes excess secretions, your sense of smell is blocked. Because smell is also associated with taste; you also lose your sense of taste.

Located around the nasal cavity are the **paranasal sinuses**, which are air-filled chambers within the facial bones. They not only lighten your skull, but aid in **phonation**, giving resonance, or a fuller sound, to your voice. These can become infected, and cause pain and pressure within these spaces.

While the upper airway begins at the nose, you can also breathe through your mouth. The roof of your mouth, called the **palate**, consisting of a hard and a soft palate, separates your nasal cavity from your mouth. When you breathe air, it is directed through a hollow muscular tube called the **pharynx**, or, in a more common term, the throat. While you can breathe either through your nose or your mouth, keep in mind that the pharynx serves as a common passageway for air, food, and liquid.

Note that this area contains pharyngeal **tonsils** that fight infections that can gain entrance into your respiratory system. In addition, notice that the *eustachian tubes* are located in this region as well, which are direct links to the middle ear. This is why ear infections, sinus infections, and airway infections can all spread through this open system of passageways. Have you ever heard the expression, "the cold settled in his or her chest"?

Do you remember that the pharynx acts as a common passageway for food, liquid, and air? What causes food to enter our stomach and not our lungs? Sitting above the opening to the trachea, or main tube into the lungs, is the **epiglottis**. This important traffic controller acts as a lid or door, allowing only air into the rest of your airway, and food and water to travel down your esophagus. When you swallow, the epiglottis closes over the glottis, thus directing the food or liquid down the only available passageway, which is now the esophagus. When you breathe, the esophagus is compressed, and the epiglottis is open and, therefore, allows the air to travel into your lungs. Below the epiglottis sits the **larynx**, or voice box, which contains your **vocal cords**.

CLINICAL CONNECTION 11.1

Your airway is also protected by your **gag reflex**, which can be decreased by many neuromuscular conditions interfering with normal epiglottic function. This can lead to an **aspiration** where food or liquid can enter the airway, causing serious obstruction and damage. This is why aspiration or choking incidents often occur in restaurants where people are drinking alcohol (neuromuscular depressant), while talking and laughing with a mouthful of food, which can all overwhelm the gag reflex. The lay phrase for aspiration is "food going down the wrong pipe."

LEARNING OBJECTIVE 11.2 Describe the pathopharmacology of the upper airway.

KEY TERMS

Acute rhinitis Symptoms of congestion and runny nose usually viral etiology, aka "a cold."

Allergic rhinitis Inflammation of the mucous membranes from an *allergic reaction*, such as ragweed or grass allergies.

Analgesics Medications to reduce pain.

Antihistamines Medications to prevent the release of histamine during an allergic response.

Antipyretics Medications to reduce fever.

Antitussive agents Reduces cough.

Apnea The cessation of breathing.

Asphyxia Extreme decrease in the amount of oxygen in the body to the point of unconsciousness and death.

Corticosteroids Medications that suppress both the inflammatory and allergic response.

Croup Inflammatory pediatric condition of viral or bacterial origin that is characterized by a barking cough.

Cyanosis Bluish tint to the skin usually due to low oxygen levels.

Decongestants Medications that constrict blood flow and inflammation, thereby, reducing passageway congestion.

Dysphagia Difficulty swallowing.

Dysphonia Difficulty speaking.

Dyspnea Difficulty breathing.

Epiglottitis Potentially life-threatening illness, mainly affecting children, of epiglottic swelling, which can obstruct the airway leading to asphyxia; caused by the bacterium *Haemophilus influenzae* type b; the Hib vaccine can help protect children from developing epiglottitis.

Expectorants Agents to help increase secretions that can then be expelled.

Laryngitis Acute or chronic inflammation of the larynx and vocal cords leading to difficulty speaking.

Obstructive Sleep Apnea (OSA) Periods of cessation of breathing during sleep due to airway obstruction.

Over-the-counter (OTC) Drugs or medications that do not require a prescription.

Pertussis Preventable vaccinated pediatric disease that is also known as *whooping cough* based on the sound the patient produces when they cough.

Prophylactic treatment Treatment to prevent the exacerbation or occurrence of a disease.

Pulse oximeter Non invasive device used to measure oxygen saturation in the blood.

Rhinorrhea Runny nose.

Sinusitis Inflammation of the mucous membranes lining the sinus cavities.

Sleep apnea Periods of cessation of breathing during sleep.

Strep throat Sore, swollen, red throat caused by the bacteria streptococcus.

Tachypnea Rapid breathing.

Upper Respiratory Infections (URIs) General term for infections of the upper airway such as the common cold.

11-2 INFECTIONS OF THE UPPER AIRWAY

An important learning hint to keep in mind is that the narrower the passageway, the harder it is to breathe because of the increased resistance to moving air through restricted areas. This is why football players wear adhesive strips across their noses. These nasal strips help open the nares in order to reduce air resistance and, therefore, make ventilation easier. Much of the pathologies related to the upper airway are due to congestion, and the narrowing of the passageways of the upper airway, which make it difficult to breathe. Of course, the pharmacologic treatment will be to keep these passageways open.

Dyspnea, or difficulty breathing, is a common sign of respiratory disease. Any blockages as a result of infections, and their associated congestion, can cause mild to severe dyspnea. In addition, faster breathing or **tachypnea** may occur in order to make up for the lack of ventilation, or ability to take a deep breath, due to obstructions. From our journey through normal A&P of the upper airway, you can see many structures that can become inflamed due to trauma or infection. The suffix, "*itis*" means "inflammation of" and is found in many of the infectious diseases of the upper airway. Normally, the pathogens are either *bacterial* or *viral* in nature. The following are common inflammatory conditions of the upper airway:

- Sinusitis
- Tonsillitis
- Pharyngitis
- Laryngitis
- Acute epiglottitis

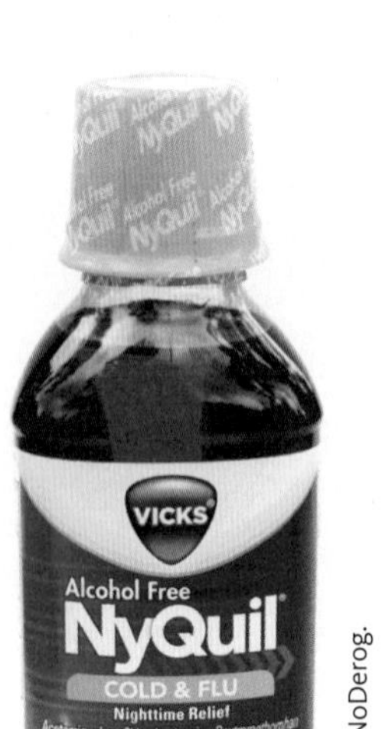

© iStockphoto/NoDerog.

FIGURE 11-2 Example of common OTC drug.

The main treatment of infectious disease in the upper airway is targeted antibiotic use on the specific bacterial infection. However, often these are viral infections and antibiotics should not be used. Many **over-the-counter (OTC)** drugs, such as NyQuil, (Figure 11-2) are used for symptomatic relief, which will be discussed soon.

11-3 UPPER AIRWAY OBSTRUCTIONS

Since the upper airway is the main entrance to the lungs, severe inflammation and swelling can lead to obstruction. Severe obstruction can cause **asphyxia**, which is an extreme decrease in the amount of oxygen in the body, to the point of unconsciousness and death. Often individuals with low levels of oxygen in the blood exhibit a bluish tint to the skin known as **cyanosis**. The percentage of oxygen in the blood can be measured with a device called a **pulse oximeter** as shown in Figure 11-3.

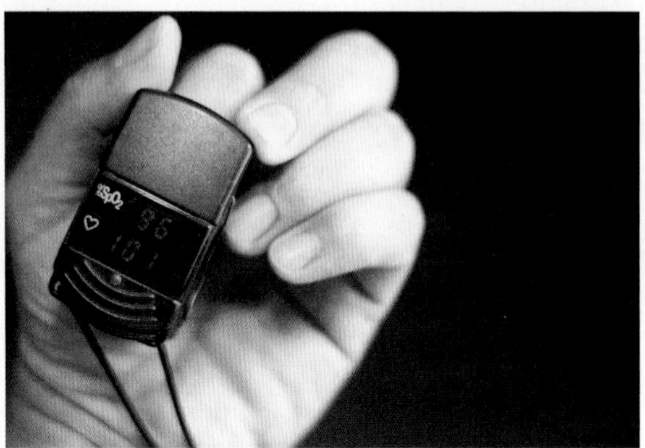

© iStockphoto/abalcazar.

FIGURE 11-3 Pulse oximetry.

Some individuals obstruct their upper airway during the normal process of sleeping, to the point where breathing actually stops. This is known as **apnea**. One form of **sleep apnea** is caused by the excessive relaxation of the muscles of the upper airway, which allows for the blockage of airflow into the lungs, even as the brain fires to make the victim try to breathe. This is called **obstructive sleep apnea (OSA)**.

CLINICAL CONNECTION 11.2

Children are especially susceptible to upper airway infections because they have a much more narrow airway than adults. A pediatric condition, **croup**, is an inflammatory process usually caused by a virus (but can also be caused by a bacteria), and is characterized by a "barking" cough. **Pertussis** is another mainly pediatric disease, which is also known as whooping cough based on the sound the patient produces when they cough. This disease had been fairly well eliminated in the United States, but is seeing a resurgence, as some parents are reluctant to immunize their children with the proper vaccine. It is now recommended that adults who are around children get booster vaccinations to prevent the spread of whooping cough to children.

11-4 SPECIFIC UPPER RESPIRATORY INFECTIONS

Some important points to keep in mind are that most **upper respiratory infections (URIs)** are not life threatening, but are highly bothersome, as in Figure 11-4. While you are highly unlikely to die from a "head cold" it is miserable with the nasal decongestion, dyspnea, lack of taste and smell, sputum production, and so on. Also, most URIs are caused by viruses, such as the very common rhinovirus, the culprit in the "common cold."

11-4a Acute Rhinitis (the Common Cold)

While technically known as **acute rhinitis**, we often call it a cold. Did you ever wonder why it is called a cold? Traditionally, it was believed that the common cold was caused by exposure to cold air, because winter was the time of the year

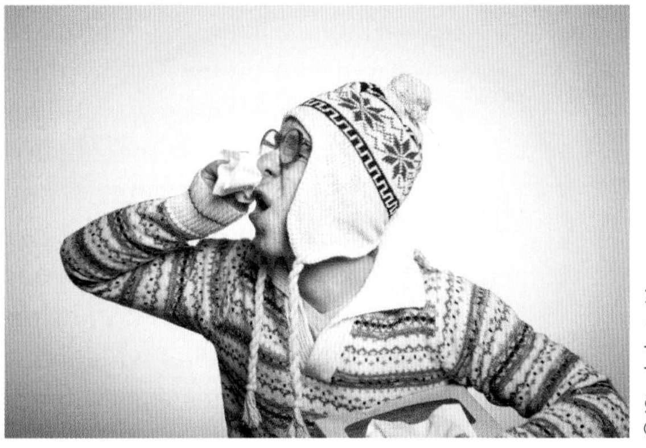

FIGURE 11-4 I think we can all relate!

that colds and flu occurred more often. Even though this myth still persists, the real reasons are the fact that the relative humidity (moisture in the air) during the winter is lower than the rest of the year. Flu and rhinoviruses prefer dryer air conditions and, therefore, become more active in winter. In addition, people are closer to each other, because they stay indoors in bad weather conditions and, thus, can spread the virus more readily.

Symptoms of the common cold can include watery eyes, running nose (**rhinorrhea**), sore throat, nasal congestion, and fever.

Pharmacologic treatment is primarily symptom relief, and often requires OTC medications in the following areas:

- **Antipyretics** to reduce fever if present.
- **Analgesics** to reduce pain if present.
- **Decongestants** to constrict the blood flow and inflammation thereby opening up the passageway.
- **Antitussive agents** to reduce bothersome non productive cough. It should be noted strongly that a productive cough should not be inhibited, as secretions that can breed infections should be expectorated.
- **Expectorants** to help increase secretions that can then be expelled.

Of course non pharmacologic treatment such as rest, drinking fluids, good hand washing, and assuring good humidification should accompany pharmacologic measures.

11-4b Allergic Rhinitis (Hay Fever)

Allergic rhinitis has many of the same cold symptoms, but is due to inflammation of the mucous membranes from an *allergic reaction*, such as ragweed or grass allergies (Figure 11-5). Since this is an allergic response, medications that inhibit the allergic or immune response can be added to the cold medications previously mentioned. These include **antihistamines** and **corticosteroids**, which both inhibit the allergic response. These medications work best when given prior to the exposure of the allergen. This is termed **prophylactic treatment**.

11-4c Pharyngitis

Inflammation of the mucous membranes lining the pharynx is called pharyngitis, or the more common, lay term: sore throat. Most commonly, this is a viral infection but can be caused by the bacteria streptococcus, and this is then called **strep throat**, as seen in Figure 11-6. Symptoms include a red swollen sore throat, tiny red dots (petechiae) on both hard and soft palates, pus, white patches, difficulty swallowing (**dysphagia**), fever, and swollen neck lymph glands. Visualization of the throat confirms the disease. A strep throat culture can be taken to determine if it is bacterial and, therefore, requires antibiotic treatment. Viral infections do not respond to antibiotics; and they should be treated for symptom relief with antiseptic gargles, throat lozenges, and analgesics for pain. Sometimes something as simple as getting a new toothbrush can prevent repeat infections!

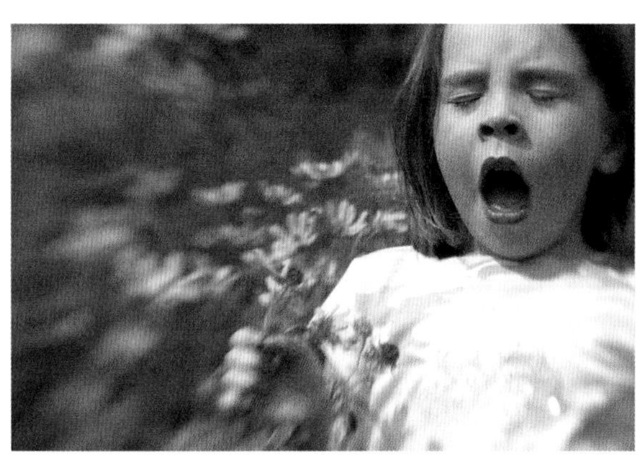

FIGURE 11-5 Allergic rhinitis, or hay fever, can be caused by various pollens.

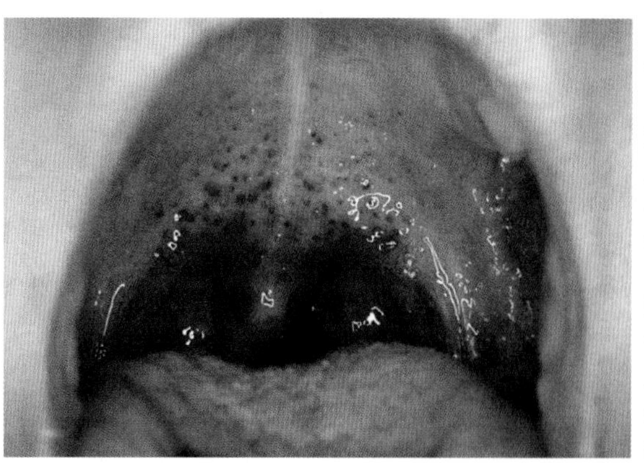

FIGURE 11-6 A severe case of strep throat caused by group A *Streptococcus* bacteria. Notice the inflammation of the oropharynx as evidenced by the small red spots called petechiae.

11-5 MEDICATIONS FOR UPPER AIRWAY DISEASE

Let's stop and take a look at the medications used for upper airway diseases discussed thus far. As you can see in Table 11-1, many of the medications are OTC for symptomatic relief.

Table 11-1 Medications for upper airway disease

MEDICATION CLASSIFICATION	DESIRED PHARMACOLOGIC ACTION	DRUG(S) EXAMPLES
Antipyretics	Reduce fever	Acetylsalicylic acid (Aspirin)
Analgesic	Reduce pain	Acetaminophen (Tylenol)
Antitussive	Reduce or prevent cough	OTC dextromethorphan; Tessalon; Codeine (requires a prescription)
Expectorant	Increase secretions and their removal	Guaifenesin
Antihistamine	Reduce inflammation caused by histamine release due to allergies	Benadryl, Zyrtec, Allegra, Clarinex
Decongestants	Reduce blood flow by vasoconstriction and, therefore, reduce congestion	Sudafed (pills), Afrin and Neo-Synephrine (Nasal spray)
Antibiotics	Fight bacterial infections	Many examples, such as penicillin, or amoxicillin to treat strep throat
Corticosteroids	Reduce immune response of inflammation, thereby, relieving congestion	Nasacort (nasal spray inhaler)

11-6 SINUSITIS

Inflammation of the mucous membranes lining the sinus cavities or **sinusitis** can often occur after acute rhinitis. Remember that we told you to keep in mind that an infection can easily spread throughout the respiratory system. When the membranes become swollen, along with producing more mucus, blockages can occur, leading to sinus headaches, dyspnea, and dizziness as in Figure 11-7. Other symptoms include cough, rhinorrhea, and congestion.

Diagnosis of sinusitis is based on patient history, physical exam, and high-resolution imaging, such as a CAT scan or MRI.

Treatment includes antibiotics, analgesics, and decongestants. Remember that antibiotics should only be used on bacterial cases. Of course non pharmacologic measures to relieve or lessen severity include proper humidification, and avoiding cigarette smoke or other pollutants and irritants.

11-7 LARYNGITIS

Laryngitis is an acute, or chronic, inflammation of the larynx and vocal cords, leading to the patient having a distinctive hoarse voice, or even a loss of voice. The etiology for laryngitis can be either viral or bacterial, resulting in an acute condition. Chronic episodes arise from excessive alcohol use, GERD, and inhaling chemical irritants or smoke. Symptoms include difficulty speaking (**dysphonia**), dysphagia, fever, and pain around the *voicebox* region, as shown in Figure 11-8.

Pharmacologic treatment includes analgesics, throat lozenges, and an antibiotic if bacterial in origin. Non pharmacologic treatment includes resting the voice and avoiding any irritants, such as cigarette smoke.

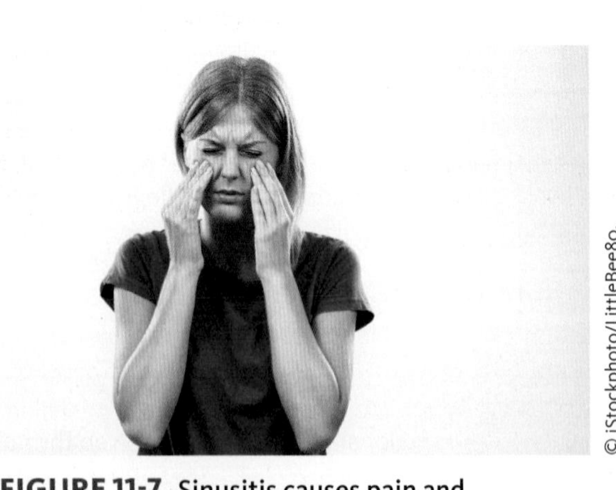

FIGURE 11-7 Sinusitis causes pain and headaches.

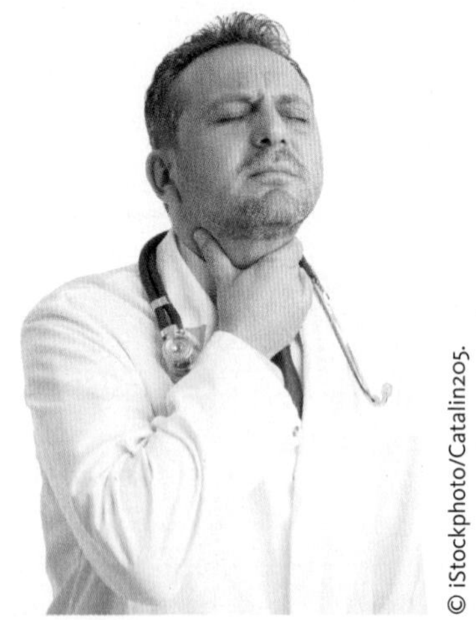

FIGURE 11-8 Laryngitis is an inflammation of the larynx or voice box, and results in pain and difficulty speaking.

11-8 EPIGLOTTITIS

The upper airway pathologies previously discussed are rarely life threatening; however, **epiglottitis** is a potentially life-threatening illness mainly affecting children. If the epiglottis swells, especially in small pediatric airways, it can obstruct the airway, leading to asphyxia. Therefore, epiglottitis is a medical emergency with a sudden onset accompanied by hoarseness, fever, sore throat, and drooling. Epiglottitis is caused by the bacterium *Haemophilus influenzae* type b. The Hib vaccine can help protect children from developing epiglottitis. Airway maintenance and antibiotics are the primary treatments.

11-9 PATHOPHARMACOLOGY OF THE UPPER AIRWAY

Now, let's put everything together in Table 11-2 to show you the complete picture of the pathopharmacology of the upper airway of the pulmonary system.

Table 11-2 Pathopharmacology of the upper airways

DISEASE	ETIOLOGY	COMMON SYMPTOMS	PHARMACOLOGIC TREATMENT
Acute rhinitis (common cold)	Usually rhinoviruses	Watery eyes, rhinorrhea, sore throat, nasal congestion, and fever	OTC medications to treat symptoms, antipyretics, analgesics, decongestants, antitussive agents, and expectorants
Allergic rhinitis (hay fever)	Many types of allergic triggers (antigens) such as grass pollen and animal dander.	Watery eyes, rhinorrhea, sore throat, nasal congestion, inflammation, and fever	Same OTC agents for cold symptom relief with addition of antihistamines and inhaled nasal corticosteroids to reduce inflammatory response
Pharyngitis	Mostly viral but can be bacterial, as in strep throat	Sore throat, dysphagia	Antibiotics if bacterial, and throat lozenges and antiseptic mouthwash
Sinusitis	Mostly viral but can be bacterial	Pain and pressure in head, dizziness, congestion	Antibiotics if bacterial, and analgesics
Laryngitis	Mostly viral but can be bacterial	Dysphonia	Antibiotics if bacterial
Epiglottitis	Bacterium *Haemophilus influenzae* type b	Can cause life threatening obstruction hoarseness, fever, sore throat, and drooling	Mostly affects children, antibiotics and airway maintenance often needed, preventable with Hib vaccine

LEARNING OBJECTIVE 11.3 Explain the normal anatomy and physiology concepts and assessment associated with the lower airways of the respiratory system.

KEY TERMS

Alveoli Lung structure where gas exchange takes place.

Antibiotic Medication to treat bacterial infections.

Arterial blood gases (ABGs) Sample of *arterial* blood to see if there are adequate oxygen and carbon dioxide levels.

Auscultation The action of listening to sounds from the heart, lungs, or other organs, typically with a stethoscope, as a part of medical diagnosis.

Bradypnea Slower than normal breathing.

Bronchi Large airways.

Bronchioles Small airways (iole = small).

Bronchospasm Narrowing of the airways due to smooth muscle contraction.

Cilia Microscopic hair-like structures that act like oars moving mucus up and out of the airways in a coordinated fashion.

Crackles Popping sound upon inspiration, representing fluid in the alveoli.

Culture and sensitivity test (sputum C&S test) A lab test that grows (cultures) the bacteria found in a sample in order to identify the type of bacteria, then tests against (sensitivity) a variety of antibiotic medications to see which are effective.

Hypoxemia Low levels of oxygen within the blood.

Mucociliary escalator The tissue layer mechanism that performs pulmonary hygiene.

Orthopnea Difficulty breathing while lying down, and the patient needs to "straighten up" in order to breathe easier.

Peak flow meter Asthma monitoring device to measure exhaled flow rates.

Pulmonary function tests (PFTs) Volume and flow tests to measure airway function.

Rales Older term for crackles (see crackles).

Rhonchi Low-pitched abnormal breath sounds, usually indicating airway secretions.

Trachea Also called the windpipe, it is the main airway of the tracheal bronchial tree.

Wheezes High-pitched abnormal breath sounds, indicating airway narrowing due to bronchospasm.

11-10 OVERVIEW OF THE LOWER AIRWAYS

The lower airways begin with the **trachea**, also called the windpipe, and end in the sac-like structures where gas exchange occurs, or **alveoli**. Review Figure 11-9 of the lower airways before we go more in depth with the terminology.

11-11 THE BRANCHING AIRWAYS

The trachea is the trunk of the *tracheobronchial tree* and, as you can see from the previous illustration, the airways actually look like an upside down tree. This tree is formed by ever smaller branching airways, beginning with a bifurcation forming the right and left main **bronchi**. Next, these two bronchi branch into lobar bronchi that reach into the five lobes of the lungs. The bronchi get smaller and smaller and divide into the smaller **bronchioles**.

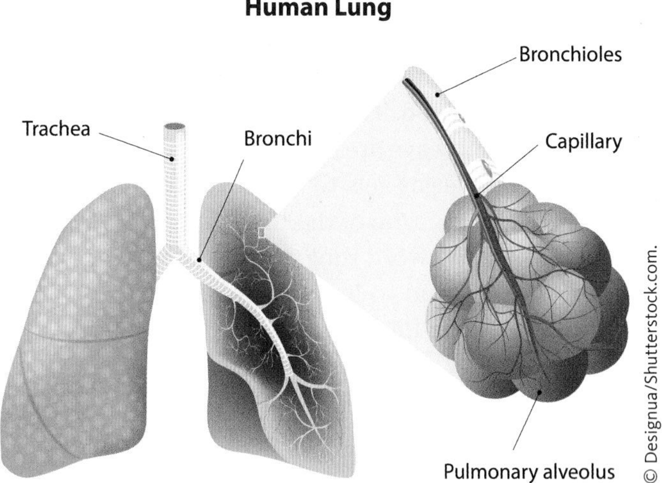

FIGURE 11-9 A representation of the lower airways from the trachea down to the alveolar region.

One of the most important functions of the airways is to perform pulmonary hygiene. This, of course, is keeping the airways clean and free of debris so that air can move in and out easily. The mechanism that performs pulmonary hygiene is called the **mucociliary escalator**.

Internally, the airways possess mucous membranes and cells that produce mucus. Mucus traps particles and pathogens just like flypaper. Mucus production is constant at approximately 100 millimeters, or a ¼ pint, daily, and must be removed to make room for fresh supplies of mucus. This is accomplished by microscopic hair-like structures called **cilia** that act as oars, moving mucus up and out of the airways in a coordinated fashion so that it can be swallowed. These cilia beat at an incredible rate of 1,500 times per minute. Smoking *paralyzes* these cilia for up to 1 hour for each cigarette smoked. This is why smokers have a lot of retained secretions—their escalators are broken. This is also why stopping (or better yet, never starting) is the most preventable measure for lung disease.

11-12 GAS EXCHANGE REGIONS

Thus far, on our journey through the respiratory system, the inhaled air has simply been transported through the airways (ventilation). Now we reach the area where vital gas exchange (respiration) takes place, oxygen is absorbed into the blood stream and carbon dioxide is removed from the blood into the lungs to be exhaled. This region is called the alveolar region, where millions of tiny air sacs called alveoli are found.

Each of these approximately 600 million alveoli can expand as air is inhaled, and return to their normal size upon exhalation. Each alveolus is wrapped with a network of pulmonary capillaries. Those alveolar walls and tightly attached capillaries form the respiratory membrane, which is where the gas exchange of oxygen and carbon dioxide occurs. Again, keep in mind that oxygen is flowing from the alveoli into the bloodstream and carbon dioxide is leaving the blood stream to be exhaled.

11-13 RESPIRATORY ASSESSMENT

You'll soon see that the pathopharmacology mirrors the A&P we have just discussed. The respiratory assessment system requires checking to make sure the airways are open and gas is moving freely (ventilation), and making sure, once the gas gets to the alveoli, that proper gas exchange can take place.

One of the first assessments is to assess the rate and quality of breathing. The word root *-pnea* means breathing. Someone breathing faster than normal is said to have *tachypnea*. Slower than normal breathing is **bradypnea**, and difficulty breathing is *dyspnea*. Some individuals have a difficult time breathing while lying down due to heart conditions that allow fluid to build up in the lungs. Have you ever heard of someone needing to prop up several pillows in order to sleep? These individuals are suffering from **orthopnea**, and need to straighten up in order to breathe easier. *Ortho* means to straighten, just like an orthodontist straightens your teeth. Of course, if a patient has *apnea*, they have stopped breathing and need CPR.

Ventilation, or the movement of air through the bronchi and bronchioles, can be assessed thorough a number of methods. A primary and immediate assessment of the respiratory system can be performed by listening to breathing with a stethoscope, and this act of listening is termed **auscultation**. Several different breath sounds can be heard, and some common abnormal breath sounds include **wheezes**, **rhonchi**, and **crackles** (a more acceptable term for **rales**). Wheezes are high-pitched musical sounds that occur due to the narrowing of the airways, as in **bronchospasm**. Rhonchi have a lower pitched musical quality, and occur as a result of air moving over secretions. Crackles are the "popping open" of the collapsed alveoli heard on inspiration, and can also be caused by a fluid buildup in the alveoli. The crackle sound is like velcro being pulled apart, or the snap, crackle, and pop of rice crispy cereal in milk.

11-14 OTHER RESPIRATORY DIAGNOSTIC TESTS

Again, constriction of the airways is called bronchospasm. The narrowing of the airway reduces the flow of air that leads to wheezing, dyspnea, and coughing. The actual amount of reduction can be measured and quantified with **pulmonary function tests (PFTs)** or a **peak flow meter**, as shown in Figure 11-10.

Chest X-rays are another valuable diagnostic tool for lung disease and can locate problems in both the airways and alveolar regions. When we get to the pathology section we will show you some specific pathologic chest X-rays.

Since a variety of bacteria can cause pneumonia and other infectious diseases in the respiratory system, we need to find out which **antibiotic** will be most effective. This is accomplished by obtaining a sputum sample in order to perform a **culture and sensitivity test (sputum C&S test)**. This test grows (cultures) the bacteria found in the sputum to identify its type, and creates a large enough growth to test against (sensitivity) a variety of antibiotic medications to see which are the best for treatment.

Arterial blood gases (ABGs), sample *arterial* blood to see if there is adequate oxygen and carbon dioxide levels. If the oxygen level is too low the patient has **hypoxemia**, and most likely needs oxygen therapy to raise the levels toward normal. If the carbon dioxide level is too high, then ventilation is

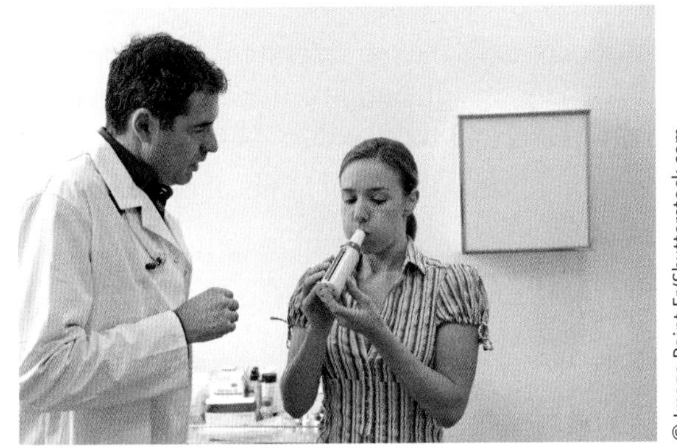

FIGURE 11-10 A patient is using a peak flow meter to measure how fast they can exhale.

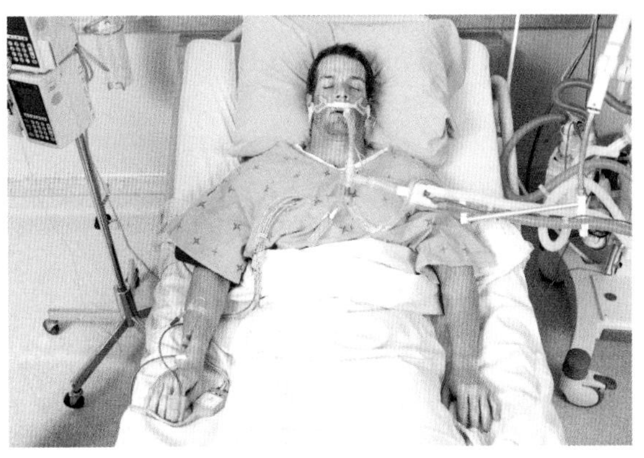

FIGURE 11-11 Intubated patient on a mechanical ventilator.

insufficient (*hypoventilation leading to respiratory acidosis*), and the patient may need help breathing. Too high levels of carbon dioxide mean respiratory failure. The patient will need *endotracheal intubation* (breathing tube placed *within* the trachea), and will need to be placed on a mechanical ventilator that will breathe for the patient and maintain normal oxygen and carbon dioxide levels (Figure 11-11).

LEARNING OBJECTIVE 11.4 Describe the pathopharmacology of the lower airway.

KEY TERMS

Acute respiratory distress syndrome (ARDS) Sudden life-threatening lung failure that develops within 24–48 hours of a major illness or injury.

Anthracosis Lung disease as result of inhaling anthracite (hard coal) dust.

Anti-fungal Agents used to treat fungal infections.

Asbestosis Lung disease as a result of the asbestos particles.

Asthma Respiratory condition where the airways go into bronchospasm and narrow due to some stimulus; patient experiences dyspnea and wheezing.

Atelectasis Lung collapse.

Black lung General term for the inhalation of all the different types of coal dust.

Bronchiectasis Area of irreversible, abnormal, and irregular enlargement of the inner diameter of an airway, usually caused by repeated infections.

Bronchogenic carcinoma Cancerous tumor, originating in an airway.

Chronic bronchitis Progressive and non reversible obstructive respiratory disease characterized by swollen airways, bronchospasm, and excessive mucus production that affects the flow of air in and out of the lungs.

Chronic Obstructive Pulmonary Disease (COPD) Category of non reversible obstructive lung disease with distinct diseases, chronic bronchitis, and emphysema, that can occur singularly or in combination.

Cystic fibrosis Is an inherited disease causing exocrine glands to malfunction; as a result, the airways produce a thick mucus that is hard to eliminate, thus, leading to repeated lung infections or pneumonias.

Dry powder inhaler (DPI) Portable inhalation device that delivers aerosolized powdered medication to the airway. Since the patient must generate high inspiratory flows for the delivery, this is only used prophylactically with maintenance medications.

Emphysema Progressive and non reversible obstructive respiratory disease characterized by the destruction of alveolar walls and the surrounding capillaries, and affects the exchange of gas between the alveoli and blood.

Hemoptysis Coughing up bloody sputum.

Influenza More commonly known as the flu; a highly contagious respiratory viral infection spread by coughing and secretions.

Lobectomy Surgical removal of a lobe of the lung.

Long-term control or maintenance agents Agents used in chronic respiratory disease to lessen or prevent exacerbations; not to be used in acute situations, examples include inhaled steroids, such as beclomethasone (Qvar) and budesonide (Pulmicort), and long term bronchodilators, such as Serevent.

Malignant Cancerous cell growth.

Metered Dose Inhaler (MDI) Pressurized inhalation device to deliver aerosolized medication to the airways.

Oxygen therapy Used in many of the diseases of the lower airway to provide adequate oxygen levels for gas exchange; therapy can include a nasal cannula or various types of oxygen masks.

Pneumoconiosis General term for *conditions* caused by the inhalation of inorganic dust particles that can produce toxic effects.

Pneumonectomy Surgical removal of entire lung.

Pneumonia Inflammation of both the airways and alveoli due to infection by bacteria, viruses, fungi, and even chemicals that create an inflammatory response.

PPD test Skin test to diagnose tuberculosis.

Pulmonary abscess General term for a collection of infectious material in encapsulated regions of the lungs.

Rescue or quick-relief inhaled bronchodilators Aerosolized medications used in acute bronchospasm, such as albuterol (Proventil, Ventolin), levalbuterol (Xopenex), and ipratropium bromide (Atrovent) to give relief of bronchospasm within minutes.

Silicosis Lung disease resulting from the inhalation of silicates, such as those found in sand, glass, ceramics, and rocks.

Small Volume Nebulizer (SVN) Special inhaled aerosol delivery device that is powered by compressed gas to deliver aerosolized medications to the airway over a several minute treatment.

Surfactant Fluid produced within lungs that helps hold the alveoli open between breaths.

Tissue infarction Tissue death due to lack of oxygen.

Tuberculosis (TB) Contagious bacterial infection that affects the lungs, but can also impair other organs and affect the bones; the causative agent is *mycobacterium tuberculosis*.

11-15 DISEASES OF THE LOWER AIRWAYS

We made a big point about the difference between ventilation and respiration. The diseases of the lower airways affect ventilation, while the diseases of the alveolar region of the lung mainly affect respiration or gas exchange. Of course if you can't ventilate properly, the gases will not reach the alveoli for exchange. Obstructive diseases narrow the airways and make it difficult to breathe. They include asthma and chronic obstructive pulmonary disease (COPD). You will note that the main pharmacologic treatment will be bronchodilators to relax and open the airways, corticosteroids to reduce inflamed airways, oxygen therapy, if the episode is severe enough, and, on rare occasions, mucolytics if the secretions are very thick and unable to be cleared with coughing.

11-16 ASTHMA

Asthma is a condition where the airways go into bronchospasm due to some stimulus. Since the airways narrow, it becomes harder to breathe, and the patient experiences dyspnea and wheezing. See Figure 11-12.

Treatment for this condition often involves the inhalation of a *bronchodilating* medication directly into the airways to cause bronchial relaxation. In other words, you give this inhaled medication in order to open the airways to make it easier to breathe. The medication is delivered via a fine mist or *aerosol* and can be created by portable devices such as a **metered dose inhaler (MDI)** or a **dry powder inhaler (DPI)**. In the hospital, or for more serious cases, a longer treatment may be delivered using a **small volume nebulizer (SVN)**. These special delivery devices were all discussed/demonstrated in Module 4: Routes of Administration.

Asthma bronchodilators can be broken down into **rescue or quick-relief inhaled bronchodilators**, such as albuterol (Proventil, Ventolin), levalbuterol

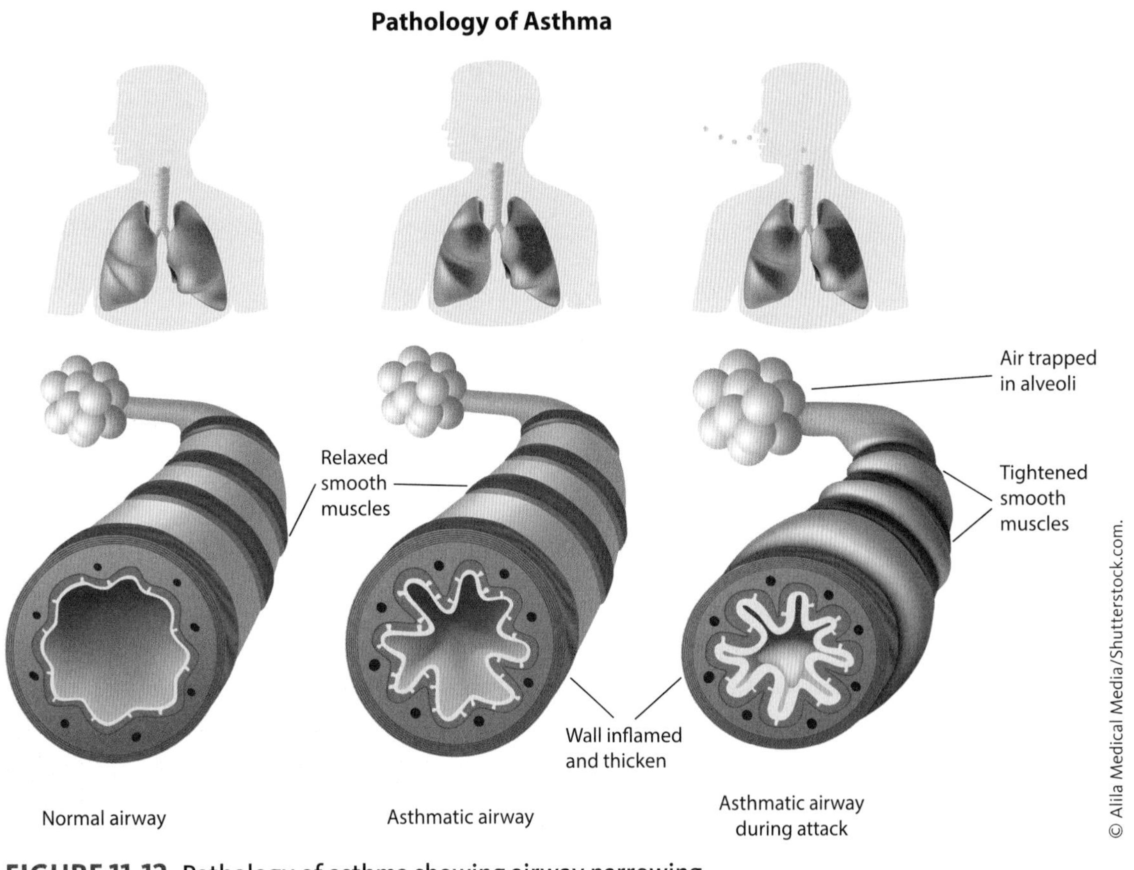

FIGURE 11-12 Pathology of asthma showing airway narrowing.

(Xopenex), and ipratropium bromide (Atrovent). These work in acute asthmatic attacks to, normally, give relief of bronchospasm within minutes.

There are several **long-term control or maintenance agents**. These consist of inhaled steroids, such as beclomethasone (Qvar) and budesonide (Pulmicort). In addition, a long-term bronchodilator, such as Serevent, can be mixed with a steroid fluticasone to make the combination maintenance drug, Advair, which is used to lessen or prevent attacks.

Other categories of drugs, such as leukotriene inhibitors (Singulair and Accolate) and antihistamines (Allegra), can be used prophylactically to block the chemical (leukotriene and histamine) that can lead to an asthma attack. Another maintenance drug stabilizes the membrane of the mast cells that, when ruptured, leads to an asthma attack by spilling its irritating chemicals. These drugs are aptly called mast cell stabilizers; Cromolyn Sodium is an example. To effectively build up in the system, Cromolyn should be inhaled two weeks before the exposure to the allergen, such as the ragweed pollen release, in order to be effective.

Important clinical note: None of the maintenance or long-term medications should be used during an acute attack—only quick acting rescue inhaler medications.

Asthma is a reversible disease and requires proper monitoring and treatment plans for a good prognosis. Asthma can become very serious and may require hospitalization, and the use of **oxygen therapy**. Oxygen therapy is needed in severe episodes as the increased work of breathing consumes much of the needed oxygen, and replacement is vital. Indeed, many of the diseases of the lower airway may require oxygen therapy, since effective gas exchange is impaired. Oxygen therapy can include a nasal cannula or various types of oxygen masks.

11-17 CHRONIC OBSTRUCTIVE PULMONARY DISEASE

Chronic obstructive pulmonary disease (COPD) is actually a combination of two distinct diseases: **chronic bronchitis** and **emphysema**. Chronic bronchitis is characterized by swollen airways, bronchospasm, and excessive mucus production that affect the flow of air in and out of the lungs. Emphysema is characterized by the destruction of alveolar walls and the surrounding capillaries, and affects the exchange of gas between the alveoli and blood. These diseases are contrasted in Figure 11-13. Since getting air out of the lungs is very difficult for these patients, it is called an obstructive disease. While asthma is also an obstructive disease, it is reversible and, therefore, not considered COPD, which is progressive and non reversible. Patients with COPD can have either chronic bronchitis or emphysema, but often the two will co-exist with one form being dominant.

Chronic bronchitis is a long-term inflammation of the airways, leading to increased cough and mucus production. This chronic inflammation of the airways can lead to **bronchiectasis**, an area of irreversible, abnormal, and irregular enlargement of the inner diameter of an airway. Bronchiectasis is usually caused by repeated infections. This condition creates large amounts of foul smelling thick sputum, which often results in the coughing up of a bloody sputum called

Chronic Obstructive Pulmonary Disease (COPD)

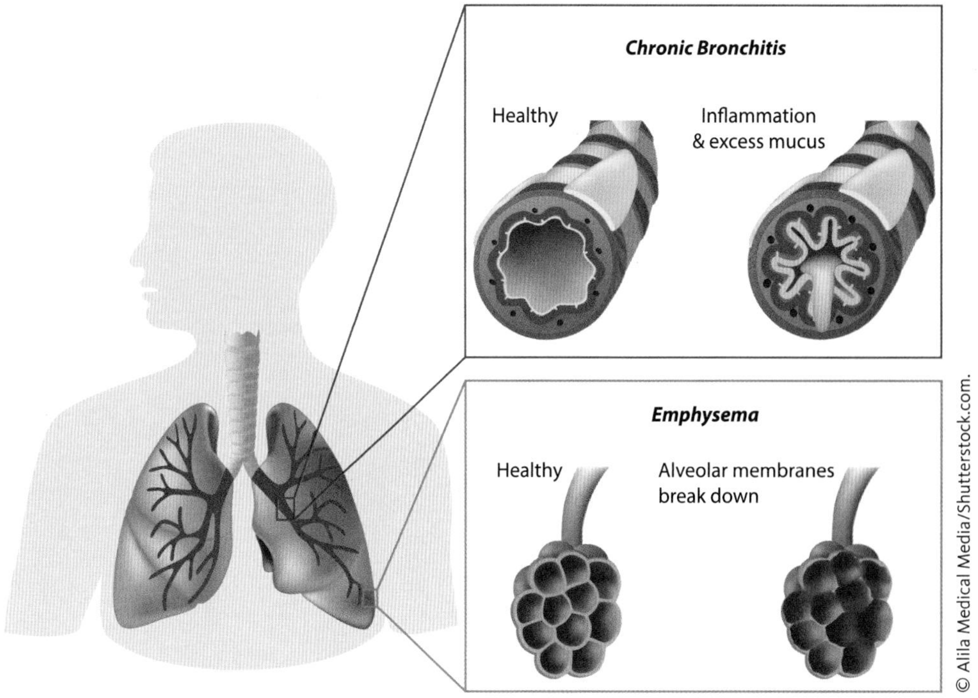

Chronic Bronchitis

Healthy

Inflammation & excess mucus

Emphysema

Healthy

Alveolar membranes break down

FIGURE 11-13 Contrasting the two COPD diseases: chronic bronchitis and empysema.

hemoptysis. Symptoms of chronic bronchitis include wheezing, rhonchi, cough, mucus production, and cyanosis if severe. Treatment includes bronchodilators to ease breathing, and mucolytics to break up thick secretions if the patient has an ineffective cough. Oxygen may be needed.

Emphysema destroys the alveolar walls and therefore affects gas exchange. Symptoms include severe dyspnea, weight loss due to the increased energy used to breathe, and often low oxygen in the blood (hypoxemia) due to poor gas exchange. Treatment includes oxygen therapy and bronchodilators to ease breathing and increase gas exchange.

A very sobering fact is that most COPD cases are caused by smoking and, are, therefore, preventable. While we will soon summarize the pharmacologic treatment for COPD, keep in mind that the best treatment for COPD is smoking prevention and, indeed, many other respiratory diseases. This module will end with smoking cessation therapy, and the very effective pharmacologic aides that help smokers quit. While smoking does cause most of the incidences of COPD, certain individuals are genetically predisposed to emphysema due to the lack of an enzyme called alpha-1 antitrypsin. For these individuals alpha-1 anti-trypsin replacement therapy is used.

11-18 PATHOPHARMACOLOGY OF DISEASES OF THE LOWER AIRWAY

Review Table 11-3 to contrast asthma and COPD diseases of the airways.

Table 11-3 Diseases of the airways

DISEASE	ETIOLOGY	MAJOR SIGNS/ SYMPTOMS	DIAGNOSTIC TESTS	TREATMENT
Asthma—bronchoconstriction due to allergen or inhaled irritant that is reversible	Many allergen triggers such as food, exercise, cold air, and smoking.	Dyspnea, wheezing, and productive cough	Patient history and pulmonary function testing	For acute attack: inhaled rescue bronchodilators, albuterol (Proventil), levalbuterol (Xopenex), ipratropium bromide (Atrovent), and oxygen if needed; For long-term control maintenance bronchodilators, salmeterol (Serevent), or tiotropium (Spiriva); inhaled steroids (QVAR, Pulmicort, or Flovent); antiasthmatic agents, such as mast cell çmembrane stabilizers, (Cromolyn Sodium), and leukotriene inhibitors (Singulair and Accolate)
COPD				
Chronic Bronchitis—chronic inflammation of the airways leading to increased mucus production, which is clinically diagnosed by a daily productive cough for three consecutive months for two consecutive years	Cigarette smoking and long-term exposure to air pollutants	Dyspnea, wheezing and rhonchi, and productive cough	Patient history and pulmonary function testing	Rescue inhaled bronchodilators, such as Ventolin, Xopenex, and Atrovent; Long-acting bronchodilators (Spiriva), and oxygen therapy; Steroids are not used early in the disease as this is not an allergic inflammation, however, they are used in the end stage of the disease after repeated flare ups have caused chronic inflammation
Emphysema—destruction of the alveolar walls leading to impaired gas exchange	Cigarette smoking and long-term exposure to air pollutants; some individuals have genetic form of alpha-1 antrypsin deficiency	Dyspnea, tachypnea, weight loss, and hypoxemia	Patient history and pulmonary function testing	Rescue inhaled bronchodilators such as Ventolin and Atrovent; Long-acting bronchodilators (Spiriva), and oxygen therapy; Alpha-1 antitrypsin therapy if this was the etiology (Prolastin, Aralast)

11-19 DISEASES OF THE LUNG

Now, we address diseases that can affect the entire lung, especially the areas of gas exchange. These include various types of pneumonias, lung cancer, lung collapse or **atelectasis**, situations and diseases that lead to pulmonary edema, pulmonary tuberculosis, and cystic fibrosis.

11-19a Pneumonia

Pneumonia is an inflammation of both the airways and alveoli due to infection. The infection can be caused by bacteria, viruses, fungi, and even chemicals that create an inflammatory response. This disease can damage lung tissue and fill the alveoli with fluid, thus decreasing the lungs' ability to exchange gas with the blood system. Since a variety of bacteria can cause pneumonia, we need to find out which antibiotic will be most effective. This is accomplished by obtaining a sputum sample in order to perform a *culture and sensitivity test (sputum C&S test)*. This test grows (cultures) the bacteria found in the sputum to identify its type, and creates large enough numbers to test against a variety of antibiotic medications to see which are best for treatment. A chest X-ray can diagnosis and locate the area most affected. The X-ray in Figure 11-14 shows an infiltrate in the left lower lung. Remember this is on the right side of the X-ray you are viewing, because it is the patient's *left* as they are facing you.

Symptoms of pneumonia can include dyspnea, fever, weakness, productive cough, and hypoxemia. Treatment is antibiotics if bacterial, oxygen therapy if hypoxemia exists, and symptomatic treatment relief for fever, cough, and pain.

The names for the different pneumonias can get quite confusing. Here is a brief list:

- Aspiration pneumonitis—pneumonia as a result of a chemical, gastric contents, or foreign object entering the lung
- Health care associated pneumonia (HCAP)—pneumonia developed while in a health-care institution
- Ventilator associated pneumonia (VAP)—pneumonia developed while on a mechanical ventilator to assist breathing

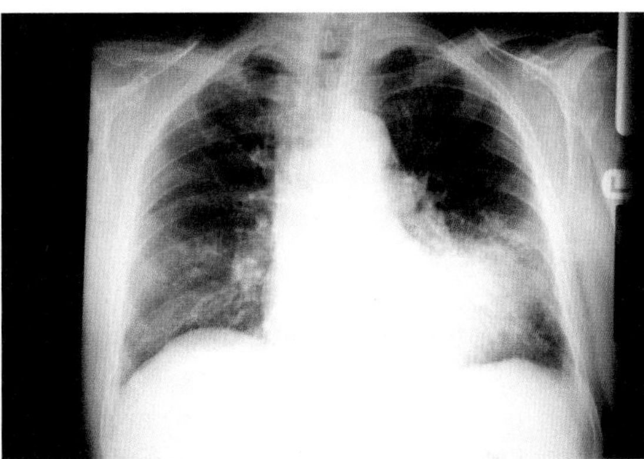

FIGURE 11-14 Chest X-ray of pneumonia of the left lower lobe.

- Community acquired pneumonia (CAP)—pneumonia developed outside of a health-care facility.
- Pneumococcal pneumonia—pneumonia caused by pneumococcal bacteria
- Lobar pneumonia—pneumonia confined to a lobe of the lung

Regardless of the name, the treatment remains in identifying the causative microorganism, and treating with antibiotics if bacterial. In addition, giving symptomatic relief and proper hydration is essential.

11-19b Cystic Fibrosis

Cystic fibrosis is an inherited disease, causing exocrine glands to malfunction. As a result, the airways produce a thick mucus that is hard to eliminate, thus leading to repeated lung infections or pneumonias, which is why it is mentioned here. Both systemic and inhaled antibiotics can be given to treat the lung infections. In addition, mucolytics can be given to break down the very thick mucus that is characteristic of this disease. Examples of mucolytics, which breakdown and dissolve thick mucus, are Pulmozyme and Mucomyst.

11-19c Fungal Lung Disease

Along with bacteria and viruses, inhaled fungi and fungal spores can cause lung disease. Histoplasmosis is a fungus from bird and bat droppings. Coccidioidomycosis, also known as dessert fever, occurs primarily in the Southwestern United States where it thrives in hot dry areas. Fungal lung disease is fairly uncommon but difficult to treat. Its symptoms are similar to pneumonia. However, since the etiology is non bacterial, the main treatment includes **anti-fungal agents**, rest, and symptomatic relief.

11-19d Atelectasis

Atelectasis is the collapse of alveoli, often a result of not taking deep enough breaths especially with fractured ribs, after abdominal or thoracic surgery, or when it hurts to take a deep breath. Deep breathing stimulates the alveoli to produce **surfactant**. Surfactant is a fluid that helps hold the alveoli open between breaths. If alveoli collapse it makes the exchange of gas much more difficult so there is a decrease in oxygen, and an increase in carbon dioxide in the blood. Diagnosis can be confirmed with a chest X-ray. Treatment is re-expanding the lung through deep breathing, patient ambulation, and treating pain so that they can take a deep breath. If untreated, atelectasis can lead to pneumonia.

11-19e Lung Cancer

When a **malignant**, or cancerous, tumor originates in an airway, it is called a **bronchogenic carcinoma**. There are two types of primary lung tumors. Small cell tumors (aka, oat cell) are less frequent but grow rapidly and have a poor prognosis. Chemotherapy and radiation treat small cell tumors.

Non-small cell tumors are often associated with smoking, and are treated by surgical removal. If large enough portions of the lung are affected, it may need to be surgically removed. This can include an entire lobe (**lobectomy**), or an entire lung (**pneumonectomy**).

Diagnosis of lung cancer is made by imaging and biopsy. Lung cancer is often asymptomatic until it has metastasized (spread). Related symptoms include cough, dyspnea, and hemoptysis. Figure 11-15 shows risk factors and symptoms of lung cancer.

11-19f Influenza

Influenza, or more commonly known as the flu, is a highly contagious respiratory viral infection spread by coughing and secretions. The flu has many strains and genetic variations; and this is why the flu vaccine, while very effective, might not cover a particular strain.

Flu is sometimes hard to differentiate from common cold symptoms, but a history that reveals sudden onset of body aches, fever, headache, and cough can confirm influenza. A rapid viral detection test can confirm definitely. Since this is viral in nature, symptomatic relief with analgesics and antipyretics, along with rest, is the main treatment. The main preventive treatment is vaccination. There are two FDA approved anti-viral medications oseltamivir (Tamiflu) and zanamivir (Relenza) that can be used for the treatment of influenza A and B

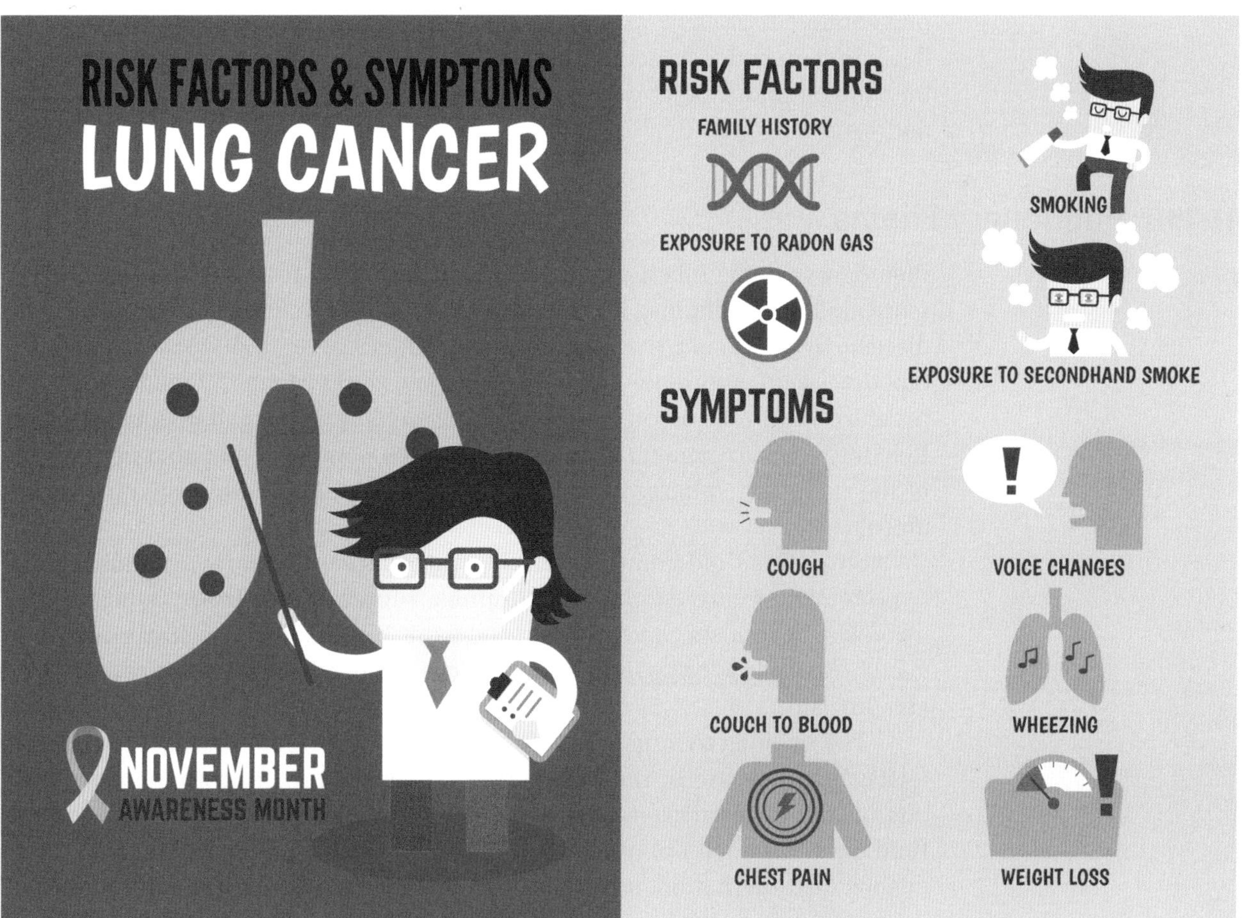

FIGURE 11-15 Lung cancer risk factors and symptoms.

viruses. These must be used within two days of symptoms to be effective. Antibiotics are only used if a secondary bacterial infection develops.

11-19g Pulmonary Abscess/Tuberculosis

Pulmonary abscess is a general term for collections of infectious material in encapsulated regions of the lungs. You can think of this as contained pockets of infection within the lung. This occurs in a number of diseases including pneumonia, lung cancer, and tuberculosis. **Tuberculosis (TB)** is a contagious bacterial infection that affects the lungs, but can also impair other organs and affect the bones. The causative agent is *mycobacterium tuberculosis*; and this microorganism has a tough outer covering that makes it difficult to kill and allows it to stay dormant for long periods of time.

The infection can be literally *walled off* by the immune system and rendered inactive for long periods of time before it reactivates. Secondary TB occurs when an individual is re-infected with mycobacterium tuberculosis, or the primary disease has been reactivated due to an immunodeficiency problem.

Symptoms include frequent coughing and hemoptysis, anorexia, and weight loss. Often times, dyspnea and night sweats accompany the active form of the disease. TB is diagnosed by skin testing (**PPD test**), chest X-ray, and sputum culture. Extensive long-term antibiotic treatment is required. Once exposed, preventative treatment with isoniazid for 6–12 months decreases the risk of it becoming an active infection. Active TB treatment takes 6–24 months of combination antibiotics that include isoniazid, rifampin, pyrazinamide, ethambutol, and streptomycin.

11-19h Pulmonary Edema

Pulmonary edema fills the alveolar region with fluid from the vascular system (surrounding capillaries), and has several etiologies that include cardiovascular disease, hypertension, pulmonary emboli (blockage or blood clot in pulmonary blood vessels), and renal failure. Notice that all these conditions increase the pressure within the blood vessels, and the small fragile capillaries can leak out fluid into the surrounding alveoli. Figure 11-16 is an X-ray of pulmonary edema of the right lung, where the white out represents fluid within the lung versus air (black).

Since this fluid greatly interferes with gas exchange, symptoms include hypoxemia, severe dyspnea, orthopnea, blood-tinged frothy sputum, and cyanosis. Diagnosis can be confirmed from a chest X-ray, and arterial blood gas showing low oxygen and high carbon dioxide levels due to impaired gas diffusion.

The obvious treatment is to try to reduce the blood pressure causing the leakage, and get rid of the excess fluid. Diuretics are given to increase urine output, and cardiac drugs are given to increase the efficiency of the heart so that fluid does not back up. In addition, morphine can be given because it causes venous dilation that opens up the vessels, thereby, reducing the pressure. The patient usually requires oxygen therapy, and might need mechanical ventilation to assist breathing.

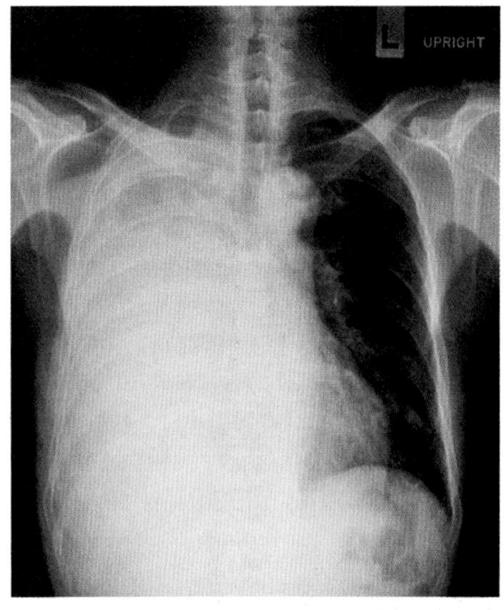

© Tewan Banditrukkanka/Shutterstock.com.

FIGURE 11-16 Pulmonary edema of the right lung.

11-19i Pulmonary Emboli

While pulmonary emboli (PE) are technically a cardiovascular complication, it severely affects the pulmonary system. A PE is a sudden blockage of an artery in the pulmonary system that disrupts the blood flow downstream of the blockage. Without blood flow, oxygen can't be delivered, and the tissue will die (**tissue infarction**). Symptoms vary due to the size, type, and location of the blockage, but can include dyspnea, cough, cyanosis, chest pain, and anxiety. Diagnosis can be confirmed by X-ray and lung scans. Treatment requires oxygen therapy, anticoagulants to prevent further clotting, and fibrinolytics or surgery to break-down, or remove, any existing clots. Anticoagulants and fibrinolytics are often confused. Anticoagulants, such as heparin and aspirin, thin the blood and help prevent blood clots from forming, but do nothing to an already existing clot. An existing clot needs to be surgically removed or dissolved by a fibrinolytic agent, such as streptokinase, that breaks down the fibrin of the clot.

11-19j Acute Respiratory Distress Syndrome

Acute respiratory distress syndrome (ARDS) is a sudden life-threatening lung failure that develops within 24–48 hours of a major illness or injury. This was previously called "shock lung," which is pretty descriptive of what happens. Conditions that can lead to shock lung are sepsis, severe chest trauma, near drowning, pulmonary emboli, aspiration pneumonia, major burns, and inhaling toxic fumes.

The symptoms include sudden dyspnea, severe hypoxemia, cyanosis, and pulmonary hypertension. Diagnosis is based on blood gases that show severe hypoxemia and respiratory acidosis (increase in carbon dioxide levels). The chest X-ray shows a bilateral white out condition.

In essence, the alveoli fill with fluid and causes severe pulmonary edema, requiring the patient to be placed on a mechanical ventilator. The underlying cause that led to the shocked lung must be treated along with maintaining adequate gas exchange until the lung recovers. This disease has a high mortality rate, between 30% and 50% and almost always requires the patient to be placed on a mechanical ventilator to assist breathing and oxygenation.

11-19k Pneumoconiosis

Pneumoconiosis is a general term for *conditions* caused by the inhalation of inorganic dust particles that can produce toxic effects. These are often occupational hazard diseases, such as coal miner's getting black lung. While **black lung** is a general term for the inhalation of all the different types of coal dust, **anthracosis** occurs as a result of inhaling anthracite (hard coal) dust. **Asbestosis** is a result of the inhalation of asbestos, and **silicosis** occurs from the inhalation of silicates, such as those found in sand, glass, ceramics, and rocks. These diseases cause progressive chronic inflammation and lung damage. They are treated as the symptoms arise and often require oxygen therapy in end stages, along with bronchodilators to assist with breathing.

11-20 PATHOPHARMACOLOGY OF THE LUNG

Review Table 11-4 for the pathopharmacology of lung conditions and disease.

Table 11-4 Conditions and diseases of the lung

DISEASE	ETIOLOGY	MAJOR SIGNS AND SYMPTOMS	DIAGNOSTIC TESTS	MAIN PHARMACOLOGIC TREATMENT
Pneumonia	Viral or bacterial; could also be from aspiration of gastric contents or other foreign bodies	Dyspnea, productive cough, fever, and weakness	Chest X-ray, blood work indicating infection, sputum culture to identify causative microorganism	Antibiotics if it is a confirmed bacterial pneumonia, symptomatic treatment for pain and fever, and rest and fluids
Influenza	Virus	Fever, cough, and body aches	History and physical exam	Symptomatic treatment of pain (analgesics) and fever (antipyretics), preventative vaccination, anti-viral medications oseltamivir (Tamiflu) and zanamivir (Relenza) used within 2 days of symptoms, and antibiotics are only used if a secondary bacterial infection develops

Table 11-4 Conditions and Diseases of the Lung—*continued*

DISEASE	ETIOLOGY	MAJOR SIGNS AND SYMPTOMS	DIAGNOSTIC TESTS	MAIN PHARMACOLOGIC TREATMENT
Cystic fibrosis	Hereditary disease transmitted from recessive gene	Excessive and thick mucus with repeated lung infections, and poor digestion	Genetic testing and chloride sweat test	Mucolytics, such as Pulmozyme and Mucomyst; inhaled and systemic antibiotics for bacterial infection; pancreatic enzyme supplements
Fungal lung disease	Inhalation of fungi or fungal spores	Dyspnea, productive cough, and hypoxemia	History and physical exam, sputum culture	Antifungal agents either IV (fluconazole) or inhaled (amphotericin B), and oxygen therapy if needed
Atelectasis	Collapse of portion of lung due to inadequate lung inflation because of pain, trauma, or surgery	Dyspnea, cyanosis, and hypoxemia	Chest X-ray and physical exam	Deep breathing and ambulation; and treat any complication that might arise, such as pneumonia; oxygen therapy if severe
Lung cancer	Cause not fully known but linked to smoking and inhalation of carcinogens	Coughing, hemoptysis, anorexia, and weight loss	Imaging and tissue biopsy	Chemotherapy and radiation to treat small-cell tumors; non-small cell tumors are treated by surgical removal
Tuberculosis (TB)	Mycobacterium tuberculosis	Coughing, hemoptysis, anorexia, and weight loss	Purified protein derivative skin testing (PPD test), chest X-ray, and sputum culture	Combination of antibiotics that include isoniazid, rifampin, pyrazinamide, ethambutol, and streptomycin
Pulmonary edema	Build-up of fluid in alveolar region due to a variety of causes, but mainly from pulmonary hypertension causing capillary leakage	Hypoxemia, severe dyspnea, orthopnea, blood tinged frothy sputum, and cyanosis	Chest X-ray and arterial blood gas showing hypoxemia and high carbon dioxide (respiratory acidosis) levels due to impaired gas diffusion	Diuretics, cardiotonic drugs are given to increase the efficiency of the heart, morphine for venous dilation to reduce vessel pressure, oxygen therapy and mechanical ventilation to assist breathing if needed

(continued)

Table 11-4 Conditions and Diseases of the Lung—*continued*

DISEASE	ETIOLOGY	MAJOR SIGNS AND SYMPTOMS	DIAGNOSTIC TESTS	MAIN PHARMACOLOGIC TREATMENT
Pulmonary emboli	Blockage of pulmonary blood flow going to the lung, usually by blood clot dislodged from the pelvic region or legs	Sudden dyspnea, cough, cyanosis, chest pain, and anxiety	X-ray and lung scans	Oxygen therapy, anticoagulants (heparin, aspirin) to prevent further clotting, and fibrinolytics (streptokinase) to dissolve existing clot, or surgery to remove any existing clots
Acute respiratory distress syndrome (ARDS)	Form of pulmonary edema with high mortality rate and stiff lungs due to many causes, such as sepsis, prolonged shock, and near drowning	Sudden dyspnea, severe hypoxemia, cyanosis, and pulmonary hypertension	Arterial blood gases that show severe hypoxemia and respiratory acidosis (increase in carbon dioxide levels); chest X-ray showing bilateral infiltrates	Mechanical ventilation, and aggressive supportive intensive therapy focused on treating the underlying cause of the ARDS
Pneumoconiosis	Prolong exposure to occupational particles, such as coal, asbestos, and silica	Dyspnea, chest pain, inability to take deep breaths due to fibrotic (stiff) lungs	Chest X-rays, PFTs showing a restrictive disease, and arterial blood gases showing hypoxemia	No cure and the major goal is to relieve symptoms with bronchodilators and oxygen therapy, and treat any complications, such as bacterial infections with antibiotics

LEARNING OBJECTIVE 11.5 Describe the physiology and pathopharmacology of the supporting structures of the lung.

KEY TERMS

Chest tube Tube inserted into the pleural space to remove the air and allow re-expansion of the lung.

Diaphragm Main breathing muscle.

Empyema Formation of pus in the pleural space, usually due to a bacterial infection.

Endotracheal intubation Inserting a tube *within* the trachea, often connected to a machine called a ventilator to help the patient breathe.

Hemothorax Collection of blood in the pleural space.

Phrenic nerve A nerve that innervates the diaphragm causing it to contract and flatten out creating more room in the thoracic space (chest cavity) and less pressure, allowing air to rush into the lungs for inspiration.

Pleural cavity Cavity where lungs are housed; contains a double layered serous membrane, which creates the visceral pleura, which surrounds each lung; and the parietal pleura, which covers the inner wall of the thoracic cage.

Pleural effusion Fluid entering the pleural space.

Pleural fluid Fluid within the pleural space needed to make the movement of the pleural layers friction free as you breathe in and out.

Pleuritis Also called *pleurisy*, is an inflammation of the pleura, which is characterized by a sharp pain when breathing.

Pneumothorax Condition that allows air into the pleural space and can collapse the lung or lungs.

Pyothorax Formation of pus in the pleural space, usually due to a bacterial infection.

Thoracentesis Procedure using a large needle and syringe to remove fluid from the pleural space.

11-21 NORMAL PHYSIOLOGY OF BREATHING

So, how do we get the lungs to fill themselves with air, and then empty for the next breath? This is done mainly by pressure changes initiated by the main breathing muscle called the **diaphragm**. When the diaphragm is stimulated by the **phrenic nerve**, the diaphragm contracts and flattens out creating more room in the thoracic space (chest cavity) and less pressure, allowing air to rush into the lungs. When the diaphragm relaxes, it goes back to its normal dome shape that takes up space in the thoracic space, thus pushing the air out of the lungs. Inhalation is an active process, and exhalation is a passive process.

Each lung is located in the **pleural cavity**. This cavity gets its name from the double layered serous membrane, which creates the visceral pleura, which surrounds each lung, and the parietal pleura, which covers the inner wall of the thoracic cage. There is a very small space between both of the pleura that contains **pleural fluid**, which is needed to make the movement of the pleural layers friction free as you breathe in and out. See Figures 11-17 and 11-18.

11-22 PATHOPHYSIOLOGY OF PLEURA CONDITIONS

So what could go wrong with the lung pleura? As stated before, the pleural space, which lies outside the lung, is normally very, very small and filled with a small amount of pleural fluid. In fact, it is called a "potential space" because normally the fluid lining leaves no space, and the parietal and visceral pleura glide friction free against each other as we breathe.

Trauma or disease can cause this space to be filled with extra fluids, such as blood or pus, and this can then compress against the lung, making it hard to breathe. Fluid entering this space is called a **pleural effusion**. **Empyema** is the formation of pus in the pleural space, usually due to a bacterial infection. This condition is also called **pyothorax**. Blood can also enter this space, and this condition would be called a **hemothorax** (Figure 11-19). Often these conditions can resolve on their own, but serious cases need you to "tap the chest" of the patient using a large needle and syringe to remove the fluid. This procedure is called a **thoracentesis**, and allows the lung to re-expand. Analgesics are

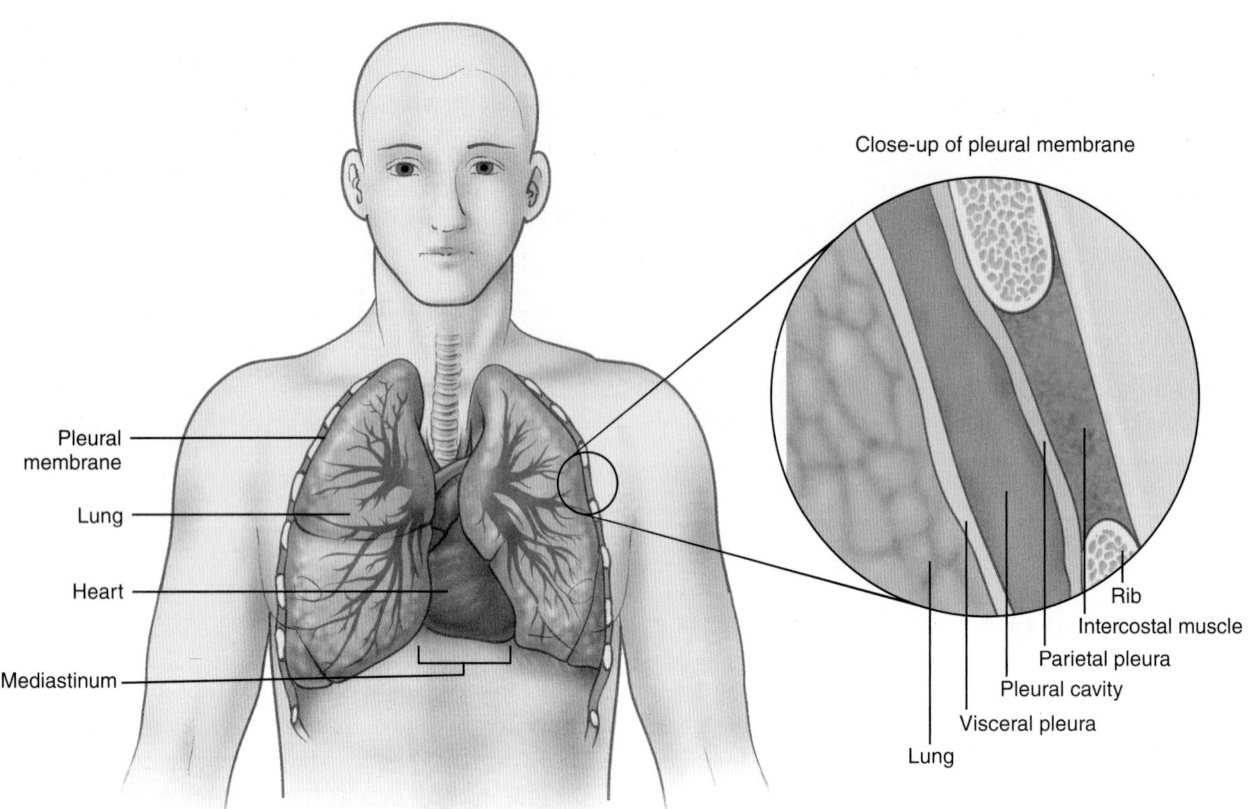

FIGURE 11-17 Each lung is located in the pleural cavity.

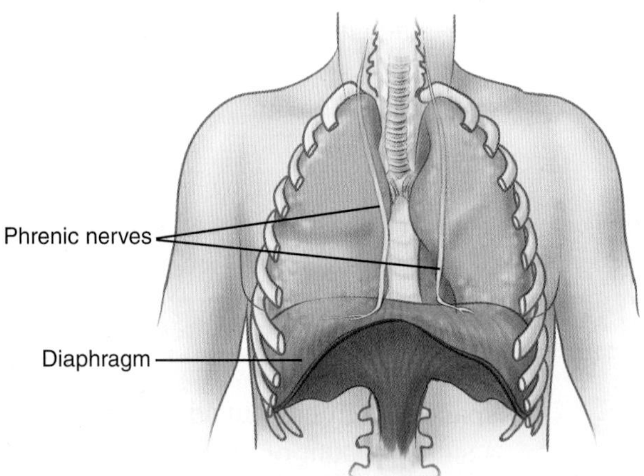

FIGURE 11-18 The phrenic nerve originates in the neck and passes down between the lung and heart to reach the diaphragm. It is important for breathing, as it passes motor information to the diaphragm and receives sensory information from it.

needed to treat pain, and numbing anesthetics are used at the puncture site. Antibiotics are indicated for bacterial infections, especially in empyema.

Not only can fluid fill this space, but extra air can also get in this region. You would think extra air in the lung space is good, but remember, this is

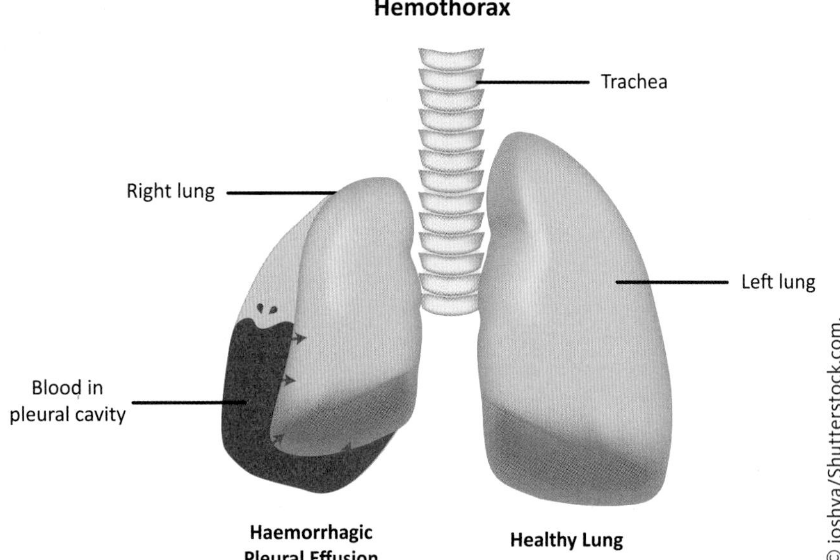

FIGURE 11-19 A hemothorax with blood in the pleural space compressing the right lung.

not within the lung but outside of the lung, thereby causing lung compression. A **pneumothorax** is a condition that allows air into the pleural space, which can collapse the lung or lungs. For example, a thoracic stab wound can allow outside air to enter this space. If severe enough, a **chest tube** must be inserted to remove the air and allow re-expansion of the lung. Analgesics are needed to treat pain and numbing anesthetics are used at the puncture site. Oxygen therapy is usually required. Often in severe trauma situations involving the chest, the patient will need help breathing. This is accomplished by inserting a tube within the trachea, which is termed **endotracheal intubation**. This tube is then attached to a machine called a ventilator to help the patient breathe.

Finally, this space can become infected or inflamed. **Pleuritis**, also called *pleurisy*, is an inflammation of the pleura, which is characterized by a sharp pain when breathing. This pain worsens with cough and can cause shallow breathing leading to atelectasis. Treatment includes pain medications and treating the underlying cause of the inflammation.

LEARNING OBJECTIVE 11.6 Compare the types of smoking cessation pharmacologic therapies.

11-23 SMOKING AND LUNG DISEASE

Smoking is the number one preventable cause for respiratory disease! COPD and lung cancer has very strong links to smoking, but so do many other diseases as well. Not only does smoking cause, or aggravate, many respiratory conditions, it also affects other systems, most notably the cardiovascular system. This is why smoking cessation therapy is critical. Just take a look at the following depiction in Figure 11-20, which shows the medical links to smoking.

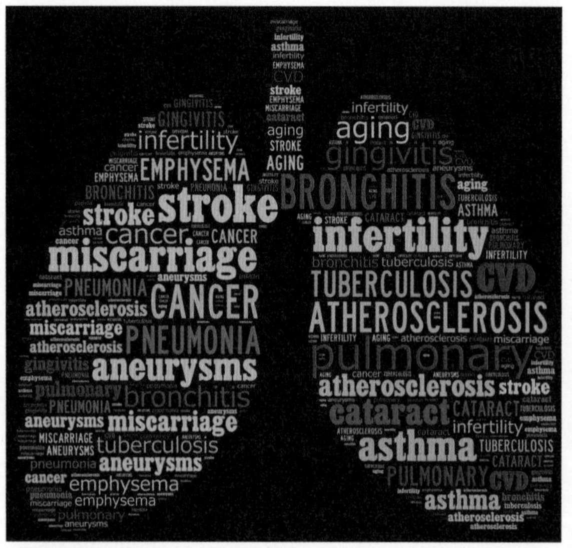

FIGURE 11-20 Various diseases and conditions that can be affected by smoking.

11-24 PHARMACOLOGY OF SMOKING CESSATION

Cigarette smoking is the leading cause of preventable death in the United States. Pharmacologic smoking cessation medication, when used in conjunction with behavior modification therapy and social support systems, can be quite effective for those who are motivated to quit.

Nicotine is a highly addictive substance. By using nicotine replacement therapy, the patient can still satisfy the nicotine craving without inhaling all the other carcinogens. In addition, using nicotine patches to satisfy their cravings will not allow other people in close proximity to inhale their damaging cigarette smoke (passive smoking). Nicotine replacement forms include Nicorette gum, Commit lozenges, Nicoderm CQ patch, Nicotrol inhaler, and nasal spray. These all can lessen the nicotine withdrawal symptoms, while the smoker focuses on behavioral modification to break the social habit of smoking. The levels of nicotine can be tapered down over time. Side effects are few but some cardiac irritability, and skin reaction with patches can occur. Overdose can be an issue, especially if a patient continues to smoke while using the nicotine replacement products.

Bupropion (Zyban) is an oral antidepressant medication used to reduce nicotine cravings. It can be used in conjunction with transdermal nicotine patches. Varenicline (Chantix) has been shown to not only reduce nicotine cravings, but to diminish the pleasurable effects associated with smoking. It does have some side effects that can include nausea, vomiting, sleep disturbances, and abnormal dreams. There have been reports of changes in behavior, agitation, depression, and suicidal ideation, so this medication should be monitored closely and any side effects should be immediately reported to the physician.

Module 12

Pathopharmacology of the Cardiovascular System

Module Introduction

As we begin our journey through the cardiovascular system, let's first take a look at the big picture. This system can be compared to a hot water heating system in a house. The furnace is the "heart" of the system and pumps the hot water throughout a series of pipes throughout the house to deliver heat. If the pump doesn't generate enough pressure, the heat will not get to all areas of the house. If the pipes are clogged with rust, the pressure will build up in the system, causing the furnace to work harder and eventually fail. You'll see how this analogy relates when we get to the pathology sections.

The heart is the body's pump, circulating blood throughout the body through a system of blood vessels (pipes). Instead of hot water being circulated, blood supplies heat, oxygen, and vital nutrients to all parts of our bodies. The blood that is circulated through our system is a form of connective tissue that is made up of many different types of cells and a fluid called plasma. The blood transports oxygen, carbon dioxide, nutrients, and waste products and also fights infection.

LEARNING OBJECTIVE 12.1 Describe the anatomy and physiology of the cardiovascular system.

KEY TERMS

Anastomoses New connections developed between vessels that serve as a backup or alternative pathways to allow blood flow if a blockage occurs.

Bundle of His Collection of cardiac muscle nerve fibers for electric conduction.

Capillaries Very tiny blood vessels that connect to form a network.

Cardiac cycle Series of heart movements that repeat for every heartbeat.

Cardiac output Amount of blood pumped by the heart in 1 minute.

Circulation Movement of blood throughout the body.

Diastole Part of the cardiac cycle in which the heart relaxes and fills with blood.

Endocardium The inner layer of the heart.

Epicardium The outer of three layers of the heart.

Inferior vena cava Large vein that brings deoxygenated blood to the heart from the lower body.

Interatrial septum Septum separating the right and left atria.

Interventricular septum Septum that separates the right and left ventricles.

Myocardium Heart muscle.

Parietal pericardium The outer layer of the pericardium.

Pericardial sac Double-walled sac that surrounds the great vessels and heart.

Peripheral resistance The resistance to blood flow from the arteries.

Pulmonary artery Artery that carries deoxygenated blood from the heart to the lungs.

Pulmonary circulation Part of the circulatory system that carries deoxygenated blood from the heart to the lungs.

Pulmonary valve Valve located between the right ventricle and pulmonary artery.

Pulmonary veins Veins that carry oxygenated blood from the lungs to the left atrium.

Purkinje fibers Collection of special fibers that send electrical impulses to the ventricles.

Rh factors Type of antigen found on the surface of red blood cells in some humans.

Sphygmomanometer Blood pressure cuff.

Stroke volume Amount of blood pumped from the left ventricle per heartbeat.

Superior vena cava Large vein that brings deoxygenated blood to the heart from the upper body.

Systemic circulatory system The part of the circulatory system that carries oxygenated blood from the heart to the tissues of the body and returns deoxygenated blood to the heart.

Systole The part of the heartbeat when contraction occurs.

Tricuspid valve Heart valve located between the right atrium and right ventricle.

Type A blood Blood that contains only A antigens on the red blood cell and B antibodies in the plasma.

Type AB blood Blood that contains both A and B antigens on the red blood cells and no antibodies for A or B in the plasma.

Type B blood Blood that contains only B antigens on the red blood cells and A antibodies in the plasma.

Type O blood Blood that does not have any A or B antigens on the red blood cells, but both A and B antibodies in the plasma.

Visceral pericardium The inner layer of the pericardium.

12-1 SYSTEMIC AND PULMONARY CIRCULATION

The technical term for the movement of blood through the body is **circulation**. The heart is actually two pumps: the right heart circulates blood to the lungs to get oxygenated, and the left heart circulates the now-oxygenated blood throughout the body. That means the body actually has two circulatory systems. **Pulmonary circulation** consists of the blood that goes from the right side of the heart to the lungs, while the **systemic circulatory system** consists of the blood flow from the heart that goes throughout your body and then back to the heart. See Figure 12-1.

12-2 STRUCTURES SURROUNDING THE HEART

The heart is between the left and right lungs and is enclosed in a protective **pericardial sac** (peri = around, cardial = heart). This sac is made up of a serous membrane that has two layers, the *fibrous pericardium* and *the serous pericardium*. The fibrous membrane is the tough outer layer that is fixed to surrounding structures for protection. Inside this covering is the serous pericardium, which has two layers, the **parietal pericardium** and **visceral pericardium**. The parietal pericardium is fixed onto the fibrous pericardium, while the visceral pericardium is fused to the surface of the heart, which is why it is also called the *epicardium* (epi = on, cardium = heart), the outer muscle of the heart.

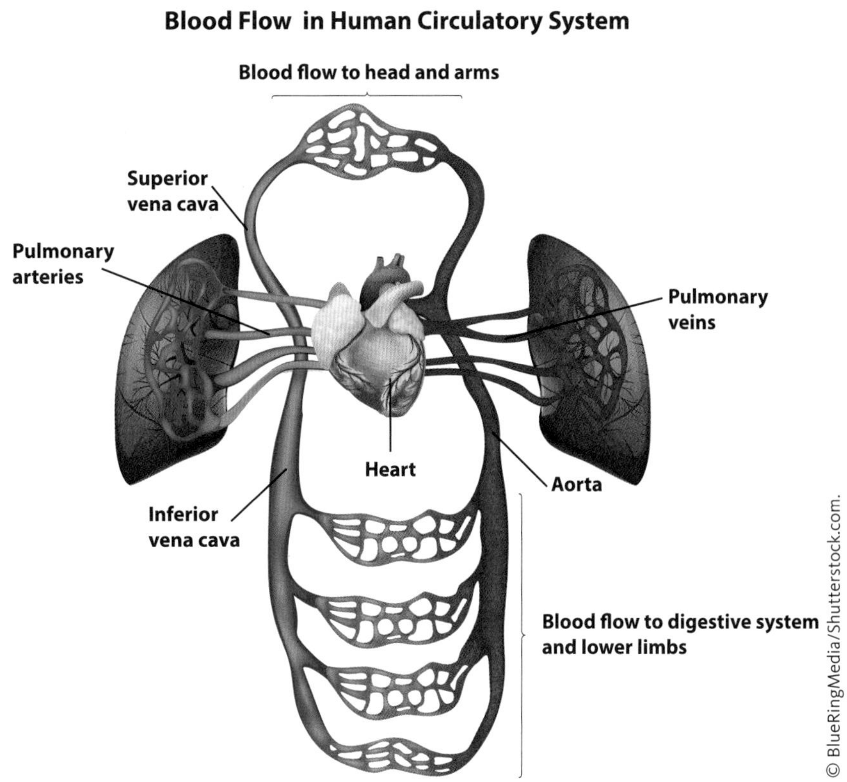

FIGURE 12-1 Pulmonary circulation: The right side of the heart pumps into the pulmonary arteries, sending the blood to the lungs to become oxygenated and returning via the pulmonary veins. System circulation: The left side of the heart pumps blood throughout the body via the aorta and returns blood to the right side of the heart via the superior and inferior vena cavae.

Between the visceral pericardium and fibrous pericardium is a space called the pericardial cavity. This cavity contains serous fluid, which is a watery substance that lubricates the layers, decreasing the surface tension or friction of the heart's movement as it pumps. An inflammation of this protective encasement is called pericarditis (Figure 12-2), which causes discomfort, chest pain, and even shortness of breath. With inflammation comes swelling, and the protective encasement puts pressure on the outside of the heart, making it more difficult for the heart to pump blood.

12-3 INTERNAL STRUCTURES OF THE HEART

The heart wall has three layers, the **epicardium** or outer layer; the **myocardium** or middle layer, consisting of actual cardiac muscle (myo); and the **endocardium** or inner layer of the heart (endo = inner), which lines the chambers of the heart and is connected to the valves.

Inside the heart are four chambers: two atrial (upper) and two ventricular (bottom). The atria are smaller and have less mass than the ventricles because they do not have to pump the blood very far, and they simply empty into their respective ventricles. So the right atrium pumps into the right ventricle, and the left atrium pumps into the left ventricle.

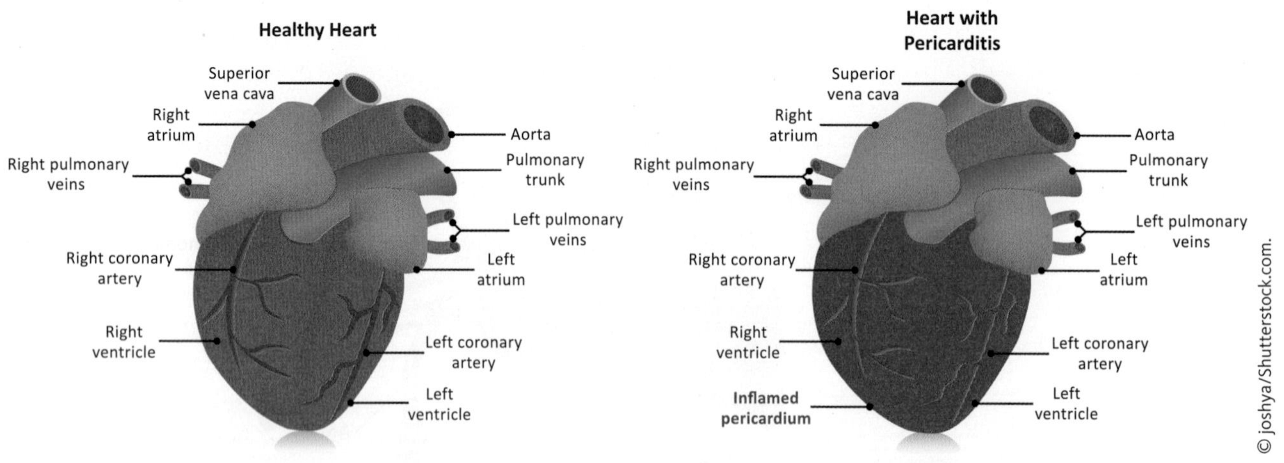

FIGURE 12-2 Inflammation of the sac enclosing the heart is called pericarditis, which is treated with NSAIDS and a drug called Colcrys (colchicines). Colcrys is used to treat gout, but it can also be used to decrease inflammation in other parts of the body and can be used for acute pericarditis or recurring episodes. However, if these drugs are not effective, corticosteroids such as prednisone might be given.

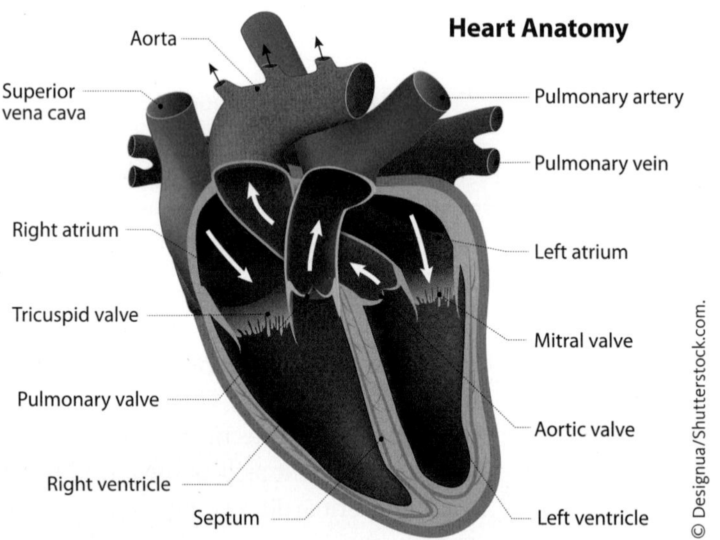

FIGURE 12-3 Shown in this cross section of the heart are the chambers of the heart and the location of the great vessels.

Just as a septum in the nose that separates the nostrils, these chambers are separated by a septum that helps prevent blood from mixing around the heart in an unorganized fashion. The two atria are separated by the **interatrial septum** (inter = between), and the two ventricles are separated by the **interventricular septum**. See Figure 12-3.

12-4 BLOOD FLOW THROUGH THE HEART

Understanding blood flow through the heart is critical in understanding the cardiac pathologies that disrupt this flow. Venous or deoxygenated blood that has fed the body's tissues with vital oxygen and nutrients returns to the right atrium via the **superior vena cava** (upper body) and **inferior vena cava** (lower body). From the right atrium, the blood passes through the **tricuspid valve**, which ensures blood is flowing in the right direction. The tricuspid valve consists of three folds known as cusps. When this valve opens, blood pours from the right atrium into the right ventricle, which pumps and opens the **pulmonary valve**, sending the blood to the lungs via the pulmonary arteries. The **pulmonary artery** splits in two, allowing blood to flow into both the right and left lung.

After blood is oxygenated by the lungs, it travels back to the heart via the **pulmonary veins**. It enters the left atrium, which contracts and pumps blood through the bicuspid or mitral valve into the left ventricle, the heart's largest muscular chamber. The left ventricle pumps the blood into the aorta and its branches, sending the oxygenated blood throughout the entire body. See Figure 12-4A, which traces these steps in order and illustrates the journey the blood takes throughout the system. Figure 12-4B shows the location of the various heart valves.

The Pathway of Blood Flow through the Heart

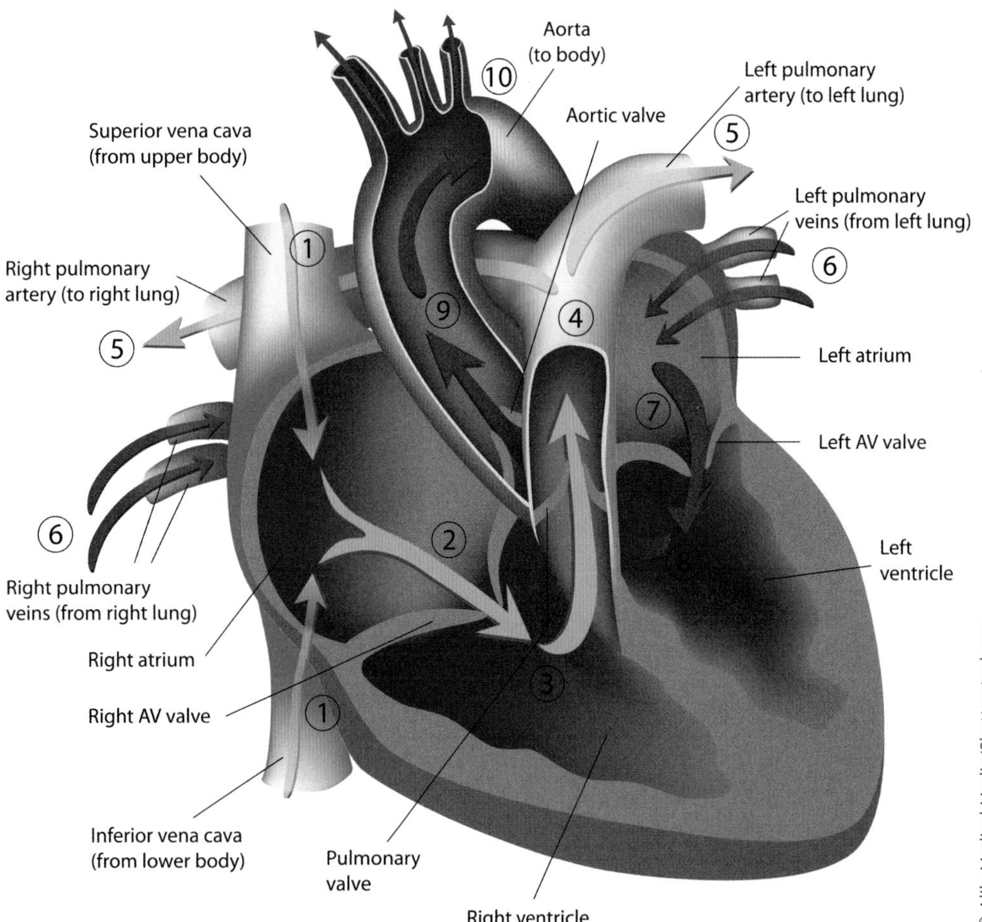

FIGURE 12-4A Blood flow through the heart. The blue areas are deoxygenated or venous blood, and the red represents oxygenated or arterial blood. The pulmonary artery is the only artery that carries deoxygenated blood; all other arteries carry oxygenated blood. It is called an artery, however, because the blood it carries is moving away from the heart. Conversely, the pulmonary vein is the only vein to carry oxygenated blood because it is returning blood back to the heart.

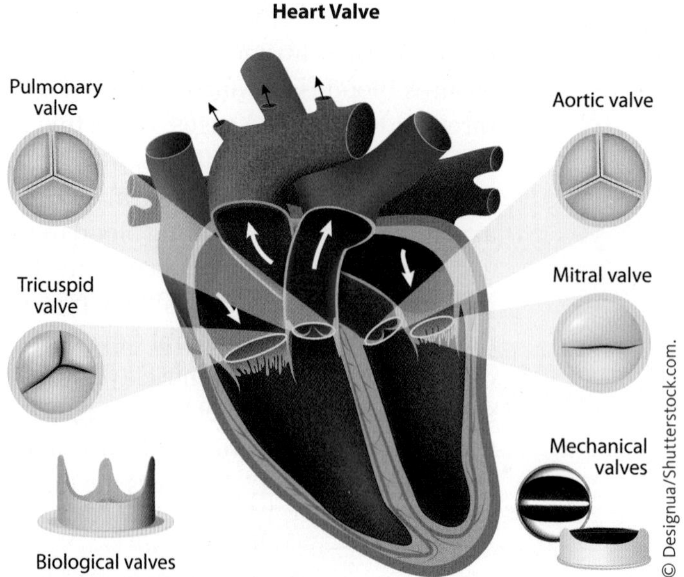

FIGURE 12-4B Location of heart valves.

12-5 CARDIAC CYCLE

The **cardiac cycle** refers to the two distinct phases of the heart: contraction and relaxation of the heart muscle. The contraction, called **systole**, is the phase that pumps or circulates the blood. **Diastole** is the relaxation phase, which allows the chambers to fill up with blood while awaiting the next contraction or systolic phase. As the chamber is filling with blood, the pressure inside that particular chamber increases, causing the closure of the one-way valves to prevent blood from backing up.

When discussing this cycle, we focus on ventricular activity. Ventricular systole is when the right and left ventricles simultaneously pump their blood to the lungs and body, respectively. During ventricular diastole, the ventricles fill with blood from the atria and await the next contraction. This must all work in synchrony, or circulatory problems would occur.

12-5a Cardiac Cycle and Blood Pressure

Blood pressure is measured by a blood pressure cuff or **sphygmomanometer**, Figure 12-5.

The cuff is placed around the upper arm just above the elbow and then inflated to stop the blood flow through the brachial artery. The pressure is then released slowly, until a squirting sound is heard through the stethoscope. That sound signals that the left ventricle pressure is now slightly higher than the cuff pressure and is forcing blood through the partially open brachial artery. This is known as the peak systolic pressure, or the maximum exertion of the left ventricle as it contracts.

As the cuff is further deflated, the throbbing pulse heard in the stethoscope decreases until it disappears because the pressure in the artery has become equal to the pressure in the blood pressure cuff. When that last sound is heard, it signals that the brachial artery is fully open. The pressure reading at that last sound is the diastolic pressure, when the heart is relaxing, or in diastole. Normal blood pressure is 120/80, which means a systolic pressure of 120 mmHg with a diastolic pressure of 80 mmHg.

Although healthy blood pressures can vary by age and gender, the ranges of the various stages of blood pressure are shown in Table 12-1.

12-5b Blood Pressure Regulation

Going back to our heating system analogy, what would happen to the pump pressure if the pipes become partially clogged with rust? The pump has to increase its pressure to push the same amount of fluid through narrower pipes. A similar situation occurs if our blood vessels become partially clogged with plaque from high cholesterol. The systolic pressure has to increase to push the blood through the now-restricted arteries. The systolic number gives an indication of how hard the heart is working and its potential for cardiovascular diseases. For example, the systolic value increases with the age of the patient from plaque build up and increased stiffness of the arteries.

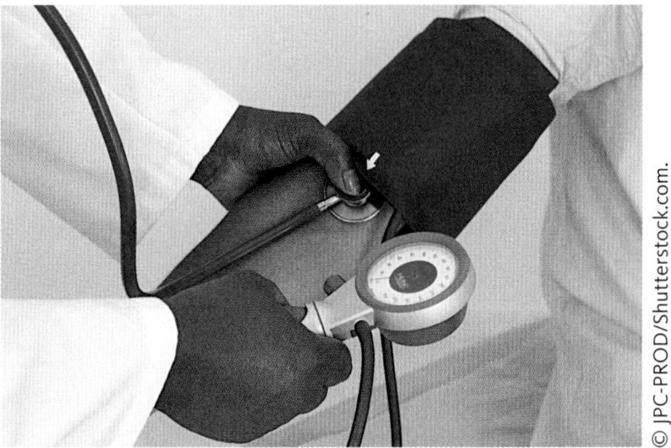

FIGURE 12-5 A sphygmomanometer (blood pressure cuff) is being used to measure a patient's blood pressure.

Table 12-1 Stages of blood pressure

BLOOD PRESSURE STAGE	SYSTOLIC (MMHG)		DIASTOLIC (MMHG)
Normal	80–120	And	60–80
Hypotension	Less than 80	Or	Less than 60
Prehypertension	120–139	Or	80–89
Stage 1 hypertension	140–154	Or	90–99
Stage 2 hypertension	160 or higher	Or	100 or higher
Hypertension crisis	Higher than 180	Or	Higher than 110

In this scenario, the diastolic pressure also would increase because it represents the resistance of the blood vessels. If the vessels are wide open, there is little resistance to flow and the pressure goes down, but with narrowing and stiffening, the resistance increases and the pressure goes up. How far open or closed the blood vessels are determines the **peripheral resistance**. The peripheral resistance is controlled by the sympathetic nervous system. If the blood pressure decreases too low, the sympathetic system will cause the blood vessels to constrict to increase your blood pressure. Patients with high blood pressure can be given medications to lower their peripheral vascular resistance by causing vasodilation or enlarging the diameter of the "pipes."

Cardiac output is the measure of the total amount of blood that circulates through the body in 1 minute. Normal cardiac output is 5–6 liters per minute, or about 5–6 quarts of blood is sent throughout the body in 1 minute. Cardiac output, therefore, is dependent upon how much the left ventricle pumps (**stroke volume**) and how many times (heart rate).

The standard normal heart rate for adults is 60–100 beats per minute. However, this value is being reconsidered and might trend lower. In addition, more importance is being placed on measuring the resting heart rate, which should be in the 50–80 beats per minute range. The stroke volume is the amount of blood pumped with each ventricular contraction. The normal range for an adult is 50–70 mL while at rest. Anything that decreases heart rate or stroke volume also decreases cardiac output and therefore the delivery of oxygen to tissues. It is also dangerous for cardiac output to be too high because it can cause too much pressure and rupture delicate blood vessels such as capillaries.

12-6 CORONARY BLOOD FLOW

We have discussed blood flow *through* the heart, but the heart muscle itself needs a blood supply in order to function properly. The blood that flows through the heart is not supplying the heart muscle with needed oxygen. So how does the heart muscle get oxygenated blood?

Oxygenated blood is redirected from the aorta via the left and right coronary arteries to supply the actual heart muscle. These arteries split up into even smaller vessels to supply blood evenly throughout the heart via a network of vessels called **anastomoses**. When coronary blood flow becomes blocked, it can result in myocardial infarction (MI) or heart attack, causing possible cardiac tissue death.

If a blockage is caught in time, the patient might undergo a heart catheterization, in which a wire mesh stent is placed at the site of the clog, as shown in Figure 12-6. This procedure is risky and is performed only if the benefits outweigh the risks. The stent forces open the once-blocked vessel, allowing blood to flow.

12-7 CORONARY CONDUCTION SYSTEM

The heart beats without our conscious effort, and therefore is connected to the autonomic nervous system. This electrical conduction must be done in a highly coordinated fashion. The heart has specialized cells that can self-excite and create and send electrical signals throughout the heart in an organized manner. Without this, the heart would contract and relax in an unsynchronized way and affect cardiac output.

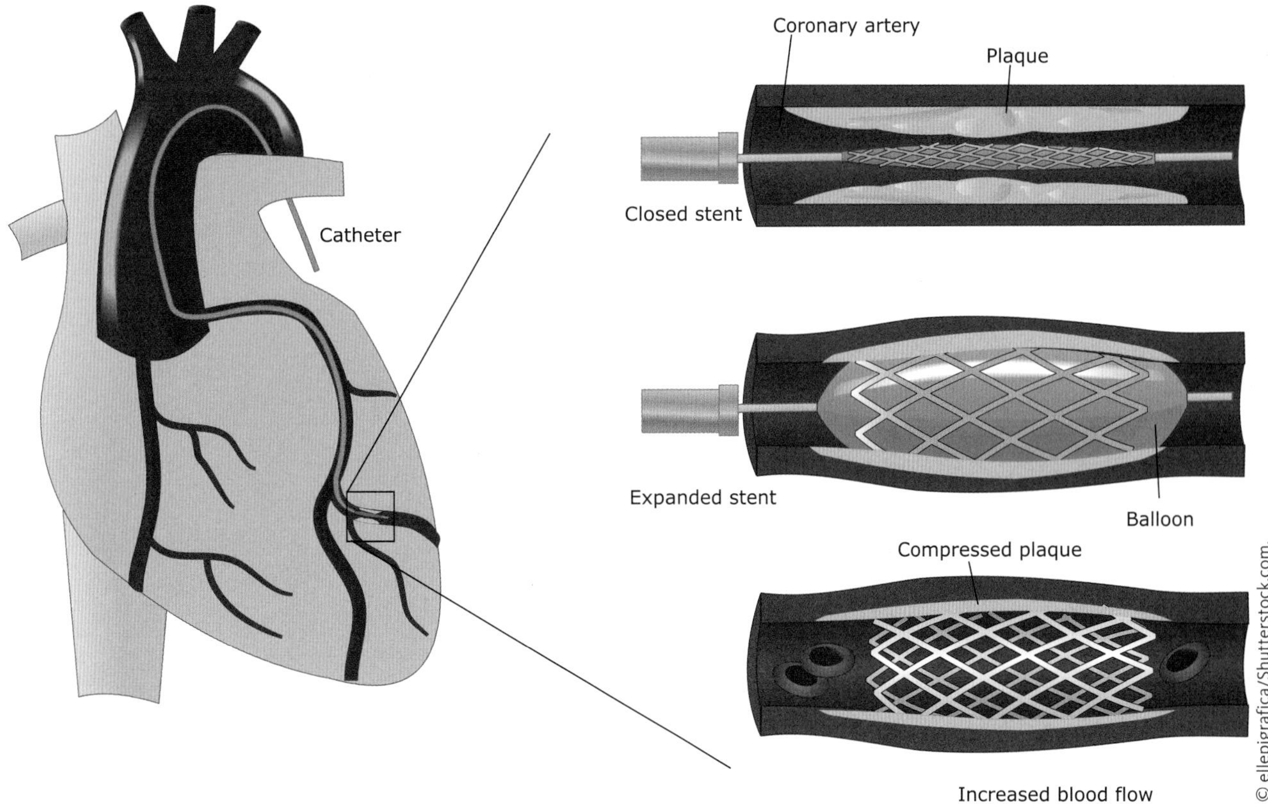

FIGURE 12-6 This illustration shows a balloon angioplasty, which is done to expand a stent where the coronary blockage occurs and allows blood to circulate to the heart muscle.

The self-generating cells that create the organized electrical impulses are known as nodal cells or pacemaker cells. There are two different groups of nodal cells; the sinoatrial node (SA node) and atrioventricular node (AV node). The SA node is the main type of pacemaker cells, creating about 70–80 electrical impulses per minute, and setting our heart rate. The node is located near the superior vena cava in the wall of the right atrium and starts the whole process of a heartbeat.

The AV node is found where the atrium and ventricle connect and produces a beat of 40–60 per minute. The AV node is also called the gatekeeper because it allows only certain electrical impulses through to the ventricle.

So how is this all coordinated? The sinoatrial node stimulates an electrical impulse causing the atriums to contract. This signal then travels to the AV node via intermodal pathways and is actually delayed slightly, so the ventricles have time to fill. From the AV node, the impulse travels down the **bundle of His**, which divides into the left and right bundle branches, which then travels out into the ventricles. The impulse then moves to the **Purkinje fibers**, sending the impulse to the contractile cells in the ventricles. Therefore, the heart's contractions start at the apex and work their way upward to the ventricles. See Figure 12-7.

12-8 BLOOD VESSELS

Your heart pumps blood throughout your body, and this distribution is made possible by many blood vessels: arteries, arterioles, capillaries, veins, and venules. Most of our vessels are made of three layers called tunics or coats, shown in Figure 12-8.

SA node
RA
LA
AV node
LV
RV
His bundle
© Blamb/Shutterstock.com.

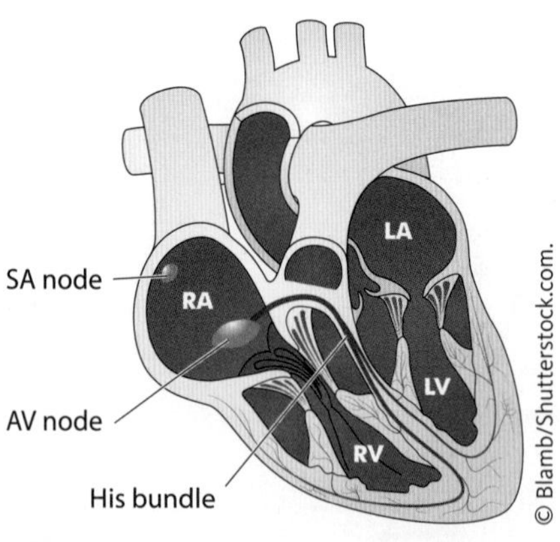

FIGURE 12-7 Location of coronary conduction.

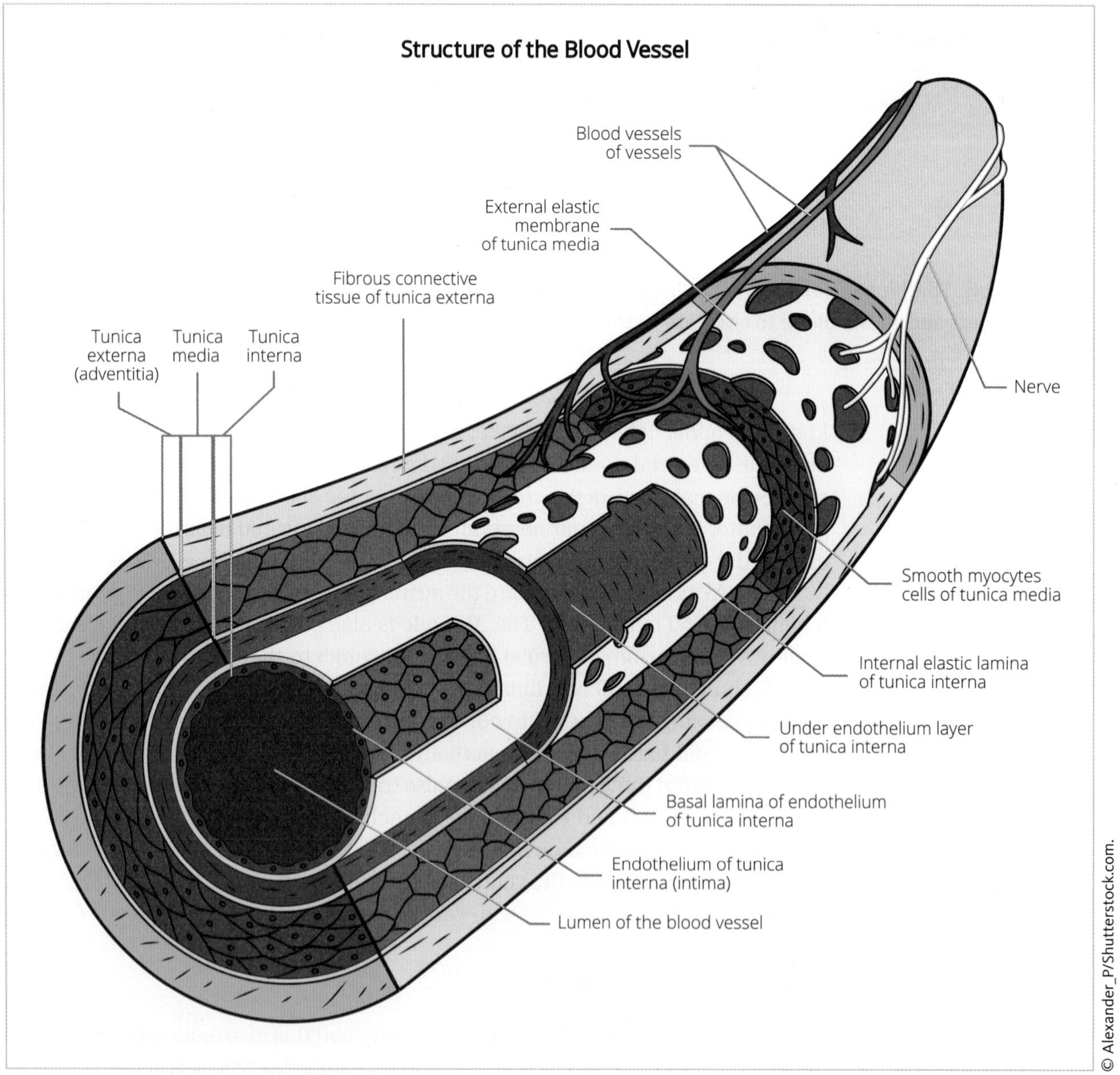

Structure of the Blood Vessel
Blood vessels of vessels
External elastic membrane of tunica media
Fibrous connective tissue of tunica externa
Tunica externa (adventitia)
Tunica media
Tunica interna
Nerve
Smooth myocytes cells of tunica media
Internal elastic lamina of tunica interna
Under endothelium layer of tunica interna
Basal lamina of endothelium of tunica interna
Endothelium of tunica interna (intima)
Lumen of the blood vessel
© Alexander_P/Shutterstock.com.

FIGURE 12-8 Anatomy of a blood vessel.

12-9 ANATOMY OF BLOOD VESSELS

The outer layer of blood vessels is called the *tunica externa*, which is constructed out of fibrous tissue that provides support and protection. The middle layer is the *tunica media*, which is made up of smooth muscle and elastic tissue giving the vessel the ability to constrict and dilate. This ability controls the size of the opening and thus the resistance within the vessel. The innermost thin layer is called the *tunica interna*, a smooth surface allowing for easy flow of blood because of its composition of squamous epithelial cells. This is the layer that can become clogged or blocked, increasing pressure and/or disrupting the flow. See Table 12-2 for a list of differences in arteries and veins.

Table 12-2 Differences in arteries and veins

Arteries	• Contain thicker walls than veins. • Deal with the high-pressure system (blood flow from the heart). • Smaller lumen than veins. • Large arteries have elastic laminae in the middle to give them added durability.
Arterioles	• Small arteries.
Veins	• Thinner vessel walls than arteries. • Larger lumen than arteries. • Large veins contain one-way valves to keep blood flowing in the appropriate direction. See Figure 12-9.
Venules	• Small veins.

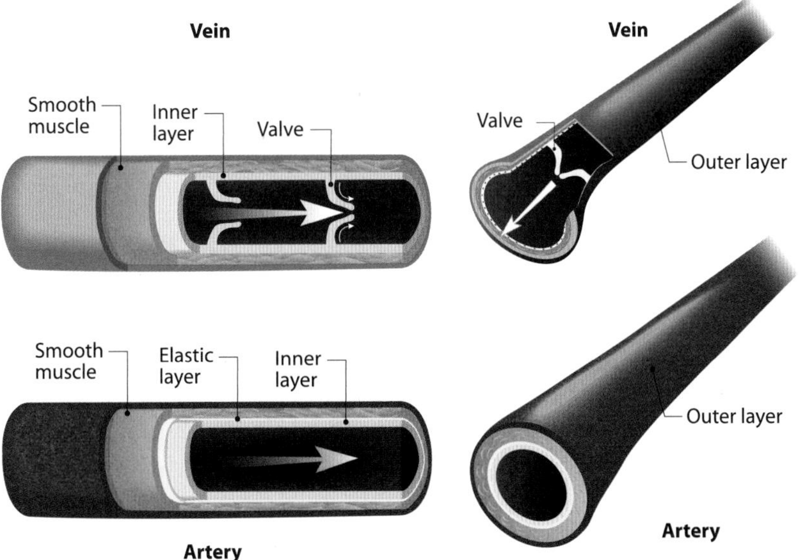

FIGURE 12-9 This image contrasts the differences between arteries and veins.

12-10 CAPILLARIES

The body also has **capillaries**, which are primarily where gas exchange takes place. These very tiny tubes have a diameter that is just larger than a red blood cell. Capillaries also have only one layer to allow for oxygen and carbon dioxide to pass through the walls easily.

The lungs have capillary networks surrounding the alveoli so oxygen can travel from the alveoli into the blood via the capillary. Carbon dioxide moves out of capillaries and into the lungs to be exhaled.

Systemic capillaries throughout the body supply the various tissues with oxygen. Here, oxygen moves into the tissue, and carbon dioxide enters the blood to eventually be sent back to the lungs.

These tiny vessels make a network of vessels referred to as a capillary bed, Figure 12-10.

12-11 BLOOD

Blood is made up of connective tissue that is composed of plasma (liquid portion) and solid elements (blood cells).

The solid or formed components of the blood are mainly the different types of cells, including red blood cells and white blood cells. Platelets or thrombocytes are the smallest of the solid blood components and are essential in the clotting process.

Plasma is mainly made up of different salts and nutrients, as well as water, oxygen, and carbon dioxide molecules. In the endocrine module, we learned about the different hormones and how they travel throughout the body in the blood. Well, those hormones are found in the plasma. Also located within the plasma are the following proteins:

- Fibrinogen and prothrombin used for clotting
- Globulin used to create antibodies to prevent infection
- Albumin plays an important role in fluid regulation. Think of it as a sponge that will not allow fluid to leak from the blood vessels and into the surrounding tissues

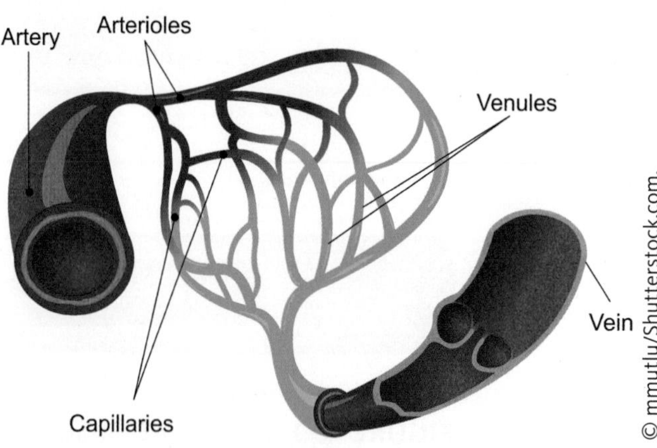

FIGURE 12-10 Capillary bed.

Blood also has the important role of keeping the body in a homeostatic state by:

- Maintaining a certain pH, acidity or alkalinity
- Regulating body temperature
- Maintaining sufficient electrolyte levels for cellular function
- Preventing and fighting infection

12-11a Red Blood Cells

Red blood cells, or erythrocytes, are made in the bone marrow and have many responsibilities, such as transporting oxygen and carbon dioxide throughout the body. They also transport nutrients, ions, and water from the digestive tract. Blood is filtered by the kidneys, and the wastes are removed by excretion. Every red blood cell contains upward of 300 million molecules of hemoglobin, which is the substance that actually binds to O_2 and CO_2 molecules. See Figure 12-11 for an illustration of the different types of blood cells.

12-11b White Blood Cells

White blood cells, or leukocytes, are also made in bone marrow. Their primary role is to prevent and fight infection. Leukocytes can be divided into two different groups.

Polymorphonuclear granulocytes consist of *basophils*, *eosinophils*, and *neutrophils*. Basophils increase the body's response to allergens, but they also prevent the blood from clotting by secreting what is known as heparin. Eosinophils fight various foreign irritants that eventually cause allergies. Neutrophils are highly aggressive white blood cells that kill foreign invaders. These cells destroy bacteria by surrounding them with special enzymes they release called lysosomes; this process is known as phagocytosis.

Mononuclear cells consist of *monocytes* and *lymphocytes* produced in the lymphatic system. Monocytes are found in higher than normal numbers when a chronic infection is present. Like neutrophils, they destroy foreign invaders with phagocytosis. Although monocytes take longer to get to the site of infection, they arrive in greater numbers than neutrophils. Lymphocytes fight infection by creating antibodies instead of by phagocytosis.

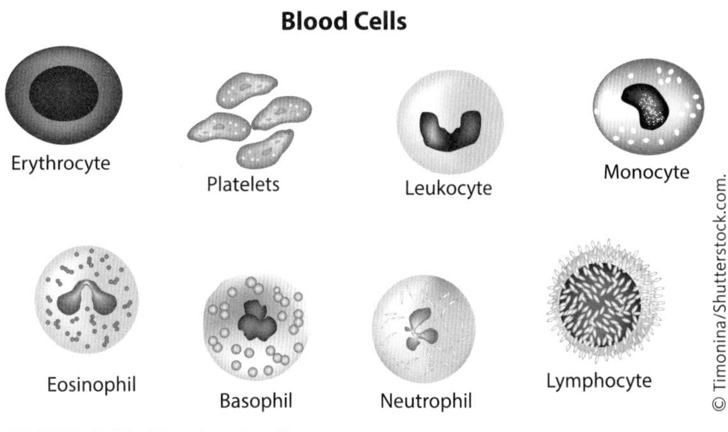

FIGURE 12-11 Blood cells.

CLINICAL CONNECTION 12.1

How do your blood and blood vessels control body temperature? When you are cold, your blood absorbs heat from your skeletal muscles and then disperses it to the rest of your body. Your blood vessels help by vasoconstricting in the peripheral regions (arms and legs) to keep warmer blood in the central region of the body around vital organs. On the flipside, if the body is too hot, the vessels in your periphery dilate to allow heat to radiate from the blood and through the skin.

12-12 CLOTTING MECHANISM

When a blood vessel is injured, it begins to bleed. What causes it to stop and heal? First, platelets on the scene stick to the damaged area. Those platelets release chemicals that attract other platelets to the site, forming a platelet plug, which prevents blood from flowing out of the injured vessel. Platelets also release a chemical called serotonin, which constricts the vessel and decreases blood flow.

Under normal circumstances, coagulation happens within 15 seconds of an injury. Plasma has 11 clotting factors, but we will mention only the most significant ones. Prothrombin is a clotting protein that is made in the liver, and when it is needed, it is converted into thrombin with the help of vitamin K. Thrombin turns fibrinogen into fibrin, which is like an interwoven mesh net. Fibrin collects more platelets and red blood cells, developing a clot in 3–6 minutes. The clot pulls together the edges of the damaged blood vessel and the edges of the epithelial tissue to create a permanent repair. When the clot is no longer needed, it dissolves away. See Figure 12-12.

12-13 BLOOD TYPES

All blood is not the same. In fact, there are four main blood types—Type A, Type B, Type AB, or Type O—and some of them are incompatible with others.

In an earlier module, we learned about antigens. Typically a foreign protein that enters the body, antigens trigger the body's immune system to make antibodies to fight off the foreign invader. This reaction also can happen with blood cells. We have antigens called self-antigens that are native to our body, and foreign antigens, such as pollen, called nonself-antigens.

An antigen–antibody reaction occurs when blood cell antibodies react to blood with antigens, causing the blood to stick together and clump in a process known as agglutination.

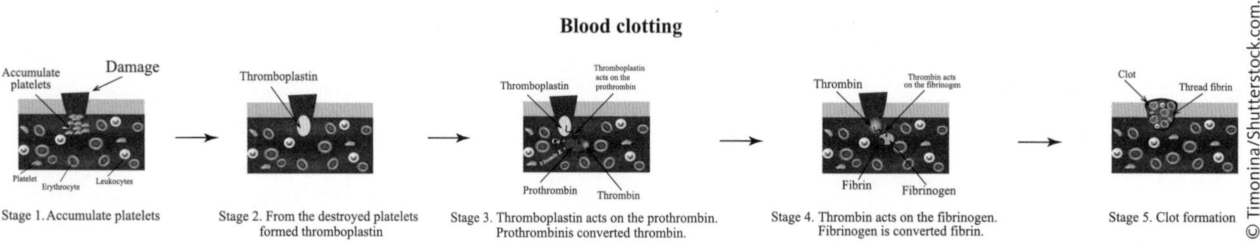

FIGURE 12-12 Blood clotting process.

Antigen–antibody reactions also occur between some different blood types. **Type A blood** has an A self-antigen and no antibodies against type A. Type A has only B antibodies. **Type B blood**, on the other hand, has a B self-antigen and no type B antibodies, but it does have A antibodies. If type A blood was administered to a type B patient, agglutination would occur because of the antigen–antibody reaction. This agglutination or clumping could cause serious harm or even death.

Type O blood does not have any A or B self-antigens, yet it still has both A and B antibodies. With no A or B antigens to react with its A or B antibodies, type O blood can be given to anyone, making it the *universal donor*.

Type AB blood, however, has both A and B self-antigens, but no A and B antibodies. With both A and B antigens, type AB blood can receive blood from anyone, making it the *universal recipient*.

See Figure 12-13.

12-13a Rh Factor

What about positive and negative blood types? The positive and negatives are from **Rh factors**, with the Rh taken from Rhesus because it was first discovered in Rhesus monkeys. This factor also is found in other primates, including about 85 percent of humans. Some people have a special antigen on the surface of their red blood cells, making them Rh positive. If they don't have the antigen, they are Rh negative. The positive or negative is attached after the blood type designation, as in AB negative or A positive. The only time this factor can become an issue is during pregnancy. For example, a mother has a negative Rh factor and a father has a positive Rh factor. Their child inherits the positive factor, causing the mother to develop Rh antibodies. If a second child with a positive Rh factor is conceived, those antibodies will attack the second fetus.

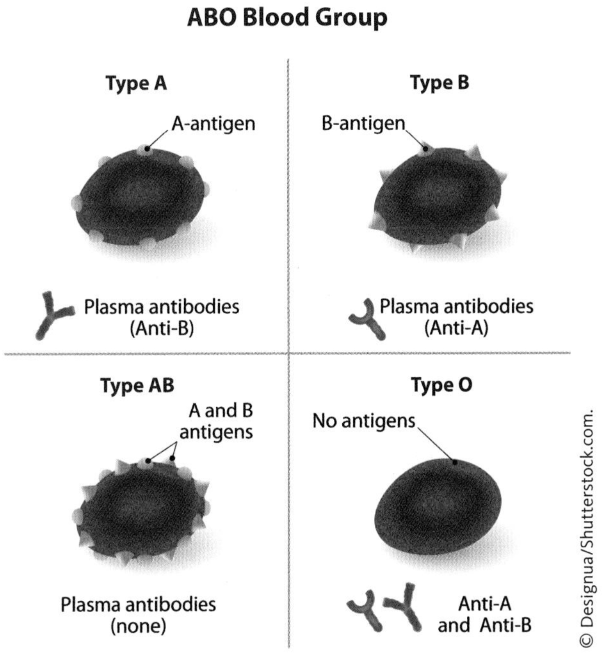

FIGURE 12-13 ABO blood group.

LEARNING OBJECTIVE 12.2 Describe assessments and diagnostics of the cardiovascular system.

KEY TERMS

Angiocardiography Examination of the vessels and chambers of the heart performed with a special dye and an X-ray.

Ankle-brachial index (ABI) Noninvasive method used to check for the presence of peripheral artery disease.

Arteriography Test that uses a special dye and an X-ray to check the inside of the arteries.

Auscultation Listening to the heart with a stethoscope to check for murmurs.

Bell Side of the stethoscope used to listen to the patient's heart.

Cardiac catheterization Invasive procedure used to treat and diagnose cardiovascular conditions.

Doppler echocardiogram Test used to study the flow of blood through the heart.

Peripheral artery disease (PAD) Narrowing of the arteries in the body other than the heart and brain.

Venography Procedure that uses special dye and an X-ray to examine veins.

12-14 COMMON SIGNS AND SYMPTOMS OF CARDIOVASCULAR DISEASE

As we learn about cardiovascular diseases, you will see that each disease has its own characteristics and different variations of signs and symptoms. Some basic signs and symptoms, however, are common to many cardiac and vascular ailments:

- *Tachycardia* (fast heartbeat): The heart has to work harder to compensate for the disease process.
- *Fatigue*: Can be caused by the heart's inability to pump oxygenated blood to the skeletal muscles and instead keeps blood near the vital organs. Patients also can feel tired because the body is not able to remove wastes.
- *Chest pain* or *angina*: Comes in different forms. Some chest pain feels like a continuous bout of indigestion, while more severe forms feel as if the patient's chest is being crushed. Pain also can be felt radiating in the neck, jaw, and left arm and shoulder.
- *Increased respiratory rate/shortness of breath (SOB)*: Because the body lacks oxygenation, the respiratory system needs to work harder to provide the body with oxygen.
- *Heart palpitations*: Some patients experience an irregular heartbeat or one that is stronger and faster than normal, so much so that the patient actually feels it.
- *Edema*: Fluid can back up into the lungs (pulmonary edema), abdomen (ascites), and peripherally (affecting the extremities) depending on the type of heart failure.

- *Distended neck veins*: If blood flow backs up in the heart, the fluid has to go somewhere so the neck veins become enlarged and the liver becomes engorged.
- *Diaphoresis*: Sweating occurring day and night without any activity is caused by your body having to exert itself to pump blood and work harder to do so. Your body sweats to try to cool your body temperature. This results in a cool, clammy skin. Women might blame night sweats on menopause, but this might not be the case, and they should consult a physician promptly.
- *Indigestion, nausea, and vomiting*: Many people blame these symptoms on their diet, but if they persist, they should check with their physician. People have reported these symptoms before having a heart attack.
- *Cyanosis*: A bluish skin color results from the lack of oxygen in the tissues.
- *Pain*: Can be caused by poor perfusion of blood.
- *Ischemia*: Caused by lack of oxygen to tissues causing tissue death.

12-15 COMMON DIAGNOSTIC PROCEDURES

Before a physician can decide on a treatment, the patient's condition must be diagnosed. Some are quick and easy, noninvasive methods, while others are very invasive and potentially dangerous.

12-15a Auscultation

A simple noninvasive technique is to listen to heart sounds. **Auscultation** is done by listening to the heart with a stethoscope. The end of a stethoscope placed on the patient has two sides: a diaphragm and a bell (Figure 12-14). To remember which side is used when: The side used to listen to the lungs is the larger side called the diaphragm, and the body's diaphragm helps the lungs work. The **bell** is the smaller side, and is used to listen to lower pitched heart sounds, such as blood flow through the valves.

Another use for auscultation, previously discussed, is blood pressure measurement. As a review, *blood pressure* is a measurement of the arterial pressure in

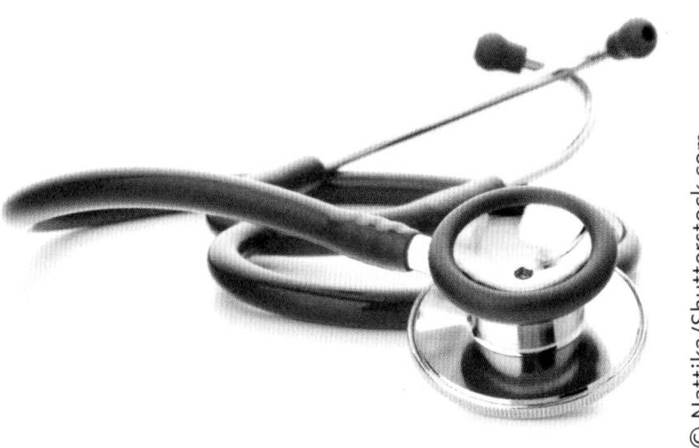

© Nattika/Shutterstock.com.

FIGURE 12-14 The smaller side of the stethoscope is the bell, while the larger side is the diaphragm.

a patient. It is measured with a blood pressure (BP) cuff, also known as a sphygmomanometer. This device obtains systolic and diastolic values. Systolic occurs when the heart contracts, and the diastolic is obtained when the heart relaxes.

12-15b ECG

An *electrocardiograph* is a machine that uses electrical leads that are placed strategically on the patient to record the heart in action. The actual recording is called an *electrocardiogram*, and the procedure is called an *electrocardiography*. The heart rhythms are recorded and printed so they can be studied. Any abnormal heartbeats, known as heart arrhythmias, can be seen and identified using this technique. See Figure 12-15.

12-15c Cardiac Imaging

An *X-ray* of the heart is used to see the size, structure, and shape of the heart and vessels. A dye can be injected to get a better image of the heart and vessels. There are four common types of X-rays used to check the chambers of the heart and the surrounding vessels. **Arteriography** is a procedure done to check the condition of the patient's arteries. **Angiocardiography** is a procedure used to check the chambers, arteries, and vessels of the heart (angio = vessel, cardio = heart, graphy = procedure). **Venography** (veno = vein, graphy = procedure) is a procedure used to inspect veins in a patient's body. See Figure 12-16.

12-15d Doppler Studies

Doppler echocardiogram, often referred to as an echo, is a type of ultrasound used to study the blood flow through the heart and to examine the function of the heart valves. The physician can see the direction and speed of the blood flow and determine if any abnormalities are present. There are different types of echocardiograms, but we will focus on an enhanced version called a color Doppler. The word Doppler often is used in conjunction with a weather forecast, with Doppler radar translating information about types of precipitation into different colors on a map. A Doppler heart echo also can be done in color to reflect the direction and speed of blood. See Figure 12-17.

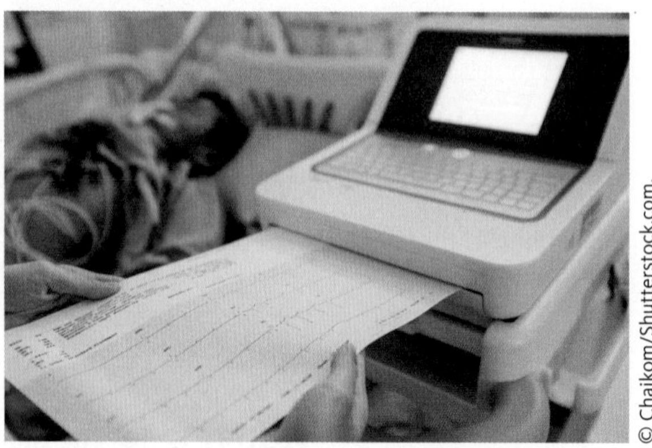

FIGURE 12-15 An electrocardiograph printing out an electrocardiogram.

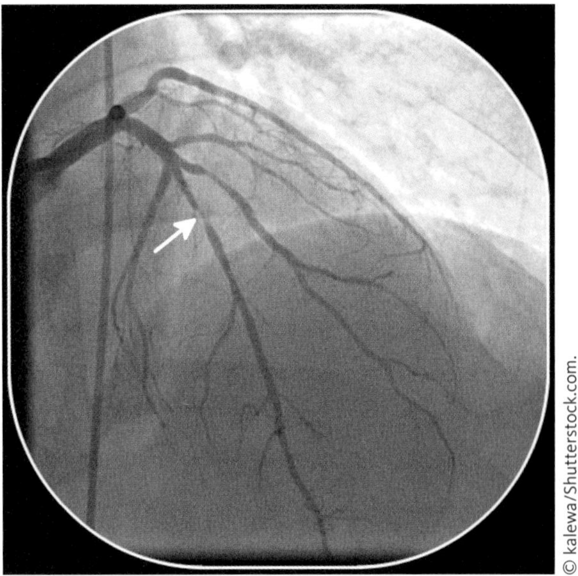

FIGURE 12-16 Image of coronary artery stenosis (narrowing) of the left anterior descending coronary artery provided by an angiography.

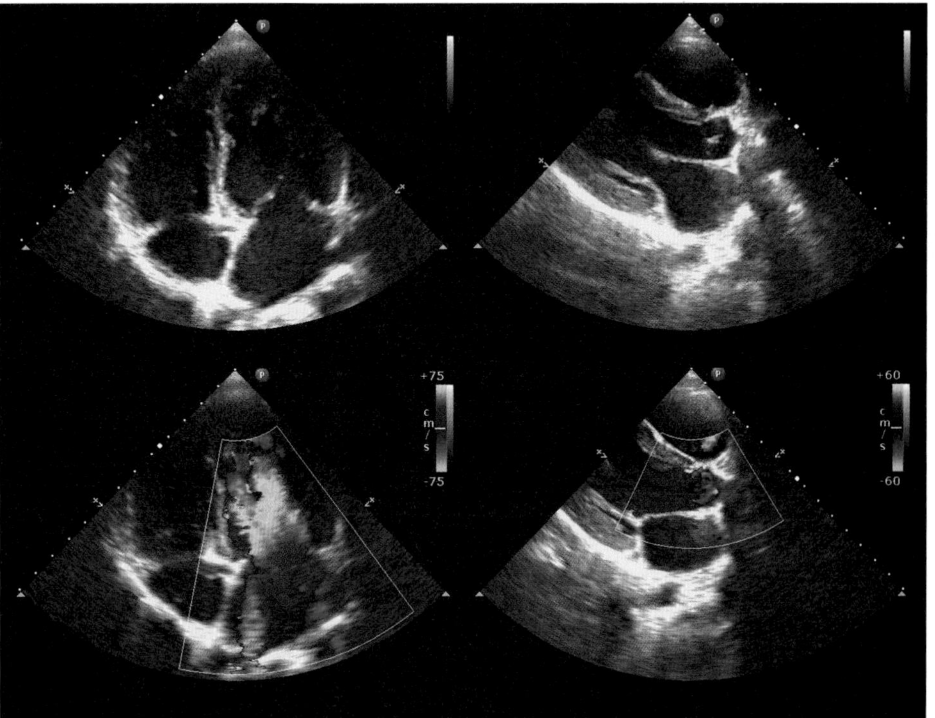

FIGURE 12-17 Images of an electrocardiogram displaying various colors. Black means no flow; yellow reflects a high velocity, and green shows the turbulence of blood flow. The red color shows the flow of blood toward the transducer (the device placed on the patient to transmit ultrasound waves), while the blue coloration is the flow of blood away from the transducer. The brighter the shade of color is, the higher will be the velocity of blood flow; for example, a bright red or yellow indicates a high speed. The slower the flow of blood is, the darker the coloration appears.

12-15e Cardiac Catheterization

Cardiac catheterization is a very invasive procedure that involves inserting a catheter into an artery until it reaches the heart. The insertion can be done either through the patient's groin or through the arm as shown in Figure 12-18; we'll describe the procedure using the groin. The catheter is inserted into the femoral artery and pushed through the circulatory system until it reaches the desired area of the heart or nearby vessels. Stents can be placed using this technique to open coronary arteries that are clogged with plaque. Cardiac catheters also can measure pressures in the heart by inflating a balloon at the tip of the catheter. For example, the catheter can be guided into the pulmonary artery to measure its pressure if pulmonary hypertension is suspected.

12-15f Ankle Brachial Index

Ankle-brachial index (ABI) is a diagnostic test used to check a patient for **peripheral arterial disease (PAD)**. The patient's blood pressure is measured at the ankle and the arm, and the two systolic pressures are compared to get the ABI. The pressure in the ankle should be the same as the arm, if not slightly greater. If the pressure at the ankle is lower than that obtained in the arm, some artery blockage is present. See Figure 12-19.

12-15g Blood Tests

Blood testing for cholesterol, low-density lipoprotein (LDL), high-density lipoprotein (HDL), and triglycerides is done to determine if the patient is at risk of developing plaque in the arteries, which eventually would cause high blood pressure or heart attack.

- Cholesterol is a substance found in all the body's cells and travels through the bloodstream as lipoproteins. The body makes cholesterol to help process food and produce hormones and vitamin D. Cholesterol also can be obtained from food, and too much of this waxy product can be harmful. A normal reading for cholesterol is below 200 mg/dL. The range between 200 and 240 is considered borderline high, while anything greater than 240 mg/dL is high cholesterol.

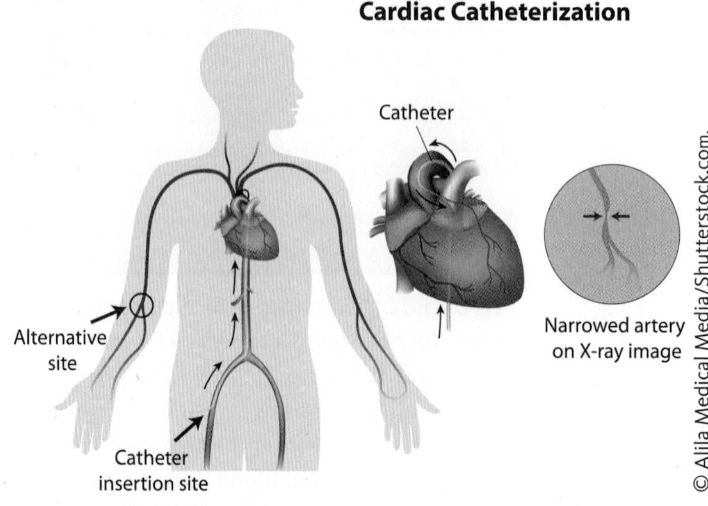

FIGURE 12-18 Cardiac catheterization.

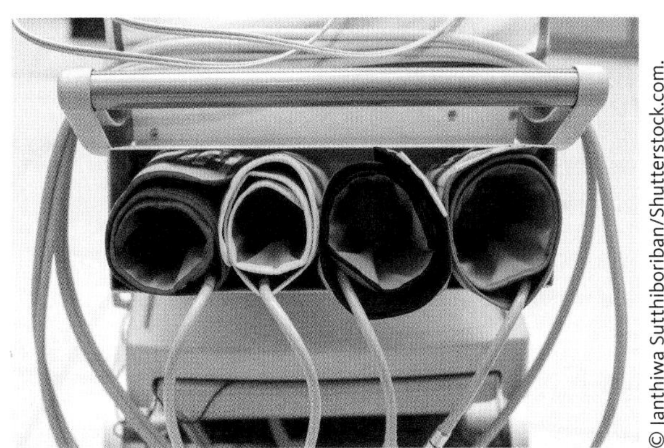
© Janthiwa Sutthiboriban/Shutterstock.com.

FIGURE 12-19 Blood pressure cuffs for an ABI machine.

- LDL, or bad cholesterol, should be lower than 100. These lipoproteins are in large part responsible for the development of plaque deposits on the walls of blood vessels.
- HDL, or good cholesterol, should be higher than 45. This lipoprotein is "good" because HDL removes LDL from the walls of arteries, transporting the LDL to the liver from which it can be excreted.
- Triglycerides are the energy stored in cells from food we eat and should be below 200. Triglycerides are stored as fat in adipose tissue until needed for energy, but when in excess from a poor diet, this lipoprotein can cause atherosclerosis.

Blood tests also can be used to determine if the patient has had a heart attack. When heart muscle dies, it releases specific substances, such as creatinine phosphokinase (CPK) and troponin lactic dehydrogenase (TnL). The appearance of these substances in the blood analysis indicates heart muscle death.

LEARNING OBJECTIVE 12.3 Explain vascular diseases and related medications.

KEY TERMS

Aneurysm Weak spot in a vessel.

Antiarrhythmics Drugs used to treat an abnormal heartbeat.

Anticoagulants Drugs that prevent the blood from clotting.

Antilipemic agents Drugs that help decrease the amount of lipids in the blood.

Antiplatelet drugs Drug class that prevents platelets from sticking together to cause a clot.

Arteriosclerosis Develops when the vessels are no longer elastic and have become stiff, can cause an increase in blood pressure, can be caused by old age.

Atherosclerosis A condition caused by plaque that builds up on the walls of the arteries causing the walls to become thicker.

Bile acid sequestrants Medications used to help lower cholesterol by binding to certain resins in the bile.

Blood thinners Drugs used to prevent clotting and to increase the time it takes for blood to clot.

Coronary artery disease (CAD) Disease caused by the buildup of plaque in the arteries of the heart.

D-dimer test Test used to measure a specific substance that would be present if a clot has been broken up.

Deep vein thrombosis (DVT) Clot that has formed within the deep veins.

Hypertension High blood pressure.

Hypertensive heart disease Group of conditions that cause high blood pressure, which in turn affect the function of the heart.

Nicotinic acid (niacin) Class of drugs used to decrease the amount of triglycerides present in the blood.

Nitroglycerin Drug that causes vasodilation; used to treat angina (chest pain).

Phlebitis Inflammation of a vein.

Statins Class of drugs used to lower cholesterol.

Thrombolytic agents Clot-busting agents dissolve an existing clot.

Thrombophlebitis Inflammation of a vein caused by a thrombus (clot).

Varicose veins Veins that are characterized by being twisted, bulging, and distorted.

12-16 ARTERIAL DISEASES

Arteries are vital to the function of the body's circulatory system. These vessels are specifically developed to handle the high pressure of blood being pumped throughout the body from the heart. Because the pressure is high, the flexible arteries do not need one-way valves to prevent blood from flowing backward. However, diseases that affect these important structures can have devastating outcomes.

12-17 HYPERTENSION

Hypertension is a chronic cardiovascular disease that also can be an indicator that another disease process, such as kidney disease and cerebrovascular disease, is present. People with hypertension are at a greater risk for a heart attack or stroke and other problems as shown in Figure 12-20.

Although normal blood pressure varies with every person, the excepted normal range is lower than 120/80 mmHg. The top number, in this case 120, is the systolic number, which occurs when the ventricles of the heart contract. The lower number, 80, is measured when the heart is at rest. When the pressure in the system is increased, those numbers will increase, too.

One factor that can cause an increased blood pressure, especially in the diastolic number, is the resistance of the vessels. If the lumen of the vessels is constricted or blocked from plaque, the baseline pressure will increase. Think about a garden hose: The water will flow out slower than if resistance is added by partially blocking the end, which causes the velocity and pressure to increase.

The body has receptors that are sensitive to pressure changes and helps control blood pressure by vasodilating or vasoconstricting. If blood pressure is too high, these sensors will cause the vessels near the kidneys to dilate so the body will create more urine (removing fluid from the blood) and decrease the blood pressure. On the other hand, if the blood pressure is too low, blood vessels will constrict, decreasing urine output to normalize blood pressure. The kidneys, therefore, play an important role in controlling blood pressure.

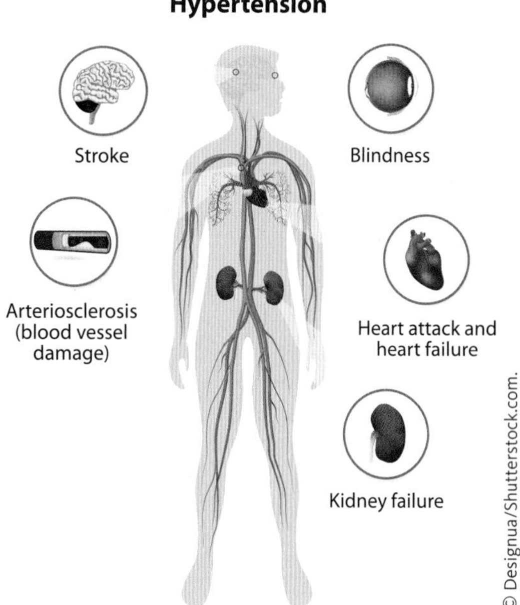

FIGURE 12-20 Possible effects of hypertension.

12-17a Types of Hypertension

Hypertension has many different causes. Primary hypertension is idiopathic, which means its cause is unknown. Factors that have been identified as contributing to the cause of hypertension include aging, obesity, diet, smoking, heredity, and stress. Individuals with a Type A personalities, who tend to lead a hyperactive, high-strung, and stressful lifestyle, often have hypertension.

Secondary hypertension occurs when another disease, such as kidney disease, is involved. Because the kidneys help control blood pressure, if they are affected by a disease, they might become unable to remove salt and water from the body. If salt and water are retained, then blood pressure will rise.

Those suffering from hypertension might not even realize it because the symptoms do not show until extensive heart or vessel damage has occurred. Eventually, the heart has to work so much harder to keep up with the body's demand that the heart's structure becomes permanently changed. The left ventricle, which is the chamber that pumps the hardest to push blood throughout the body, will become enlarged, in a condition known as left ventricular hypertrophy. In weight lifting, to get larger muscles, a person needs to work out by lifting weights. As a person continues to work his or her muscles, they get larger. This might be good for skeletal muscles, but not for heart muscle.

If the heart muscle becomes enlarged, its ability to function properly alters and causes problems. Even though the heart muscle becomes larger, its blood supply is not increased, so the extra tissue will not get enough blood. The result can be chest pain or angina from ischemia. This condition can cause a heart attack or myocardial infarction (MI), heart failure, and death. Damage to the blood vessels also can occur from the constant high pressure, losing their elasticity and becoming hardened. This is termed arteriosclerosis (sclerosis = hardening or stiffening).

12-17b Diagnosing and Treating Hypertension

Diagnosing blood pressure can be done by having it checked regularly via routine physical examinations. Because hypertension is hereditary, the physician also will look at the patient's family history. The physician also can order an electrocardiogram (EKG, ECG) to check the heart rate and rhythm. A blood sample can be taken to examine:

- Cholesterol
- Triglycerides
- Low-density lipoprotein (HDL)
- High-density lipoprotein (LDL)

The treatment of hypertension varies, depending on how high the blood pressure is and what factors are causing the condition. Since there are many contributing factors, hypertension has a host of medication strategies that can be tailored to the patient's circumstances. Common medications that can be used in treating **hypertensive heart disease** are:

- Nitroglycerin
- Antilipemic agents/statins
- Bile sequestrants
- Nicotinic acid
- Beta blockers
- Diuretics (covered in Module 10: Urinary Disease and Medication)
- Angiotensin-converting enzyme (ACE) inhibitors
- Angiotensin receptor blockers (ARBs)
- Calcium channel blockers

12-17c Nitroglycerin

Nitroglycerin temporarily vasodilates coronary arteries, allowing more blood flow and oxygen delivery to decrease the work of the heart and stopping chest pain (angina). Nitrates come in various forms, including patches, tablets, and sprays. Examples include:

- Nitro-Bid (Nitroglycerin ointment USP 2%)
- Nitro-Dur, Minitran (transdermal nitroglycerin patch)
- Nitrolingual spray
- Nitrostat tablets (sublingual tabs for under the tongue)

12-17d Antilipemic Agents/Statins

Antilipemic agents (cholesterol medications) help increase good cholesterol (HDL) while decreasing the bad cholesterol (LDL). This helps prevent the buildup of harmful clogging plaque in the arteries. These medications can slow or stop the progression of the disease, and even reverse the condition to a degree. **Statins** are drugs used to block the enzymes responsible for making cholesterol in the liver (see Table 12-3).

Table 12-3 Common types of statins

BRAND NAME	GENERIC NAME
Zocor	Simvastatin
Mevacor, Altoprev	Lovastatin
Lipitor	Atorvastatin
Pravachol	Pravastatin
Lescol	Fluvastatin
Crestor	Rosuvastatin

Table 12-4 Common bile acid sequestrant medications

BRAND NAME	GENERIC NAME
WelChol	Colesevelam
Questran, Locholest, Prevalite	Cholestyramine
Colestid	Colestipol

12-17e Bile Sequestrants

Bile acid sequestrants also are used to help lower high cholesterol. They work by inhibiting bile acids from being reabsorbed into the bloodstream from the intestines. This might not seem like a big deal, but by doing so, the liver must produce more bile, and to make more bile, the liver needs cholesterol. This causes the liver to consume the cholesterol floating around in the bloodstream, decreasing the LDL in the blood. Examples of such drugs are shown in Table 12-4.

12-17f Nicotinic Acid

Nicotinic acid (niacin) lowers cholesterol by a different mechanism. Triglycerides known as very low-density lipoproteins (VLDLs) become LDL. Nicotinic acids decrease the amount of triglycerides produced and increase the HDL level. The drug niacin comes in three different forms of release as shown in Table 12-5.

12-17g Beta-Adrenergic Blockers

The drugs in this class are **antiarrhythmics**, which prevent heart arrhythmias by blocking the adrenergic (sympathetic) nerve receptors. They reduce the heart rate and cause vasodilation, reducing the amount of pressure within the system.

Table 12-5 Types of nicotinic acid drugs

FORM OF RELEASE	BRAND NAME	GENERIC NAME
Immediate release	Niacor	Niacin
Sustained release	Slo-Niacin	Niacin
Extended release	Niaspan	Niacin

Table 12-6 Examples of beta blockers

BRAND NAME	GENERIC NAME
Tenormin	Atenolol
Inderal	Propranolol
Lopressor	Metoprolol

Beta receptors in the heart, when stimulated, cause an increase in heart rate and vasoconstriction. By giving a beta blocker, the opposite effect occurs, causing vasodilation and a decrease in heart rate and therefore decrease blood pressure. Beta blockers help alleviate signs and symptoms such as chest pain, making this class great for coronary artery atherosclerosis. Examples of beta blockers are found in Table 12-6.

12-17h Angiotensin-Converting Enzyme (ACE) Inhibitors (ACEIs)

Angiotensin is a chemical that causes the blood vessels to constrict. If a medication inhibits this chemical, vasoconstriction will not occur. These drugs decrease blood pressure by increasing the diameter of the vessels and the amount of blood to the heart without causing considerable changes in the patient's heart rate as do the beta blockers discussed in the previous section.

ACEIs are both the first and second line of defense against hypertension, but they can be used in conjunction with other drugs, such as calcium channel blockers or even diuretics, to create a synergistic effect. ACEIs work great to treat diseases that cause hypertension and other major diseases, as they help to decrease the progression of those diseases. See Table 12-7 for examples.

12-17i Angiotensin Receptor Blockers

An alternative to ACEIs are angiotensin receptor blockers (ARBs). Angiotensin receptors cause vasoconstriction when they are stimulated by angiotensin II. By blocking the receptors, the process is blocked, and vasodilation is favored.

Table 12-7 Examples of angiotensin-converting enzyme (ACE) inhibitors (ACEIs)

BRAND NAME	GENERIC NAME
Altace	Ramipril
Accupril	Quinapril
Aceon	Perindopril erbumine
Capoten	Captopril
Lotensin	Benazepril
Marik	Trandolapril
Monopril	Fosinopril
Prinivil, Zestril	Lisinopril
Univase	Moexipril
Vasotec	Enalapril maleate

Table 12-8 Commonly used angiotensin receptor blockers (ARBs)

BRAND NAME	GENERIC NAME
Atacand	Candesartan
Avapro	Irbesartan
Benicar	Olmesartan
Cozaar	Losartan
Diovan	Valsartan
Edarbi	Azilsartan
Micardis	Telmisartan
Teveten	Eprosartan

These drugs work similar to ACEIs to decrease blood pressure by blocking the angiotensin, while also not causing a significant change in the patient's heart rate. ARBs are known to have fewer side effects than ACEIs. See Table 12-8 for examples.

Table 12-9 Examples of various calcium channel blockers

BRAND NAME	GENERIC NAME
Dynacirc	Isradipine
Plendil	Felodipine
Norvasc	Amlodipine
Cardizem, Tiazac, Dilacor, Dilt-cd	Diltiazem
Sular	Nisoldipine
Adalat, Procardia	Nifedipine
Cardene	Nicardipine
Calan, Verelan, Isoptin	Verapamil

12-17j Calcium Channel Blockers

All muscles, including the heart, need calcium to contract. By blocking calcium channels, contraction is reduced, thus reducing blood pressure. These drugs also slow the conduction of the AV node, which causes a decrease in blood pressure.

Various calcium channel blockers are available, but two drugs, verapamil (Calan) and diltiazem (Cardizem), stand out as having the most impact on controlling arrhythmias. For a list of calcium channel blockers, see Table 12-9.

12-18 ARTERIOSCLEROSIS AND ATHEROSCLEROSIS

These two words are very similar in appearance and are often used interchangeably, but they are not the same. **Arteriosclerosis** is a group of diseases that result in thickened and stiff artery walls, often called hardened arteries. This condition can restrict blood flow to vital organs, causing ischemia or tissue death. **Atherosclerosis** is the term used when plaque builds up on the inside of the vessel. It is a *type* of arteriosclerosis. This sticky accumulation of fats and cholesterol (shown in Figure 12-21) causes a decrease in blood flow, possibly resulting in tissue death. The plaque can even break away from the side of the vessel and travel through the cardiovascular system, causing a blockage known as an embolism.

The thickening, stiffness, and plaque build up of these conditions all can cause an increase in blood pressure because the vessels are not able to expand when needed. This in turn increases the workload on the heart and diminishes blood supply to the heart.

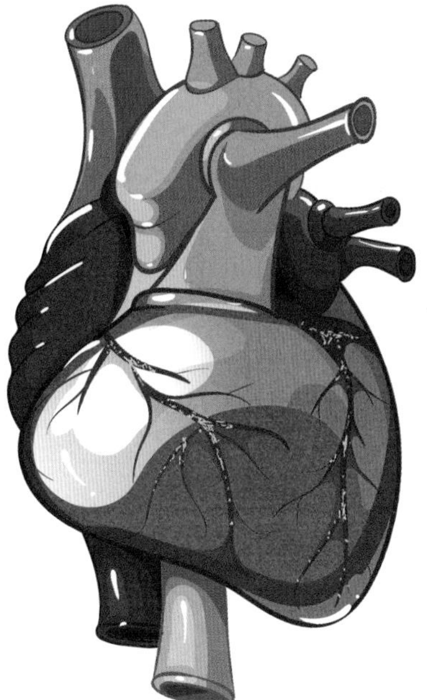

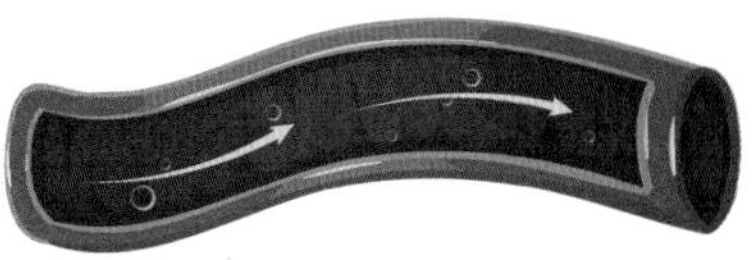

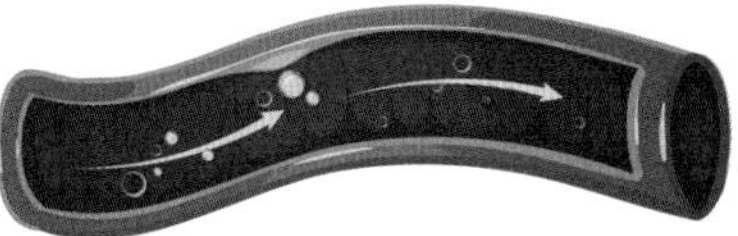

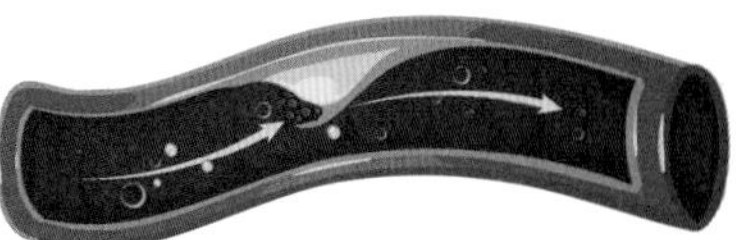

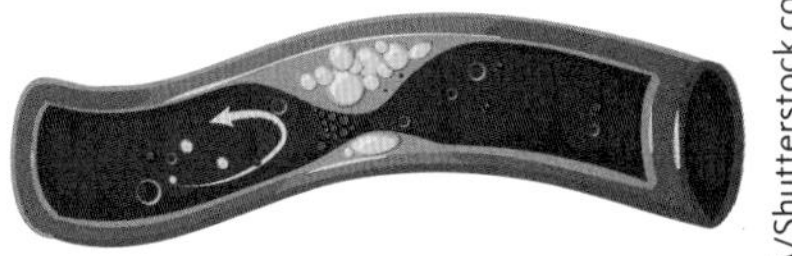

FIGURE 12-21 Atherosclerosis.

12-18a Locations of Atherosclerosis

While atherosclerosis can occur anywhere in the body, it is most commonly found in:

Coronary arteries: Since these arteries supply the heart muscle with the oxygen it needs, plaque buildup in the coronary arteries is very serious and given its own classification called coronary artery disease (CAD).

Cerebral arteries: These arteries supply the brain with blood and oxygen, and if blood cannot travel through these arteries, it could cause a stroke or cerebral vascular accident (CVA).

Peripheral arteries: These arteries supply your extremities (arms and legs) with blood and oxygen. This condition is called peripheral vascular disease (PVD).

Aorta: This vessel, the largest artery in the body, takes all of the blood from the heart and carries it throughout the body. As with the other three areas, plaque buildup can be devastating, and in this case, it could result in an aneurysm.

12-18b Causes of Atherosclerosis

The exact cause of atherosclerosis is unknown, but various factors are known to increase the odds of developing this disease. These factors can be broken down into two categories: uncontrollable and controllable factors. Some uncontrollable factors are:

- Heredity: People with family members with atherosclerosis have a better chance of developing the disease.

- Gender: Men have more plaque buildup than women until menopause, then both male and female have about the same amount of atherosclerosis.
- Age: Everyone has some plaque buildup by age 30; however, the older the person is, the more plaque is present.
- Type 1 Diabetes: Those with this condition have a greater chance of developing more plaque.

Below is a list of controllable factors:

- Smoking is a major cause of disease, and atherosclerosis is no exception. Smoking also increases blood pressure.
- Sedentary lifestyle: People who sit for long periods of time, such as at work, or those who lack a proper exercise regime are at much greater risk in the development of plaque.
- Diet: People who are overweight have a greater risk of developing atherosclerosis.
- High blood pressure: While high blood pressure can be caused by the stiffening of the arterial walls because of age, it can be amplified by the buildup of plaque because of disease or poor lifestyle choices.
- Stress: Also might be linked because it can cause high blood pressure, which can result in atherosclerosis.

Signs and symptoms occur slowly over time. Patients with mild atherosclerosis might not present any signs or symptoms until the condition worsens. The signs and symptoms experienced also depend on which arteries are affected. See Table 12-10 for signs and symptoms of mild to severe cases.

12-18c Diagnosis and Treatment of Atherosclerosis

To diagnose this condition, patients have their blood pressure measured for signs of high blood pressure, and lipid blood profiles are done. In addition, vascular

Table 12-10 Mild to severe signs and symptoms of atherosclerosis

LOCATION	SIGNS/SYMPTOMS
Coronary arteries	• Angina (chest pain), pressure in chest
Cerebral arteries	• Sudden tingling, numbness, or weakness in arms and legs • Difficulty speaking • Facial drooping • Temporary vision loss • Transient ischemic attack (TIA) is an indicator that a stroke is likely to occur. • Cerebral vascular accident (CVA) or stroke
Peripheral arteries	• Leg pain, especially when walking

studies, in this case, arteriograms, are done to discover where the problem is located, as well as Doppler studies to determine the flow of blood.

There are two main surgical procedures that can be performed:

- Coronary bypass surgery to insert a vessel from another part of the body to bypass the blocked coronary vessel or vessels.
- Insertion of a stent to open up the blocked artery.

Various medications can be used to treat atherosclerosis along with the resulting hypertension:

Treat resulting hypertension:

- Diuretics to reduce fluid volume and therefore blood pressure
- Angiotensin converting enzyme (ACE) inhibitors (ACEIs)
- Angiotensin receptor blockers (ARBs)
- Beta-adrenergic blockers
- Calcium channel blockers

To prevent further plaque build up:

- Antilipemic agents
- Bile acid sequestrants
- Nicotinic acid (niacin)

To treat formed clots:

- Fibrinolytic therapy in which agents are given to dissolve an existing clot causing the vessel to be blocked.

12-19 PERIPHERAL VASCULAR DISEASE

Any disease affecting the circulatory system (arteries, veins, and lymph vessels) outside of the heart is known as peripheral vascular disease (PVD).

PVD is caused by the waxy plaque buildup seen with atherosclerosis, but the vessels affected are in the peripheral circulation, especially the arteries in the legs. This condition can be either acute or chronic; however, in either case, the blood supply to the affected extremity is decreased.

Those with PVD might not experience any signs or symptoms with minimal activity, but they occur during physical exertion. When this happens, the patient will experience muscle cramps from the lack of blood and oxygen to the extremity. After the patient stops and rests, the cramps should subside. This is termed intermittent claudication.

Other symptoms are pain in the feet or toes, a sore on the foot or leg, cold feet or legs, or color changes such as cyanosis. In addition, the affected limb can have poor hair or nail growth.

To diagnose, the following can be used:

- Ankle-brachial index (ABI) after a treadmill test
- Doppler
- Check for a pulse in the feet

- Treadmill test in which the patient walks on a treadmill until symptoms occur
- Angiography
- MRI

Drugs used to treat PVD are:

- Statins to decrease cholesterol
- Beta blockers to decrease blood pressure and slow heart rate
- Angiotensin converting enzyme (ACE) inhibitors (ACEIs) to decrease blood pressure
- Angiotensin receptor blockers (ARBs) to decrease blood pressure
- Calcium channel blockers to decrease blood pressure by slowing the conduction of the AV node
- Blood thinners such as anticoagulants and antiplatelets to prevent blood from clotting at the site of the plaque buildup. An example available over the counter is aspirin for its antiplatelet effect. Pletal (cilostazol), a vasodilator that increases circulation and also prevents platelets from sticking together, is used to treat leg pain experienced from intermittent claudication

12-20 CORONARY ARTERY DISEASE

Coronary artery disease (CAD) develops over a long period of time. Plaque builds up on the walls of the arteries, causing a partial or complete blockage of blood flow causing coronary atherosclerosis. The occlusion blocks oxygen supply to the myocardium, the heart muscle itself. As the condition persists, signs and symptoms begin to show including:

- Shortness of breath occurs because the heart is not able to work efficiently to pump blood around the body to meet oxygen demand.
- Fatigue because the body has to work much harder to meet oxygen demands.
- Chest pain (angina) is pain experienced in the middle and left side of the chest that can present as chest tightness or a feeling of pressure on the chest.
- Myocardial infarction (MI) or heart attack is the result of occluded blood flow.
- Blood clot (thrombus) occurs if plaque breaks free from two walls. This condition can be caused by:
    - High blood pressure because of increasing thickening and hardening of blood vessels, making it difficult for blood to travel through the vessel.
    - High cholesterol from an increase in LDL and the lowering of HDC causes a higher risk for plaque to form.
    - Diabetes can cause CAD by causing high blood pressure and obesity

Other risk factors for CAD include:

- Gender: Men are more likely to be affected than women, but the risk for women developing CAD increases after menopause.
- Family history: CAD tends to run in the family.
- Age: Aging increases the odds of developing CAD.

12-20a Diagnosis of Coronary Artery Disease

To diagnose CAD, the physician starts by taking the patient's personal and family histories. The symptoms experienced by the patient can help narrow down the disease, along with an electrocardiogram (ECG).

Another diagnostic method is an exercise stress test, in which the patient is placed on a treadmill so the heart can be monitored during exertion. If the patient is unable to walk on the treadmill, physical exertion can be chemically induced.

An echocardiogram can check the blood flow through the heart to see how well the heart is performing. If an area of the heart is not functioning as it should, it might be deprived of oxygen.

An angiogram can be done by injecting dye into the coronary arteries to determine if there are any narrow spots indicating an occlusion. A CT scan of the heart also uses dye to get a better look at the structures, including the arteries.

12-20b Treatment of Coronary Artery Disease

To treat CAD, surgical procedures can be performed. A coronary artery bypass graft (CABG), pronounced "cabbage," can be done to bypass the occluded vessel with a vessel harvested from the patient's leg or breast. Another method used is a coronary artery angioplasty (angio = vessel, plasty = repair), in which a catheter is inserted with a balloon on the distal tip into the affected artery. The balloon is inflated at the site of plaque to dilate the vessel. A cardiac catheterization can be done to insert a wire mesh stent to prevent the vessel from reclosing.

The following drug classes can be used:

- Nitroglycerin to dilate coronary arteries
- Beta-blockers to reduce the heart workload
- Antilipemic agents to reduce plaque build up
- Angiotensin-converting enzyme inhibitors (ACEI) to reduce blood pressure/heart workload
- Angiotensin II receptor blockers (ARBs) to reduce blood pressure/heart workload
- Nonsteroidal anti-inflammatory drugs to reduce resulting inflammation

12-21 ANEURYSM

Another major complication of an artery and a potentially life-threatening condition is an **aneurysm**. An aneurysm is a weak spot in the wall of an artery causing it to have a balloon-like bulge. Aneurysms often are caused by atherosclerosis,

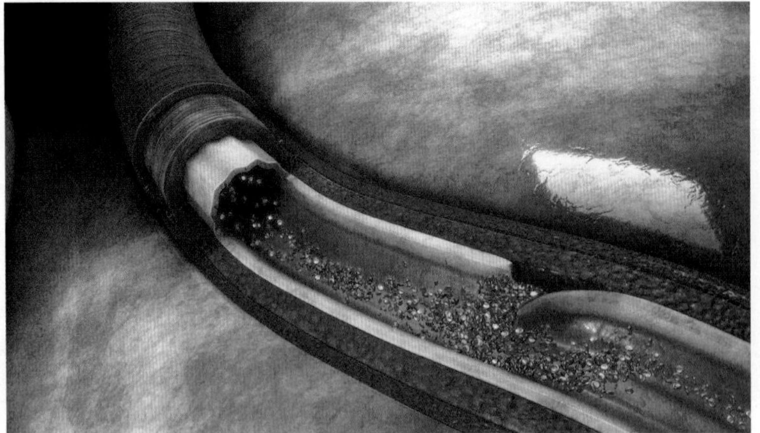

FIGURE 12-22 Dissecting aneurysm.

but they also can be from a congenital birth defect or the result of an injury. There are three types of aneurysms:

1. Saccular: One side of the vessel is bulged out
2. Fusiform: Distorted structure throughout the vessel
3. Dissecting: Blood leaves the vessel by separating the layers that comprise the vessel walls, as shown in Figure 12-22. A characteristic that makes this condition especially deadly is that the patient might not even be aware of the condition until it ruptures, resulting in a sudden medical emergency

If an aneurysm is in the aorta, a diagnosis can be made by listening to blood flow through a stethoscope. Other locations can be checked with the help of a CT, MRI scan, and angiogram.

Treatment of an aneurysm entails surgery to correct the weak vessel before it can rupture. Also controlling blood pressure and statin treatment to prevent plaque can help prevent this condition from occurring.

12-22 DISEASES OF THE VEINS

Diseases affecting veins range in severity, but generally become increasingly common with age because veins become weaker as a person ages.

12-23 PHLEBITIS

Phlebitis, or inflammation of a vein, is a common condition often occurring in the patient's arms or legs. Phlebitis can occur in deep veins; however, it is most often used in reference to veins close to the surface of the skin. While some causes are unknown, the known causes of phlebitis include:

- Injury
- Infection
- Sedentary lifestyle
- Prolonged inactivity
- Poor circulation

- IV medications
- Pregnancy
- Obesity
- Blood clot (thrombophlebitis)

Symptoms include warmth and red coloration at the affected site, which also can feel hardened and tender, as well as swelling, pain, and a burning sensation. Women can experience what is known as "milk leg," which is phlebitis of the lower leg after giving birth and milk production begins.

12-23a Diagnosing and Treating Phlebitis

Phlebitis can be diagnosed with an ultrasound to find any blockage present. A venogram might be performed to inspect small vessels, such as those in distal regions of the body. Another way to look for clots is by using a **D-dimer test** to check the patient's blood for the presence of a fibrin degradation product (FDP), which would be present in the blood as a blood clot is broken down (fibrinolysis).

Superficial (surface) vein phlebitis can be treated by taking analgesics for pain and NSAIDs for inflammation, while a warm compress can be placed on the site to increase blood flow to that area. The patient should keep the affected extremity elevated above the heart to prevent edema and increase venous return to the heart with the help of gravity. Patients might be given compression stockings to help improve venous return from the legs.

12-24 DEEP VEIN THROMBOSIS

If the inflammation of phlebitis forms into a clot, it is called **thrombophlebitis**. It is not likely for a clot to break loose in superficial phlebitis, but it is more likely to occur in deep veins. When a clot develops there, it is called a **deep vein thrombosis (DVT)** as shown in Figure 12-23. This can be serious because the

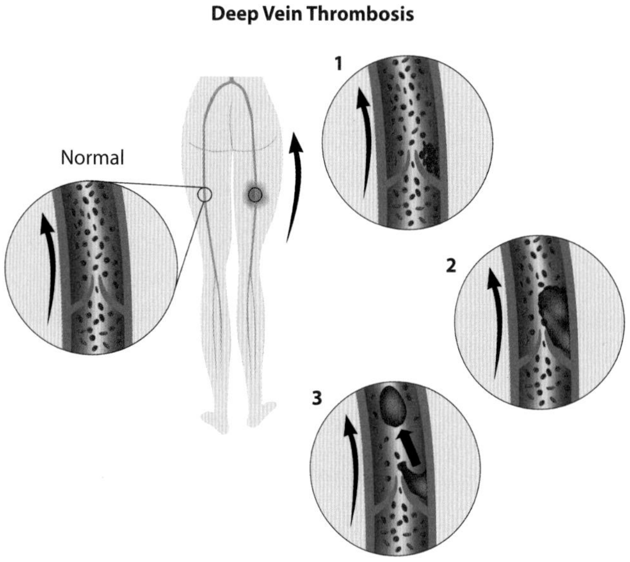

FIGURE 12-23 Deep vein thrombosis (DVT).

clot can break fee (embolus) and travel throughout the bloodstream and lodge in the lungs (pulmonary embolus) or brain (cerebral embolus).

Many factors increase the odds of forming a DVT and include many that also cause phlebitis. The causes of a DVT are as follows:

- Varicose veins: Veins that have a distorted appearance commonly seen on the surface of the legs. These veins are more likely to develop a thrombus because of their abnormal structure.
- Dehydration: When the body's fluid volume is low, the blood becomes more viscous or thicker.
- Prolonged immobility: One of the reasons a postsurgical patient begins walking as soon as possible is that ambulation (walking) helps to decrease the likelihood of a clot developing. Even sitting in a vehicle or plane for long periods of time increases the risk.
- Obesity: Obesity causes changes in the patient's venous blood flow because of increased pressure put on the veins.
- Pregnancy: Pregnancy causes changes in the patient's venous blood flow because of increased pressure in the veins.
- Smoking: Alters circulation and clotting ability.

Goals in treating DVTs are to stop the clot from becoming larger and to keep the clot from breaking loose causing an embolism. After treatment, the next goal is to prevent this condition from recurring. Various agents such as platelet inhibitors, anticoagulants, and thrombolytics are used to treat and prevent clots from occurring.

12-25 BLOOD THINNERS

Blood thinners do not actually make the blood thinner, but they increase the time it takes for blood to clot. Blood thinners can be broken down into two main groups, anticoagulants and antiplatelets.

12-25a Anticoagulants

Anticoagulants prevent the blood from coagulating by chemically altering the clotting factors. They also increase the time it takes for clotting to occur. Different types of anticoagulants work in different ways.

Coumarins and *indandiones* inhibit vitamin K from playing its role in clotting blood. Patients are told not to eat leafy green vegetables that are high in vitamin K because it would reverse the effect of these drugs. An example drug of this group is Coumadin (warfarin).

Factor Xa inhibitors block the ability of the clotting Xa factor to initiate the prothrombin and thrombin that cause a clot. This group does not interfere with vitamin K, so leafy greens are not contraindicated.

Drugs in this group are:

- Xarelto (rivaroxaban)
- Savaysa (edoxaban)
- Eliquis (apixaban)
- Arixtra (fondaparinux)

Heparin is another type of anticoagulant that works by interfering with factor Xa and thrombin through the activation of antithrombin III. There are two types of heparin: high molecular weight and low molecular weight. High-molecular-weight heparin requires daily monitoring to check the patient's activated partial thromboplastin time (aPTT) or clotting time. Low-molecular-weight heparin does not need to be monitored daily. Two common examples of heparin agents are:

- Lovenox (enoxaparin)
- Fragmin (dalteparin)

Thrombin inhibitors are anticoagulants that bind to thrombin in the blood and take away its ability to form clots. Examples are:

- Pradaxa (dabigatran)
- Angiomax (bivalirudin)

12-25b Platelet Inhibitor Therapy

These agents inhibit the ability of the blood's platelets to clump together, which is known as platelet aggregation. **Antiplatelet drugs** inhibit the release of thromboxane, which is the substance that signals platelets to stick together in a certain area to form a clot. By blocking thromboxane, the platelets can no longer stick together. Antiplatelet drugs are given to patients during and after certain procedures, such as angioplasty and coronary stenting, to prevent clot and emboli formation.

Antiplatelet medication is administered to patients who have diseases that increase the risk of clots developing, such as coronary artery disease or peripheral vascular disease. Table 12-11 lists examples of antiplatelet drugs.

12-25c Thrombolytic Drugs (Clot Busters)

Thrombolytic agents are used to dissolve existing clots by liquefying the fibrin that forms the clot. In the body, a natural peptide known as tissue plasminogen activator (t-pa) triggers fibrinolysis, or clot breakdown. Thrombolytic drugs increase this action. They do nothing to prevent clot formation, but will dissolve clots that are already formed.

Table 12-11 Commonly used antiplatelet drugs

BRAND NAME	GENERIC NAME
Ecotrin, Fosprin, others	Aspirin
Plavix	Clopidogrel
Persantine	Dipyridamole
Ticlid	Ticlopidine

Examples of these medications are:

- reteplase (Retavase)
- alteplase (Activase)

12-26 VARICOSE VEINS

To many people, **varicose veins** are an unsightly cosmetic issue, but there is more to this condition than meets the eye. Appearing blue because they carry dark deoxygenated blood, varicose veins are distorted, dilated vessels that usually occur in the legs and feet, but can affect any vein. This deformity slows blood flow back to the heart and allows it to pool or stagnate, increasing the chances of developing a blood clot. For blood to flow efficiently, the veins must be able to close the small one-way valves to keep blood from going backward. See Figure 12-24.

Varicose veins can be caused by pressure being put on the veins, such as by an occupation that requires standing for long periods of time. Another potential cause is obesity since the extra weight adds more pressure on the veins.

During pregnancy, the mother has more blood for the fetus and the body sends less blood to the legs, enhancing the chance of developing varicose veins. Heredity is another cause, as is the process of aging, which makes the veins less elastic and therefore weaker and not able to push the blood forward in the correct direction. This pooling of blood stretches out the veins.

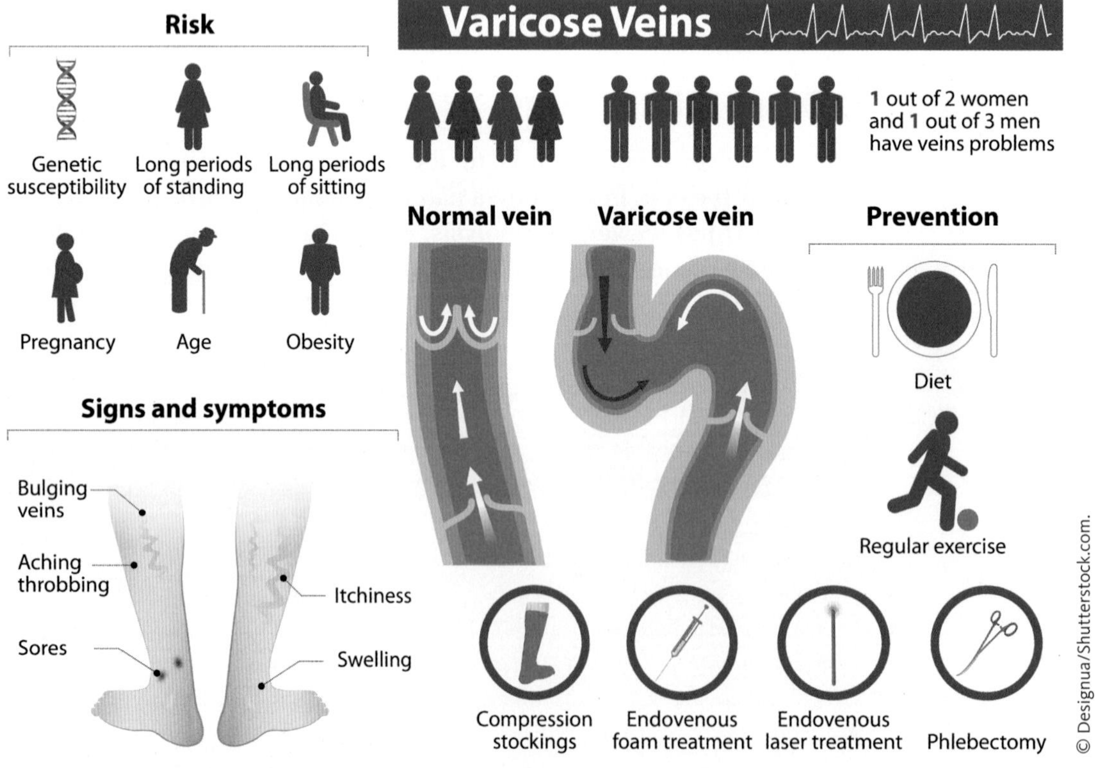

FIGURE 12-24 Varicose veins.

12-26a Diagnosis and Treatment of Varicose Veins

A patient notices changes in his or her veins gradually. The veins might become harder and thicker than normal, and the person might have a fatigue feeling in his or her legs. What many people associate with varicose veins is the distorted shape and bluish-purple coloration. Unfortunately, patients might develop other signs and symptoms, including different forms of pain and irritation such as burning, itching, throbbing, and aching.

As the contorted veins have trouble allowing blood to flow easily, the blood becomes congested and fluid begins to accumulate in the area of the varicose veins. This causes *stasis dermatitis* to develop, which is a thickening of the skin that appears to be a dark, scaly, and dry skin patch. As tiny hemorrhages occur under the skin, blood leaks out into the surrounding connective tissue giving the skin a brown color. Patients can develop ulcerations from this condition that are difficult to heal, and ultimately might result in amputation.

Diagnosing varicose veins is rather simple because they can be seen easily, but to determine how well blood flows through these veins, a Doppler ultrasound is used.

Varicose veins have many treatment options, starting with self-care to reduce the pressure. Options include:

- Weight loss by dieting and exercising
- Elevating the feet
- Not standing or sitting for long periods of time
- Wearing compression stockings to help assist blood flow.

If self-care techniques are not enough, specific procedures can be done. Laser therapies can seal off the affected veins. Sclerotherapy involves injecting a substance into the vein, causing a scar that seals it off. Injecting a foam solution into the varicose vein also can close it off.

There is no medication to correct the distorted vessels. However, analgesics and NSAIDs may be used to control pain and inflammation.

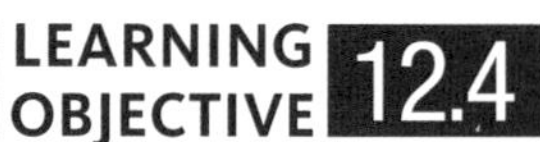

Explain diseases of the heart and related medications.

KEY TERMS

Angina pectoris Chest pain caused by decreased oxygenation to the heart muscle.

Arrhythmia Abnormal heartbeat.

Asystole Condition with no electrical heart activity and therefore no heart beat.

Bradycardia Heartbeat that is slower than normal.

Cardiomyopathy Disease of the heart muscle.

Carditis Inflammation of the heart.

Congestive heart failure (CHF) Fluid builds up in tissues around the heart because of heart failure.

Cor pulmonale Lung disease that leads to right-sided heart failure.

Dilated cardiomyopathy The left ventricle becomes stretched and enlarged, causing the heart not to beat properly.

Hypertrophic cardiomyopathy Condition in which a chamber of the heart becomes enlarged without a specific cause.

Inotropic agents Drugs that change the heart's contraction. Positive inotropic agents increase the heart's contractility, while negative inotropic agents cause the heart to have a weaker contraction.

Myocardial infarction (heart attack) Also known as a heart attack; can be caused by a blockage of blood flow to the heart muscle.

Polycythemia Increased number of red blood cells in the blood.

Restrictive cardiomyopathy Disease in which the ventricle walls are too stiff, not allowing the heart walls to expand as it should.

Rheumatic heart disease Heart disease caused by rheumatic fever that damages the heart valves.

Stable angina Stable and predictable chest pain caused by exertion and relieved with medication or rest.

Tachycardia Faster than normal heart rate.

Unstable angina Chest pain that has a longer duration than a stable angina and is not caused by exertion. It is not likely to be relieved by medicine.

Valvular heart disease Any condition or disease that affects the heart valves.

Variant angina (Prinzmetal's angina) A severe pain brought on by the temporary spasm of a coronary artery; treated with medicine.

12-27 INTRODUCTION TO THE HEART

Now that we have covered the anatomy of the cardiovascular system and discussed the various diagnostic tests and the many diseases that are known to affect the veins and arteries, let's take a look at the heart itself.

Carditis is a basic term used to describe inflammation of the heart. Various types of inflammation that affect the heart are pericarditis, myocarditis, and endocarditis. They can be caused by viruses, bacteria, and other diseases.

- Pericarditis: Inflammation of the pericardium, the sac covering the heart. Signs and symptoms associated with this condition are chest pain, decreased heart rate, or low-grade fever.
- Myocarditis: Inflammation of the heart muscle. Signs and symptoms include chest pain, fever, lightheadedness, edema in the lower extremities, tachycardia, arrhythmias, and fatigue.
- Endocarditis: Inflammation of the inner lining of the heart, including the outside surface of the heart valves. Signs and symptoms include shortness of breath; edema of the legs, feet, and abdomen; chest pain, nausea, fever, sweating at night, achy joints, and heart murmur.

Diagnosis starts with a history and physical. During auscultation of the heart, a murmur might be heard, indicating a backflow of blood. An EKG might uncover the presence of an arrhythmia; blood can be tested to determine levels of chemicals, enzymes, and proteins; and imaging studies, such as a chest X-ray, echocardiogram, CT, and MRI scan, can be done.

Carditis is treated with pain relievers such as aspirin and ibuprofen, antibiotics if an infection is present, and antipyretics to reduce any fever.

12-28 ANGINA PECTORIS

Angina pectoris is chest pain that is experienced from lack of oxygen to the heart muscle because of a blockage of blood flow as by atherosclerosis. Anginas can be acute or chronic and might be an indicator that a heart attack or myocardial infarction (MI) is pending.

Symptoms of angina are:

- Chest pain
- Pain radiating into the arms, neck, shoulder, jaw, and back
- Fatigue
- Dizziness
- Shortness of breath
- Diaphoresis
- Nausea
- Chest pain during exertion, stress, and digestion after a big meal

The three different types of angina have their own characteristics.

Stable angina occurs after exertion and is similar or the same as previous chest pain the patient might have experienced in the past. Stable angina usually lasts about 5 minutes and dissipates after using medication such as nitroglycerin, or after the patient stops the exertion.

Unstable angina lasts longer than 5 minutes, in fact, it can last up to a half-hour. This pain occurs without exertion. Unstable angina is not similar to other chest pain felt before, and medication is not likely to stop the pain. If this type of angina occurs, the person should seek medical attention immediately because a heart attack is likely to occur soon.

Variant angina (Prinzmetal's angina) is severe and can happen without exertion. It is caused by a sudden coronary artery spasm, causing the artery to narrow momentarily. This angina can be treated with medication.

12-28a Diagnosis and Treatment of Angina

Diagnosis begins with a physical examination. Procedures and tests used are an EKG, echocardiogram, CT scan of the heart, chest X-ray, blood tests, and coronary angiography, to list a few.

Invasive procedures can be done, such as inserting a stent to prevent the vessel from narrowing or closing or coronary bypass surgery to correct the cause of decreased blood flow to the heart muscle.

Medications that can be used are:

- Nitroglycerin to vasodilate coronary arteries to increase blood flow and decrease the work of the heart
- Antiplatelet agents to prevent platelets from sticking together forming a clot
- Beta blockers to decrease blood pressure and heart workload
- Calcium channel blockers to decrease blood pressure by slowing the conduction of the AV node
- Statins to decrease cholesterol

12-29 MYOCARDIAL INFARCTION

In order to function properly, a continuous supply of blood must carry nutrients and oxygen to the heart muscle. This is accomplished by two coronary arteries that split into smaller branches. When these branches or arteries become blocked, that region of the heart is starved of oxygen and nutrients and will die. The dead tissue, called an infarct, will never be regenerated or replaced with new tissue. See Figure 12-25.

12-29a Diagnosis and Treating Myocardial Infarction

Symptoms of **myocardial infarction (heart attack)** vary based on the extent of the heart attack and the patient's gender. Men experience the classic signs and symptoms more often than women. Classic signs and symptoms are chest pain (angina), crushing or pressure sensation in the chest, diaphoresis (sweating), shortness of breath, light-headedness, and nausea. Women tend to note pain in their left arm and shoulder, neck, and jaw.

To discover if a patient had a heart attack, an EKG is taken, and a patient history and physical are done. Blood is drawn to check for certain enzymes that are released during a heart attack, such as troponin and creatinine phosphokinase.

Treatment can involve a stenting procedure of the affected coronary artery or, if needed, open heart surgery to perform a coronary bypass. Drugs are also a large part of treating a heart attack. They are as follows:

- Oxygen is used to decrease the work of the heart and decrease the respiratory rate.
- Nitroglycerin is used to vasodilate blood vessels and decrease the work of the heart.

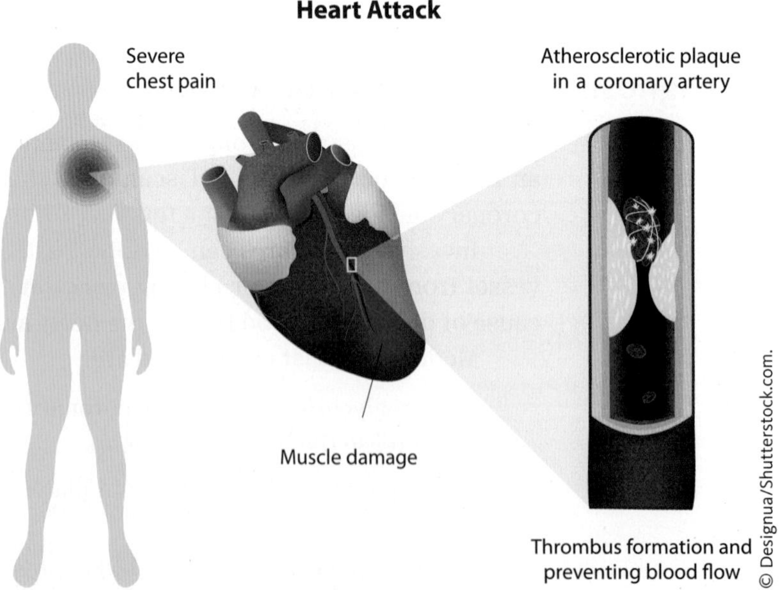

FIGURE 12-25 This image shows a blockage of a coronary artery leading to a lack of blood and oxygen to heart tissue causing a heart attack.

- Beta blocker is used to decrease blood pressure.
- Angiotensin-converting enzyme inhibitors (ACEIs) are used to decrease blood pressure.
- Anticoagulants are used to prevent clotting.
- Antiplatelet agents are used to prevent platelets from sticking together to form a clot.
- Thrombolytic drugs are used to dissolve existing clots.

12-30 RHEUMATIC HEART DISEASE

Rheumatic heart disease is a condition caused by a complication of the *streptococcus* bacteria that cause rheumatic fever. The body makes antibodies to fight this infection, but the antibodies cause an inflammatory disorder that attacks the heart valves. This causes the heart to work harder to compensate and eventually can lead to heart failure. Symptoms might not develop until 10–20 years after the initiating illness.

Symptoms vary by individuals; however, signs and symptoms include:

- Shortness of breath
- Fever
- Swollen, achy joints
- Chest pain
- Weakness
- Lattice-like rash

12-30a Diagnosis and Treatment of Rheumatic Heart Disease

A patient history and physical, coupled with a blood test to check for the presence of tropomyosin, which is a cardiac antibody, can lead to this diagnosis. A chest X-ray can be done to check the size of the heart, along with an echocardiogram to check the flow of blood through the heart to look for leaky valves. An MRI also can check the heart's valves. An EKG can be check for any discrepancy in the heart's electrical activity. Auscultation of the heart will reveal a murmuring sound caused by the leaky valves.

Treatment involves antibiotics, such as penicillin or erythromycin. Surgical procedures can be done to help correct the damaged valves.

12-31 VALVULAR HEART DISEASE

Valvular heart disease refers to any disease that causes one of the four heart valves to malfunction, see Figure 12-26. The four valves are the tricuspid and pulmonary valve on the right side of the heart, and the mitral and aortic valves on the left. These valves are supposed to prevent the blood from flowing backward in the wrong direction. If blood deviates, even just a little bit, it will cause the heart to work harder than it should to pump blood. When this is present, an abnormal heart sound called a murmur can be heard with a stethoscope.

In addition to rheumatic fever, congenital malformations are another common cause of valvular disease.

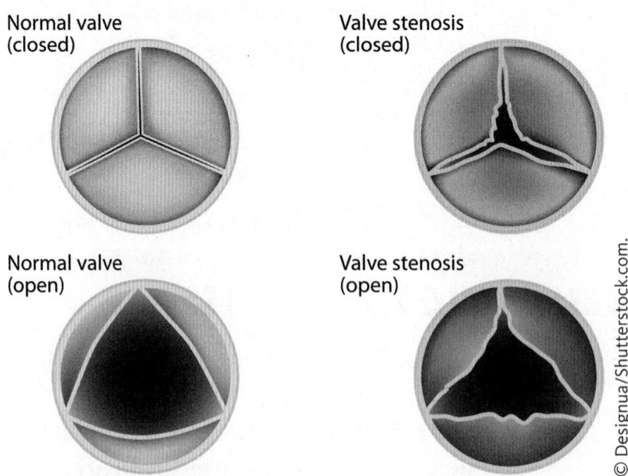

FIGURE 12-26 Comparison between a normal valve and a valve with stenosis.

Valvular stenosis (stenosis = narrow) occurs if blood flow is restricted by a valve that does not open as it should and instead is narrowed, see Figure 12-26. On the other hand, a valve might be opening too much and not be able to close right away, which also causes problems with blood flow. When valves do not operate properly, the heart has to work much harder and might begin to fail, resulting in congestive heart failure or allowing blood clots to develop.

Some patients affected by valvular heart disease might not have any signs or symptoms, while others notice signs and symptoms that develop over time. The signs and symptoms might not indicate the severity of the condition. Some of the possible signs and symptoms are:

- Lightheadedness
- Fatigue
- Fever
- Shortness of breath
- Chest pain
- Palpations
- Murmur
- Syncope (fainting)
- Edema in the abdomen, ankle, and feet

12-31a Diagnosis and Treatment of Heart Valve Disease

Diagnosis is made, first by auscultation for any abnormal heart activity. An electrocardiogram can be taken to study the rhythm of the heart. A chest X-ray can give clinicians an idea about the shape of the structures, such as an enlarged heart. Calcium deposits, which can occur with valvular insufficiency, can be seen on the radiograph.

The best way to check for any valve issues is to have an echocardiogram, which will show the direction and speed of blood flow through the heart. If there is a valvular dysfunction, the severity of the condition can be determined with a CT scan. Another method to check the heart's valvular dysfunction is with a cardiac catheterization. Finally, a stress test can be used to study the heart valve function with exertion.

Treatment varies depending on the severity of the condition. If it is severe and interfering with the function of the heart, surgical repair or replacement will be required. However, the condition might only need to be observed and treated with medication. If caused by a bacterial infection as with rheumatic fever, for example, antibiotics are given. In addition, to prevent blood clots, anticoagulants are given. See Figure 12-26.

12-32 HEART FAILURE AND CONGESTIVE HEART FAILURE

Heart failure can occur on the left or right sides. Left heart failure occurs when the left side of the heart cannot pump blood out to the body as well as it should, as shown in Figure 12-27. This results in the left ventricle (LV) becoming enlarged and stiff, causing poor function.

Right-sided heart failure usually occurs as a result of left-sided heart failure because of increased fluid that backs up into the lungs. This causes the right ventricle, which has to pump into the now congested lungs, to fail and causes blood to back up throughout the body.

Congestive heart failure (CHF) occurs when blood flow leaving the heart has been slowed, and veins taking blood back to the heart back up. This results in congestion of the body's tissues, which presents as edema or swelling in the lower extremities and lungs (pulmonary edema). With proper care and ongoing treatment, this congestion can be resolved.

Symptoms are:

- Shortness of breath
- Tachypnea (high respiratory rate)
- Tachycardia (high heart rate)

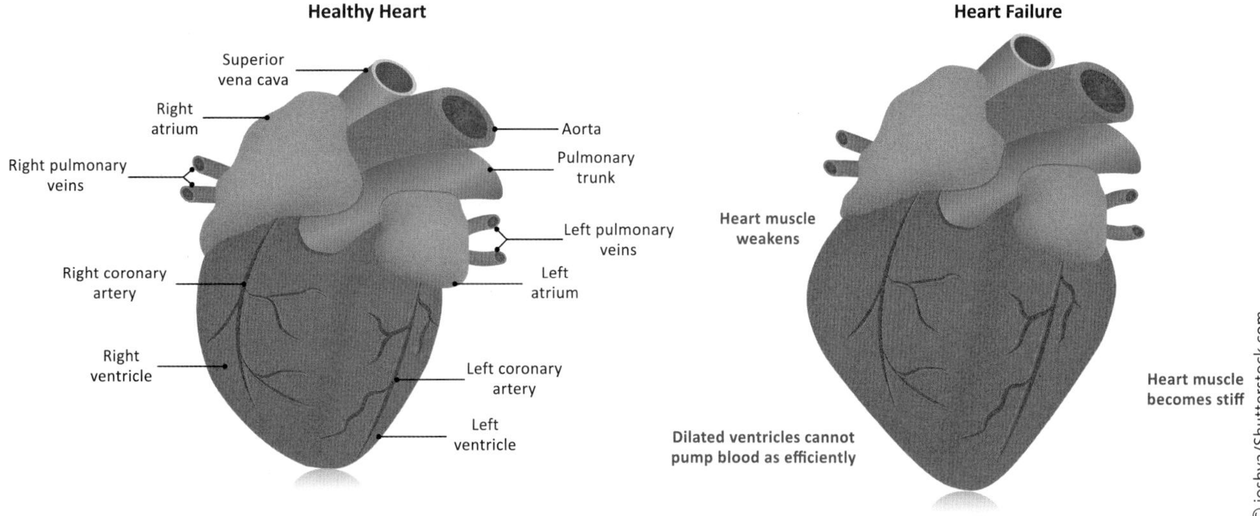

FIGURE 12-27 Heart failure.

- Neck veins distended from fluid back-up
- Liver engorged from fluid backing up (when right heart failure is present)
- Ascites from fluid accumulated in the abdomen
- Pulmonary edema (when left heart failure is present)
- Frothy white- or pink-colored secretions

The congestion subsides with medical intervention, and the patient receives additional treatment to prevent the heart failure condition from worsening again.

12-32a Diagnosis and Treatment of Heart Failure

History and physical are often enough to diagnose the patient as being in heart failure. However, after the patient is stabilized, further testing can be done to confirm the diagnosis. A chest X-ray will show heart enlargement and congestion (fluid) around the heart, vessels, and in the lungs. An EKG is used to check for arrhythmias, and an echocardiogram can check the valve function.

For CHF, the patient is given diuretics such as Lasix to remove the accumulated fluid. In addition, oxygen is given to help decrease the work of the heart as well as beta blockers to help slow the heart rate. **Inotropic agents** such as Lanoxin (digoxin) increase the strength of the heart's contraction to make it beat more efficiently. In addition, angiotensin-converting inhibitors can be used to cause vasodilation and decrease the work of the heart.

12-33 COR PULMONALE

Cor pulmonale (cor = heart and pulmonale = lungs) is literally a heart condition caused by bad lungs. Other terms used for this condition are pulmonary heart disease and right heart failure.

This condition occurs when the right side of the heart fails from an acute or chronic pulmonary disease that causes increased pulmonary pressure against which the right heart must pump. This causes hypertrophy or enlargement of the right ventricle, making it function improperly. In addition, the existing lung disease causes low levels of oxygen in the blood. The body responds by making more red blood cells because the tissues are not getting enough oxygen. However, this increased production of RBCs makes the blood thicker (increased viscosity) and causes a condition called **polycythemia**. This makes the heart have to work harder to pump the extra cells throughout the body. The blood eventually will back up into the veins in the patient's neck, and the liver will become engorged with blood.

People with this disease may experience the following signs and symptoms:

- Cyanosis (bluish coloration) of the lips and fingertips
- Chest pain
- Edema (swelling) of the lower extremities
- Syncope (fainting)
- Shortness of breath
- Headaches

12-33a Diagnosis and Treatment of Cor Pulmonale

Diagnosis can be made by:

- Patient history of prior lung disease
- CT scan
- MRI
- Electrocardiogram
- Echocardiogram
- Chest X-ray
- Arterial blood gas (ABG), in which a sample of blood is taken from the artery to check the patient's oxygen and carbon dioxide levels

Drugs used to help treat this disease are:

- Blood thinners used as a prophylactic measure to prevent blood clots
- Diuretics to remove excess fluid
- Vasodilators to increase blood flow
- Inotropic agents such as digoxin (Lanoxin) to increase the strength of heart contractions

12-34 CARDIOMYOPATHY

Cardiomyopathy means any disease of the heart muscle and refers to conditions that affect the heart's muscle. These diseases make it very difficult for the heart to function properly and come in two main types.

Primary cardiomyopathy is idiopathic, or, in other words, the patient does not have existing conditions that would cause a diseased heart muscle. Secondary cardiomyopathy is caused by a disease or substance (drug). Secondary cardiomyopathy has three main types: dilated, hypertrophic, and restrictive.

- **Dilated cardiomyopathy** is when a heart chamber is dilated or stretched. When the heart's left ventricle is enlarged and weakened, it cannot function efficiently, eventually leading to heart failure. Dilated cardiomyopathy is the most common of the secondary cardiomyopathies.
- **Hypertrophic cardiomyopathy** is present when the heart muscle has become thicker and might cause the heart valves to leak in time. Hypertrophic cardiomyopathy is the most uncommon form of secondary cardiomyopathy.
- **Restrictive cardiomyopathy** is present when both the left and right ventricles become less compliant or stiff.

See Figure 12-28 for an illustration of heart muscle diseases.

Symptoms of cardiomyopathy include:

- Shortness of breath
- Weakness
- Fatigue
- Swelling of the lower extremities

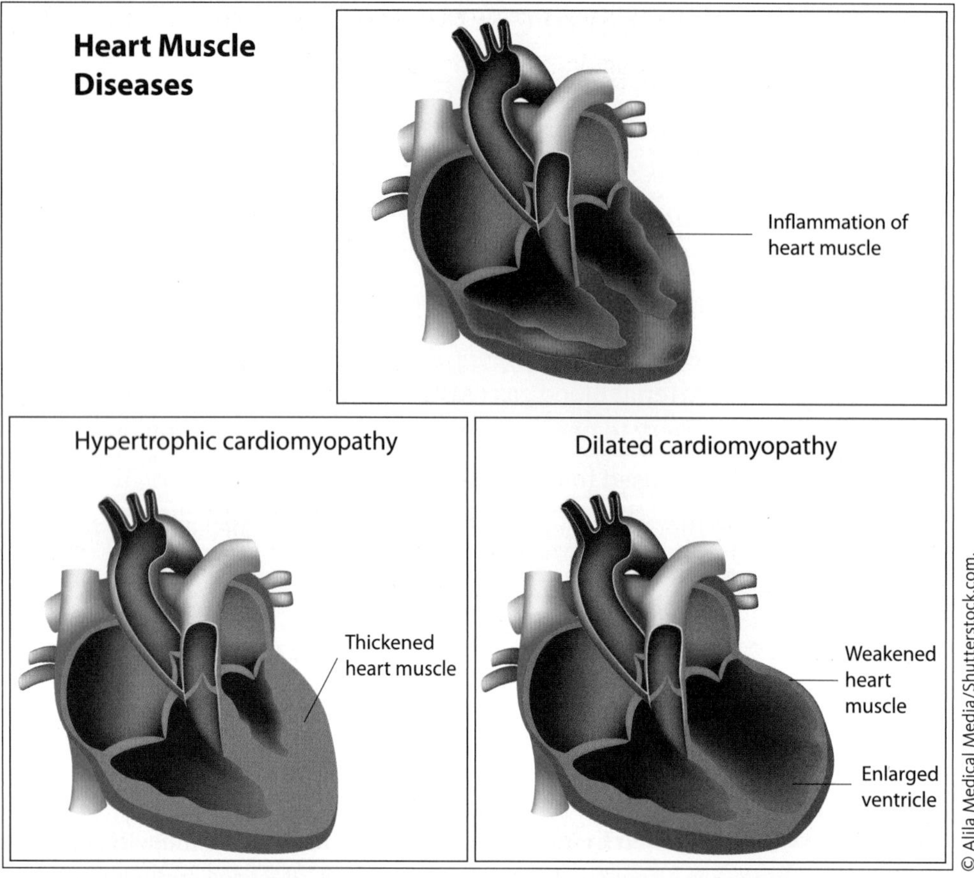

FIGURE 12-28 This image shows the difference between hypertrophic cardiomyopathy and dilated cardiomyopathy.

- Chest pain
- Palpitations
- Syncope (fainting)

12-34a Treatment and Diagnosis of Cardiomyopathy

To diagnose cardiomyopathy, certain procedures can be done to evaluate the patient. Common methods are as follows:

- History and physical
- Blood testing
- EKG
- CXR
- MRI
- CT
- Ultrasound
- Nuclear imaging
- Cardiac catheterization

Common drugs that can be used to treat cardiomyopathy include:

- Anticoagulants to prevent clotting
- Diuretics to decrease excess fluid
- ACEIs to decrease blood pressure/workload
- Beta blockers to decrease blood pressure/workload
- Calcium channel blockers to decrease blood pressure by slowing conduction of the heart
- Corticosteroids to decrease inflammation
- Angiotensin II receptor blockers to decrease blood pressure/workload

12-35 ARRHYTHMIAS

An **arrhythmia** is when the heart does not beat as it should because of an abnormal electrical impulse. When this occurs, the heart is out of synch and cannot pump blood efficiently. Arrhythmias can be caused by cardiovascular disease, ischemia, and medications.

Before discussing some common types of arrhythmias, let's look at a normal heart rate, which is 60–100 beats per minute. Athletes who train and exercise on a regular basis can condition their body to work more efficiently, so a heart rate of 50 beats per minute might be their normal.

Tachycardia is when the heart beats faster than it should while at rest. With activity, a faster heart rate is normal but an arrhythmia is present if it occurs at rest. A tachyarrhythmia means that the heart is not only out of its normal conduction rhythm, but also is beating too fast at rest (greater than 100 beats per minute). If not treated promptly, complications such as stroke or a heart attack might arise. Drugs that can be used to control tachycardia are beta blockers, calcium channel blockers, and antiarrhythmic agents (used to treat abnormal heart activity).

Bradycardia is present when the resting heart rate is less than 60 beats per minute. While bradycardia might not cause any problems with some people, it can have an effect on how well the body is being oxygenated. If the heart is unable to pump fast enough, a pacemaker might be inserted into the patient to correct the issue. The drug atropine sulfate is an injection that is used to increase the patient's heart rate. Atropine is an anticholinergic medication that works by inhibiting the vagus nerve in the parasympathetic nervous system. Stimulation of the vagus nerve slows the heart; blocking it speeds up the heart rate.

Asystole is when the heart is not producing any electrical activity and has stopped working (no heart beat is present). This life-threatening event requires quick action to get the heart pumping to circulate oxygen throughout the body. To help the heart begin pumping again, cardiopulmonary resuscitation (CPR) and electrical defibrillation can be used, as well as medication. Epinephrine is used to stimulate both the rate and the force of contraction of the heart to help increase the blood flow to the heart and brain.

Module 13

Pathopharmacology of the Nervous System

Module Introduction

The nervous and endocrine systems are the body's control center. Unlike the endocrine system, however, the nervous system works at lightning speed. The nervous system must continuously monitor the body and the environment and make the needed changes to maintain homeostasis, often at a level of which we are not even aware.

The nervous system is composed of the **central nervous system (CNS)** and the **peripheral nervous system (PNS)**. The CNS is composed of the brain and spinal cord; the PNS represents all the nerves lying outside of the brain and spinal cord as shown in Figure 13-1.

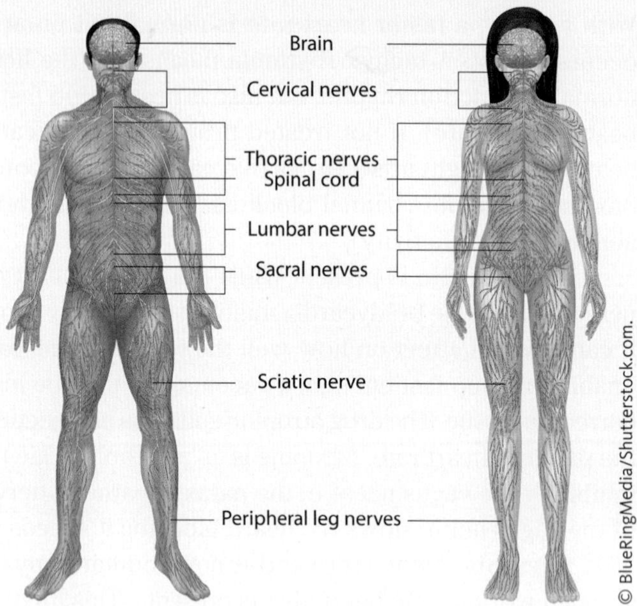

FIGURE 13-1 The central nervous system consists of the brain and spinal cord. The peripheral nervous system consists of all nerves outside the brain and spinal cord.

LEARNING OBJECTIVE 13.1 Explain the normal anatomy and physiology of the nervous system.

KEY TERMS

Autonomic nervous system Involuntary portion of peripheral nervous system whose output controls cardiac muscle, smooth muscle, and glands.

Axon Long portion of the neuron that transmits the received signal.

Brain stem Stalk-like structure inferior to the cerebrum that contains the medulla oblongata, midbrain, and pons.

Central nervous system (CNS) The portion of nervous system composed of the brain and spinal cord.

Cerebellum Located posterior to the brain stem; plays an important role in sensory and motor coordination and balance.

Cerebral spinal fluid (CSF) Specialized fluid that bathes and protects the brain and spinal cord.

Chemical neurotransmitter Chemical substance such as acetylcholine that can carry the signal on to the next nerve, gland, skeletal, smooth, or cardiac muscle.

Cranial nerves 12 pairs of nerves associated with the brain that conduct information to (sensory) and from (motor) the brain.

Dendrites Branching portions of neuron that receive information from the environment or from other cells.

Frontal lobes Section of the brain responsible for motor activities, conscious thought, and speech.

Glial cells Support tissue for the nervous system that lines cavities and provides functions such as producing myelin.

Insula Section of the brain located deep inside the temporal lobe that coordinates information from the autonomic nervous system.

Limbic system Series of nuclei in the cerebrum and superior brain stem involved in mood, emotion, and memory.

Medulla oblongata Section of the brainstem continuous with the spinal cord that controls heartbeat, breathing, and blood pressure.

Meninges Protective membranes of the brain and spinal cord.

Meningitis Viral or bacterial inflammation of the protective coverings of the brain and spinal cord.

Midbrain Superior section of brain stem that acts as a two-way conduction pathway to relay visual and auditory impulses to the cerebrum.

Motor system Portion of the nervous system that sends orders to skeletal, smooth, and cardiac muscles and to the body's glands.

Multiple sclerosis Neural disease that causes destruction of myelin sheath of neurons.

Myelin Lipid insulation produced by Schwann cells that line the neurons.

Neuroglia Support tissue for the nervous system.

Neurons Nerve fibers that transmit signals in the nervous system.

Occipital lobes Section of the brain responsible for vision.

Parasympathetic branch Division of the autonomic nervous system dedicated to maintenance activities of normal body functions.

Parietal lobes Section of the brain involved with body senses and speech.

Peripheral nervous system (PNS) The portion of the nervous system composed of all the nerves outside of the brain and spinal cord.

Pons Section of brainstem that plays a role in regulating breathing.

Reticular system Diffuse network of nuclei in the brain stem responsible for bringing the cerebral cortex to conscious awareness of the surroundings.

Sensory system Input portion of nervous system that receives information about the immediate environment.

Somatic nervous system Voluntary portion of peripheral nervous system that controls movements of skeletal muscle.

Spinal cord Structure in the CNS that represents the neural highway upon which nerve signals are transmitted to and from the brain and all parts of the body.

Spinal nerves 31 pair of nerves named for their corresponding vertebrae that travel to various parts of the body.

Sympathetic branch Division of autonomic nervous system known as the fight-or-flight response system; prepares the body for high stress and emergency situations.

Synapse Gap at the end of an axon, also known as the synaptic gap, where the nerve signal can continue on via a chemical neurotransmitter.

Temporal lobes Section of brain involved in hearing, taste, and integration of emotions.

13-1 SENSORY AND MOTOR SYSTEMS

To properly respond to both the external and internal environments, the nervous system relies on its **sensory system**. The sensory system will be covered in more depth in Module 14 with a focus on hearing and seeing. The sensory input comes into the CNS, where it is interpreted by the brain to determine the appropriate response. After the response is determined, the CNS must activate the output or **motor system** to carry out the desired change or action. For example, one of the authors foolishly sniffed an unmarked bottle of fluid while cleaning out a shed. The bottle contained muriatic acid, also known as hydrochloric acid. The sensory system, via the olfactory nerve, sent signals to the brain. The signals were interpreted immediately, and motor output was sent to cough and breathe out forcibly to minimize further damage to the lungs and contain the irritant to the nasal region. The nasal passages healed over time, but if the sensory and motor systems did not coordinate their efforts, severe and permanent lung damage could have occurred.

The motor system relays response orders to skeletal, smooth, and cardiac muscles and to the body's glands telling them how to respond. The motor system is divided into the **somatic nervous system**, whose output controls the voluntary movements of skeletal muscle, and the **autonomic nervous system**, whose output controls cardiac muscle, smooth muscle, and glands. Although the somatic portion is a voluntary system under conscious control, the autonomic system is involuntary and not under conscious control, alleviating, for example, the need to think each time the heart should beat.

13-2 THE AUTONOMIC NERVOUS SYSTEM

The autonomic nervous system has two branches: one dedicated to everyday maintenance activity and the other for emergency situations. The **parasympathetic branch** can be thought of as your "resting and digesting" system, controlling normal body functioning. The **sympathetic branch** is known as the "fight-or-flight" response system, and activates in times of emergency.

Let's use a real-life event to demonstrate the organization of the nervous system. You are walking along the street, and a large dog comes running at you, snarling and barking viciously. Your sensory system quickly gathers information and sends signals to the CNS (through the spinal cord to the brain) that you are in danger. The brain interprets the danger, and the PNS activates the sympathetic nervous system to gear you for "fight or flight." Your cardiac muscles are stimulated to increase heart rate to deliver more oxygen to the skeletal muscles, your pupils dilate to let in more light, the smooth muscle in your airways relaxes so you can breathe faster and deeper, and your mental acuity sharpens. All this is done immediately and without any conscious control on your part. Your motor system is now fully ready for fight or flight. However, the dog's owner miraculously appears and restrains it. You cannot remain in this hyper alert state for long, so now that the danger has passed, the parasympathetic (para means working alongside) brings you "back down" to normal. The parasympathetic responses are the opposite of the sympathetic, and your heart rate slows to normal, your pupils constrict to a normal state, and your lungs return to normal breathing.

13-3 NERVOUS TISSUE

That's a look at the big picture; now let's go to the tissue level. The body has two types of nervous tissues; neuroglia and neurons. **Neuroglia** or **glial cells** can be thought of as the "glue" that holds the nervous system together and supports its functions. The glial cells line cavities and support and protect structures. There are several types of glial cells, but one, in particular, is important to discuss. Schwann cells make a lipid insulation called **myelin** that lines neurons. This insulation, called the *myelin sheath*, is like insulation around a wire carrying electricity. If a crack were to occur in the insulation, the current would short circuit and not be carried through the wire efficiently.

CLINICAL CONNECTION 13.1

MULTIPLE SCLEROSIS

Multiple sclerosis (MS) is a neural disease that causes scarring and destruction of the myelin sheath as shown in Figure 13-2. The nerves, which are now exposed, can "short out" and prevent the current from passing farther down the nerve fiber. The disruption of the myelin insulation inhibits the electrical charge, and impulse conduction is slowed or even stopped. Symptoms of multiple sclerosis differ depending where the myelin damage occurs. Patients can have disturbances in vision, balance, speech, or movement. MS is more common in women than in men.

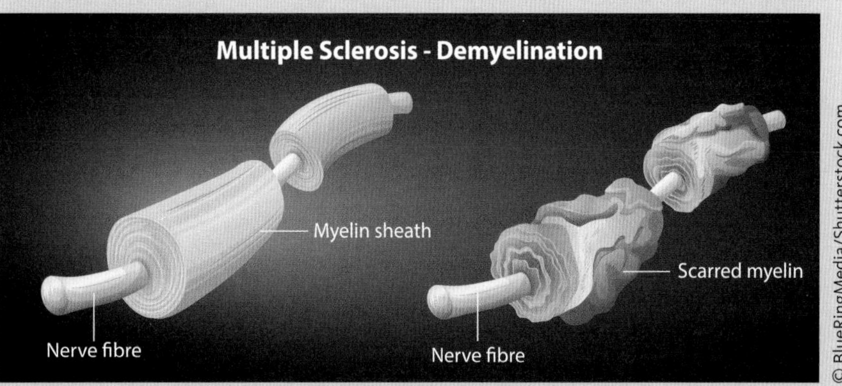

FIGURE 13-2 Normal nerve fiber contrasted to a nerve fiber with myelin sheath damage.

13-4 NEURONS

While glial cells act in a support capacity, **neurons**, or the actual nerve fibers, are signal senders and receivers within the nervous system. A neuron has a special property that makes it an *excitable cell*, meaning it carries a small electrical charge when stimulated. The tiny electrical current that moves through the cell is what sends and receives signals.

Neurons are bizarre-looking cells with many branches and what appears to be a long tail (see Figure 13-3). The neuron cell body deals with support and cell metabolism. The branches or **dendrites** receive information from the environment or other cells, and the cell body of the neuron then generates and sends electrical signals that travel down the **axon**, or long portion of the neuron, until it reaches the *axon terminal.* The axon terminal ends in a gap; a receiving cell is on the other side of the gap.

13-4a Neurochemical Transmission

This combination of axon terminal and receiving cell is called a **synapse** or *synaptic gap.* If the receiving cell is a skeletal muscle cell, then this particular synapse is called the *neuromuscular synapse* or *junction* as discussed in Module 6. A **chemical neurotransmitter** must now carry the signal across the synapse to the receiving cell to elicit a response. Using the angry dog example, the parasympathetic neurons send electrical impulses down the axon that cause the release of the neurochemical acetylcholine (Ach) to bind with receptors in the cardiac muscle to slow the heart rate back to normal after the danger had passed.

Like every process, neurotransmitter release must be regulated and "cleaned" from the synapse, or it will continually bind with the receiving cell and

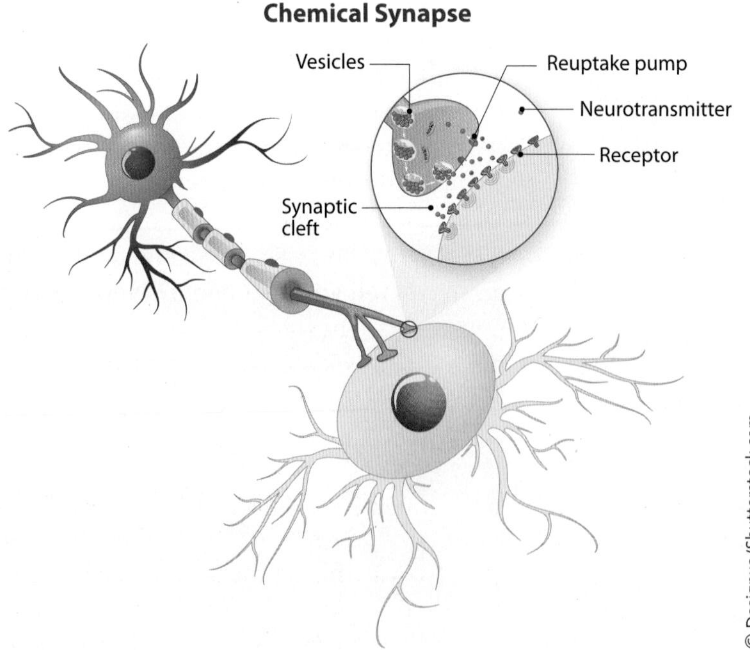

FIGURE 13-3 A neuron and chemical synapse. Chemical neurotransmitters vary according to location in the body.

cause a continual response. Some chemical neurotransmitters, such as norepinephrine, are cleaned up by recycling the neurochemical back into the terminal axon to be stored and awaiting the next electrical stimulus. Some neurotransmitters are cleaned up by being broken down by an inactivator enzyme, as when acetylcholine (ACh) is is broken down by acetylcholinester*ase* (AChE).

CLINICAL CONNECTION 13.2

ANTIDEPRESSANTS

The understanding of chemical synapses has led to several breakthroughs in treating mental illness by modifying neurochemicals at the synapses. One example is the neurotransmitter serotonin. Serotonin elevates your mood, and therefore having more of it can help treat depression. Selective serotonin reuptake inhibitors (SSRIs) are medications that prevent the cleanup of serotonin from synapses, allowing it to stay around longer and in greater concentrations, thereby increasing its effects. Many antidepressants and medications to treat obsessive compulsive disorder and anxiety are SSRIs.

13-5 THE SPINAL CORD AND SPINAL NERVES

All nerve signals need to be routed to the appropriate area, and the main highway these signals travel is the **spinal cord**, which has many exits depending on the area that needs information or action. Ascending tracts of nerves lead up the spinal cord to the brain and carry sensory information about touch, temperature, pain, posture, and position. Descending nerve tracts take motor orders, such as those needed for skeletal muscle movement, from the brain to its respective target. The relatively delicate spinal cord is located in a hollow tube called the vertebral cavity, which surrounds it by bony vertebra for protection The spinal cord is divided into 31 segments, each with a pair of **spinal nerves** named for their corresponding vertebrae, as shown in Figure 13-4a and b.

13-5a Spinal Innervations

These spinal nerves are like a large network of wires, transporting information or orders to the appropriate parts of the body, depending on what vertebrae the wires exit. This neural information superhighway is shown in Figure 13-5. The connections of the nerve to the spinal cord are called innervations, and their location can tell you a lot about where the root of a problem might be. Looking at Figure 13-5, can you tell which vertebral nerves might be affected if someone complains of neck and shoulder pain?

13-6 BRAIN AND CRANIAL NERVES

Sitting on top of the spinal cord, the brain and its associated nerves (aptly called **cranial nerves**) represent the major control system of the nervous system. The brain acts as the main processor and controller of information, while the cranial nerves are the conduits for that information.

The 12 cranial nerves are much more specialized than spinal nerves and are named based on their specialty. Some cranial nerves carry sensory and motor information for the head, face, and neck, whereas others carry visual, auditory,

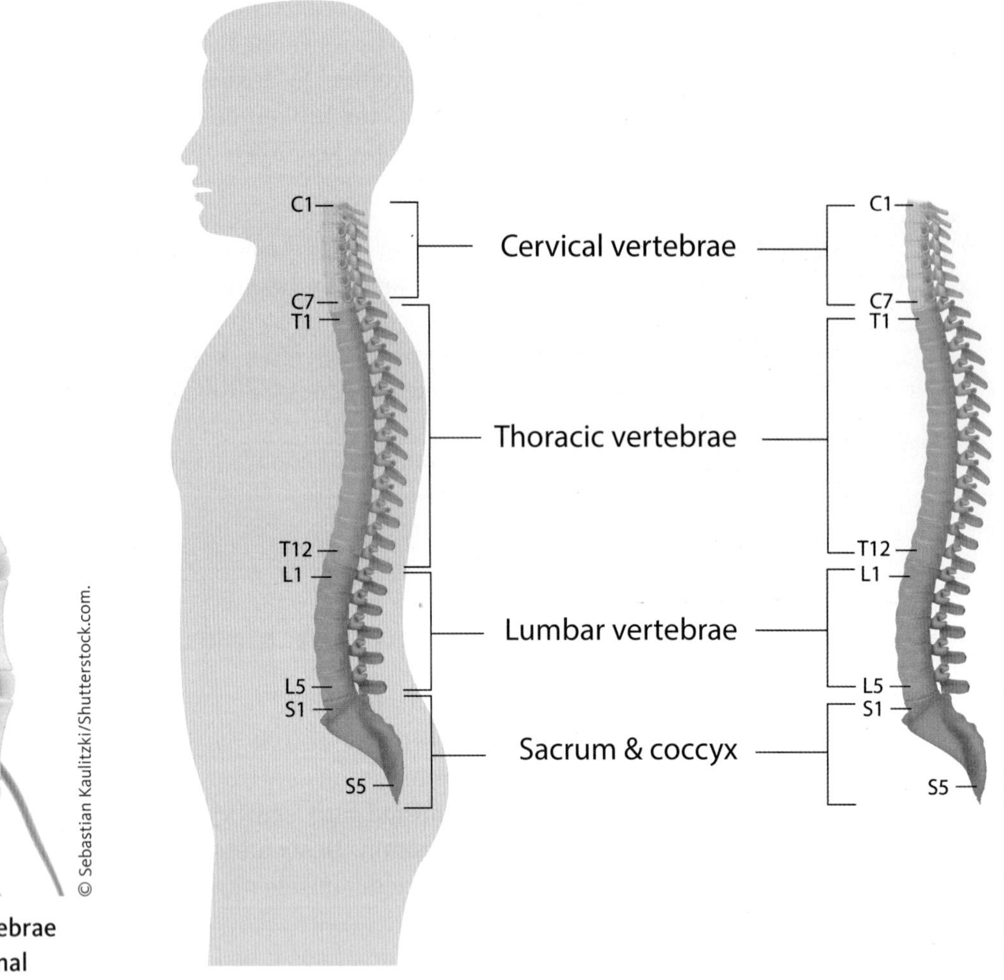

FIGURE 13-4A Vertebrae showing exiting of spinal nerves.

FIGURE 13-4B The various spinal vertebrae and corresponding number.

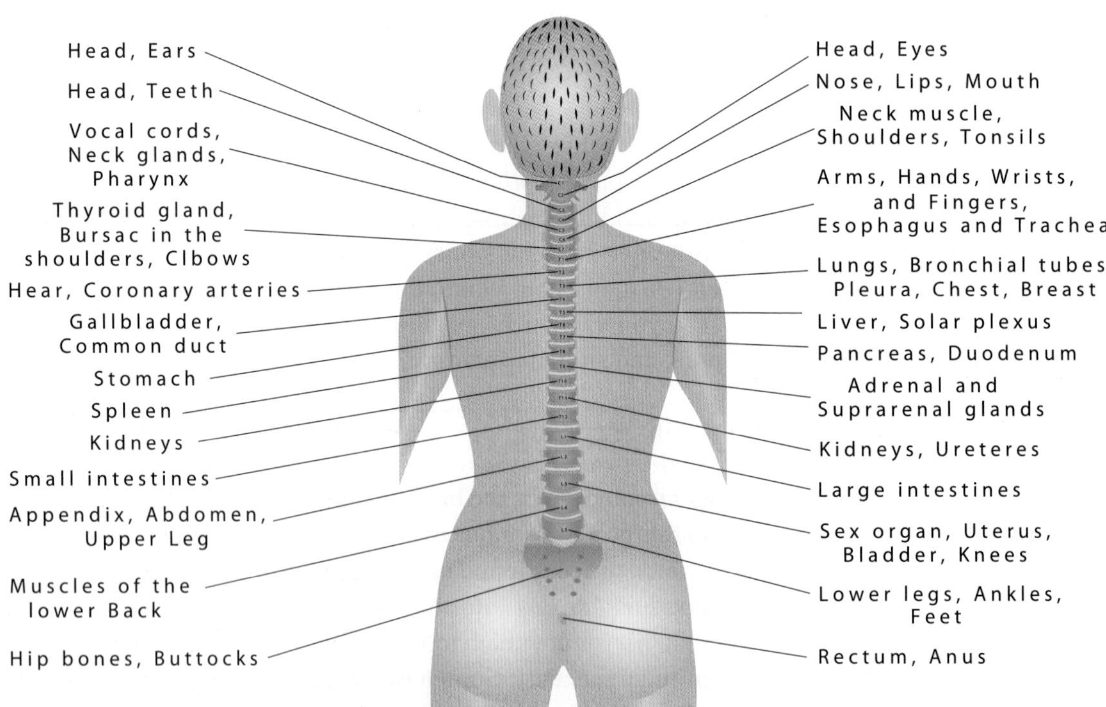

FIGURE 13-5 The nervous innervations of the spinal cord to specific body areas.

Table 13-1 Cranial nerves and their functions

NAME OF NERVE	FUNCTION
Olfactory (I)	Sensory for smell
Optic (II)	Sensory for vision
Oculomotor (III)	Motor for eye movements
Trochlear (IV)	Motor for eye movements
Trigeminal (V)	Sensory for face and motor for chewing
Abducens (VI)	Motor for eye movements
Facial (VII)	Motor for facial movements, sensory for taste
Vestibulocochlear (VIII)	Sensory for hearing and balance
Glossopharyngeal (IX)	Motor for tongue and throat, sensory for taste
Vagus (X)	Motor for heart, lungs, and organs; main parasympathetic nerve
Accessory (XI)	Motor for larynx
Hypoglossal (XII)	Motor for tongue movements

smell, or taste sensations. Table 13-1 lists the cranial nerves and their corresponding functions.

13-7 BRAIN LOBES

The brain consists of several areas and lobes that have specialized functions. For example, Figure 13-6 shows that the brain consists of a cerebrum (main brain), cerebellum, and the brain stem (top portion of the spinal cord).

13-7a Cerebrum

The cerebrum is the largest part of the brain. Its folds and ridges form convolutions to increase the surface area of the brain and still allow it to fit into a relatively small space. Certain deep grooves called *sulci* divide the brain into four large sections called *lobes*. The lobes are named for the skull bones that cover them, and they occur in pairs, one in each hemisphere. The **frontal lobes** are responsible for motor activities, conscious thought, and speech. A major portion of the frontal lobes control personality and impulsiveness, and therefore damage to the frontal lobes can cause personality disorders. The **parietal lobes** are involved with body senses and speech. The **occipital lobes** are responsible

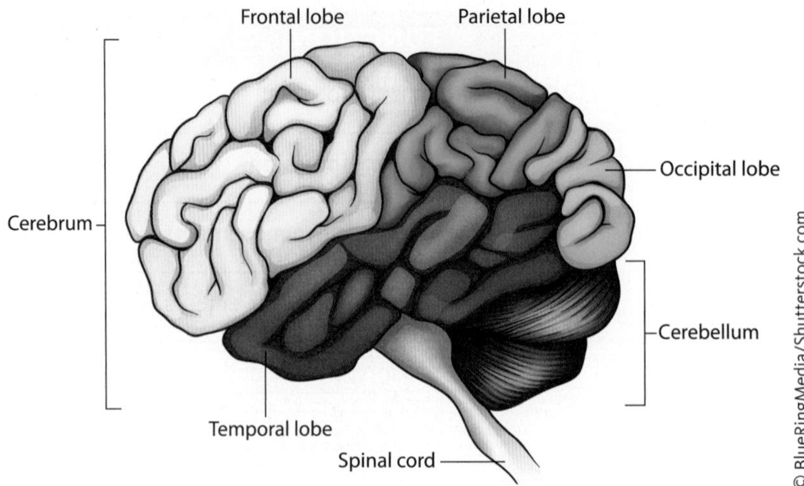

FIGURE 13-6 Human brain anatomy showing the cerebral lobes, cerebellum, and spinal cord.

for vision. The **temporal lobes** are involved in hearing, taste, and integration of emotions. The **insula** is a section of the brain located deep inside the temporal lobe and helps coordinate autonomic functions. Much of the information coming into the brain is *contralateral.* That is, the left side of the body is controlled by the right side of the brain, and the right side of the body is controlled by the left brain. You'll see how important this is when we discuss strokes.

13-7b Cerebellum

The **cerebellum** is posterior to the brain stem and plays an important role in sensory and motor coordination and balance. Just like the cerebrum, it has a convoluted surface, giving it the appearance of a "little brain" within the brain. Table 13-2 and Figure 13-7 summarize the cerebrum and cerebellum

Table 13-2 Cerebral Lobes and Cerebellum

STRUCTURE	FUNCTION
CEREBRUM	
Frontal lobe	Motor function, behavior, and emotions, memory storage, thinking, and smell
Parietal lobe	Body sense, perception, and speech
Occipital lobe	Vision
Temporal lobe	Hearing, taste, language comprehension, and integration of emotions
Insula	Autonomic functions
Cerebellum	**The "little brain"; sensory and motor coordination and balance**

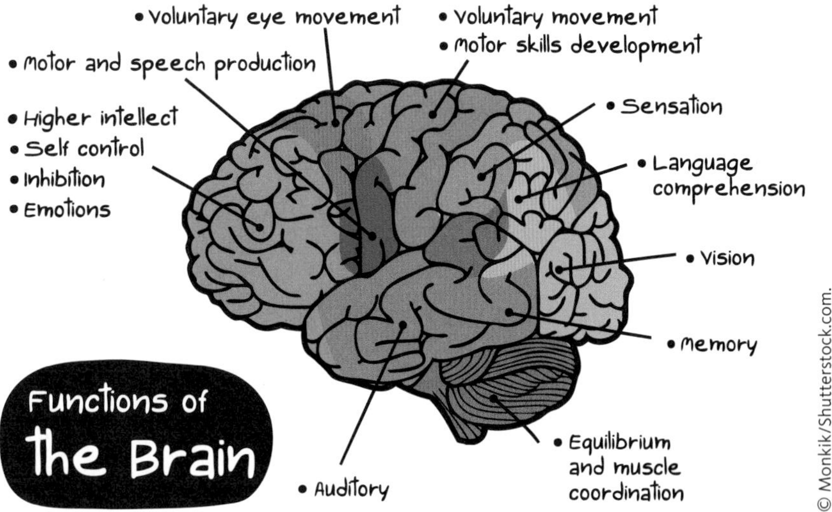

FIGURE 13-7 Sections of the brain and the corresponding functions they control.

functions. Damage to certain areas of the brain will cause clinical manifestations that will correlate to certain symptoms. For example, vision loss or disturbance can occur with occipital damage, and coordination would be affected greatly in any disease process, such as Parkinson's disease, that affects the cerebellum.

13-7c Brain Stem

The brain stem controls the vital functions of life, and injuries to it can be catastrophic. The **brain stem** is a stalk-like structure inferior to the cerebrum. It is divided into three sections as shown in Figure 13-8. The **medulla oblongata** is continuous with the spinal cord and sends impulses that control the body's vital signs: heartbeat, breathing, and the muscle tone in blood vessels, which control blood pressure. The **pons** lies just above the medulla oblongata and also plays a role in regulating breathing. The **midbrain** or most superior portion of the brain stem acts as a two-way conduction pathway to relay visual and auditory impulses to the cerebrum.

Patients with severe brain injuries but with an intact brain stem can continue in a coma or a vegetative state as long as they are supported nutritionally. Table 13-3 summarize its functions.

13-8 BRAIN AND SPINAL CORD PROTECTION

The brain and spinal cord are surrounded by a series of protective membranes called **meninges** and a cushioning fluid called **cerebral spinal fluid (CSF)**. The meninges and CSF protect the delicate structures of the brain and spinal cord much like airbags can protect your body from trauma in a motor vehicle crash. In the brain, CSF is contained within *ventricles*, which allow for its circulation to help nourish and cushion the brain from injury.

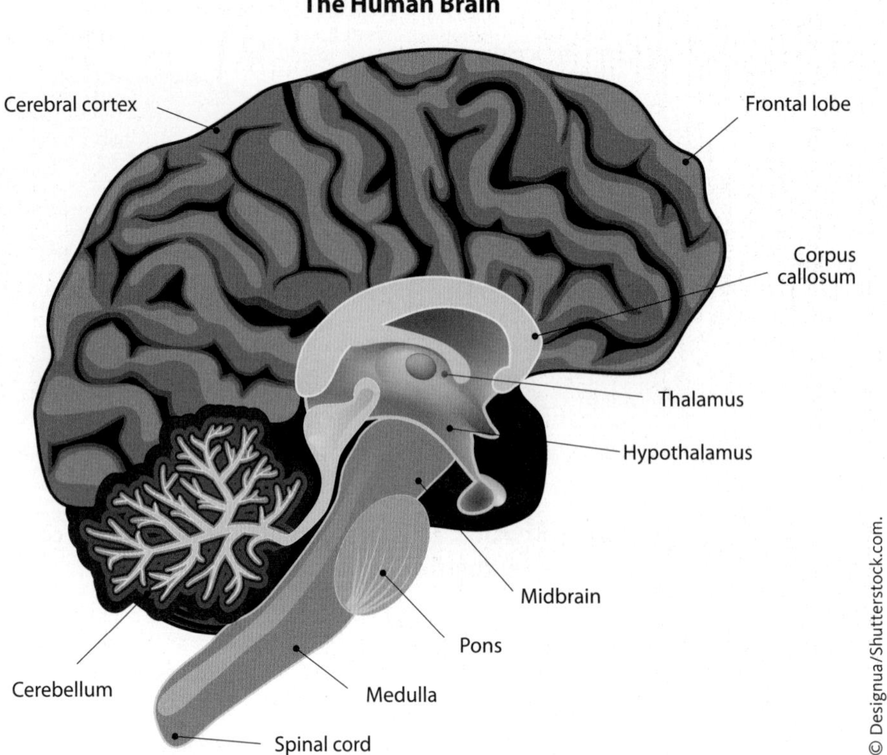

FIGURE 13-8 Brain anatomy showing the structures of the brain stem.

Table 13-3 The Brain Stem

BRAIN STEM STRUCTURE	BRAIN STEM FUNCTION
Midbrain	Relays sensory and motor information between brain and spinal cord
Pons	Relays sensory and motor information; plays a role in breathing
Medulla oblongata	Regulates vital functions of breathing, heart rate, blood pressure; reflex center for coughing, sneezing, vomiting, and swallowing

One of the most obvious protections of the brain and its structures is the skull, or cranium. Although the skull bones provide vitally needed protection, their rigidity can cause problems. For example, if you twist your ankle, the resulting bleeding and swelling cause discomfort and pressure, but the elasticity of the skin keeps the pressure down.

Now picture that same amount of blood and swelling within the brain. The bones of the skull cannot expand and stretch to dissipate the pressure, which is why small intracranial bleeds can cause high-intracranial pressures and related symptoms. Bleeding in the brain stem can affect the body's vital signs, and pressure in the occipital lobe can affect vision. This is one reason why concussions can be so dangerous.

CLINICAL CONNECTION 13.3

MENINGITIS

Meningitis is an inflammation caused by an infection, usually from viruses or bacteria, of the protective linings of the brain and spinal cord. Bacterial meningitis is a potentially fatal infection that first infects the upper respiratory tract and then travels to the meninges. High-risk groups include older adults, people with suppressed immune systems, very young children, and college students who live in dorms. Viral meningitis is a milder disease caused by viruses that enter the mouth and then travel to the meninges.

13-9 OTHER BRAIN SYSTEMS

Two other systems that do not have a single, specific location but are found throughout the brain are the limbic system and reticular system. The limbic system is a series of nuclei in the cerebrum and superior brain stem. Nuclei are clusters of densely clustered and packed neurons in the CNS. The nuclei in the limbic system are involved in mood, emotion, and memory. Damage to the limbic system can lead to changes in mood as well as emotional and memory impairments.

The reticular system is a diffuse network of nuclei in the brain stem. Some of these nuclei are responsible for "waking up" your cerebral cortex. This activity is crucial for the maintenance of conscious awareness of your surroundings. When your alarm clock wakes you in the morning, your reticular system is responsible for nudging your cortex out of slumber. General anesthesia inhibits the reticular system, rendering surgical patients unconscious. Injury because of ischemia, mechanical damage, or drugs can damage the reticular system and lead to a coma.

LEARNING OBJECTIVE 13.2 Describe the pathopharmacology of infectious and vascular disorders of the nervous system.

KEY TERMS

Carotid endarterectomy Surgical removal of the plaque within the arteries supplying the brain.

Cerebrovascular accident (CVA) Neurological condition caused by disruption of adequate blood flow to the brain, affecting its ability to function.

Electroencephalography (EEG) Measures the electrical activity of the brain; used to locate an abnormal area.

Encephalitis Inflammation of the brain tissue caused by a variety of microorganisms.

Insula Section of the brain located deep inside the temporal lobe that coordinates information from the autonomic nervous system.

Intracranial pressure (ICP) Measure of pressure within the cranial cavity.

Lumbar puncture Procedure performed to obtain CSF fluid for analysis.

Meningitis Viral or bacterial inflammation of the protective coverings of the brain and spinal cord.

Photophobia Light sensitivity.

Poliomyelitis Major crippling viral disease affecting children prior to development of a polio vaccine in the 1960s.

Post-polio syndrome (PPS) Syndrome developed by polio survivors 10–40 years after the initial disease.

Rabies Often fatal viral encephalomyelitis caused by an infected animal bite.

Shingles Herpes zoster viral disease causing itchy, painful rash with blisters along the pathway of the affected nerve.

Tetanus Life-threatening bacterial condition, also known as lockjaw, that can cause respiratory failure by paralyzing muscles needed to breathe.

Transient ischemic attacks (TIAs) Mild mini-strokes.

13-10 INFECTIOUS NERVOUS SYSTEM DISEASES

Given the importance of the nervous system and its control on all the other body systems, infectious diseases of the nervous system can wreck havoc on the entire body. While infections of the nervous system can occur at any age, they are more common in younger patients. Early diagnosis and proper treatment are critical to prevent any long-term neurologic problems.

Neurologic exams include testing both sensory and motor functioning, along with an assessment of the patient's mental status. The main laboratory test is an analysis of the cerebrospinal fluid (CSF), which is obtained by a lumbar puncture. The fluid is microscopically examined to determine the presence of microorganisms and abnormal blood cells.

Imaging studies such as X-rays, CT scans, and MRIs are valuable diagnostic tests to view the brain and spinal cord for abnormalities. Finally, **electroencephalography (EEG)** measures the electrical activity of the brain and can be used to to locate abnormal areas. See Figure 13-9.

13-10a Encephalitis

Encephalitis, or inflammation of the brain tissue, can be caused by a variety of microorganisms. Bacteria and viruses are often the culprits, and this disease can occur as a result of complications of childhood diseases such as measles, mumps, or chicken pox. Viruses spread by mosquitos also can cause some forms of encephalitis.

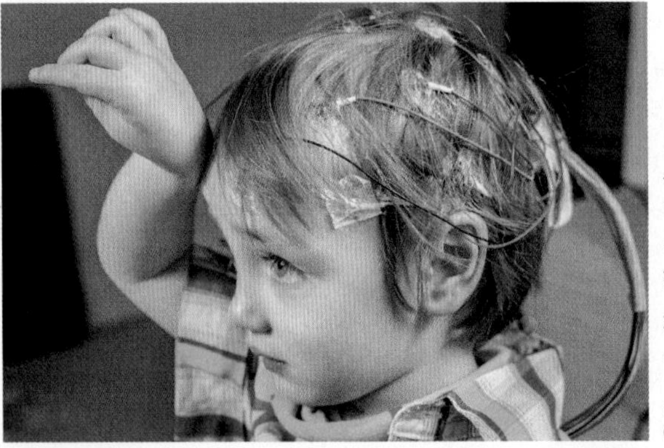

FIGURE 13-9 Child receiving an EEG exam has electrodes placed on his head to record electrical brain patterns.

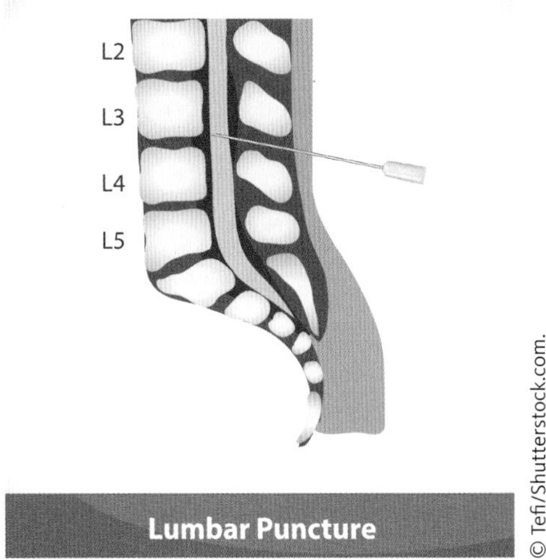

FIGURE 13-10 Lumbar puncture to obtain CSF fluid for analysis.

Symptoms can include a severe headache, fever, and muscle stiffness, primarily in the neck and back in the early stages. Lethargy, mental confusion, and even coma can result in later stages of the disease if untreated.

Diagnosis is confirmed via a **lumbar puncture** and identifying the causative microorganism in CSF fluid. See Figure 13-10. The proper antibiotic treatment for bacterial infection or antiviral agent for a viral infection is often effective if used early in the disease process.

Prevention is also a key factor, especially via vaccination of the young for childhood diseases that can lead to encephalitis. In addition, preventing mosquito bites by wearing repellant and proper protective clothing is another effective preventative measure.

13-10b Meningitis

Meningitis is an inflammation of the protective coverings of the brain and spinal cord. The causative agents can be microorganisms such as bacteria, viruses, fungi, or even toxins such as arsenic. Because the coverings are so diffuse, the infection can spread easily throughout the nervous system. Bacteria such as *Neisseria meningitides* can reach the meninges from an infection in the middle ear, sinuses, or upper respiratory tract. Infection also can be carried to the meninges by the blood in a patient who has a septicemia (infection within the bloodstream).

Symptoms include sudden onset of high fever, severe headache, light sensitivity (photophobia), and stiffness in the neck, Figure 13-11. The **photophobia** can be severe enough that the patient must be kept in a dark room. The neck can become so stiff that the patient cannot turn sideways or bend the neck forward. With disease progression, drowsiness, mental stupor, seizures, and coma can result.

Diagnosis is confirmed with a lumbar puncture and analysis of the CSF. Treatment depends on the causative agents; antibiotics such as penicillin and cefotaxime are effective against the more commonly caused bacterial infection.

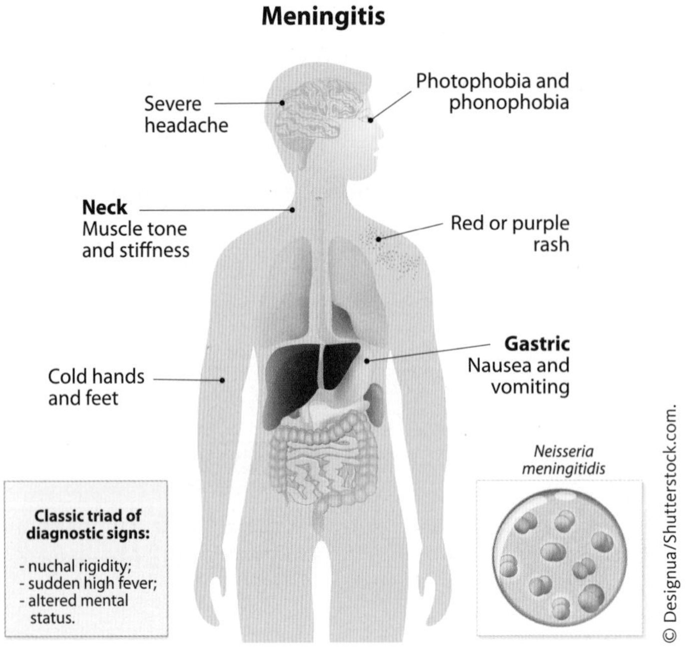

FIGURE 13-11 Signs, symptoms, and causative agent of meningitis. The CSF fluid, which is normally clear, will be milky and contain the *Neisseria* bacteria.

Other treatments include antipyretics for fever and anticonvulsants in cases of associated seizures. Handwashing as always is a good preventative measure, along with isolation of infected patients.

13-10c Rabies

Rabies is an often fatal encephalomyelitis (inflammation of the brain and spinal cord) caused by a virus that can be found in animals such as dogs, cats, foxes, raccoons, squirrels, and skunk. A bite from an infected animal can transmit the disease to a human. The incubation time for this slow-moving virus is 1–3 months, although bites to the neck or face have a faster onset because of their close proximity to the brain.

Symptoms can include pain, fever, paralysis (especially in throat), and convulsions. In the final stages, rage can manifest itself in the individual or animal, although wild animals can actually become friendly and more docile. This is why seeing a nocturnal animal such as a raccoon nearby during the day should promote caution as this animal should naturally run away.

CLINICAL CONNECTION 13.4

RABIES

Rabies also was called *hydrophobia*, which literally means fear of water. This term was coined because animals and people infected with rabies refused to drink water because of throat paralysis and severe pain associated with swallowing.

Diagnosis is based on a physical exam and patient history, which obviously would include an animal bite. Any bite from an animal should immediately be cleansed and disinfected. The animal should be

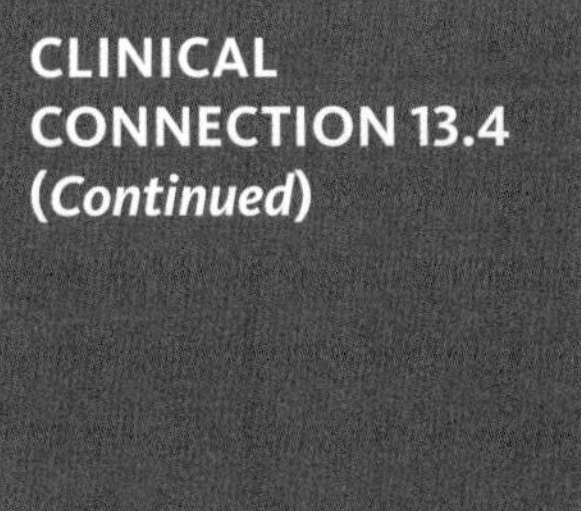

confined and placed under observation for rabies symptoms along with viral blood studies. If the animal cannot be found, the patient should be given a series of anti-rabies shots. If the animal is dead, its brain can be tested for presence of the disease.

There is no cure for rabies, and treatment is palliative, meaning the patient is given pain medication and muscle relaxants to reduce convulsions. Death usually ensues.

Prevention involves vaccinating family pets and avoiding wild animals, and learning what to do if a bite occurs. Figure 13-12 shows signs and symptoms of rabies.

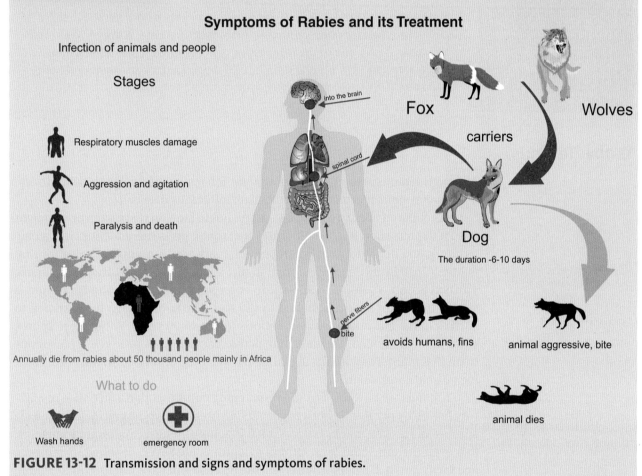

FIGURE 13-12 Transmission and signs and symptoms of rabies.

13-10d Poliomyelitis

Poliomyelitis, or simply polio, was a major crippling and life-threatening disease affecting mainly children before development of a polio vaccine in the 1950s. The poliomyelitis virus entered the body through the nose or mouth and then entered the GI system, eventually spreading to the blood and from there the brain and spinal cord. The disease has been virtually wiped out because of effective vaccination programs. The most-effective treatment is to continue to vaccinate children to prevent its re-emergence.

Symptoms of polio include muscle weakness, stiff neck, nausea, and vomiting in the early stages. Later stages included muscle atrophy and paralysis of the respiratory system, requiring mechanical ventilation. Diagnosis is made from throat, feces, or CSF cultures.

Although it no longer is prevalent as a disease, many people who survived polio as children experience **post-polio syndrome (PPS)** 10–40 years later. Symptoms include further muscle weakening, joint pain, fatigue, and skeletal deformities such as scoliosis. PPS is not an infectious condition and is rarely life-threatening, but symptoms must be treated for the quality of life issues.

CLINICAL CONNECTION 13.5

POLIO VACCINE

Dr. Jonas Salk of the University of Pittsburgh (where both authors teach) developed the first polio vaccine in 1955. Salk's vaccine, however, was effective against only one of the three types of polio viruses, making it a monovalent vaccine. Dr. Albert Sabin in 1961 developed the trivalent oral polio vaccine (TOPV), which was effective against all three forms of the virus.

13-10e Tetanus

Although tetanus was covered in Module 6 because of its relationship to the muscular system, it is also a neurological, infectious disease.

As children, we are told to be careful not to step on rusty nails or we might need a tetanus shot. It is not the rusty nail that causes the infection, but a bacterium found in nature that could be on a rusty nail—or anything else for that matter. *Clostridium tetani* is found in dirt and even in the GI tract of animals. The nail is only a vehicle to allow it to enter your body where the bacterium is spread by way of spores attached to the nail. The spores have been known to survive in the dirt and remain infectious for up to 40 years. After these spores enter an open wound, they become active bacteria that produce a poisonous toxin that interferes with the signaling between the brain and spinal cord, causing muscle contraction.

Tetanus, or lockjaw, is a life-threatening condition that can cause respiratory failure by paralyzing muscles needed to breathe. Symptoms include muscle spasms in the jaw, neck, back (causing aching), chest, abdominal muscles, and even the arms and legs. Others symptoms are fever, drooling, dysphasia, and tachycardia. If a person survives, the disease will have run its course within 6–8 weeks.

No laboratory studies can diagnose this condition, so physicians must rely on a patient's history, physical examination, and bedside tests, such as the spatula test. The spatula test involves using a tool to touch the back of the throat. People without tetanus will gag, but patients who have no gag reflex and instead bite down on the spatula are positive for tetanus.

Supportive treatment, such as mechanical ventilation if the patient is not breathing, is carried out until the toxins are resolved. Treatment includes cleaning out the wound and providing muscle relaxants and antibiotics, such as penicillin and metronidazole. A tetanus shot is given every 10 years to prevent bacteria from progressing to the infectious stage. Figure 13-13 shows a word cloud related to tetanus.

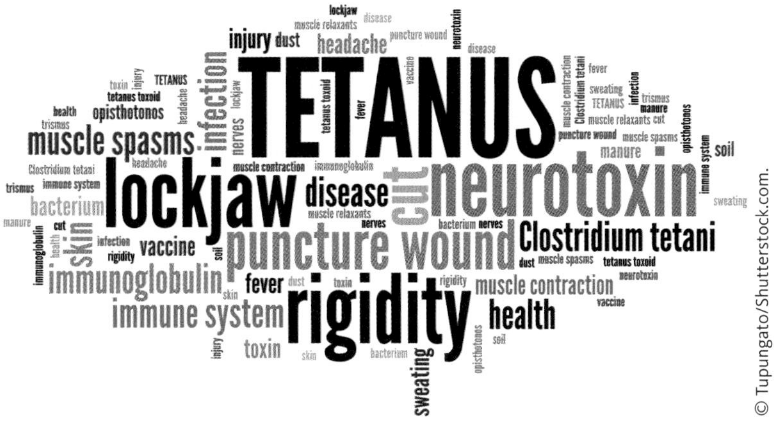

FIGURE 13-13 Tetanus is a life-threatening condition that can cause respiratory failure by paralyzing muscles needed to breathe.

13-10f Shingles

Shingles is a viral disease that is common in older adults. The causative viral agent is herpes zoster, which is the same virus that caused the person to have chicken pox as a child. The virus lays dormant for years, reappearing later in life during periods of high stress or immunosuppression from trauma, other diseases, or the aging process. It is estimated that approximately 50 percent of adults older than 80 years of age will have an episode if they were exposed to the chicken pox virus as a child.

Symptoms occur as an itchy, painful rash with blisters that develops along the pathway of the affected nerve, Figure 13-14. The neuritis causes a sharp stabbing pain that often gets more severe at night. Symptoms can last for weeks. The rash often appears in the trunk of the body but also can affect the face and eyes, causing severe conjunctivitis.

Diagnosis is based on the rash appearance and patient history. A viral culture or blood test can be used to confirm the presence of the herpes virus. Treatment involves antiviral agents, analgesics for pain, and antipruritics for itching. While not a treatment for existing shingles, the Zostavax vaccine is recommended for older adults to prevent development of the disease.

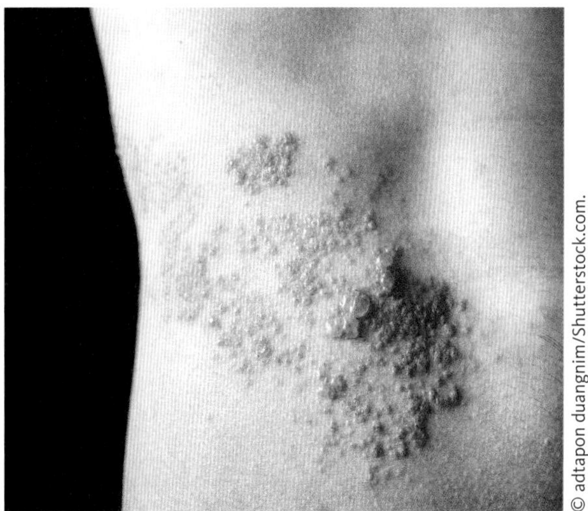

FIGURE 13-14 Characteristic rash associated with shingles.

13-11 INTRODUCTION TO VASCULAR DISORDERS OF THE NERVOUS SYSTEM

If a person twists an ankle, the resulting swelling from bleeding and inflammation is painful but not serious or life-threatening. The skin around the ankles can handle the increased pressure of bleeding and inflammation by stretching. Its elasticity helps reduce the pressure around the ankle. That is not the case with a head injury or brain infection, however, because the skull is rigid and does not expand with pressure. Small bleeds in the brain can lead to large increases in **intracranial pressure (ICP)**, which can impair vital brain function depending upon the affected area. If pressures become too high, the brain will herniate, and be displaced downward through the only opening available, the foramen magnum. If this occurs, coma and death can occur because of the pressure on the brain stem, which controls vital functions such as breathing and heart rate.

13-11a Cerebrovascular Accident

A **cerebrovascular accident (CVA)**, or stroke, is caused by inadequate blood supply to the brain. Just like a disruption of blood flow to the heart can cause a heart attack and therefore heart malfunction; a CVA can result in a disruption of adequate flow to the brain and affect its ability to function.

The disruption of blood can come from the following three sources:

Cerebral thrombus: Brain clot from a thrombus (clot) that forms where a blood vessel has narrowed by arteriosclerosis. This narrowing occurs over time, and symptoms appear and progress gradually.

Cerebral embolism: Small clot or piece of arterial plaque breaking away from the vascular wall and entering the bloodstream. Eventually the matter wedges in a cerebral vessel, blocking blood flow. This occurs acutely, and onset of symptoms happens quickly.

Cerebral hemorrhage: Cerebral bleeding can be caused by trauma or rupture of weakened cerebral vessels. The weakening can occur because of hypertension, arteriosclerosis, or an aneurysm. Symptoms occur quickly with cerebral hemorrhage.

Symptoms can include impairment or loss of consciousness and vary according to the area of the brain affected. Some common symptoms of CVA include dysphasia (difficulty speaking), dysphagia (difficulty swallowing), paralysis, and poor coordination. See Figure 13-15.

13-11b Diagnosis and Treatment of Stroke

Diagnosis is made by physical exam, EEG, CT, and MRI scanning, Figure 13-16. Early detection can involve carotid artery screening by auscultating for a bruit, or the sound of blood rushing through a narrowed vessel. Ultrasound can be used to get a better view of the actual vessels. If the carotid arteries are severely blocked, surgical removal of the plaque within the arteries can be performed in a procedure known as a **carotid endarterectomy**.

Treatment depends on the severity of stroke symptoms and the underlying cause of the CVA. Anticoagulants can be given to prevent further clots from forming and hypertensive agents given to lower blood pressure. If a disability persists, rehabilitation will be required.

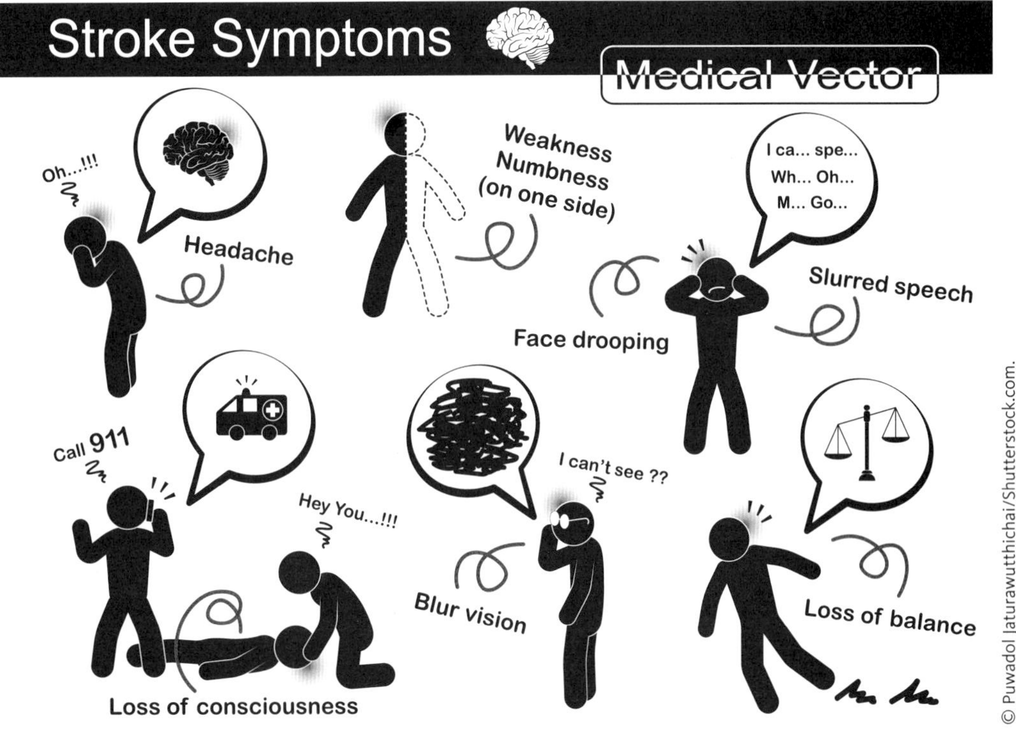

FIGURE 13-15 Stroke symptoms.

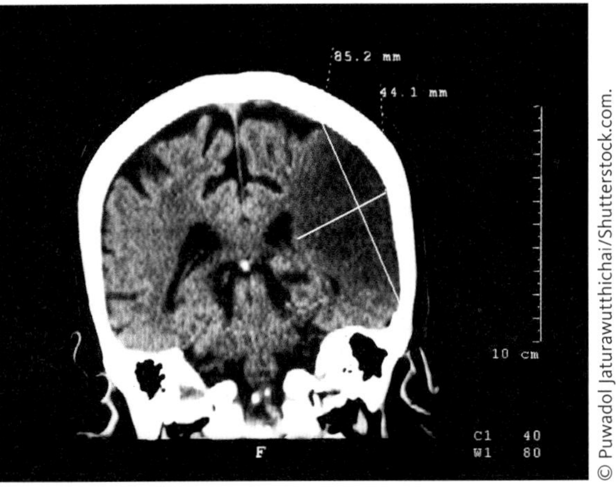

FIGURE 13-16 CT Image of brain with stroke in patient's left cerebral hemisphere.

Prevention is a key treatment in any disease but becomes critical with strokes because of their potential for long-term disability. Avoiding risk factors such as smoking, obesity, and high-fat diets not only helps reduce the risk of stroke but also reduces arteriosclerosis.

CLINICAL CONNECTION 13.6

The brain is *contralateral* meaning the right hemisphere controls the left side of the body, and the left hemisphere controls the right side of the body. Therefore, hemiparalysis of the left side would indicate a right brain injury.

13-11c Transient Ischemic Attacks

Some people consider small earthquakes to be a warning sign of a large earthquake to come. **Transient ischemic attacks (TIAs)** are similar, in that they are sudden, mild ministrokes that, if not treated, will lead to a CVA (the big one). Ischemia means insufficient blood supply, and while it might not be significant enough to fully disrupt blood supply as in a CVA, the lack of supply often builds gradually to a point where symptoms appear. The symptoms again depend on the area of the brain affected, but some common symptoms include muscle weakness, slurred speech, dizziness, and possible mild loss of consciousness. These symptoms usually go away in a few minutes or within hours.

Since the symptoms are usually gone by the time medical help is sought, diagnosis is initially made with patient history and imaging studies to see if vessels are narrowed. Arteriograms can be performed to show actually blood flow and can reveal narrowed areas.

Often TIAs are the result of narrowing of the carotid arteries supplying the brain. If this is the case, a carotid endarterectomy can be performed. Patients should be taught to avoid risk factors, have proper nutrition, and exercise to reduce plaque buildup and arteriosclerosis.

LEARNING OBJECTIVE 13.3 Describe the pathopharmacology of functional disorders of the nervous system.

KEY TERMS

Bell's palsy Disease affecting the facial nerve causing (one-sided) facial paralysis leading to face drooping.

Cauterization Electrical burning of tissue to prevent or stop bleeding.

Cluster headache Headache type occurring upon awakening with throbbing pain behind the nose and eyes.

Concussion Traumatic head injury usually accompanied by temporary loss of consciousness.

Contusion Physical bruising of brain tissue.

Degenerative disc disease Skeletal disease usually caused by aging that wears away the intervertebral disc, resulting in compression and damage to spinal nerves.

Epidural hematoma Collection or pooling of blood between the skull and dura membrane that covers the brain, often resulting in increase in intracranial pressure.

Epilepsy Chronic disease characterized by periodic episodes of abnormal electrical conduction resulting in seizures.

Glasgow coma scale (GCS) Objective standarized scale used to measure the extent of a brain injury.

Migraine headache Most severe form of headache with incapacitating pain, visual disturbances, nausea, and vomiting.

Paraplegia Paralysis of the lower body.

Parkinson's disease Slow progressive degeneration of the brain because of deficiency of the brain neurochemical transmitter dopamine.

Post-lumbar puncture headache Headache that results after lumbar puncture procedure because of leakage of CSF from the puncture site.

Quadriplegia Paralysis of all four limbs and resulting in loss of bladder and bowel control.

Spinal stenosis Narrowing of the spinal nerve root pathways.

Tension headache Type of headache caused by high levels of stress and tension.

13-12 FUNCTIONAL DISORDERS OF THE CNS

This section will cover the functional disorders of the nervous system, in which normal functioning is impaired because of trauma or disease process. Module 6 talked about the interconnection between the nervous and muscular systems. The major neuromuscular diseases of Guillain-Barre, muscular dystrophy, and myasthenia gravis were discussed in Module 6. These diseases dealt mainly with a functional disorder of the neurotransmitter substances at the neuromuscular junction.

13-13 DEGENERATIVE DISC DISEASE

Although **degenerative disc disease** is technically a skeletal disease because of the wearing away of the intervertebral disc, the resulting compression and damage to the spinal nerves that exits the vertebrae cause nerve impairment and damage. The narrowing of the nerve root openings is called **spinal stenosis**. Figure 13-17 shows types of disc degenerations.

Common symptoms depend on which vertebrae are affected, but can include difficulty walking, leg and back pains, and numbness. Diagnosis is made based on clinical history and imaging studies such as X-ray, CT scan, or MRI.

Treatment involves physical therapy and rehabilitation. If this isn't successful, surgery is probably needed. A *laminectomy* procedure can remove part of the vertebrae and widen the nerve root opening to relieve the pressure on the nerve. In severe cases, the vertebra can be fused and supported with rods to free the nerve root.

Pharmacologic treatment includes:

- Analgesics for pain
- Anti-inflammatory agents such as NSAIDs and corticosteroids to reduce swelling and inflammation

Since this is primarily a disease of aging, there are few preventative measures. However, regular exercise, especially walking coupled with good nutrition, can help slow or stop painful symptoms and slow the progression of the disease.

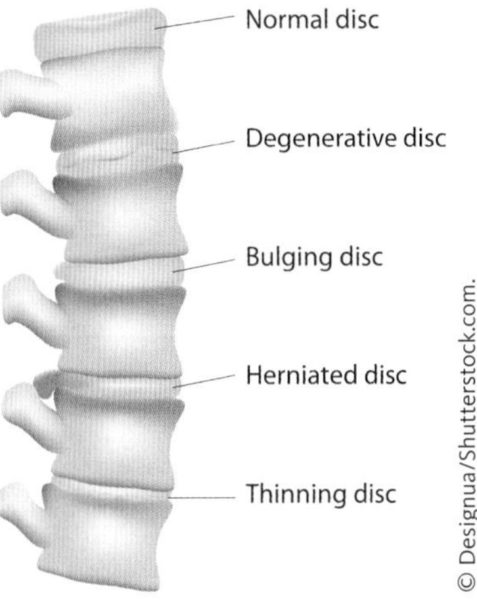

FIGURE 13-17 Types of degenerative disc disease.

13-14 HEADACHE

Headaches are among the most common problems people have, but they are not actually disorders themselves, as much as being symptomatic of another disease. A few of many disorders that typically have a headache as a common symptom are:

Sinusitis

Encephalitis

Meningitis

Hypertension

This list all has the common outcome of producing "increased pressure" in the head, therefore contributing to the *cephalgia* or "pain in the head." Obviously, the "itis" diseases need treatment with an anti-infective medication depending on the microorganism and also may benefit from corticosteroids to reduce inflammation. Hypertension would need treatment with the correct antihypertensive agent as described in Module 12.

Two situations that lead to most headaches are tension in the facial, neck, and scalp muscles, and vascular changes in blood vessels within the head that increase intracranial pressure. Many factors can lead to headaches, such as high levels of stress, lack of sleep, alcohol or drug use, nutritional reactions, and allergies.

13-14a Types and Treatments of Headaches

Headaches can be grouped under three specific types. A **tension headache** is caused by high levels of stress and tension in the facial, neck, jaw, and scalp muscles. Pain is typically in the occipital region.

A **cluster headache** also can be caused by stress and emotional trauma, but some causes are unknown. This type of headache occurs at night after falling asleep and upon awakening, usually exhibiting as throbbing pain behind the nose and eyes. For both cluster and tension headaches, OTC pain medication such as acetaminophen (Tylenol) or ibuprofen usually work well, along with diet and lifestyle changes to reduce stress.

A **migraine headache** is the most severe form of a headache, with incapacitating pain, nausea, and vomiting. Visual disturbances, such as wavy vision, dim vision, or photophobia, often precede or accompany a migraine headache. The visual disturbance that precedes or forecasts a headache is known as an *aura*. Migraine headaches occur more often in women and often the cause is unknown, but they do tend to run in families. Some foods can trigger these headaches, and prime offenders include chocolate, wine, and cheese.

Migraines, also called vascular headaches, have several treatment options because medications that cause cerebral vasoconstriction can be an effective treatment. The first option is usually a triptan medication such as sumatriptan (Imitrex). Another drug such as Cafergot that alters serotonin levels has success in some patients For severe pain, Tylenol with codeine can be used, but narcotics should be used cautiously.

Anti-nausea medications such as prochlorperazine (Compazine) and promethazine (Phenergan) can be given. In very severe cases of more than 15 migraine headaches per month, Botox therapy can be used to relax (actually paralyze) the facial muscles. Botox has several side effects and should be used only for frequent severe migraine cases.

CLINICAL CONNECTION 13.7

MEDICALLY INDUCED HEADACHES

A type of headache that can be induced in the hospital is called a **post-lumbar puncture headache**. This headache occurs after a lumbar puncture to obtain CSF fluid is performed because of leakage from the puncture site. This headache can usually be prevented by keeping the patient lying flat without any pillows for at least 2–3 hours post-puncture procedure. This helps prevent a buildup of pressure at the lower back or lumbar site that would occur while sitting up. Figure 13-18 shows the location of the lumbar puncture.

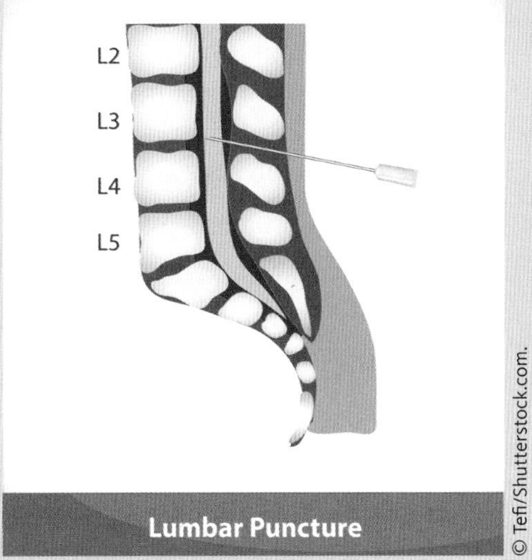

FIGURE 13-18 Location of lumbar puncture procedure.

13-15 EPILEPSY

Like the heart, the brain requires an intricate electrical conduction system to function optimally. **Epilepsy** is chronic disease characterized by periodic episodes of abnormal electrical conduction or activity within the brain, similar to an arrhythmia in the heart.

Epilepsy sometimes is caused by damage to the brain from a tumor, disease, or scar tissue from trauma or a stroke. Often the cause cannot be confirmed. The most common symptom of epilepsy is a *convulsive seizure*. The word convulsion means an abnormal muscle contraction and seizure means sudden attack, and the distinction is important.

The first type of seizure, now known as *absence seizure*, was previously called petit mal seizures. *Absence seizures* commonly occur in children and consist of a brief change in the level of consciousness, without a convulsive episode. Often the individual will have a blank stare, eye twitch or blink, and not be consciously aware of their surroundings. Episodes last only a few seconds but can occur often throughout the day.

The second type or *grand mal* is what most people associate with epilepsy. Grand mal seizures involve convulsions, loss of consciousness, tongue biting, and possible urinary and fecal incontinence. Often auras or warning signals occur such as visual disturbances, ringing in ears, or finger tingling. Contractions can last for minutes, and consciousness returns slowly with the individual weakened, confused, and having no memory of the event.

The most severe form of epilepsy is *status epilepticus*. This situation is a medical emergency with the victim in a continual convulsive seizure that does not stop. If not treated, it can lead to cerebral tissue damage, coma, and possible death.

13-15a Diagnosis and Treatment of Epilepsy

Diagnosis can be made with patient history, along with diagnostic tests such as an EEG to assess electrical brain activity. CT scans and cerebral angiograms assess blood flow throughout the brain and can identify any brain tumors that could be causing epilepsy.

Anticonvulsive medications are the treatment of choice. Some of the common anticonvulsants are:

- Carbamazepine (Tegretol or Carbatrol)
- Eslicarbazepine (Aptiom)
- Ethosuximide (Zarontin)
- Gabapentin (Neurontin)
- Levetiracetam (Keppra)
- Phenobarbital
- Phenytoin (Dilantin or Phenytek)
- Diazepam (Valium) and similar tranquilizers for sedation/calming, such as lorazepam (Ativan), Tranxene, and clonazepam (Klonopin)

The type of medication depends on several factors, such as the type of seizure and patient's age and tolerance level. Close monitoring and adjustment of medications are needed to maximize the effect and reduce side effects. The goal is to return the individual to a normal lifestyle with proper medication and disease education and emotional support.

Because one cause of epilepsy is head injury, it is important to prevent head injuries, by wearing seat belts in automobiles, and safety helmets when riding ATVs and motorcycles, as well as skateboarding and riding bicycles.

CLINICAL CONNECTION 13.8

What should you do if you see someone having a seizure? First, it is always good to call 911 for medical assistance, but you can do certain things while waiting for help to arrive. Look for a medical ID bracelet and loosen any tight clothing that might cause a choking hazard. Protect the convulsing person by clearing away nearby hazards and place a

CLINICAL CONNECTION 13.8 (*Continued*)

pillow or any kind of padding under the head to prevent further injury. Turn the person on her or his side to prevent aspiration. DO NOT put a tongue blade, hard object, or your fingers in the person's mouth (something many people were once taught). Finally, reassure them after consciousness returns.

13-16 BELL'S PALSY

Bell's palsy affects the 7th cranial nerve, also known as the facial nerve. The cause is idiopathic or unknown, but it is thought to be triggered by a viral infection or an autoimmune response. The classic sign is unilateral (one-sided) facial paralysis causing one-half of the face to droop or sag as shown in Figure 13-19.

Another symptom of Bell's palsy, which commonly occurs from ages 20 and 60, is drooling of saliva because of partial paralysis of one side of the mouth. Diagnosis is made on clinical history and the characteristic drooping symptoms.

Bell's palsy usually resolves by itself between 2 and 8 weeks after onset. Pharmacologic treatment is to address the inflammation with an anti-inflammatory, such as NSAIDs or corticosteroids, and treat any pain with analgesics. Warm moist heat and facial muscle exercise and massage, along with electrical nerve stimulation, can help lessen the facial paralysis. Artificial tear medication might be needed for the affected eye.

13-17 PARKINSON'S DISEASE

Parkinson's disease is a slowly progressive degeneration of the brain that usually develops when a person is in his or her late 50s or 60s, but can occur earlier as was the case with actor Michael J. Fox, who was diagnosed with the disease when he was 30 years old. This disease is more prevalent in men than women.

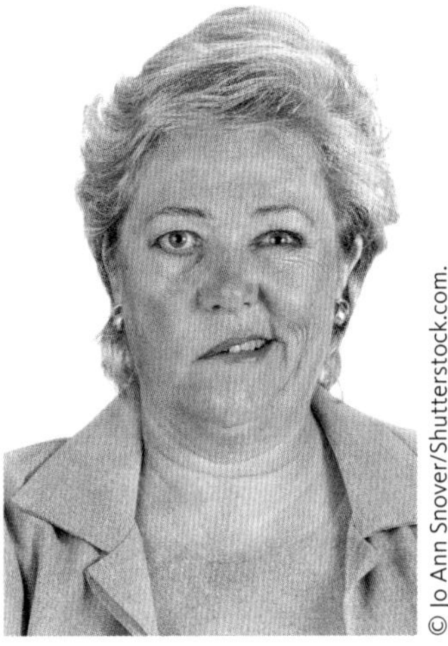

FIGURE 13-19 Woman who has Bell's palsy gives a one-sided smile.

The cause is unknown, but affected individuals have a deficiency of the brain neurochemical transmitter dopamine. Symptoms of Parkinson's include rigidity of muscles with a bent-forward or slouching posture and a bowed head. A fine tremor, described as a pill-rolling motion with the finger, can begin in the hands. The face is often expressionless and the person might have a fixed stare as if looking "off into space." The walking pattern or gait is also characteristic with short, fast-moving steps that make the person have frequent falls.

There is no cure, and the disease keeps progressing, but dopamine replacement medications can help reduce some of the symptoms. Common dopamine agonists include:

- Sinemet (Levodopa/Carbidopa)
- Requip (ropinirole)
- Mirapex (pramipexole)
- Neupro (rotigotine)

Psychological support and counseling for both patient and family members are needed to cope with this disease.

13-18 NERVOUS SYSTEM TRAUMA

Trauma to the nervous system, that happens with head injuries, can affect the brain by causing swelling and edema, along with bleeding and potential for infection. This in turn creates an increased intracranial pressure (ICP) that further inhibits brain function to the area affected. Injury to the neck and spinal cord can lead to temporary or permanent paralysis.

13-18a Brain Injuries

The National Football League, facing lawsuits and public backlash, has established concussion protocols for its players. Many other sports organizations and leagues have followed, acknowledging the danger for brain injury in many sports. A **concussion** is a traumatic injury to the brain, which can result from a blow to the head, accident, fall, or even violent shaking. A **contusion**, or actual physical bruising of brain tissue, can follow a concussion.

Symptoms of a concussion and resulting contusion include temporary unconsciousness, lasting from a few seconds or for several hours, and often resulting in memory loss. Other symptoms are confusion, headache, blurred vision, nausea, and irritability.

Diagnosis is made by taking a history of the event, a neurological exam to assess neurological function as seen in Figure 13-20, and cranial imaging with CT scans and MRI to determine the extent of the injury. Treatment consists of bed rest, with the person being assessed every few hours for level of consciousness and mood changes, and examining the pupils in his or her eyes.

Pharmacologic treatment includes mainly analgesics for pain. Sedatives or stimulants are NOT recommended because they can mask symptoms and make an assessment and proper treatment difficult.

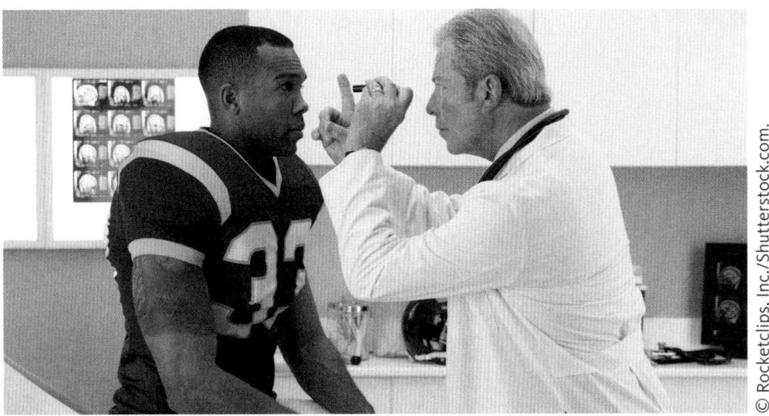

© Rocketclips, Inc./Shutterstock.com.

FIGURE 13-20 Neurological exam performed on potential concussion patient.

Additional procedures might be required for serious head trauma that causes severe damage and bleeding. The bleeding can lead to an **epidural hematoma**, which is a collection or pooling of blood between the skull and dura membrane covering the brain. A special craniotomy procedure might be required in cases of dangerously high ICP readings. The procedure involves drilling *burr holes* to allow for drainage of blood and to reduce pressure. Also, **cauterization**, or electrical burning of the tissue to stop bleeding, is often needed. If a skull fracture or break in the cranium occurs, surgical repair might be needed.

Prevention is key, and protective gear and proper concussion protocols in sports are essential because, as we know now, repeated concussions can lead to serious brain impairment and disease.

13-18b Glasgow Coma Scale

The **Glasgow coma scale (GCS)** is a standardized scoring method to describe the level of consciousness (LOC) of neurologically injured patients, most notably traumatic brain injury (TBI). This objective scale correlates well to the extent of brain injury involved.

The scale measures and assigns a number to three functions:

Eye Opening

4 - Can spontaneously open eyes

3 - Opens eyes to voice command

2 - Opens eye to pain stimuli

1 - Does not open eyes

Verbal Response

5 - Normal conversation

4 - Disoriented

3 - Speaking, but not coherent

2 - No words, only sounds

1 - No sounds

Motor Response

6 - Normal movement

5 - Movement localized to pain

4 - Withdraws to pain

3 - Decorticate posture (rigid, clenched fists with legs straight out and arms bent inward)

2 - Decerebrate posture (rigid with arms and legs straight out and toes pointed downward)

1 - No motor movement

The lower the score is, the more serious will be the injury. A total score between 3 and 8 signifies severe injury; between 9 and 12 is moderate; and between 13 and 15 is mild.

13-19 SPINAL CORD INJURIES

When the vertebral column suffers injury, the enclosed spinal cord also can be damaged. The spinal cord might be partially or completely severed, crushed, or bruised. Bruises to the spinal cord might resolve with time and rehabilitation, but a severed or crushed spinal cord usually results in a permanent injury.

The location of a spinal cord injury dictates the area of functional loss, which, with a severe injury, is often temporary or permanent paralysis. **Paraplegia** is paralysis of the lower body; **quadriplegia** is paralysis of all four limbs. The exposed area of the neck and and cervical vertebrae causes this area to be most vulnerable. The leading causes of spinal cord injury are automobile accidents, but other causes are diving and and other sporting accidents, and severe wounds, such as in gunshot or knife wounds.

Spinal cord injuries result in varying degrees of loss of feeling or movement below the area of injury. If the damage is severe, permanent paralysis can result.

Please see the brief animation on spinal cord injuries.

Symptoms are related to location; Figure 13-21 shows this relationship. Note that quadriplegia not only paralyzes the four limbs but also causes loss of bowel, bladder, and sexual functions. In addition, temperature regulation can be affected, and hypothermia, bradycardia, and respiratory function are often impaired. Actor Christopher Reeve, best known for portraying Superman in several movies, suffered a high-cervical injury from a horseback riding fall that left him a quadriplegic and dependent on a mechanical ventilator to breathe.

13-20 BRAIN TUMORS

Primary brain tumors originate in the brain, and secondary brain tumors metastasize from other areas of the body. Figure 13-22 shows the common sites of primary brain tumors. Brain tumors, like any other tumor, can be benign or malignant. However, because of the confined space and inflexible skull, even benign tumors can be very dangerous because blood vessel blockages and increase in intracranial pressure can damage vital brain tissue and functions. The cause of brain tumors is often unknown.

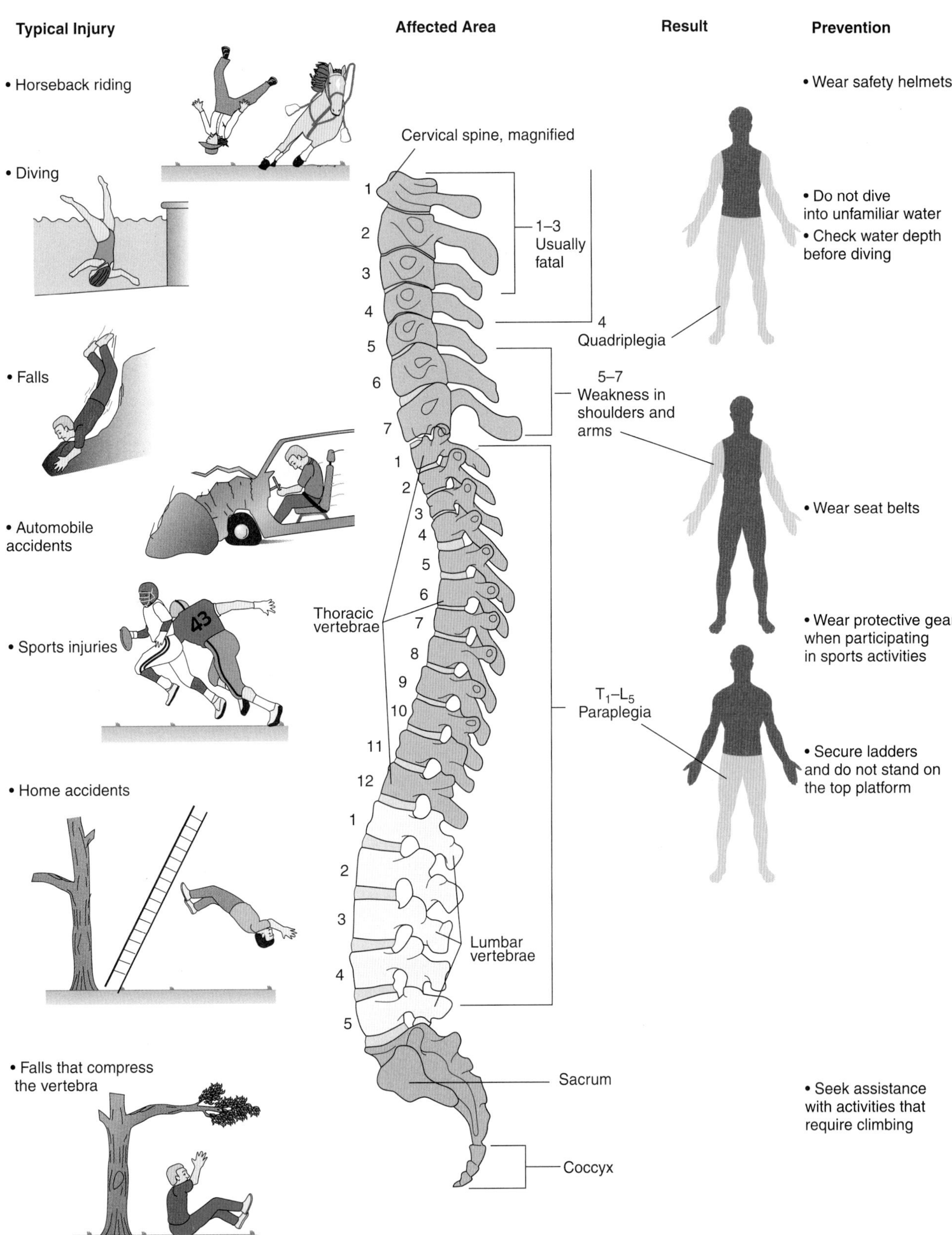
Typical Injury
Affected Area
Result
Prevention
• Horseback riding
• Diving
• Falls
• Automobile accidents
• Sports injuries
• Home accidents
• Falls that compress the vertebra
Cervical spine, magnified
1–3 Usually fatal
4 Quadriplegia
5–7 Weakness in shoulders and arms
Thoracic vertebrae
T_1–L_5 Paraplegia
Lumbar vertebrae
Sacrum
Coccyx
• Wear safety helmets
• Do not dive into unfamiliar water
• Check water depth before diving
• Wear seat belts
• Wear protective gear when participating in sports activities
• Secure ladders and do not stand on the top platform
• Seek assistance with activities that require climbing

FIGURE 13-21 Spinal cord injuries.

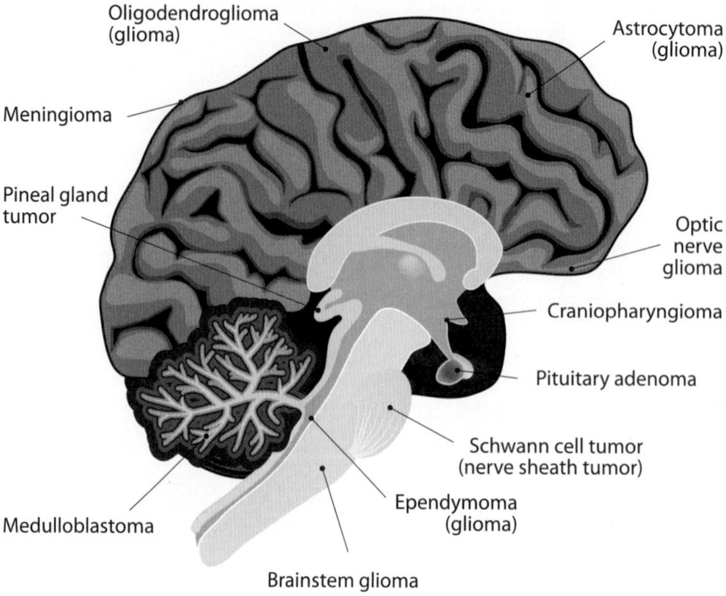

The Most Common Primary Brain Tumors

FIGURE 13-22 Common primary tumor location and corresponding name.

Symptoms vary according to tumor type, location, and area involved. Common symptoms include a headache, nausea/vomiting, seizures, visual disturbances, and changes in mood and memory loss. Diagnosis is made on clinical history and imaging studies, mainly CT scans and MRIs. Biopsies often are needed to identify the type of tumor to guide proper treatment. Treatment can include radiation, chemotherapy, and surgery, depending on the type, extent, and location of the tumor.

LEARNING OBJECTIVE 13.4 Describe the pathopharmacology of mental health disorders of the nervous system.

KEY TERMS

Anxiety disorder Mental health condition in which anxiety becomes chronic and exaggerated or inappropriate for the given situation.

Attention deficit hyperactivity disorder (ADHD) Mental health disorder that has hyperactivity along with the inability to concentrate and impulsive behaviors.

Binge eating disorder (BED) Eating disorder characterized by eating large quantities of food often very quickly to the point of discomfort on average at least once a week for three months.

Bipolar disorder Mental health condition with extreme mood changes that include emotional highs (mania) and emotional lows or depressive states.

Bulimia Eating disorder of binge eating followed by vomiting or purging the body of food.

CNS stimulant Medication that stimulates the central nervous system, usually causing tachycardia, increased respirations, and high levels of energy and alertness.

Dementia Progressive deterioration of mental abilities because of changes in the brain.

Dependency Psychological need for the drug that might or might not be accompanied by a physical need.

Generalized anxiety disorder (GAD) Anxiety disorder characterized by excessive worrying.

Major depressive disorder (MDD) Clinical term for depression that affects quality of life.

Narcotics CNS depressants such as morphine that are used primarily as prescribed painkillers (analgesics).

Obsessive compulsive disorder (OCD) Anxiety disorder with both obsession or the repetition of a thought or emotion along with compulsion to do a repetitive act.

Phobia disorder Most common anxiety disorder that exhibits an intense and irrational fear of an object, event, situation, or thing.

Post-traumatic stress disorder (PTSD) Mental health condition that develops after an intense psychological event that is outside the range of normal human experience, such as combat, rape, child abuse or incest, acts of violence/terrorism, or natural disasters.

Schizophrenia Type of psychosis with drastic personality changes and loss of reality.

Seasonal affective disorder (SAD) Type of depression associated with winter months because of lack of natural sunlight.

Sedatives Medications that have a calming affect, such as the benzodiazepines (BDZs) and valium.

Selective serotonin reuptake inhibitors (SSRIs) Drugs that increase the utilization of serotonin; used to treat depression.

Serotonin and norepinephrine reuptake inhibitors(SNRIs) Medication to increase serotonin production to treat depression.

Tolerance Need for increasing levels of drugs to get the same effect.

Withdrawal Unpleasant side effects and symptoms associated with abruptly stopping a substance to which one is addicted.

13-21 OVERVIEW

Although this section will constitute a concise pathopharmacologic discussion about common mental health diseases, entire books have been written about each specific mental condition. Mental disorders are some of the most difficult diseases to diagnose and properly treat. Behavioral therapy and counseling constitute the two main nonpharmacologic treatments in all these conditions. The hallmark sign in mental health conditions is behavioral change. Although diagnostic tests such as EEGs and MRIs can determine physical abnormalities that can cause mental health disease, the testing often involves psychological testing and written test assessments. This is especially true when no organic cause of the mental health condition can be determined.

13-22 MOOD DISORDERS

Mood disorders affect many people throughout the world. The three most common mood disorders are depression, seasonal affective disorder, and bipolar disorder, which formerly was known as manic depression. Like all mental health conditions, the main therapeutic interventions are behavioral counseling or talk therapy in addition to medications to address any chemical imbalances.

13-22a Depression

It is estimated that 350 million people worldwide and about 20 million people in the United States suffer from **major depressive disorder (MDD)**, also known simply as *depression*. Famous people including John Lennon, Abraham Lincoln, Ludwig Beethoven, Ernest Hemingway, and Vincent Van Gogh all suffered from this condition.

Depression is sometimes hard to assess because it gets confused with normal sadness and grief. The main difference is that depression is a profound, long-term feeling of extreme sadness and despair with the loss of hope. Everyone feels sadness or loss at some time, however, when these feelings become so intense and that they inhibit one's ability to eat, sleep, work, or function, they can be diagnosed as depression. A clear indication of depression includes feelings of hopelessness, emptiness, and being unworthy that lasts for weeks, months, or even years.

Signs and symptoms can vary, but general aches and pains, digestive issues, restlessness, irritability, loss of energy, eating issues, and thoughts of suicide can be added to the previously mentioned feelings. See Figure 13-23. The cause of

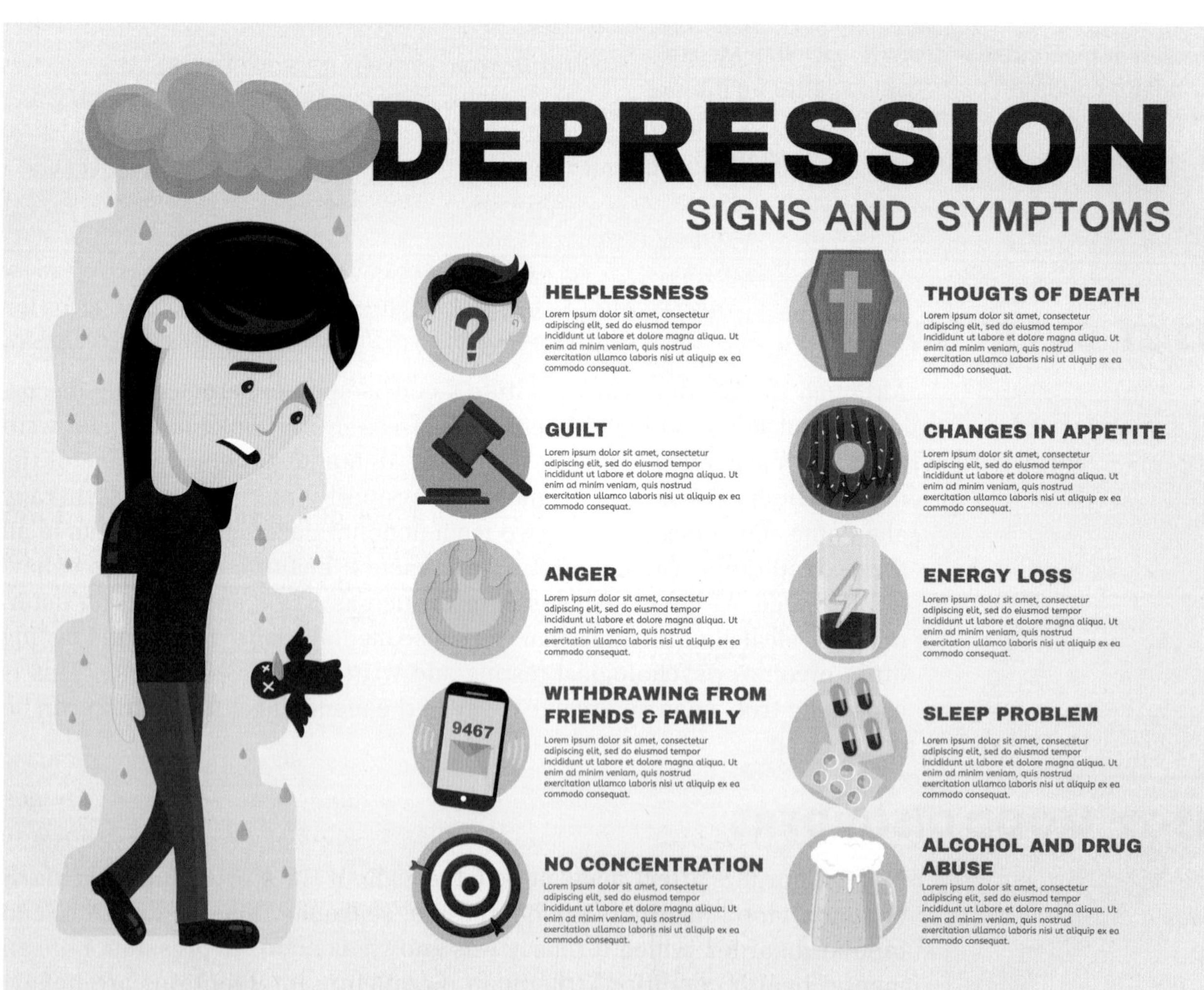

FIGURE 13-23 Depression Symptoms.

depression is not exactly known, but genetics seem to play a factor, along with functional changes in the brain such as the size of the hippocampus, which organizes our emotions and memories. Many illnesses co-exist with depression, such as substance abuse, anxiety disorders, and post-traumatic stress disorder (PTSD).

Although many men get depression, the disorder is more common among women because of the wider fluctuation in hormones in their menstrual cycle and during pregnancy. Postpartum depression is a very serious depressive condition that follows birthing and requires treatment, not only for the mother, but also for the health and protection of the infant.

13-22b Treatment of Depression

While all this information can be depressing, the good news is that this condition is 100 percent treatable with proper assessment, psychotherapy, medication, and lifestyle changes. The key factor is that the individual must seek proper help, which sadly often does not occur. Therapy alone can help with mild to moderate cases, with medication needed for severe cases of depression.

Selective serotonin reuptake inhibitors (SSRIs), such as Prozac, Celexa, and Zoloft, help the brain better utilize serotonin by keeping it around longer. **Serotonin and norepinephrine reuptake inhibitors (SNRIs)**, such as Cymbalta and Effexor, not only make serotonin use more efficient, they actually increase its production.

These medications take time to work and should be used at least 4–6 weeks to ascertain their full effect. Patients should be counseled not to stop taking the medication abruptly unless approved by their physician, as this can cause serious depressive and suicidal thoughts.

In addition, antianxiety medications, such as Xanax, can be prescribed for the associated anxiety levels. Lifestyle changes include finding support groups, regular exercise, good nutrition, healthy sleep, and reduction of stress by using relaxation techniques such as yoga or meditation.

13-22c Seasonal Affective Disorder

Seasonal affective disorder (SAD) is a type of depression associated with the winter months because of lack of natural sunlight. Although medications such as SSRIs and SNRIs can be used to treat the disorder, light therapy and getting outdoors during the winter are often very effective. Figure 13-24 shows light therapy treatment of SAD.

13-22d Bipolar Disorder

Bipolar disorder is a mental condition resulting in extreme mood changes, from emotional highs that are referred to as *mania* and emotional lows or depressive states. Depending on the severity of the disease, these mood swings from pole to pole can occur only a few times a year or as often as several times a week. See Figure 13-25.

The cause is unknown, but genetics, along with a biochemical brain deficiency, is highly suspected. A diagnosis can be made with extensive psychological testing, such as the Mood Assessment Questionnaire (MDQ) test.

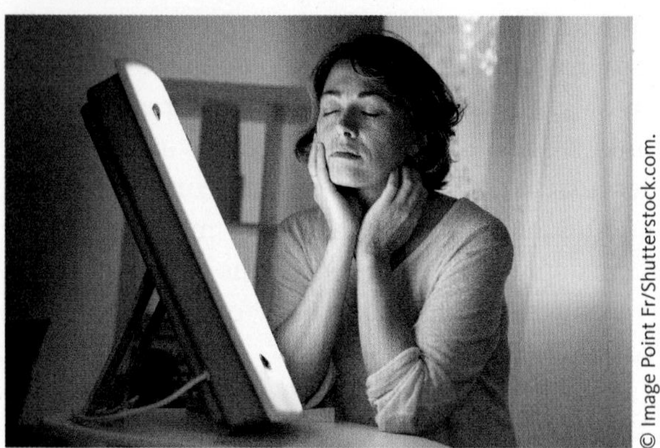

FIGURE 13-24 Light therapy treatment for seasonal affective disorder.

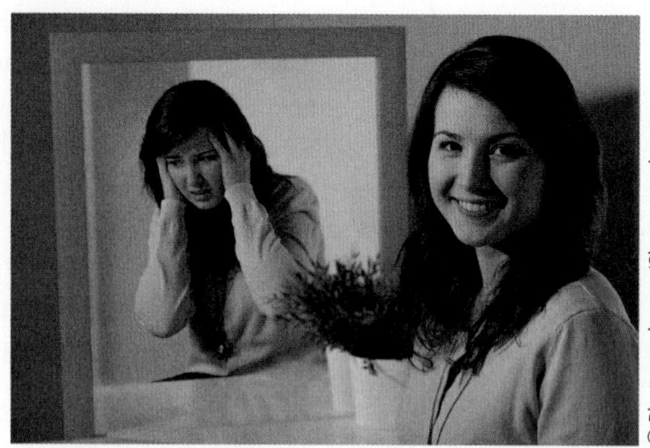

FIGURE 13-25 A person with bipolar disorder has severe mood swings from happy to sad.

Although there is no cure, psychotherapy along with supportive medications can help the patient have a high quality of life. Some examples of prescribed medication include the following:

- Mood stabilizers such as lithium to control the mania phases of the disease.
- Antidepressants such as Prozac and Effexor to treat the depressive stages.
- Antipsychotic medication such as Latuda (lurasidone HCl) is effective in combination with mood stabilizers to reduce episodes.
- Antianxiety medication such as the Benzodiazepines, Xanax, and Valium to calm patients.

As always, psychotherapy and support groups are important for successful treatment.

13-23 ANXIETY DISORDERS

It is normal to get anxious as a temporary response to a life stressor. However, when anxiety becomes chronic and exaggerated or inappropriate for the given situation, the individual likely has an **anxiety disorder**. The causes of anxiety disorders can be related to genetic factors, severe stress, biochemical brain imbalances, and even physical cause or disease such as hyperthyroidism.

Generalized anxiety disorder (GAD) is excessive worrying in which a person has an almost continuous state of anxiety and constant worrisome thoughts. A peak attack of anxiety known as a panic attack comes on suddenly and is accompanied by feelings of doom and the need for escape. Figure 13-26 shows some related terms to general anxiety disorders.

Post-traumatic stress disorder (PTSD) develops after an intense psychological event that is outside the range of normal human experience. This is commonly associated with combat situations, but also can include rape, child abuse or incest, acts of violence/terrorism, or natural disasters. Symptoms can occur immediately or not for months or even years after the event. Flashbacks are a common occurrence, with the victim reliving the traumatic event. Other symptoms can include relationship difficulties, depression, substance dependency, social withdrawal, and suicidal thoughts.

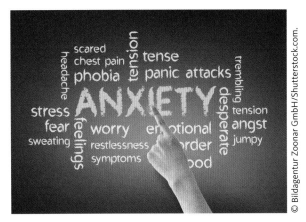

FIGURE 13-26 Descriptive associated terms of general anxiety disorder.

Table 13-4 Types of phobias

PHOBIA	FEAR
Arachnophobia	Spiders
Claustrophobia	Enclosed places
Iatrophobia	Physicians
Ophidiophobia	Snakes
Zoophobia	Animals
Triskaidekaphobia	Fear of No. 13
Acrophobia	Heights
Glossophobia	Fear of public speaking—The No. 1 phobia

13-23a Phobia Disorder

Phobia disorder is the most common anxiety disorder. A phobia is an intense and irrational fear of an object, event, situation, or thing. The individual often realizes it is irrational but still has little or no control over it. There are more than 700 different types of phobia; a few are listed in Table 13-4.

13-23b Obsessive Compulsive Disorder

Obsessive compulsive disorder (OCD) is an anxiety disorder with both obsession and compulsion. The obsession is the repetition of a thought or emotion. The compulsion is the repetitive act a person is unable to stop doing. The person becomes very ritualistic and must have certain thoughts or do certain behaviors repetitively, or extreme anxiety will build. These actions, including hand-washing, cleaning, checking object such as a stove, or locking and unlocking locks, can take up large chunks of their day.

Pharmacology treatment for anxiety disorders depends on the severity and type, but can include antidepressants and antianxiety medications. Nonpharmacological treatment includes psychological therapy, hypnosis, biofeedback, relaxation therapy, and support groups.

13-24 ATTENTION DEFICIT DISORDER

Attention deficit hyperactivity disorder (ADHD) is a mental health disorder that manifests as hyperactivity with the inability to concentrate and high levels of impulsive behavior, Figure 13-27. The cause is unknown but does appear to have genetic factors. ADHD is often diagnosed in children younger than 8 years old. Symptoms include the inability to remain seated, squirming, inability to wait for one's turn, disorganization, and inability to complete assigned work or tasks. Diagnosis is made upon observation of these behaviors, which often are more pronounced in group situations, such as attending school.

Treatment with amphetamines such as Adderall and Dyanavel has shown varying success rates.

13-25 DEMENTIAS

Dementia, formerly called senility, is a progressive deterioration of mental abilities because of changes in the brain. Dementia is not part of normal aging, but rather is caused by a variety of medical conditions. Contributing factors to dementia development can include substance abuse, medication side effects (drug-induced dementia), endocrine disorders, malnutrition, infectious neurological disease, head injuries, epilepsy, and cardiovascular disease (vascular dementia).

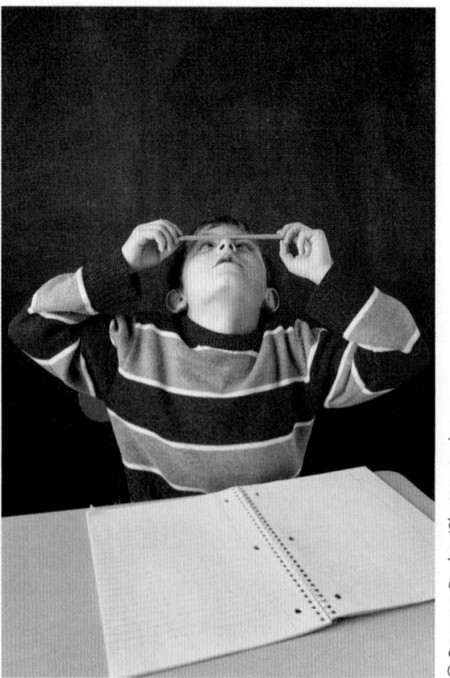

FIGURE 13-27 A child diagnosed with ADHD is unable to pay attention or perform work in class.

Symptoms often develop gradually with the loss of cognitive abilities, such as severe memory loss, impaired judgment, and disorientation. Someone with dementia might get lost driving in familiar territory or lose the ability to do common tasks such as balancing a checkbook. The symptoms can progress from highly bothersome to affecting the quality of life or the individual's ability to care for themselves.

Diagnosis is based on history and physical and neurological exams. The American Psychiatric Association lists two criteria for dementia: memory loss and loss of one of the major cognitive functions, including language, motor activity, recognition, and decision-making processes.

Treatment focuses on first identifying the etiology to see if correctible. For example, if the dementia is drug induced or caused by interactions of medications, it can be corrected with medication adjustments. In addition, malnutrition, substance abuse, and endocrine gland disorders can be reversed if diagnosed and treated properly.

13-26 ALZHEIMER'S DISEASE

Although **Alzheimer's disease** often is used synonymously with dementia, it is actually one type of dementia, albeit the most common type accounting for about 60 percent of all dementia cases. Alzheimer's is a progressive and irreversible form of dementia, commonly occurring about age 65, but it can occur as early as 40. While the cause is unknown, patients with Alzheimer's have been shown on autopsy to have higher aluminum levels in their brain and increased areas of brain plaques (buildup of fatty deposits). Also, people with head injuries, such as repeated concussions, have a higher incidence of developing Alzheimer's later in life.

Symptoms begin with memory loss. Simple memory loss, such as losing your keys, as one gets older is normal. However, Alzheimer's involves more severe memory loss, such as finding your keys in the refrigerator.

Memory loss eventually worsens and progresses to severe mental impairment, including personality changes, depression, dysphonia, and hallucinations. Later stages require personal care, and death usually ensues 10–15 years after onset. Treatment is aimed at relieving the presenting symptoms and making lifestyle changes, such as nutrition and physical and mental exercises, to slow the progression. Preventing head injuries is a good preventative measure.

13-27 EATING DISORDERS

Eating disorders are compulsions to eat or avoid eating that affects the person's physical and mental well-being. Two common disorders are **anorexia nervosa** and **bulimia**. The word anorexia by itself means "lack of appetite" and is a common symptom in many patients that can present because of a variety of reasons. However, anorexia nervosa is a mental health condition of self-imposed starvation because of a distorted body image of seeing oneself at all times as being overweight even when severely underweight, Figure 13-28. Bulimia is an eating disorder in which binge eating is followed by vomiting or purging the body of food. The exact cause is not known, but the societal emphasis on unrealistically super thin bodies as the ideal is greatly to blame.

Symptoms vary in severity but can include fatigue, growth impairment, menstrual irregularity, delayed puberty, personality changes, cardiac arrhythmia, and even death. While not 100 percent accurate, the typical profile of an

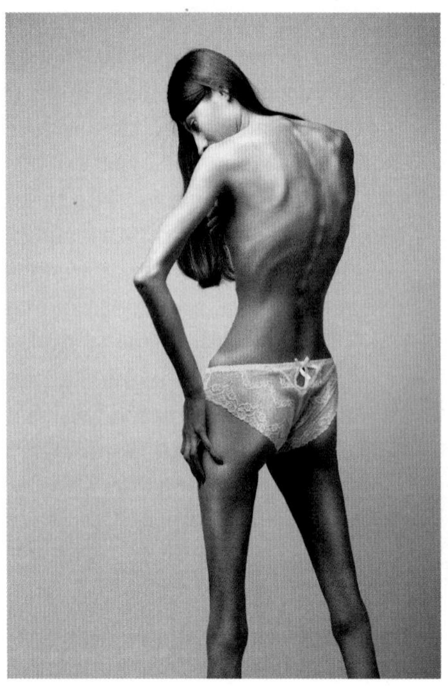

FIGURE 13-28 Severely underweight woman suffering with anorexia nervosa.

anorexia nervosa patient is of an adolescent girl who is a high achiever with an intense fear of becoming fat. She often exercises excessively.

Bulimic sufferers are usually older and have wider weight fluctuations. Because of their self-induced vomiting and excessive laxative use, they often develop electrolyte imbalances that can be dangerous to their health. In addition, frequent vomiting of acidic stomach contents often causes tooth erosion.

Another eating disorder on the other spectrum is **binge eating disorder (BED)**. This is characterized by eating large quantities of food often very quickly to the point of discomfort. This is not just overdoing it at Thanksgiving. Diagnosis is made by binge eating that occurs at least once a week for three months.

Treatment involves extensive psychological and nutritional counseling. The use of antidepressant medications is often beneficial.

13-28 SCHIZOPHRENIA

The word **schizophrenia** literally means split mind. However, schizophrenia is NOT the same thing as a split personality. Schizophrenia is a type of psychosis in which one has drastic personality changes and loses touch with reality.

Although the cause is unknown, schizophrenia has been shown to have a strong genetic component. It often develops between the ages of 16 and 25, and is more common in women and children who felt unwanted or unloved. People with this mental disorder often live in fantasy worlds and suffer from delusions, hallucinations, bizarre behavior/speech, and unresponsiveness.

Antipsychotic drugs are the main group used to manage schizophrenia. They do not cure the mental illness, but they can greatly reduce the symptoms and improve quality of life. Examples of antipsychotic drugs include chlorpromazine (Thorazine), fluphenazine (Prolixin), haloperidol (Haldol), loxapine (Loxapine), and trifluoperazine (Stelazine).

13-29 SUBSTANCE ABUSE

The annual cost of substance abuse in the United States is estimated at well over $180 billion per year. Some of the common terms used in substance abuse are tolerance, dependence, addiction, and withdrawal. **Tolerance** is the need for increasingly higher levels of drugs to get the same effect. This is why people might start off smoking only a few cigarettes per day to get a "nicotine high," but over time might work themselves up to multiple packs to achieve the same feeling. **Dependency** is the psychological need for a drug, a need that might or might not be accompanied by a physical need. A person might think she needs her morning coffee to get going, but physically she doesn't. Tolerance and dependency can lead to **addiction**, which is the physical and/or psychological dependence upon a substance. Finally, **withdrawal** is the unpleasant side effects and symptoms associated with abruptly stopping a substance to which one is addicted.

There are several types of addiction that can have a psychological and/or physical need, Figure 13-29.

13-29a Alcoholism

Alcoholism represents the most common form of substance abuse, with approximately 10 percent of the population affected. Associated mental disorders include anxiety and depression, as well as insomnia, sexual dysfunction, and amnesia. Resulting diseases from chronic alcoholism include heart disease, hypertension, cirrhosis, pancreatitis, peripheral neuropathy, and gastrointestinal disease. See Figure 13-30. Alcoholism severely affects families and relationships, along with causing serious and tragic accidents.

Intoxication occurs when the blood alcohol level reaches 0.10 percent or more. Four to six hours after intoxication, the individual usually feels a hangover effect that includes nausea, vomiting, headache, and fatigue. Chronic alcoholics can experience severe withdrawal symptoms 24–48 hours after abstaining from alcohol use. Symptoms include hallucinations, hand tremors, and mild seizures. A grouping of symptoms of memory loss, hallucination, anorexia, and agitation are called delirium tremens (DTs). DTs can last 1–5 days and can be fatal if not

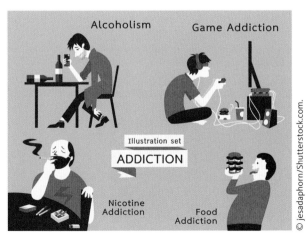

FIGURE 13-29 Examples of some various types of addictions.

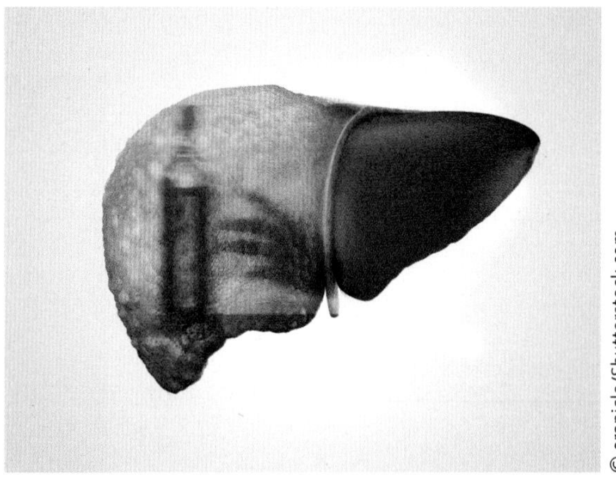

FIGURE 13-30 Alcohol-damaged portion of liver hardens and turns yellow (cirrhosis). Here it is superimposed on normal healthy red liver.

properly treated because they can lead to seizures. Treatment for withdrawal symptoms includes anticonvulsive medications, tranquilizers for calming, and antiemetic agents for nausea and vomiting.

An interesting treatment of chronic alcoholism is prescribing the drug disulfiram (Antabuse), which produces an acute sensitivity and causes immediate hangover-like effects if alcohol is consumed.

13-29b Narcotics

Narcotics are CNS depressants that are used primarily as prescribed painkillers (analgesics). Physical and psychological tolerance and dependence, however, can develop quickly. Examples of narcotics that have high-abuse potential are Demerol, methadone, morphine, heroin, and opium. See Figure 13-31.

Overuse of narcotics can severely depress the CNS and cause slurred speech, confusion, coma, and respiratory arrest. Opium is the dried milky residue from the pod of the poppy plant and has been used for centuries. Morphine is derived from opium and is a powerful analgesic. Heroin is derived from morphine, but is eight times stronger and highly addictive. Heroin can be injected, snorted, or smoked. Withdrawal symptoms include sweating, shaking, diarrhea, vomiting, sharp stomach pain, and leg cramps.

Methadone is a slow-acting opioid that can be taken orally to help prevent withdrawal symptoms. Buprenorphine (Subutex) also relieves narcotic drug cravings without producing the high or dangerous side effects of other opioids. Suboxone is the formulation of buprenorphine that is taken orally or sublingually and contains naloxone (an opioid antagonist or blocker). Naloxone (Narcan) can be used in emergency narcotic overdoses to prevent or reverse serious outcomes such as respiratory arrest.

13-29c Cocaine

Cocaine originates from the coca plant leaves of South America, but is now primarily synthetically produced as a white powder. Cocaine is a highly addictive CNS stimulant that produces euphoria and increased energy expenditure. It is abused by sniffing or snorting, IV injection, or inhalation (smoking crack). It can be addictive even after short-time use. Cocaine crosses the placental barrier and causes irritability, anorexia, and seizures in babies.

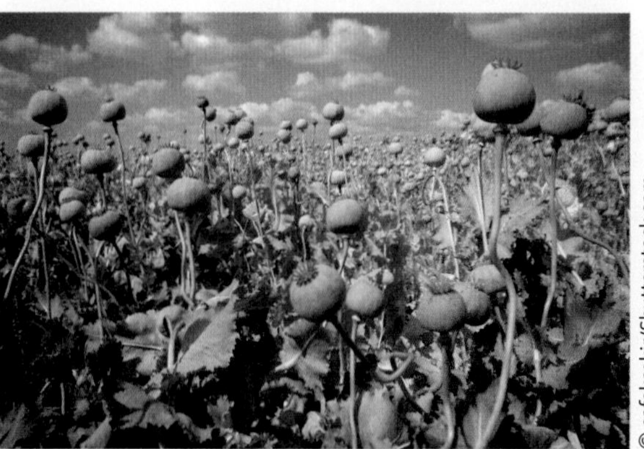

FIGURE 13-31 Plants with poppy pods, from which a milky residue containing opium is obtained.

CLINICAL CONNECTION 13.9

COCAINE

Although cocaine use has caused many deaths and led to many crimes, it does have an approved medical use. Cocaine is approved applied topically only to mucous membranes of the laryngeal, nasal, and oral cavities as a local anesthetic agent.

13-29d Methamphetamine and Amphetamines

Methamphetamines are a CNS stimulant and one of the fastest-growing abused drugs. It is relatively cheap and produced in home laboratories known as meth labs. The drug, also known as crystal meth, crank, glass, or ice, can be injected, smoked, or sniffed, Figure 13-32. Methamphetamines are highly addictive, and users develop a tolerance for it.

The effects of meth use, which can last up to 8 hours, include decreased appetite, high-energy levels, anxiety, and a general euphoric feeling. Sudden withdrawal from chronic use often leads to the opposite effects of drowsiness, depression, and suicidal thoughts.

Amphetamines are stimulant drugs that increase alertness, heart rate, and respiratory rate and were called speed, uppers, or pep pills on the street. These drugs are often used by truck drivers to stay awake and college students to pull all-nighters. Benzedrine and Adderall are two examples of amphetamines.

13-29e Sedative and Depressants

Sedatives, such as benzodiazepines (BDZs), can be abused, as can barbiturate depressants, such as phenobarbital. Examples of prescribed sedatives that can be abused are Xanax and Valium. Barbiturate street drugs are called downers, and they often are mixed with alcohol to potentiate their effect. Addiction and tolerance to barbiturates develop rapidly, leading to higher doses and addiction. Since this is a combination of CNS depressants, heart rate and breathing can be dangerously slowed or even stopped. Sudden withdrawal is also dangerous and should be medically supervised to prevent severe nausea, seizures, or delirium.

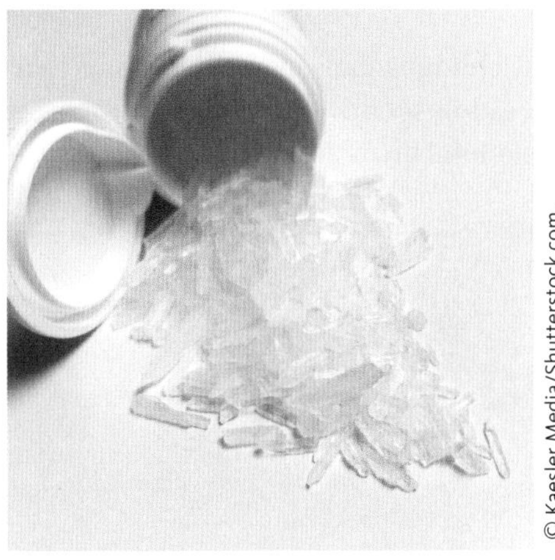

FIGURE 13-32 Crystal meth.

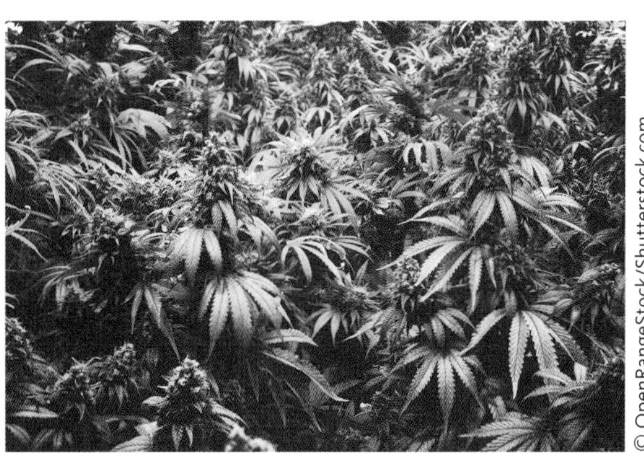

FIGURE 13-33 Marijuana plants.

13-29f Marijuana

The *Cannabis* plant that produces marijuana is grown throughout the world, Figure 13-33. The active ingredient is tetrahydrocannabinol (THC). Although technically classified as a depressant, it has properties of a euphoric, sedative, and hallucinogen. Several states have legalized its use for medical purposes, and currently, a few states have legalized it for recreational use. THC is absorbed by fatty tissue in the body and slowly released. This factor causes it to be found in urine for weeks after its use.

Physical tolerance to marijuana does not develop, but psychological dependence does occur. Short-term effects can include memory loss, slowed ability to learn, distorted perception, tachycardia, and loss of coordination.

Medical marijuana is approved for prevention of chemotherapy-induced nausea and vomiting. It also is used as an appetite stimulant for the cachexia or wasting because of anorexia that occurs in cancer patients. Glaucoma patients use it to reduce intraocular eye pressure.

13-29g Inhalants and Anabolic Steroids

Inhalants are chemicals in vapor form that can be inhaled into the pulmonary system to produce mind-altering effects. This very dangerous activity is often done by young people searching for a cheap high. The intentional breathing of inhalants such as glue, nail polish, gasoline, paint, or hair spray is called huffing or bagging. Bagging is the most dangerous because the user places a plastic bag over his or her head to get a longer effect.

Use of inhalants can cause permanent brain, heart, liver, and kidney damage, often leading to death. Inhalants are the third-most abused substances by teenagers, following only nicotine and alcohol. Symptoms of someone using inhalants include glassy eyes, mouth sores, anxiety, loss of appetite, and the smelling of fumes on the breath and clothing.

Anabolic steroids are synthetically produced forms of testosterone widely abused by athletes for performance enhancement. Steroids can be taken orally or injected and promote an increase in muscle size and strength and a leaner body mass in the short term. The long-term effects, however, far outweigh these temporary gains—and they are illegal. The side effects include shrinkage of the testicles for men, and infertility, baldness, and menstrual changes and deepening of voice in women.

A variety of extreme behavioral changes can occur, including increased aggressiveness known as "roid" rage. Adolescents or preteenagers can experience increased puberty changes and skeletal growth stoppage, along with mood swings and depression.

Module 14

Pathopharmacology of the Eyes and Ears

Module Introduction

So far, you have learned about many bodily processes and diseases in the various modules that discussed the various regions of the body. When an individual does not encounter a problem with a bodily system, many of these functions might be taken for granted. Therefore, you might realize its importance only when a function is compromised. Nowhere is this truer than with our senses, specifically our eyes and ears. Although when something goes wrong with our eyes and ears, it might not be life-threatening, it can, however, make life much more difficult.

An **optometrist** can be seen for basic eye care such as an eye exam or for medications to treat an infection. An **ophthalmologist** is a specialist who performs surgical procedures on the eye. If hearing impairment is the problem, an **audiologist** can determine if you might benefit from hearing aids. For medical and surgical treatment of the ear, an **otolaryngologist**, more commonly known as an ear, nose, and throat (ENT) specialist, should be consulted.

LEARNING OBJECTIVE 14.1 Explain the anatomy of the eye.

KEY TERMS

Aqueous humor Gelatinous fluid found in both anterior and posterior chambers between the lens and cornea of the eye.

Audiologist One who specializes in hearing impairments and disorders.

Choroid The vascular layer of the eye found between the retina and the sclera.

Ciliary muscles Muscles that flatten the lens to assist focusing.

Cones Provide central vision and the ability to see color.

Eyelids Skin folds located on the top and bottom of the eye that cover the eye when closed.

Iris Controls size and diameter of the pupil and therefore controls the amount of light allowed into the eye.

Lacrimal apparatus Consists of lacrimal glands and ducts, which secrete and drain lacrimal fluid.

Lacrimal glands Glands that produce lacrimal fluid.

Ophthalmologist One who specializes in treating disease of the eye.

Optometrist One who practices optometry.

Orbital cavity Two sockets located in the anterior portion of the skull that house the eyes.

Otolaryngologist One who treats conditions of the ears, nose, and throat.

Pupil The opening in the center of the iris.

Retina The light-sensitive portion of the eye that sends signals to the brain via the optic nerve.

Rods Provide side vision and the ability to see at night or in a dimly lit room.

Sclera Outer layer of the eye made of connective and fibrous tissues; the white of the eye.

Sebaceous glands Glands located around the eyes that secrete an oily substance to lubricate the eyes; known as meibomian glands.

Vitreous humor A clear jelly-like substance that fills the area between the lens and the retina.

14-1 EXTERNAL ANATOMY OF THE EYE

Your eyes are spheres that measure approximately one inch in diameter and rest in a cone-shaped cavity called the **orbital cavity**, which is lined with fatty tissue to protect the eyeball. Nerves and blood vessels attach to the eye through small holes in the orbital cavity. Each eye is connected to six different muscles to allow them to move in many different directions and to give it support.

The **eyelids** are skin folds found on the top and bottom of the eyes that protect them from debris and injury. On the eyelids are the eyelashes, tiny hairs that prevent large debris from entering the eyes. When an object gets close to your eyes, the eyelashes act as a trigger to close your eyes as a means of protection. They also help protect the eyes from bright lights.

Found near the outer edge of the eyelids are **sebaceous glands**, also known as meibomian glands, which secrete a type of sebum called meibum. An oily substance that lubricates the eyes and keeps them soft, meibum also comes in handy for trapping foreign particles. The outside of the eyeball, or conjunctiva, acts as a protective cover.

Each eye has a **lacrimal apparatus**, which is made up of various structures and ducts that produce, store, and drain tears. The **lacrimal glands**, Figure 14-1, are exocrine glands (remember, exo = outside) because these glands secrete

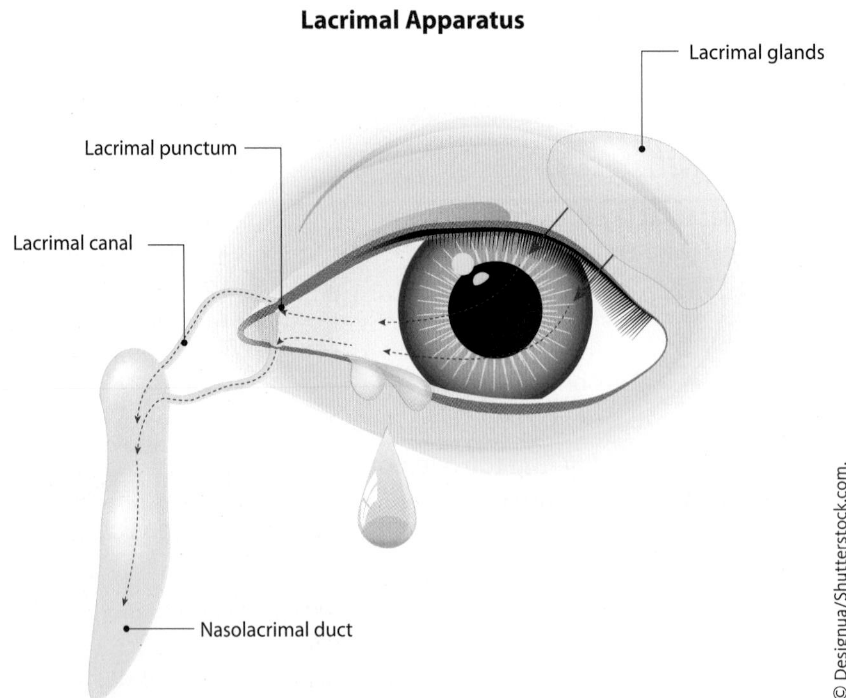

FIGURE 14-1 The lacrimal apparatus and lacrimal glands.

tears outside the body. Lacrimal glands create tears to clean and lubricate the eyes, while also acting as an antiseptic to fight infection.

14-2 INTERNAL ANATOMY OF THE EYE

The eyes are bathed in protective fluids known as humors. There are two types of humors: the **aqueous humor** and **vitreous humor**. Aqueous humor is found throughout the eye in both the anterior chamber (behind the cornea and in front of the iris) and the posterior chamber (the area between the outer portion of the iris and in front of the suspensory ligament), Figure 14-2. This watery substance also covers the lens and pupil. The vitreous humor is a jelly-like substance that fills the remaining cavity (virtuous body) of the eye behind the lens.

14-2a Layers of the Eye

The eyeball itself has three different layers, starting outward and working our way in is the **sclera**, **choroid**, and **retina**, Figure 14-3. The sclera, or white of

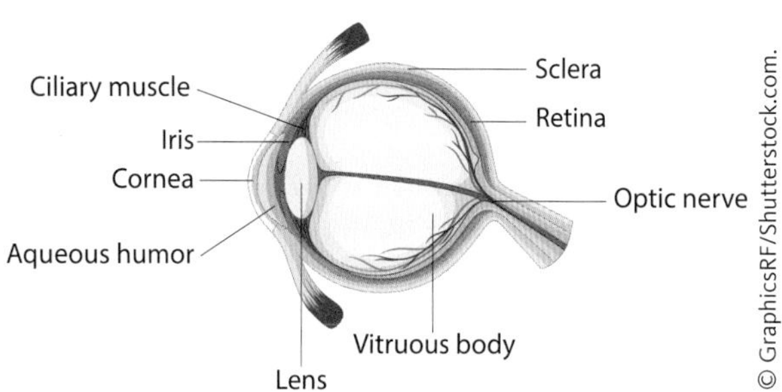

FIGURE 14-2 Location of the aqueous and virtuous humors with other structures.

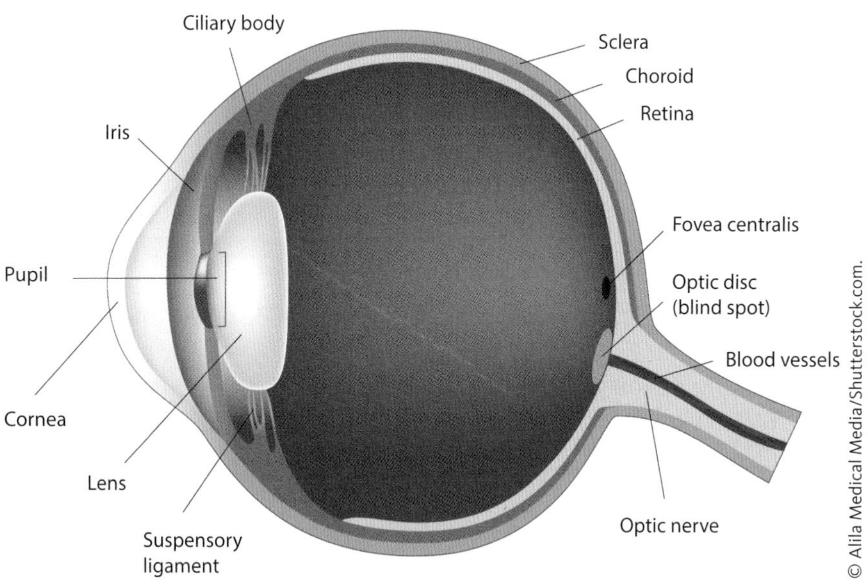

FIGURE 14-3 Anatomy of the eye.

the eyes, is the outermost layer of the eyeball. It is made of durable fibrous tissue that protects the eyeball. On the anterior portion of the eye is a six-layered transparent area, called the cornea, which allows light into the eye.

14-2b The Choroid Layer

The middle layer is the choroid. The choroid is a pigmented area of the eye with a plentiful blood supply providing nutrients to the eye. Also in this middle layer is the **iris**, the color portion of the eye, giving us blue or brown eyes, etc. The iris also controls the size of the **pupil**, which is the opening in your eyes that allows in light and can dilate or constrict in varying light conditions. For example, in a dark room, your pupil will get large to allow more light in the eye to get a better image. Conversely, the pupil will vasoconstrict in bright sunlight to prevent too much light from entering and damaging the eye.

Behind the pupil is the lens, which is surrounded by **ciliary muscles**. These muscles adjust the shape of the lens, making it thinner or thicker to allow light rays to go through the eye and focus on the retinal region. This process is known as accommodation, which combines the lens curvature and the size of the pupil to ensure the image meets at the same place on the retina so that it is properly focused.

14-2c Retinal Layer

The third and innermost region of the eye is the retina. The retina contains all the nerve ends needed to help your brain interpret the rays of light into images. The retina is a fragile membrane that eventually meets the optic nerve in the back of the eye. The retina contains receptors called cones and rods. **Rods** are active in dim light and do not perceive color, while **cones** work best in bright light and can perceive color. Rods and cones have photo pigments that cause a chemical change to occur when light hits them.

Light rays enter the pupil and accommodation occurs to adjust the lens so the light correctly meets and is focused on the retina. The retinal image or signal is then sent through the optic nerve to the brain, where the signal is interpreted, and you visualize the objects that you see.

LEARNING OBJECTIVE 14.2 Discuss the pathopharmacology of the eye.

KEY TERMS

Alpha-agonists (ophthalmic) Decrease the production of aqueous humor while increasing the outflow of aqueous humor from the anterior chamber to lower intraocular pressure.

Astigmatism A refractive error condition that causes light to be unevenly scattered over the retina.

Beta-adrenergic blockers (ophthalmic) Used to relieve the pressure of glaucoma by decreasing the fluid in the eye.

Blepharitis Inflammation of the eyelid that results in redness, crusty dandruff-like skin flakes on the eyelashes, and itchiness.

Carbonic anhydrase inhibitors Agent used to decrease intraocular fluid production to decrease the pressure in the eye.

Cataract An opaque clouding of the lens of the eye resulting in vision impairment.

Conjunctivitis Inflammation of the lining of the eye known as the conjunctiva, commonly known as pink eye.

Diabetic retinopathy Vascular changes on the retina; a complication from either Type I or Type II diabetes.

Glaucoma An eye condition that affects the optic nerve and overtime may result in blindness.

Hyperopia A refractive error condition known as farsightedness, meaning objects at a distance can be seen clearly while objects nearby are blurry.

Keratitis Inflammation of the cornea.

Macular degeneration A condition in which the macular region of the retina degrades, causing central vision impairment or loss.

Miotics Agent used to constrict the pupil of the eye.

Myopia A refractive condition known as nearsightedness, meaning objects that are close by are seen clearly, while objects at a distance are blurry.

Nystagmus A condition of involuntary eye movements.

Presbyopia Hyperopia caused by old age.

Prostaglandin analogs (ophthalmic) A group of agents used to lower intraocular pressure by increasing the outflow of aqueous humor from the anterior chamber.

Refractive errors Symptoms of a group of conditions that prevent light rays from properly reaching the retina at a correct focal point.

Strabismus A condition of abnormal eye alignments; also known as a lazy eye.

Sty Inflammation of the top or bottom eyelid from a blocked gland resembling a pimple or boil. Also called stye.

14-3 REFRACTIVE ERRORS

One of the more common eye problems deals with **refractive errors**. Refraction occurs when light bends as it moves from one object to another and again as light moves through the cornea and then the lens. The lens must adjust and focus the light rays properly on the retina for a good image to be interpreted by the optic nerve.

A refractive error can occur when the eye is misshapen, which means light does not land correctly on the retina. For example, if the eye is a little shorter or longer than it should be, light can be prevented from hitting the retina properly. The causes of refractive errors are unknown, but hereditary is a strong factor. The most common types are myopia, hyperopia, presbyopia, and astigmatism.

14-3a Myopia

Myopia, also known as nearsightedness, is when a person can see objects close by clearly while objects far away appear blurry. To keep up with the refractory theme, the light entering the eye does not focus on the retina because of the longer-than-normal distance from the front to the back of the eye, Figure 14-4.

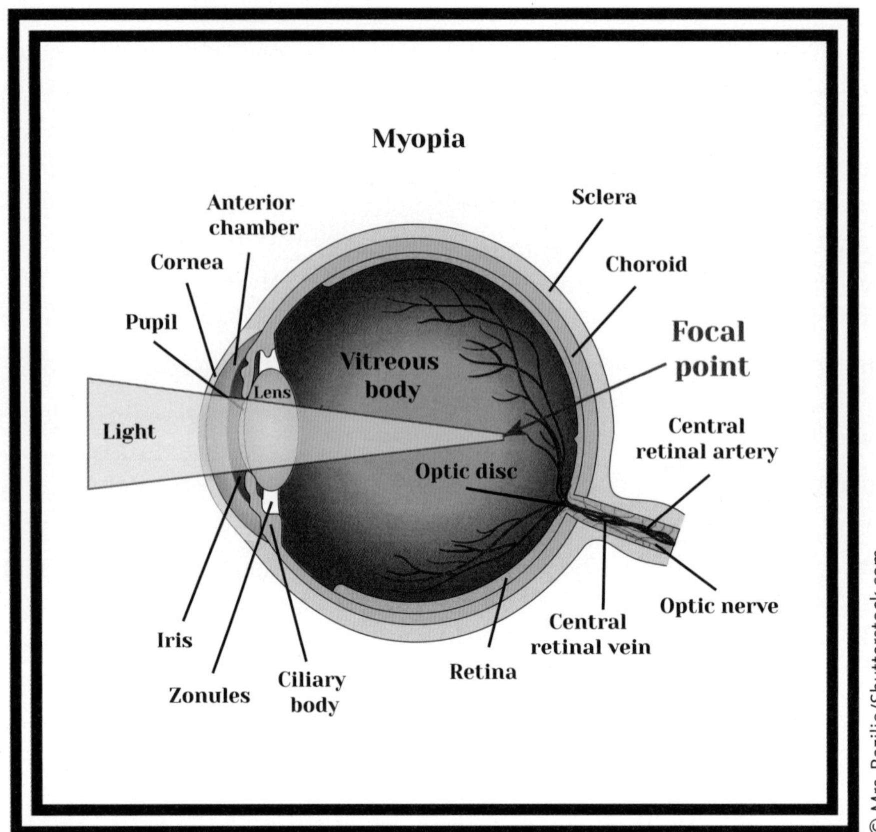

FIGURE 14-4 Image showing the focal point of light in an eye with myopia.

14-3b Hyperopia

Hyperopia, also known as farsightedness, is when objects far away will appear clear while objects up close look blurry. The light entering the eye does not focus on the retina because of the shorter-than-normal distance from the front to the back of the eye, Figure 14-5.

14-3c Presbyopia

Presbyopia is hyperopia that is caused by old age, hence the medical term "presby" meaning old age. Presbyopia usually occurs around age 40 and is why reading glasses become a needed item. This form of hyperopia is caused by the inability of the aging lens to focus light rays, not from a misshapen eyeball, Figure 14-6.

14-3d Astigmatism

Astigmatism is caused by an irregular corneal surface, which causes light rays to be unfocused and spread over the retina, Figure 14-7. This results in blurry vision that many patients describe as seeing halos around objects.

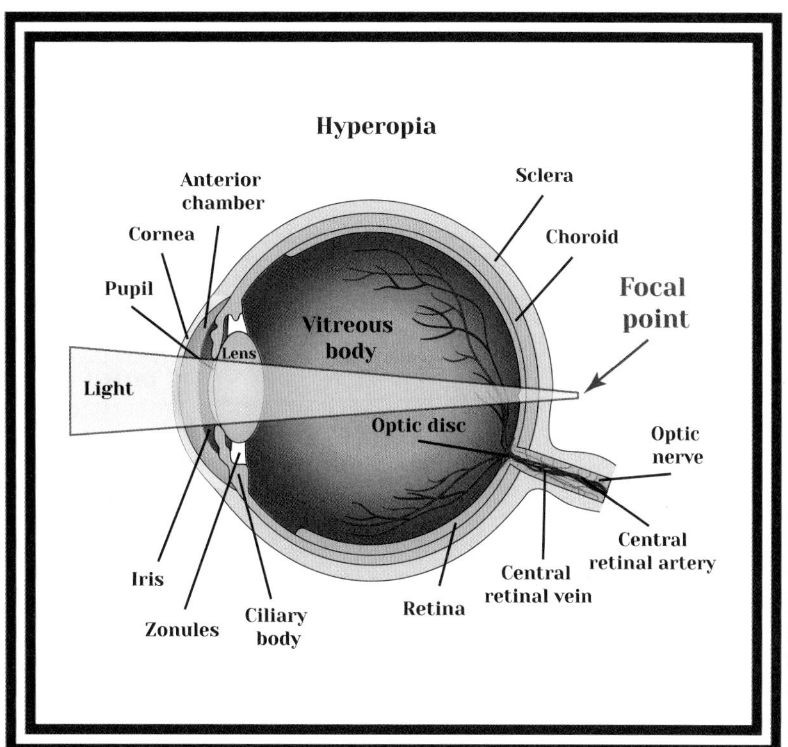

FIGURE 14-5 Image showing the focal point of light in an eye affected by hyperopia.

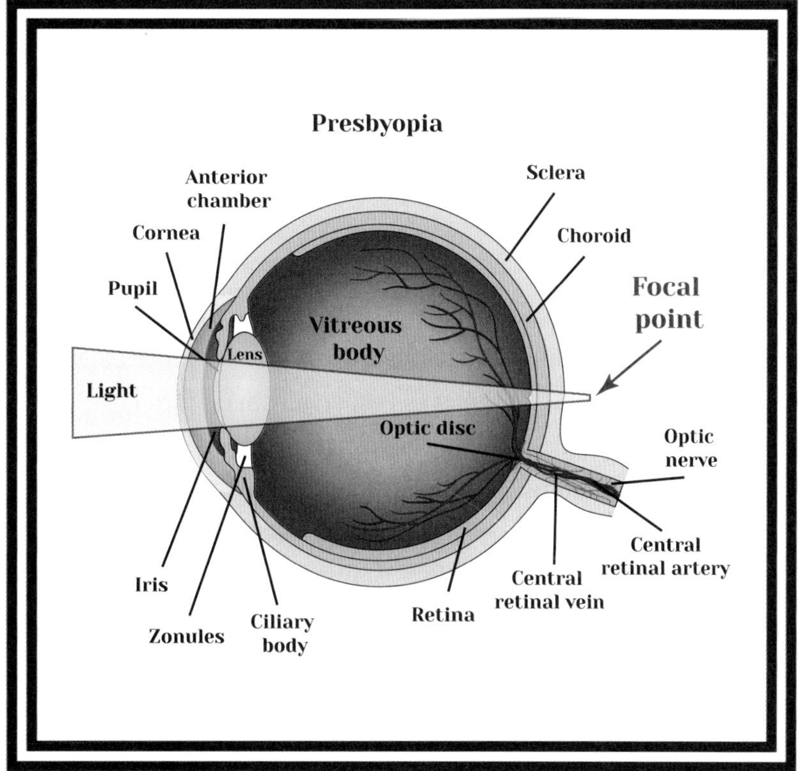

FIGURE 14-6 Image showing the focal point of light in an eye affected by presbyopia.

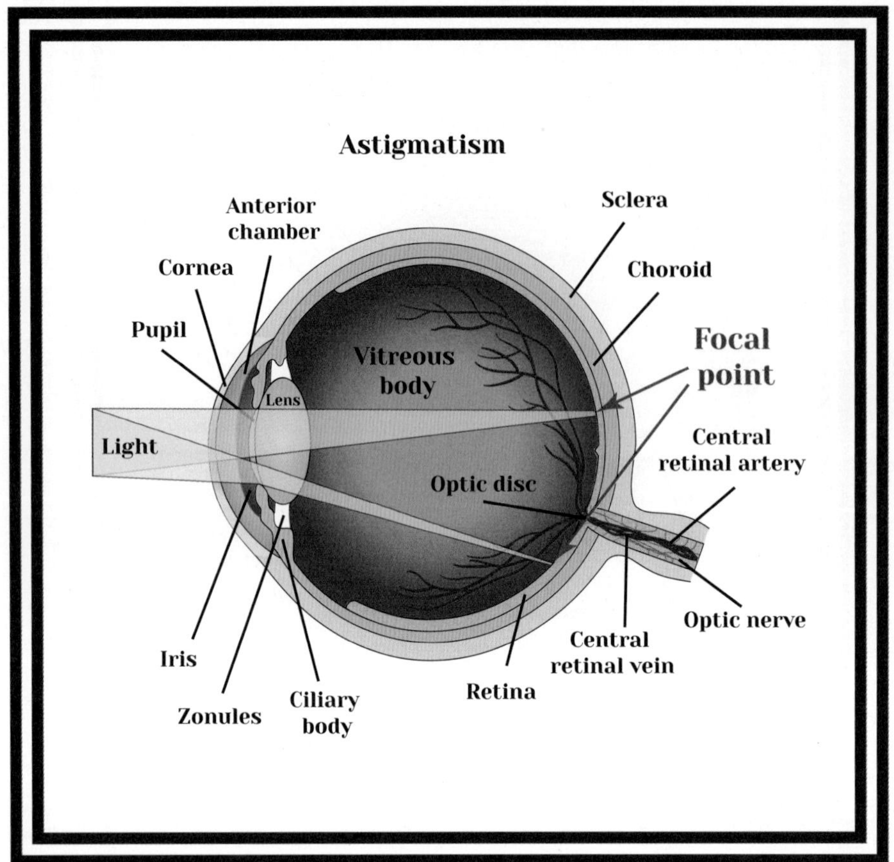

FIGURE 14-7 Image showing the focal point of light in an eye with astigmatism.

14-3e Diagnosing Refractive Errors

To assist in diagnosing one of these conditions, the physician will get a vision history from the patient. The physician might suspect a refractive error if the patient describes any of the following common signs and symptoms.

- Blurry vision
- Squinting or straining the eyes to see more clearly
- Rubbing of the eyes (especially in children)
- Headaches (from squinting)
- Difficulty reading up close
- Children who are unable to see clearly a chalkboard or whiteboard at the front of the classroom

To diagnose a refractive disorder, an ophthalmologist will complete a comprehensive eye exam. To study the patient's visual acuity, while one eye is covered, the physician will use a Snellen chart, which has letters arranged in a pyramid with a large "E" on the top. The patient is asked to read aloud the smallest line he or she can see clearly without squinting, Figure 14-8. The process is repeated with the other eye, and the patient's vision is compared to the standard of what is considered normal vision when reading at that distance.

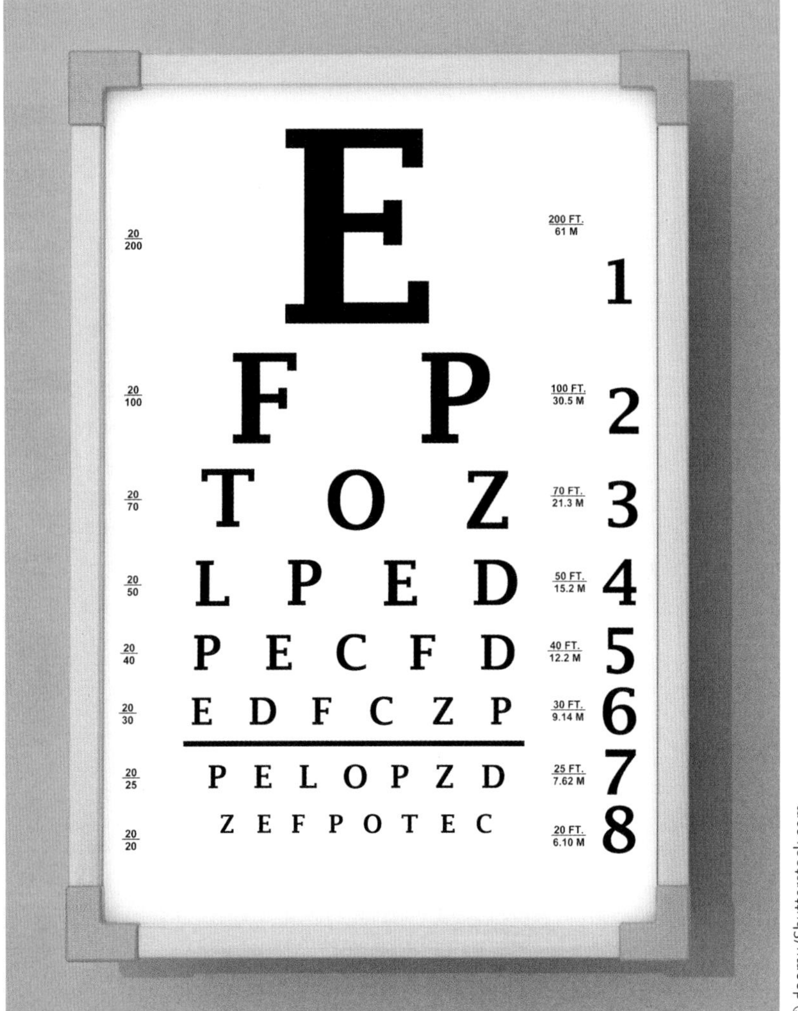

FIGURE 14-8 Snellen chart.

14-3f Surgical Procedures to Treat Refractive Errors

An ophthalmologist can prescribe corrective lenses or contact lenses for treatment of refractive disorders. More permanent solutions, however, can be done with various surgical procedures. A few examples can be found in Table 14-1.

14-4 COMMON INFECTIONS OF THE EYE

Infections of the eye are more common on the surface than the inside of the eye. Bacteria, viruses, allergies, and trauma are among the most common causes of eye infections. Conjunctivitis, blepharitis, keratitis, and sty (shown in Figure 14-9) will be explained, but first let's look at some eye medications, starting with anti-infective agents.

14-5 ANTI-INFECTIVE MEDICATION

Anti-infective agents, which come in both solutions and topical ointments, are indicated to treat superficial eye infections. Ointments are preferred to treat

Table 14-1 Examples of surgical procedures used for refractive errors

PROCEDURE	DEFINITION
Radial keratotomy (RK)	Used to correct myopia. Radial incisions are made in the cornea, shortening the length of the eye and correcting the refractive error.
Automated lamellar keratoplasty (ALK)	An instrument called a microkeratome is used to separate a thick layer of the cornea. By reducing its thickness, the refractive error is corrected.
Laser-assisted in-situ keratomileusis (LASIK)	A laser is used to cut and remove a portion of the cornea to make it flatter and lessen the curve.
Implantable contact lenses (ICL)	A contact lens is surgically implanted into the eye.
Conductive keratoplasty (CK)	This procedure tightens up the cornea with heat produced by radio waves, which shrink the tissue around the outside of the cornea.

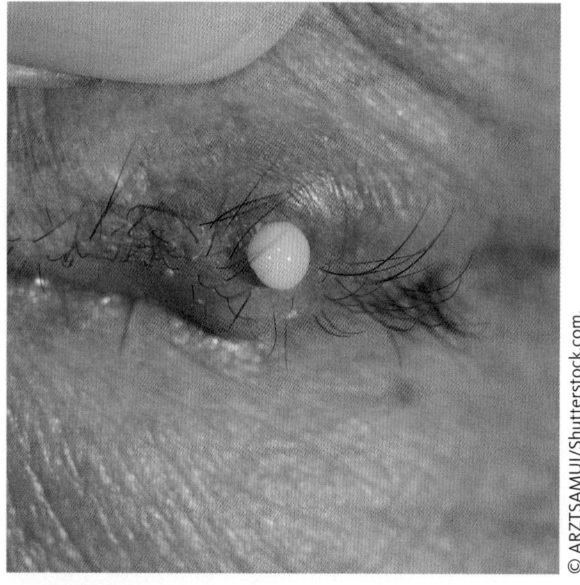

FIGURE 14-9 Ruptured sty.

children instead of drops, because patient cooperation is likely to be poor. For adults, however, drops are preferred over topical ointments because ointments cause blurred vision for 20 minutes after application.

To maintain the effectiveness of anti-infective agents and prevent drug-resistant bacteria from developing, the pathogen responsible for the infection must be identified. Ophthalmic antibiotic preparations can be used by themselves or in combination with another drug. Commonly used ophthalmic antibiotic preparations include:

- Macrolides
- Bacitracin
- Fluoroquinolones

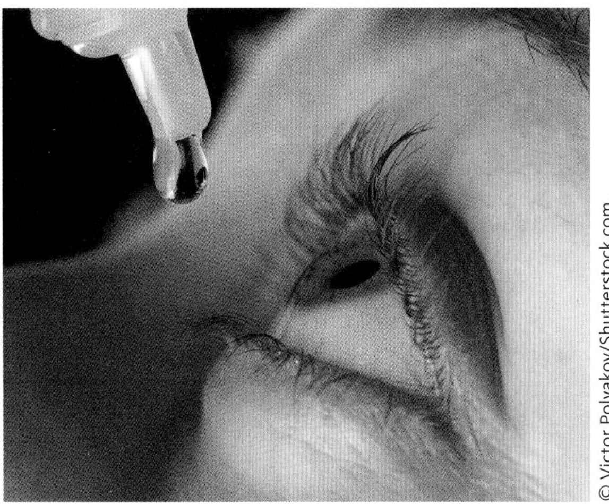

FIGURE 14-10 Instillation of eye drops to the left eye.

- Sulfonamides
- Bacitracin–polymixin
- Trimethoprim–polymyxin

Note: Aminoglycosides are not often used because they can be toxic to the corneal epithelium.

Topical therapy is generally used for seven to ten days. If used longer, opportunistic microorganisms such as fungi might grow.

14-5a Antiviral Medications

Although bacterial infections are treated with antibiotics, they have no effect on viruses such as herpes simplex, keratitis, and viral conjunctivitis. An example of an antiviral preparation is trifluridine (Viroptic) ophthalmic solution. One dose usually equals one drop to the lower conjunctival sac (the small space between the lower eyelid and the eye) of the infected eye. These drops can be instilled every two hours for a maximum of nine times a day while awake, Figure 14-10.

CLINICAL CONNECTION 14.1

If there is no improvement in the infection in two to three days, suspect microbial resistance, wrong drug choice, or wrong diagnosis. If this should occur, the antibiotic should be changed to another class, and the patient might have to return to the physician's office for a follow-up appointment.

14-6 ANTI-INFLAMMATORY AGENTS

Anti-inflammatory ophthalmic agents relieve inflammation caused by foreign objects, burns, or allergic reactions or after a surgical procedure (postoperatively). One such type of anti-inflammatory agent is corticosteroids shown in Table 14-2.

Many different types of corticosteroids are administered in the acute stages of an eye injury to help decrease the likelihood of scarring. Other reasons for

Table 14-2 Anti-Inflammatory ophthalmic drugs: corticosteroids

GENERIC NAME	TRADE NAME	DOSAGE
fluorometholone	FML	Oint, susp; varies with condition
prednisolone	Omnipred, Pred Forte	Sol, susp; varies with condition
	Many combinations with antibiotics	Oint, sol, susp; varies with condition
dexamethasone	Maxidex	Sol, susp, implant; varies with condition
	Many combinations with antibiotics	Oint, sol, susp; varies with condition

using corticosteroids are when severe symptoms are present, or if the eye does not respond to other drugs. Although corticosteroids have many side effects, ophthalmic corticosteroids have minimal side effects because they are topically applied and the effects remain local and not systemic.

Corticosteroids should not be used for longer than needed because they cause the eye to heal slower than normal and might only mask the symptoms of the infection. Also, if not used appropriately, these drugs can threaten the patient's vision.

Combination drugs that consist of both corticosteroids and antibiotics are used to treat steroid-responsive bacterial infections. Examples of such drugs are Tobradex (tobramycin and dexamethasone) and Blephamide (sulfacetamide and prednisolone).

14-7 NONSTEROIDAL ANTI-INFLAMMATORY DRUGS

Nonsteroidal anti-inflammatory agents are not usually the first-line of defense against inflammation but they are used if corticosteroids are contraindicated. For example, these drugs can be used to treat inflammation after cataracts are removed. Examples of NSAIDS include flurbiprofen (Ocufen) and ketorolac (Acular).

Caution applies to those who may be allergic to aspirin and other NSAIDs. While topical NSAIDs are relatively safe and have a few local or systemic side effects, patients allergic to aspirin should use with caution. Ketorolac can sting or burn during application, but keeping the solution refrigerated can help prevent this from occurring. See Table 14-3.

Table 14-3 Nonsteroidal anti-inflammatory drugs

GENERIC NAME	TRADE NAME	DOSAGE
flurbiprofen	Ocufen	Sol; varies with condition
ketorolac	Acular, Acular LS	Sol; varies with condition

14-8 OPHTHALMIC IMMUNOLOGIC AGENT

Topical cyclosporine (Restasis) increases tear production in patients whose tear production is suppressed because of ocular inflammation. Cyclosporine is an immunosuppressive agent for organ transplant rejection prophylaxis when administered systemically, but the risk of systemic toxicity is minimal when given topically. Topical cyclosporine has demonstrated long-term efficacy and safety in the treatment of dry eye disease.

14-9 ANTIHISTAMINES OR DECONGESTANTS FOR THE EYES

Antihistamines administered to the eye block histamine receptors in the conjunctiva, relieving ocular pruritus (itching) associated with allergic conjunctivitis. Decongestants administered to the eye cause vasoconstriction of blood vessels, thereby providing relief from minor eye irritation and redness, Figure 14-11.

These two classes of drugs are also used in combination in Naphcon-A and Visine-A. The most common use of ophthalmic antihistamines is from seasonal allergies that precipitate symptoms such as itchiness, redness, and irritation of the eyes.

Manufacturers recommend that these products should not be used for more than 72 hours. If the redness or irritation of the eye continues or patients experience eye pain or changes in vision, they should stop using the product and see a physician.

14-10 OPHTHALMIC LUBRICANTS

Ocular lubricants such as artificial tear solutions help protect the conjunctival mucosa by providing a barrier and helping to remove irritants and allergens by flushing them off the surface of the eye. Ophthalmic lubricants are very safe and can be used as often as needed. Artificial tear products that contain preservatives, however, can cause allergic reactions; in such events, use should be stopped immediately.

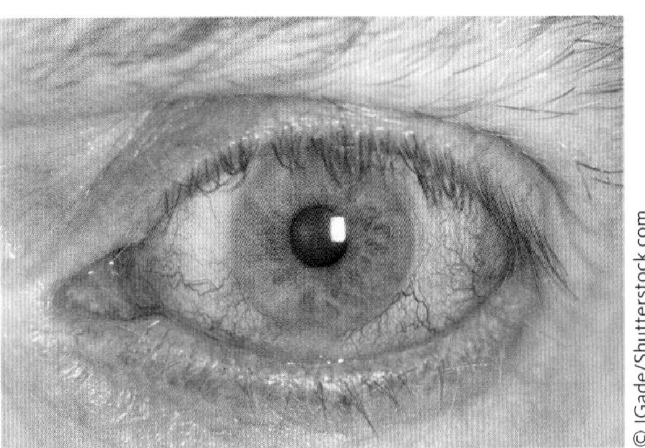

FIGURE 14-11 Irritated eyes.

14-11 LOCAL ANESTHETICS

Local ophthalmic anesthetics are used topically to assist in diagnostic procedures, minor surgical procedures, removal of foreign debris, or if a painful injury has occurred. See Table 14-4 for some ophthalmic anesthetics.

14-12 MYDRIATICS

Mydriatics, shown in Table 14-5, are used topically to dilate the pupil for ophthalmic examinations. Atropine also acts as a cycloplegic, which paralyzes the muscles of accommodation. It is the drug of choice in eye examinations for children. Other mydriatics, such as cyclopentolate, are commonly used for adults because of their faster action and faster recovery time.

CLINICAL CONNECTION 14.2

Have you ever wondered why some people wear sunglasses after an eye exam? If the physician instills mydriatic eye drops into the eye to assist in the examination of its structures, the pupil will become dilated and unable to shrink in response to bright light until the medication wears off. Therefore, to protect the eyes from bright light, the patient wears eye protection in the form of disposable sunglasses.

Table 14-4 Optic medications: local anesthetics

GENERIC NAME	TRADE NAME	DOSAGE
tetracaine	TetraVisc	Sol, 0.5% Note: Apply eye patch
proparacaine	Alcaine	Sol, 0.5% Note: Apply eye patch; store product in refrigerator

Table 14-5 Optic medications: mydriatics

GENERIC NAME	TRADE NAME	DOSAGE
atropine	Isopto Atropine	Oint, sol 1% Note: Administered 60 min before eye exam
cyclopentolate	Cyclogyl	Ophthalmic sol, 0.5%, 1%, 2% Note: Available in many different strengths
phenylephrine	Mydfrin	Ophthalmic sol, 2.5%, 10%

14-13 CONJUNCTIVITIS

Conjunctivitis, also known as pink eye, is inflammation of the conjunctiva (the outer mucous layer of the eye and eyelids) that causes the eye to become red or pink and swollen. Conjunctivitis can be caused by the sun and the wind, or from temperature extremes of cold and hot. If caused by bacteria, pink eye is very contagious. Symptoms include:

- Eye pain
- Itching
- Burning sensation
- Excessive watery eyes
- Pink or red color
- Inflammation

Diagnosis is made with a patient history and eye examination. If a bacterial infection is suspected, secretions or tears can be swabbed and tested for bacteria. Treatment includes analgesics for pain while a warm compress and anti-inflammatory agents are used to decrease inflammation. If caused by bacteria, antibiotic eye drops or ointment might be prescribed. See Figure 14-12.

14-14 BLEPHARITIS

Inflammation occurring around the edge of the eyelid, glands, and eyelashes is called **blepharitis**. This condition can be caused by irritants such as chemicals or smoke, allergens such as dust and pollens, and microorganisms such as bacteria. Seborrheic blepharitis is caused by a condition that causes the skin of the eyelids to flake off. If the flakes fall into the eye, they can cause irritation. See Figure 14-13.

Signs and symptoms of blepharitis are:

- Pain
- Redness
- Swollen eyes

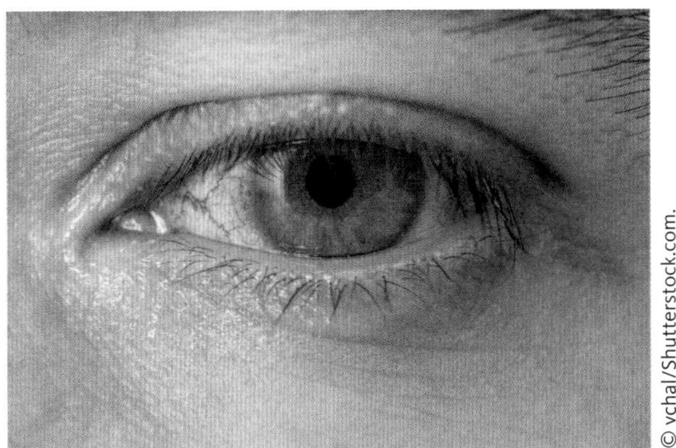

FIGURE 14-12 Conjunctivitis can be caused by bacteria, viruses, or stressful environmental conditions.

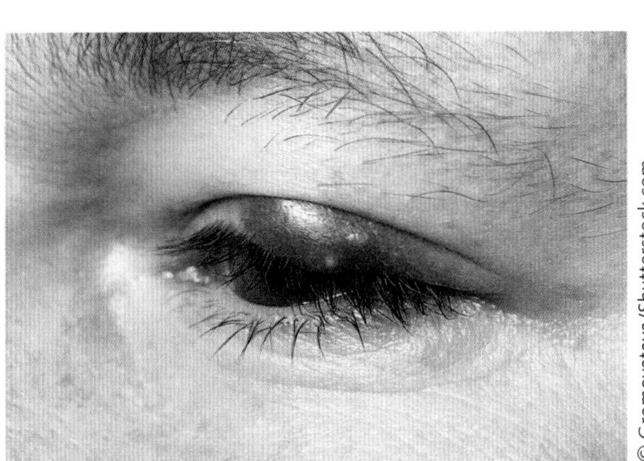

FIGURE 14-13 Left eye with blepharitis.

- Dry eye
- Itchiness
- Blurred vision
- Eyelashes might touch eye
- Eyelashes might fall out
- Watery eyes
- Burning sensation
- Flaky skin around eyelashes
- Crusted eyes

Diagnosis is made with an eye examination, which includes using a slit-lamp with a bright light and magnification. The physician also might test secretions or crust found at the eye for an infection. If bacteria are the cause, an antibiotic will be used, while a steroid will help reduce inflammation. An allergy medication might be needed if the condition is caused by an allergic reaction.

14-15 KERATITIS

Keratitis is inflammation of the cornea (the clear tissue in the exterior of the eye) and usually does not affect both eyes, making it a unilateral condition. Keratitis can be caused by an infection caused by bacterium, virus (herpes simplex or herpes zoster), fungus, or parasite. Noninfectious causes include a slight trauma or injury such as a scratch from wearing contact lenses too long, or a noninfectious autoimmune disease. Those with keratitis experience:

- Pain
- Redness
- Discharge or tears
- Feeling like something is in the eye
- Light sensitivity
- Blurred vision

This condition can be diagnosed with a routine eye examination. The physician might perform a penlight exam, which entails shining a bright light into the eye to check the reaction of the pupils. A stain can be used to help identify if any abrasions or other abnormal characteristics are present. A slit-lamp might be used to shine a bright light into the eye to examine the lens and iris, with magnification helping evaluate the structures of the eye. A sample of the patient's tears or corneal cells can be sent to a lab for further analysis.

After the cause is identified, treatment can be given. If it is caused by a bacterium or parasite, an antibiotic is used. If viral, an antiviral medication will be selected. Antifungal agents are used for fungal infections. See Figure 14-14.

14-16 STY

Shown in Figure 14-15, a **sty** (hordeolum) is inflammation of the sebaceous gland (the oil-secreting gland of the eyelid at the base of the eyelashes or inside

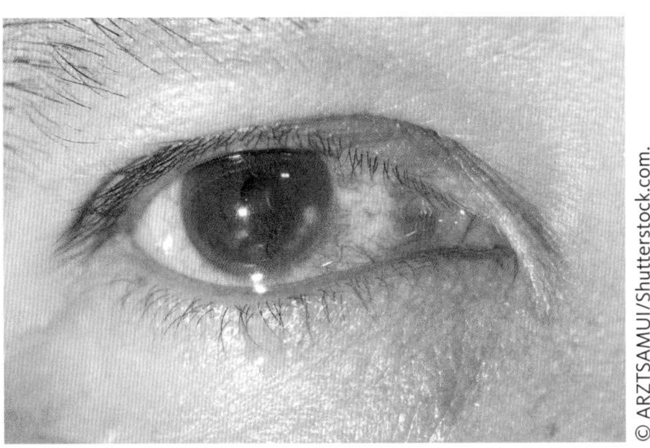

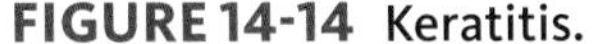
FIGURE 14-14 Keratitis.

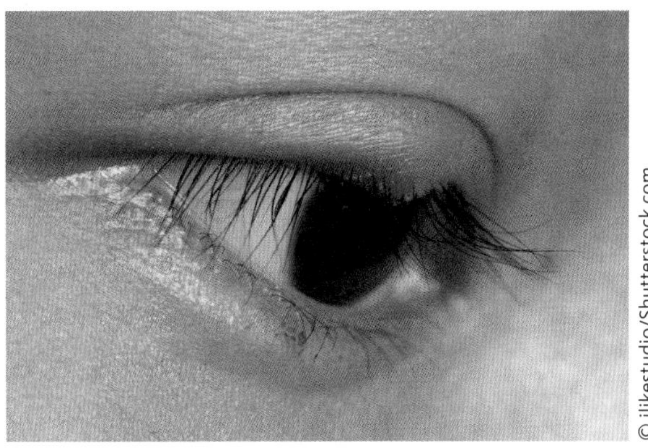

FIGURE 14-15 Sty located on upper right eyelid.

the eyelid). A sty, which resembles a pimple when irritated, is commonly caused by a staphylococcus bacterium and causes:

- Red pimple-like appearance on eyelid
- Pain
- Swelling of the eyelid
- Purulent (pus) discharge

Diagnosis is done by examining the patient's eyelid. A sty usually does not require any treatment. However, if the condition does not subside with a warm compress, antibiotic eye drops or ointment may be used. If the condition does not totally resolve, then antibiotics can be given orally. Also, an incision on the sty might be needed to relieve the buildup of pus.

14-17 NONINFECTIOUS CONDITIONS OF THE EYE

There are also many noninfectious conditions of the eye such as cataract, glaucoma, macular degeneration, and diabetic-related eye issues. These conditions require specialized diagnostic testing and treatment.

14-18 CATARACT

A **cataract** is clouding of the lens of the eye and is typically caused by changes in the nutrition and metabolism of the eye's lens as a person ages, Figure 14-16. The eye lens becomes less pliable and becomes thicker. When a cataract is in its early stages, it might not interfere with a patient's vision. As the condition slowly progresses, however, the once-clear lens becomes cloudy, and it is like looking through a haze or fog. When the patient can no longer see well enough to perform basic daily activities, surgery is required to remove the cataract. Although cataracts are most often caused by increasing age, they also can be caused by diabetes mellitus, long-term steroid use, and genetic disorders.

Signs and symptoms include, but are not limited to:

- Blurry vision
- Difficulty seeing at night
- Double vision in only one eye

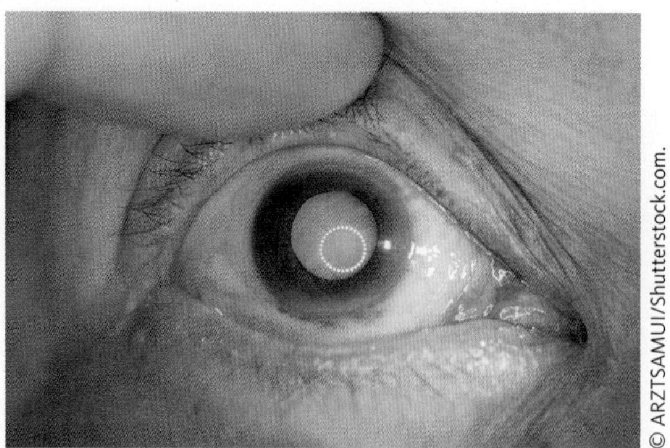

FIGURE 14-16 Shown is a thicker, cloudy lens caused by a cataract.

- Seeing a halo around objects
- Requiring bright light to see clearly

To diagnose cataracts, an eye examination is performed along with a visual acuity test to check how well the patient can read letters from a chart. A slit-lamp exam can be used to inspect the structures of the eye, and a retinal exam is completed by dilating the pupils using eye drops to examine the retina with an ophthalmoscope.

To correct a cataract, surgery is required to remove the cloudy lens and insert an artificial lens in its place. The procedure begins with eye drops or an injection around the eye before surgery to help it relax. The surgeon enters the eye via small incisions in the cornea, breaks apart the lens, and removes the pieces through these tiny incisions. After the lens has been removed, the new artificial lens is inserted. The small incisions will close on their own as the eye heals. The eye is covered to protect it from light and medicated eye drops are used. The drops include a steroidal anti-inflammatory such as Pred Forte (prednisolone) to reduce inflammation and antibiotics such as Azasite (azithromycin) to prevent or treat infection. A third type of eye drop such as Acular (ketorolac), a nonsteroidal anti-inflammatory agent to treat pain, can be indicated post-surgery.

14-19 GLAUCOMA

While rarely affecting people younger than 40, glaucoma is a condition caused by excessive pressure in the eye from the aqueous humor fluid. Aqueous humor is secreted by the ciliary epithelium, circulates throughout the eye, and is then reabsorbed back into the bloodstream. Pressure in the eye is caused by either too much fluid in the eye or the inability for the fluid to drain properly from the eye.

Glaucoma tends to be an inherited condition that will show up later in the patient's life. If not treated within a couple of years, this condition will result in permanent blindness from damage caused to the optic nerve from increased intraocular pressure. See Figure 14-17.

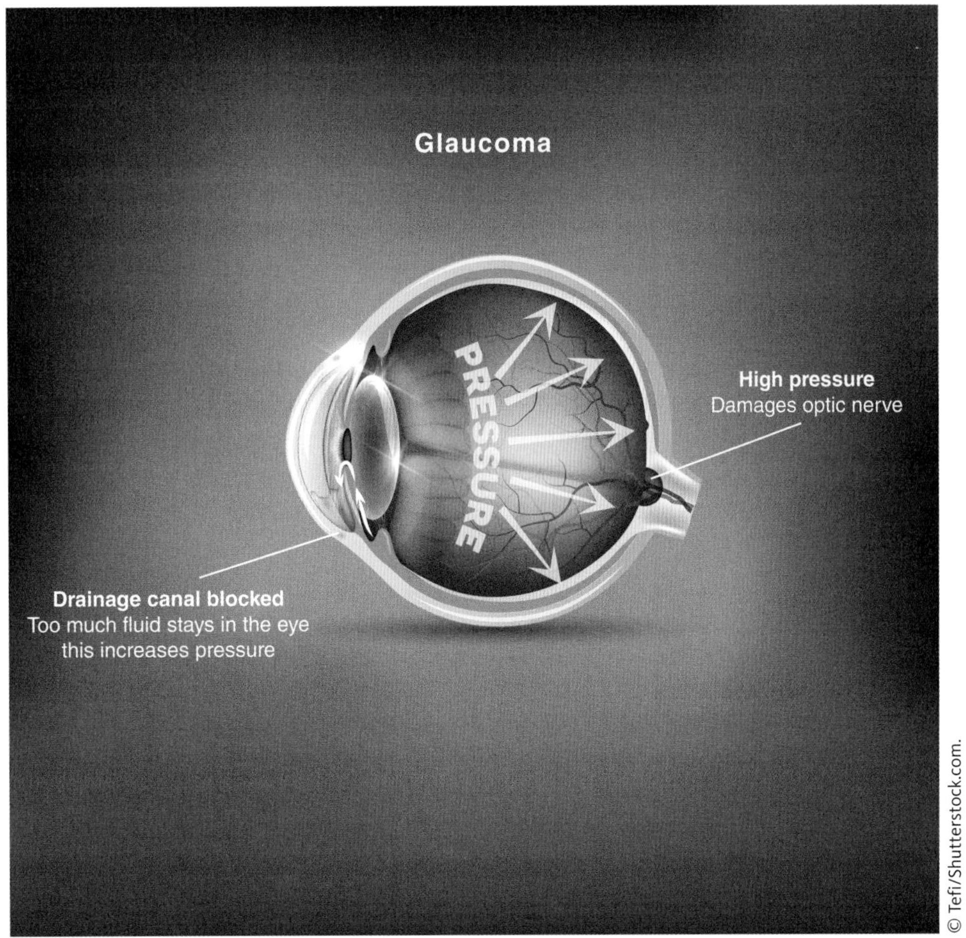

FIGURE 14-17 Glaucoma caused by pressure buildup from a blockage in the eye.

14-19a Types of Glaucoma and Diagnosis

The two main types of glaucoma are open-angle glaucoma and angle-closure glaucoma, of which the more common is open-angle glaucoma.

Open-angle glaucoma, also known as wide-angle glaucoma, is caused by the eye not draining as it should, causing increased pressure. Open-angle glaucoma occurs slowly, so patients might not recognize any damage or signs and symptoms.

Angle-closure glaucoma is caused by a sudden increase in pressure inside the eye (intraocular) or a blocked drainage canal. Angle-closure glaucoma develops quickly, and the patient notices signs and symptoms. This type causes a narrowing or closing angle between the cornea and iris of the eye.

Signs and symptoms of glaucoma are:

- Peripheral vision loss
- Eye pain
- Seeing halos
- Narrowed vision
- Nausea

The physician will use drops to dilate the pupils before examining the eye and inspecting the optic nerve for damage. A routine vision test is done to check the patient's peripheral vision, and a test called tonometry is done to check the pressure in the eye. Noncontact tonometry or pneumotonometry is done by shooting a puff of air at the eye to flatten the cornea to measure its resistance. This method does not require eye drops to numb the eye because there is no actual contact.

14-19b Treatment of Glaucoma

Treating glaucoma depends on the type. Treatment can include eye drops and surgery such as laser trabeculoplasty to help correct open-angle glaucoma or laser iridotomy to treat closed-angle glaucoma. Medicated eye drops can decrease the pressure in the eye by reducing the amount of fluid or by facilitating fluid out of the eye by way of the drainage canal.

Antiglaucoma drugs work in different ways and can be divided into five main categories based on their actions.

14-19c Carbonic Anhydrase Inhibitors

Carbonic anhydrase inhibitors such as dorzolamide (Trusopt) decrease the formation of aqueous humor and have a diuretic effect to clear fluid from the eyes. Oral acetazolamide (Diamox Sequels) in large part has been replaced by topical preparations, because they have fewer side effects. However, it is occasionally used in the adjunctive treatment of open-angle glaucoma or short-term preoperatively (IV or regular-release tabs) to reduce intraocular pressure (IOP) in angle-closure glaucoma and is given with miotics. See Table 14-6.

14-19d Miotics

Miotics increase the aqueous humor outflow, which reduces IOP. These drugs also cause the contraction of the ciliary muscles, which can cause blurred vision. Miotics such as pilocarpine, shown in Table 14-7, are indicated in the treatment of open-angle glaucoma if both first- and second-line drugs do not work. Pilocarpine is the third line of therapy because of the associated side effects. However, pilocarpine can be used in the short-term treatment of angle-closure glaucoma before surgery.

Table 14-6 Antiglaucoma agents: carbonic anhydrase inhibitors

GENERIC NAME	TRADE NAME	DOSAGE
acetazolamide	Diamox	Tab, IV, 125–250 mg two to four times per day (max 1 g per day)
	Diamox Sequels	ER cap 500 mg PO BID (max 1 g per day)
dorzolamide	Trusopt	Ophthalmic sol 1 drop TID

Note: Diamox is no longer marketed, but the name is still commonly used.

Table 14-7 Antiglaucoma agents: miotics

GENERIC NAME	TRADE NAME	DOSAGE
pilocarpine HCl	Isopto Carpine	Ophthalmic sol 1%, 2%, 4%[c]; 1 drop up to four times per day
pilocarpine gel	Pilopine HS	Ophthalmic gel 4%[c] at bedtime

Table 14-8 Antiglaucoma agents: beta-adrenergic blockers

GENERIC NAME	TRADE NAME	DOSAGE
timolol	Timoptic	Ophthalmic sol 0.25–0.5%, 1 drop BID
	Timoptic-XE	Ophthalmic gel 0.25–0.5%, 1 drop daily
timolol 0.5% with dorzolamide 2%	Cosopt	Ophthalmic sol 1 drop BID
betaxolol	Betoptic-S	Ophthalmic susp 0.25%, 1 drop BID

Pilocarpine can be used in glaucoma patients to constrict the pupil and counteract the mydriatic (pupil-dilating) effects of other drugs. Drugs that are usually given with miotics are acetazolamide and/or timolol. Because of its increased duration and less-frequent administration, pilocarpine hydrochloride gel (Pilopine HS) is given for its advantages over ophthalmic medications, especially for long-term use with noncompliant patients.

14-19e Beta-Adrenergic Blockers

Beta-adrenergic blockers such as timolol (Timoptic) lower pressure in the eye by decreasing the production rate of aqueous humor. Timoptic is a topically applied nonselective beta-adrenergic blocker that lowers the IOP in open-angle glaucoma. See Table 14-8.

14-19f Alpha-Agonists

Alpha-agonists such as brimonidine (Alphagan-P), which is a selective alpha2-agonist, increase the outflow of aqueous humor while decreasing the production of aqueous humor. Since it is a selective agent, it works without causing mydriasis and has minimal effects on cardiovascular or pulmonary hemodynamics. Brimonidine is an alternative for whom topical beta-blocker therapy is contraindicated. See Table 14-9.

Table 14-9 Antiglaucoma agents: alpha-agonists

GENERIC NAME	TRADE NAME	DOSAGE
brimonidine	Alphagan-P	Ophthalmic sol 0.1%, 0.15%, 0.2%; 1 drop TID (8 h apart)
brimonidine 0.2% with timolol 0.5%	Combigan	Ophthalmic sol 1 drop q12h

Table 14-10 Antiglaucoma agents: prostaglandin analogs

GENERIC NAME	TRADE NAME	DOSAGE
latanoprost	Xalatan	Ophthalmic sol 0.005%, 1 drop at bedtime
travoprost	Travatan-Z	Ophthalmic sol 0.004%, 1 drop at bedtime

14-19g Prostaglandin Analogs

Prostaglandin analogs such as latanoprost (Xalatan) and travoprost (Travatan Z) are first-line agents in treating IOP by increasing aqueous outflow to decrease IOP. These drugs can be used with other topical ophthalmic drugs to lower IOP, but they should be used at least five minutes apart. See Table 14-10.

14-20 NYSTAGMUS

Nystagmus is constant involuntary movement in circular, vertical, or horizontal directions of one or both eyes as shown in Figure 14-18. The patient might not even realize it is happening. This condition can be caused by a congenital neurological defect or the result of a stroke or trauma later in life.

Abnormal eye movement is the major sign of this condition. Diagnosis is made by looking at the patient's medical history, an eye examination to check the patient for a refractive error that needs to be corrected, or other imaging methods such as an MRI or CT scan.

Nystagmus can decrease over time, and surgery is rarely used because it does not cure the condition. It would help patients see better only by not having to turn their head to see. Corrective lenses might also help decrease this unwanted eye movement.

14-21 STRABISMUS

Often referred to as a lazy eye, **strabismus** is a condition in which the patient's eye or eyes are unable to look in the same direction at the same time because of a weak muscle in the affected eye. If the eye points inward toward the nose, it is called convergent strabismus; when the eye points outward, it is called a divergent strabismus. This condition requires early intervention to prevent

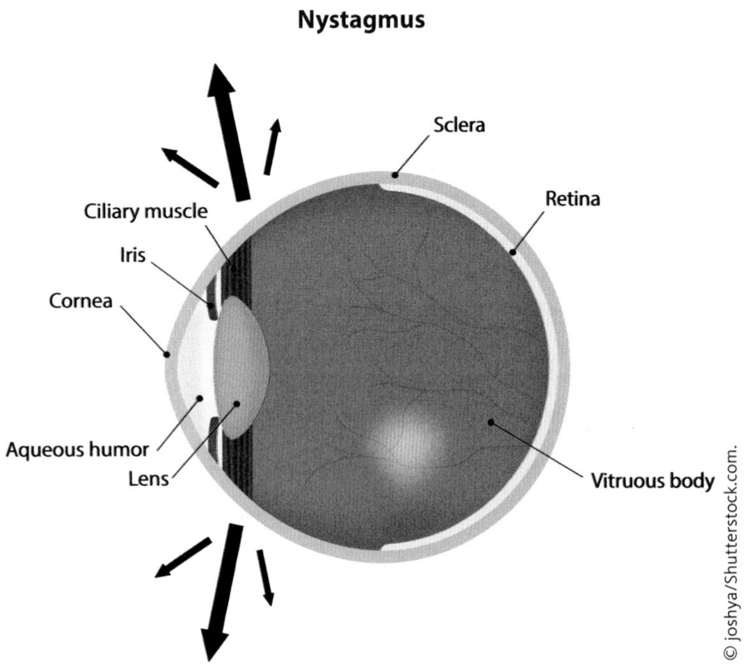

Nystagmus
Sclera
Retina
Ciliary muscle
Iris
Cornea
Aqueous humor
Lens
Vitruous body
© joshya/Shutterstock.com.

FIGURE 14-18 The various directions the eye can move when nystagmus is present.

© Julia Kuznetsova/Shutterstock.com.

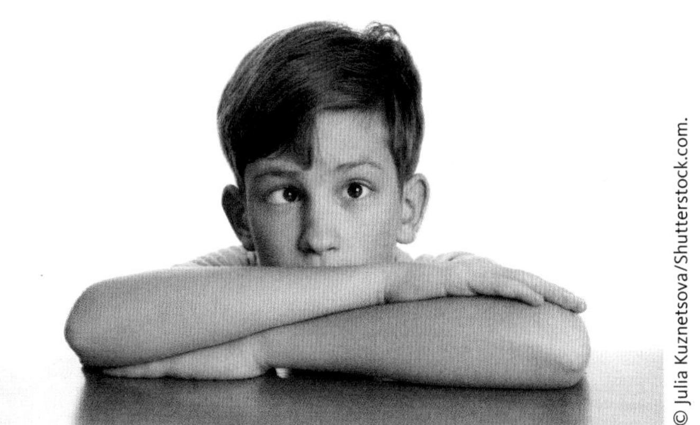

FIGURE 14-19 Young boy with strabismus.

amblyopia, a decrease in vision in the affected eye. The most prominent sign is double vision (diplopia). See Figure 14-19.

To diagnose, the patient is instructed to focus on an object with his or her unaffected eye. That eye is then covered, and the affected eye will straighten out to focus on the object.

Treatment involves eye exercises and covering the unaffected eye to force the lazy eye to function appropriately. If this does not work, surgery will be required.

14-22 MACULAR DEGENERATION

Macular degeneration is the degeneration of the macular area (central region of the retina) of the eye. The macular region is responsible for sending images to the brain via the optic nerve. The condition is irreversible and permanent.

The two types of macular degeneration are dry and wet (exudative). Dry macular degeneration is caused by the accumulation of yellow deposits called drusen, which lessen the thickness of the macula causing it to dry out and begin to lose function. The amount of function loss is in direct correlation with the amount and location of the drusen.

Wet or exudative macular degeneration is caused by the leakage from abnormal blood vessels into the macula of the eye. This blood has cellular debris such as red blood cells and white blood cells known as exudate that damage the macula, resulting in central vision loss.

Macular degeneration is commonly caused by old age and often is called age-related macular degeneration (AMD). There are three stages of AMD. During the early stage of the disease, the patient might not have any vision impairment. However, as it progresses to the intermediate stage, patients might experience

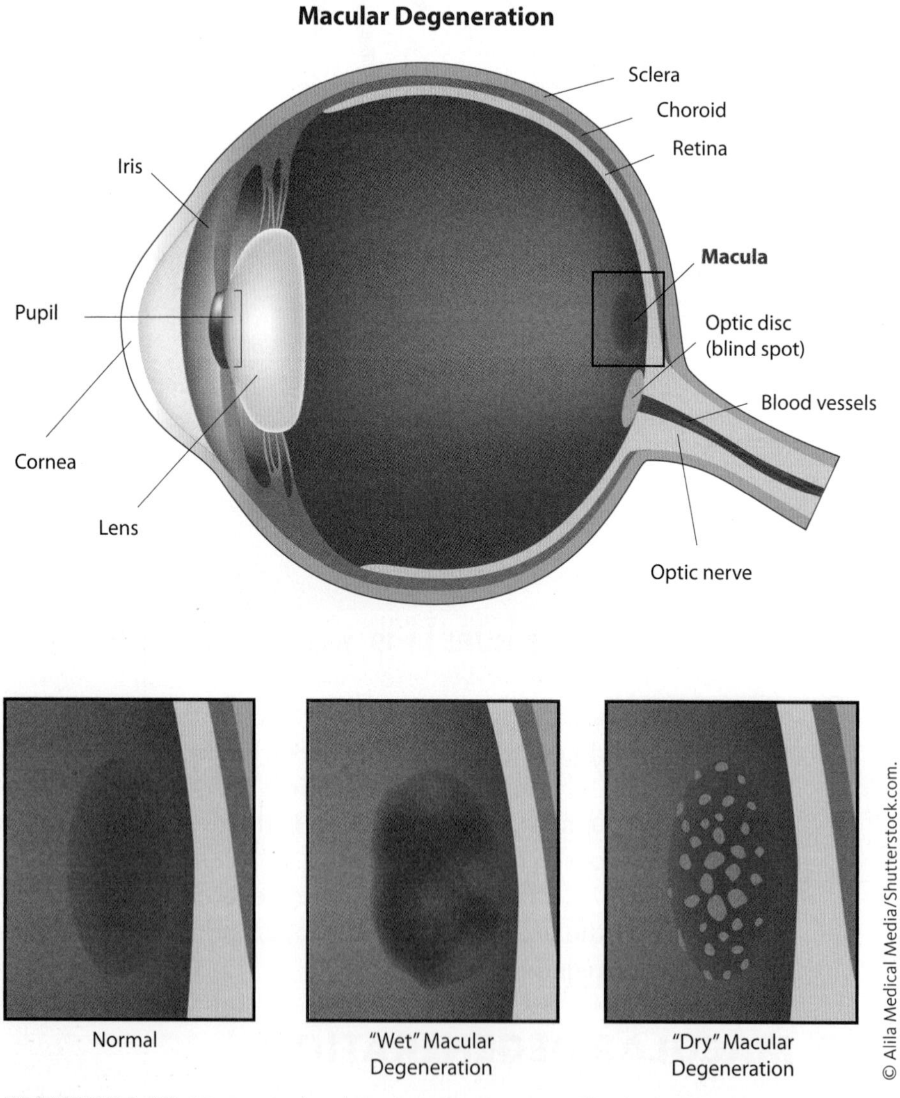

Macular Degeneration

FIGURE 14-20 Wet macular degeneration is caused by leaky blood vessels under the retina. Dry macular degeneration occurs when the center of the retina deteriorates.

a wavy and blurred area in the center of their vision. Even then, some patients still might not notice any changes in vision. During AMD's advanced stages, however, patients see only peripherally because the center of their vision is gone. See Figure 14-20. When in the advanced stages of the disease, the patient is often legally blind.

The risk of developing the condition increases with smoking, genetics, and race. Although there is no cure, laser surgery might help improve the patient's vision.

14-22a Diagnostic Testing for Macular Degeneration

Tests used to diagnose this disease are:

- Fluorescein angiography. This procedure requires a dye to be injected into a vein in the arm. After the dye travels through the bloodstream and to the retina of the eye, if macular degeneration is present, blood can be seen leaking out of vessels in the macula.
- Optical coherence tomography (OCT). This takes a three-dimensional picture of the retina to check its layers for any damage.
- Amsler grid. A card with straight lines on it that look like a checkerboard can be used. If the patient sees that these straight lines are wavy or even missing, macular degeneration might be present.

14-23 DIABETIC RETINOPATHY

Diabetic retinopathy, shown in Figure 14-21, is a complication of either Type I or Type II diabetes. Diabetes mellitus can cause changes in the vasculature of the retina, decreasing the patient's visual acuity. The vessels affected tend to bleed and produce scar tissue on the retina. This condition not only impairs vision but also can cause permanent blindness in the affected eye.

Signs and symptoms:

- Might not appear early in the disease
- Poor vision at night

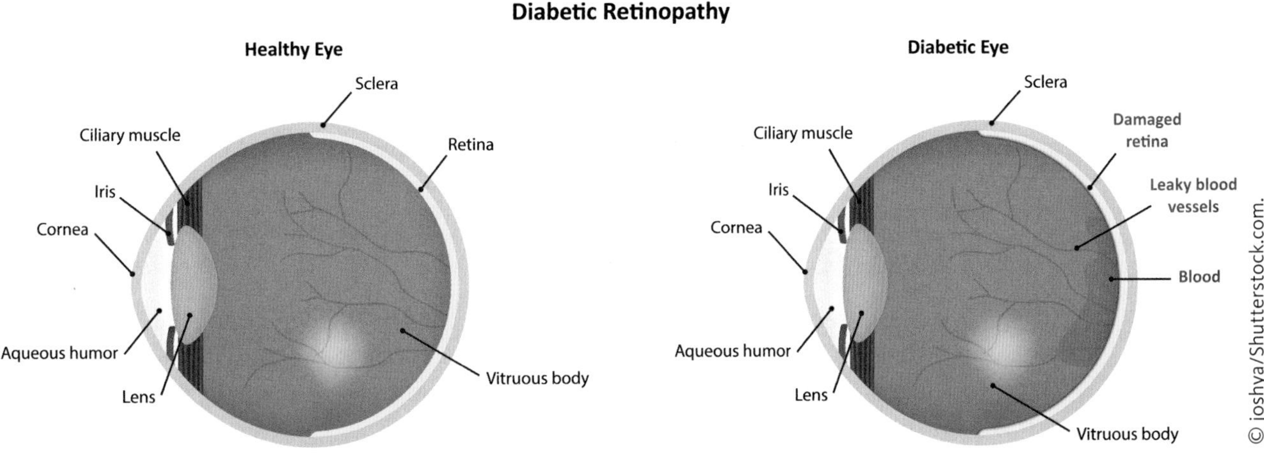

FIGURE 14-21 Comparison between a healthy eye and one with diabetic retinopathy.

- Blurred vision
- Floating spots in the eye
- Loss of vision

A dilated eye exam is performed to check for abnormal vessels in the eye, fatty deposits in the retina, and nerve tissue damage. Laser photocoagulation therapy is done to treat this condition, but it is in large part unsuccessful and requires repeated treatment.

LEARNING OBJECTIVE 14.3 Describe the anatomy of the ear.

KEY TERMS

Auricle Part of the external ear, the portion you can see. Also known as the pinna.

Cerumen Earwax.

Cochlea Spiral cavity found in the inner ear that plays a major role in hearing.

Endolymph fluid Fluid found in the labyrinth.

Eustachian tube A tube that acts as a passageway in between the middle ear and nasopharynx.

Incus Anvil-shaped bone in the middle ear; located between the malleus and stapes.

Inner ear Innermost section of the ear.

Labyrinth Bony outer wall of the inner ear.

Malleus The outermost small hammer-shaped bone in the middle ear.

Organ of Corti A structure located in the cochlea that produces nerve impluses in response to sound.

Oval window An opening covered by a membrane that leads from the middle ear to the inner ear.

Semicircular canals Passageways in the bony labyrinth that help to control equilibrium.

Stapes A bone in the middle ear between the incus and oval window; also called the stirrup bone.

Tympanic membrane Eardrum.

Vestibule chamber An oval-shaped cavity in bony labyrinth.

Vestibulocochlear nerve The nerve in the ear is responsible for transmitting information from the inner ear to the brain; responsible for balance and hearing.

14-24 OVERVIEW OF THE EAR

Your ears, through the sense of hearing, also provide you with great insights of the world. They do more than hearing, however, because they also play a critical role in your sense of balance. The ears have three parts as shown in Figure 14-22: the external ear, the middle ear, and the inner ear.

14-25 EXTERNAL EAR

The external ear, called the **auricle** or pinna, is the part of the ear you can see. It helps direct sound into the external ear canal, which is also part of the outer ear. Earwax or **cerumen** helps keep this canal clean and protected. Cerumen is secreted by glands called ceruminous glands. The external auditory canal leads to the middle ear and meets with the tympanic membrane, also known as the eardrum.

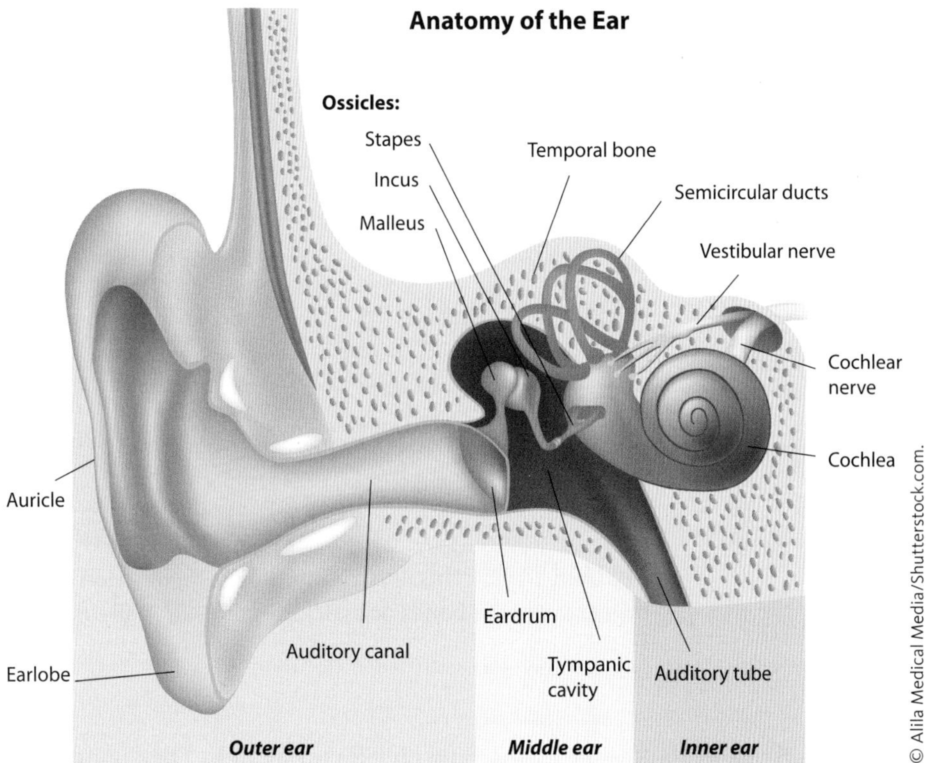

FIGURE 14-22 This illustration breaks down the anatomy of the ear into three sections.

14-26 MIDDLE EAR

Inside the middle ear are three of the smallest bones in the human body. They are joined together to help amplify sound waves received by the **tympanic membrane**. The sound is then transmitted to the inner ear via the fluid found there. Shown in Figure 14-23, these bones (also called ossicles) are named after their shapes. The first is the **malleus** or hammer, which is attached to the tympanic membrane. The **incus** or anvil is attached to the hammer, while the **stapes** or stirrup is connected to a membrane called the **oval window**.

The **eustachian tube** is also located in the middle ear and is connected to the pharynx. The eustachian tube equalizes air pressure on both sides of the eardrum, which consists of the pressure in the inner ear and the atmospheric pressure coming from the nose and throat. The equalization of pressure allows the eardrum to vibrate properly with sound waves.

14-27 INNER EAR

The oval window is the beginning of the **inner ear**, which consists of the **labyrinth**, or bony labyrinth, which looks like a maze of winding channels. The labyrinth consists of three parts: the **cochlea**, **vestibule chamber**, and **semicircular canals**. The cochlea looks like a snail and is connected to the oval window. Inside the cochlea is a tube called the cochlear duct that contains fluid known as perilymph. Perilymph fluid assists in the transmission of sound to the

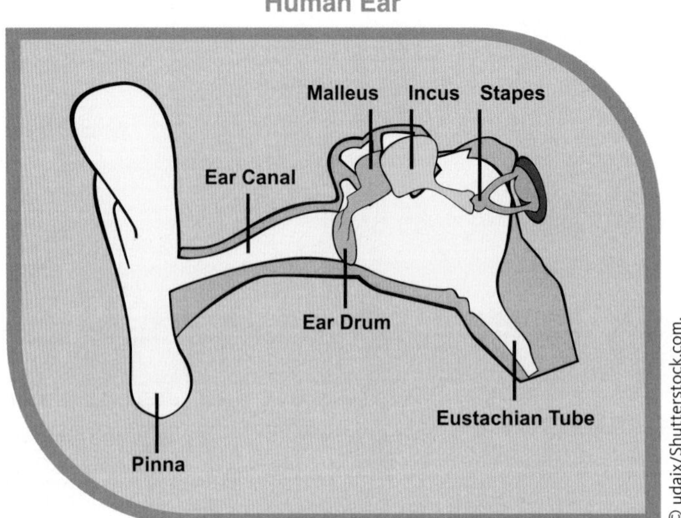

FIGURE 14-23 This illustration shows the location of the three connected bones or ossicles in the ear: malleus, incus, and stapes.

back of the cochlea via a fluid called endolymph. The sound is sent to hair-like receptors of the organ of Corti, which picks up the vibrations and sends the signal through the vestibulocochlear nerve (cranial nerve VIII) to the brain.

The vestibule chamber maintains balance while stationary and determines your head position in relationship to gravity such as laying down or getting up in bed. The semicircular canals have receptors that help you keep your balance based on the change of your head rotation such as making a quick turn. Three loops in the inner ear make up the semilunar canals that are filled with endolymph fluid just like the cochlea. Each canal contains a sensory receptor to help move fluid around when you change body positions. Movement of the body is received by a sensory receptor and triggers the nerve impulse that sends the signal to the brain stem and cerebellum by way of the vestibulocochlear nerve. The signal is then interpreted as the position your body is in and helps maintain muscle coordination and body equilibrium.

LEARNING OBJECTIVE 14.4 Describe the pathopharmacology of the ear.

KEY TERMS

Audiogram A graph that gives a detailed description of how well a patient can hear.

Impacted cerumen A blockage of earwax.

Mastoiditis Inflammation of the mastoid bone located behind the ear.

Otitis externa Inflammation of the external ear canal.

Otitis media Inflammation of the middle ear.

Otosclerosis A condition of abnormal hardening of the bones in the ear that reduces vibrations producing sound.

Otoscope A device used to look into the ear.

Presbycusis Hearing loss because of old age.

Sensorineural deafness Permanent loss of hearing caused by damaged nerves or cochlea in the inner ear.

Serous fluid Clear fluid in the ear caused by pressure or allergy.

Suppurative fluid Pus accumulation in the ear from an infection.

14-28 COMMON EAR MEDICATIONS

Because the ear is connected to the respiratory system (nasopharynx) via the eustachian tube, microorganisms can easily travel into the ear and cause an infection. In addition to pathogenic organisms invading the ear, pressure, impacted wax, trauma, and old age all can cause undesired effects. The following tables list common medications used to treat ear infections, inflammation, and pain described in the various conditions of this section. See Table 14-11.

Table 14-11 Otic preparations and medications

TOPICAL ANTIBIOTICS		
GENERIC NAME	**TRADE NAME**	**DOSAGE**
ciprofloxacin	Cipro	Otic sol, 0.2%, 3–4 drops BID for 7 to 14 days
Ofloxacin	Floxin	Otic sol, 0.3%, 10 drops BID for 7 to 14 days
COMBINATION TOPICAL ANTIBIOTICS AND STEROIDS		
ciprofloxacin and dexamethasone	Ciprodex	Otic sol, 0.3%/0.1%, 4 drops BID for 7 days
ciprofloxacin and hydrocortisone	Cipro HC	Otic sol, 0.2%/0.1%, 3 drops BID for 7 days
polymixin B, neomycin, and hydrocortisone	Cortisporin	Otic sol, 4 drops q6-8h
TOPICAL ANALGESICS AND ANTI-INFLAMMATORY AGENTS		
acetic acid and hydrocortisone Note: Combination corticosteroid and antibacterial agent	Vosol HC	Otic sol, 1%/2%, 3–5 drops 4 to 6 times daily prn
benzocaine and antipyrine Note: analgesic and anesthetic (currently not being manufactured)	Auralgan	Otic sol, 2–4 drops TID prn

14-29 OTITIS MEDIA

Otitis media, or inflammation of the middle ear, is commonly seen in infants and children. Under normal circumstances, the middle ear is filled with air, but when fluid accumulates there, inflammation will occur. Children are predisposed to having otitis media because their eustachian tube is narrower, shorter, and more horizontal than an adult's. As children age, the eustachian tube becomes more vertical, and they grow out of having ear infections. Acute otitis media is caused by a bacterial infection that lasts for a short time, usually no longer than six weeks; a chronic case of otitis media can last up to three months and usually causes a perforated eardrum.

The two different types of otitis media are classified based on the type of fluid in the ear.

The first type has **serous fluid** accumulation. Serous fluid is clear and builds up in the middle ear from a blocked eustachian tube or a change in pressure or allergy; it is not from an infection. Signs and symptoms include:

- A slight discomfort in the ear or feeling of fullness
- Hearing impairment or conductive hearing loss

Suppurative fluid is pus accumulation caused by a bacterial infection of the middle ear, caused when bacteria ascend to the ear from an upper respiratory infection via the eustachian tube. Signs and symptoms include:

- Ear pain or otalgia, which varies per case
- Dizziness or vertigo
- Nausea
- Fever
- Chills
- Vomiting
- Hearing impairment or conductive hearing loss

14-30 DIAGNOSING OTITIS MEDIA

An **otoscope**, shown in Figure 14-24, is a valuable diagnostic tool to view inside the ear. If otitis media is present, the eardrum will be bulging from the accumulation of fluid on the other side, and it will be red and inflamed.

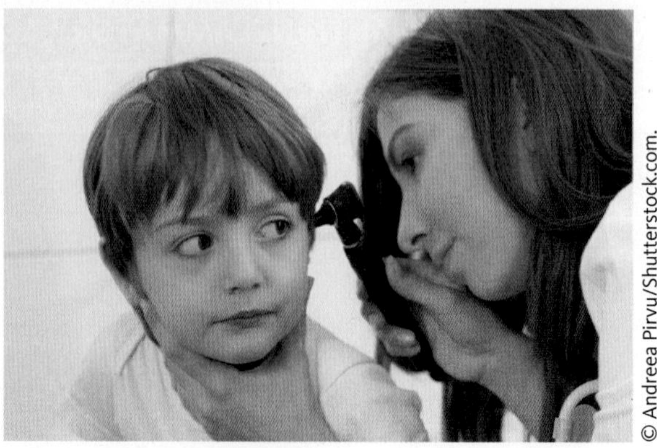

FIGURE 14-24 Otoscope.

Both types of otitis media can be treated with a decongestant to help facilitate the drainage of fluid and an analgesic to treat the pain. If an infection is present, however, an antibiotic will be needed. If the patient is experiencing chronic otitis media, other interventions can be done. See Table 14-12.

14-31 OTITIS EXTERNA

Otitis externa or swimmer's ear is an inflammation of the external ear canal, shown in Figure 14-25. This condition commonly occurs in swimmers who spend a long time in the water or swim in contaminated water. It is most commonly caused by bacterial or fungal microorganisms.

Table 14-12 Procedures for chronic otitis medias

PROCEDURE	DEFINITION
Myringotomy	Incision into the eardrum to remove fluid accumulation to prevent complications such as an eardrum rupture, permanent loss of hearing, and mastoiditis.
Tympanostomy	Creating a new opening through the tympanic membrane to relieve pressure and fluid with tubes. Tubes will eventually fall out of the ear on their own in a few months or can be removed surgically after 6 to 12 months.
Tympanoplasty	A procedure used to surgically repair the tympanic membrane in the event of a perforated eardrum from a chronic ear infection.

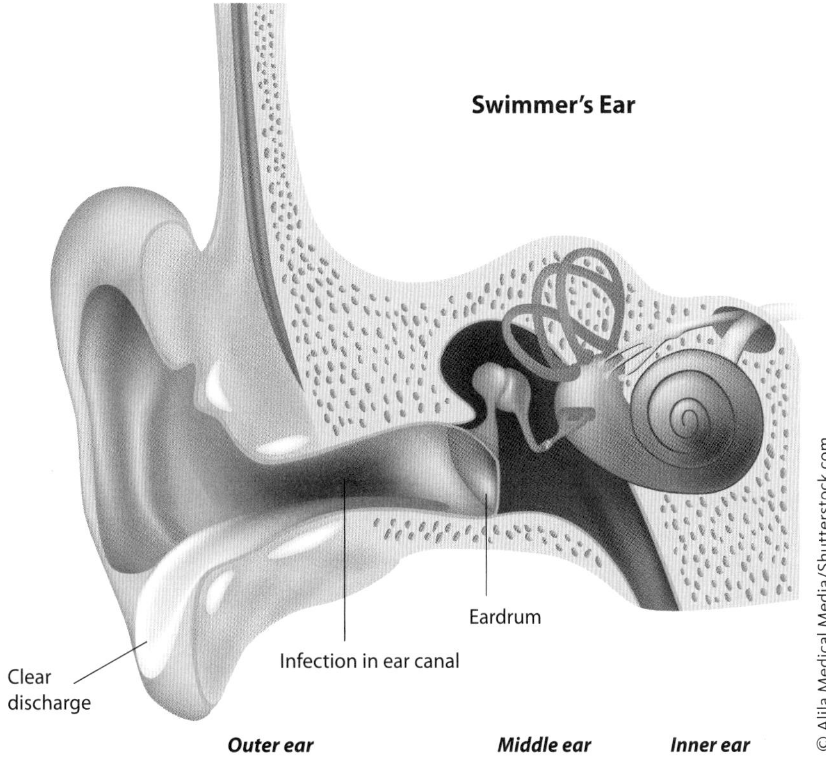

FIGURE 14-25 Illustration showing the location of inflammation with swimmer's ear.

Signs and symptoms include:

- Swelling of the external ear canal
- Intense pain
- Pruritus (itching)
- Fever
- Hearing loss
- Possible fluid discharge from the ear

To diagnose, an ear exam is required, and, if present, a fluid discharge might be cultured. Treatment includes analgesics to control the pain, and antibiotics if there is an infection.

14-32 MASTOIDITIS

Mastoiditis is inflammation of the honeycomb-like bone called the mastoid behind the ear. The common cause for this type of inflammation is a middle ear infection caused by streptococcus bacteria. Because middle ear infections are common in children, mastoiditis is mainly seen in pediatric patients. Before the advent of antibiotics, mastoiditis was the most common cause of death in children.

Signs and symptoms of mastoiditis include:

- Pain in the ear (otalgia)
- Fever
- Tinnitus (ringing in the ears)
- Discharge from the ear
- Swollen mastoid bone
- Mastoid bone pain

To diagnose, the drainage or discharge from the ear might be collected and sent to the lab for testing. The physician will look into the ear using an otoscope, and imaging such as X-rays and CT scans can determine if the mastoid bone is swollen. Mastoiditis is primarily treated by antibiotics for causative infection and analgesics for pain. If the condition recurs, surgery can be done to remove the mastoid bone with a procedure known as a mastoidectomy.

14-33 IMPACTED CERUMEN

Impacted cerumen occurs when earwax is pushed and packed within the ear canal. Using a cotton swab or a finger to remove earwax, as shown in Figure 14-26, can cause the earwax to form a blockage. The condition also can occur from a narrow auditory canal, dry skin, or excessive dust or hair in the ear canal. Common signs and symptoms are:

- Tinnitus (ringing in the ears)
- Pain in the ear
- Itchiness in the ear
- Temporary hearing loss

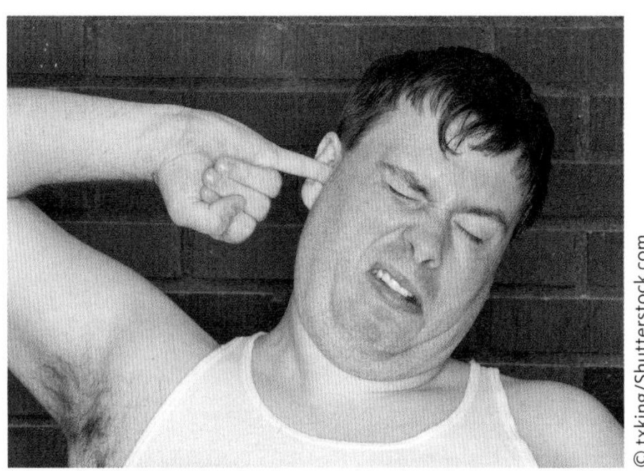

FIGURE 14-26 This man is putting himself at risk of impacting earwax.

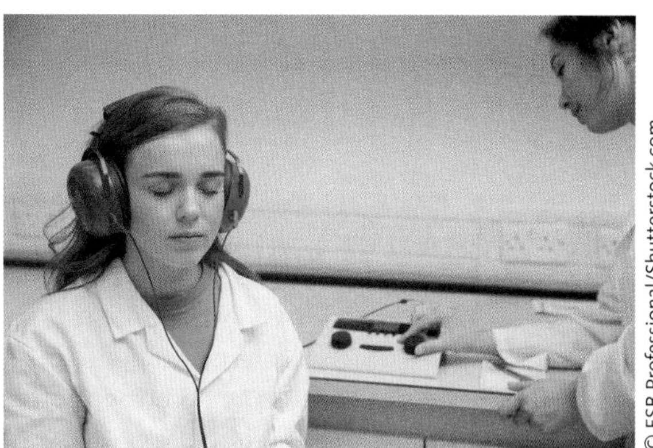

FIGURE 14-27 Audiogram.

Table 14-13 Otic preparations and medications: agents for earwax buildup

GENERIC NAME	TRADE NAME	DOSAGE
carbamide peroxide	Debrox	Otic sol, 6.5% and 10%, 5–10 drops BID, max of 4 days

Note: Keep drops in ear for several minutes by tilting head sideways and placing cotton in ear.

To confirm this diagnosis, a routine otologic exam is performed. Treatment involves irrigating the ear canal with drops to help flush out the cerumen buildup. See Table 14-13.

14-34 OTOSCLEROSIS

Otosclerosis causes the three small bones in the middle ear to become fixed, preventing the bones from conducting vibrations from the eardrum and to the inner ear. When this occurs, hearing loss will result. This condition has no known cause, but it seems to trend in families. Symptoms manifest as slow progression of hearing loss.

Otoscopy and an **audiogram**, Figure 14-27, can aid in diagnosis. An audiogram shows on a graph the lowest volume of sound a patient can hear and compares it to what a person with no hearing loss can hear.

To treat otosclerosis, the physician will perform a stapedectomy, in which the stapes bone is removed and an artificial bone put in its place.

14-35 SENSORINEURAL DEAFNESS

Sensorineural deafness is caused by permanent damage to the auditory nerve or cochlea. It might be from a congenital defect, inherited trait, or acquired through being exposed to loud, continuous noises, medications, or conditions such as stroke and tumors. Infections and traumatic injuries can also cause sensorineural deafness.

The major symptom associated with sensorineural deafness is the progression of hearing loss. To diagnose a patient, the physician uses audiometry to measure the patient's hearing in regard to both sensitivity and range. Hearing aids might be useful in helping to improve the patient's hearing. Cochlear implants might be surgically placed into the patient's ear to stimulate the auditory nerves to improve hearing.

14-36 PRESBYCUSIS

Presbycusis is hearing loss caused by old age. This progressive condition usually occurs in people 50 years of age and older. At first, the patient might not be able to hear high-pitched sounds, but as the condition progresses, the patient also might lose the ability to hear lower-pitched sounds.

Diagnosis is made with an audiogram. For a time, hearing aids help improve hearing for those with presbycusis, but eventually, the hearing loss will worsen to the point where hearing aids are no longer as useful.

14-37 MENIERE'S DISEASE

Meniere's disease usually affects people ranging from 20 to 50 years of age. The actual cause is unknown, but it is thought that allergies, viral infections, head trauma, genetics, and migraines are predisposing factors. Patients with Meniere's disease experience dizziness and the feeling that their head is spinning (vertigo). They also might have ringing of the ears (tinnitus), a sensation of fullness in the ear, and progressive hearing loss.

Those affected by this disorder report having acute attacks that last anywhere from a few hours to even days. When an attack occurs, the patient might encounter symptoms of nausea, vomiting, diaphoresis (sweating), and vertigo.

Treatment can include taking antihistamines if allergies are thought to be the cause of the problem; antinausea medications such as promethazine are used to stop nausea and vomiting. To help stop vertigo, motion sickness medications such as Antivert (meclizine) are given. If the condition does not respond to medications, the patient can undergo surgery of the inner ear. Surgery has its dangers, however, because permanent deafness can result.

Module 15

Pathopharmacology of the Reproductive System

Module Introduction

The reproductive system, shown in Figure 15-1 is an amazing system without which none of us would not exist. In all of the modules, the anatomy and physiology of the various body systems are the same in both women and men. However, that is not the case with the reproductive system. The reproductive organs for both are called genitals, but they have different names and functions. The primary genitalia are both called gonads and they both produce gametes or sex cells. The primary genitalia in women are the ovaries, which produce eggs, and in men they are testicles, which produce the sperm. The female reproductive system is more complex than that of males, and with this complexity come many different pathologies. While some diseases might only be nuisances, others are life-threatening.

LEARNING OBJECTIVE 15.1 Discuss female anatomy and physiology.

KEY TERMS

Ampulla Wide section of the fallopian tube.

Cervix Lower portion of the uterus.

Corpus luteum What remains of the follicle after ovulation.

Endometrium Innermost layer of the uterine wall.

Fallopian tube Two tubular structures that transport the egg to the uterus.

Fimbria Finger-like projections that direct an egg from the ovary to the fallopian tube.

Gametes Germ cells (sperm from the male; ovum from the female) that unite to form a fetus during reproduction.

Genitals External parts of the reproductive system.

Gonads Organs (testicles in males and ovaries in females) that produce germ cells or gametes for reproduction.

Graafian follicles The name of the mature follicle that ruptures and releases an egg.

Infundibulum Funnel-shaped end of the fallopian tube is proximal to the ovary.

Isthmus Narrow section of the fallopian tube.

Mammary glands Glands that produce milk in the female breast.

Menstrual cycle A series of changes a woman's body undergoes in preparation for pregnancy.

Myometrium Middle layer of the uterine wall.

Ova Eggs released from the ovaries; singular: ovum.

Ovarian cycle Monthly release of eggs from the ovary.

Ovary Female reproductive organ.

Perimetrium Outer layer of the uterus.

Uterine cycle Monthly sloughing of the uterus lining.

Uterus Muscular, hollow organ that carries a fetus; also known as the womb.

Vagina Hollow canal that receives the penis during intercourse and acts as the birth canal during childbirth.

15-1 INTERNAL STRUCTURES OF THE FEMALE REPRODUCTIVE SYSTEM

Ovaries are the primary genitalia in women that produce eggs or ova. One ovary on each side of the uterus is held in place by special ligaments. The ovaries are not only part of the reproductive system, but because of their ability to secrete hormones, they are also part of the endocrine system. The hormones produced by the ovaries are progesterone and estrogen, which are secreted as a response to the follicle-stimulating hormone (FSH) and luteinizing hormone (LH) from the anterior pituitary gland. Not only does estrogen help to facilitate secondary sex characteristics at puberty, but it also causes changes in the endometrium, which helps develop the placenta, mammary glands, and breasts during pregnancy.

The ovaries produce **ova** within the **Graafian follicles**, which are microscopic sacs where eggs can mature. After maturity, the follicle ruptures, and the egg travels from the ovary to the uterus via a duct called the **fallopian tube**. This process is termed ovulation, Figure 15-2.

The egg remains viable for 12–24 hours and can be fertilized if viable sperm is present. Fertilization takes place when a sperm penetrates the egg. At that time, the ruptured follicle left behind in the ovary becomes the **corpus luteum** and secretes hormones to maintain a nourishing tissue (thickened endometrium) for the growing fetus. Progesterone and estrogen are released by the corpus luteum.

While the ovary is the primary genitalia, accessory female genitalia includes the fallopian tubes, uterus, vagina, and vulva.

15-2 FALLOPIAN TUBES AND UTERUS

The fallopian tubes, also called uterine tubes and oviducts, transport the ova to the uterus. These 4-inch tubes are not directly attached to the ovary, but they are connected to the uterus as shown in Figure 15-3. The tubes start off as a large funnel called the **infundibulum** to capture the released egg. The infundibulum is surrounded by finger-like, ciliated projections called **fimbria**, which help move

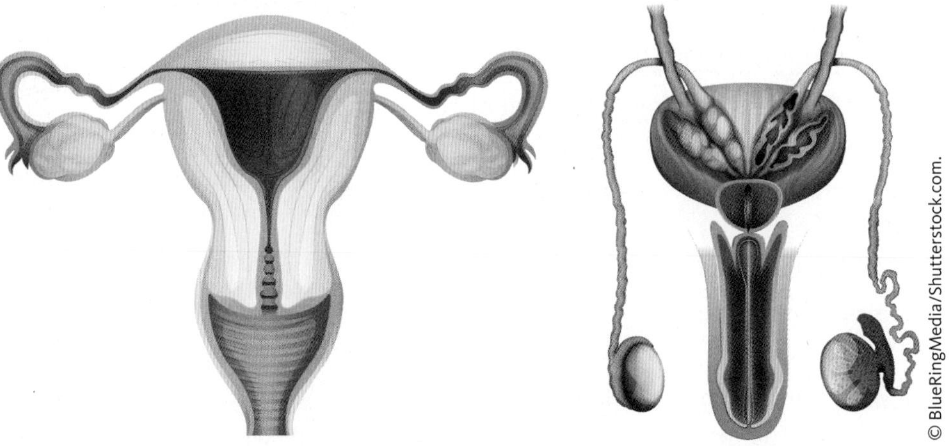

FIGURE 15-1 Female reproductive system (left) and the male reproductive system.

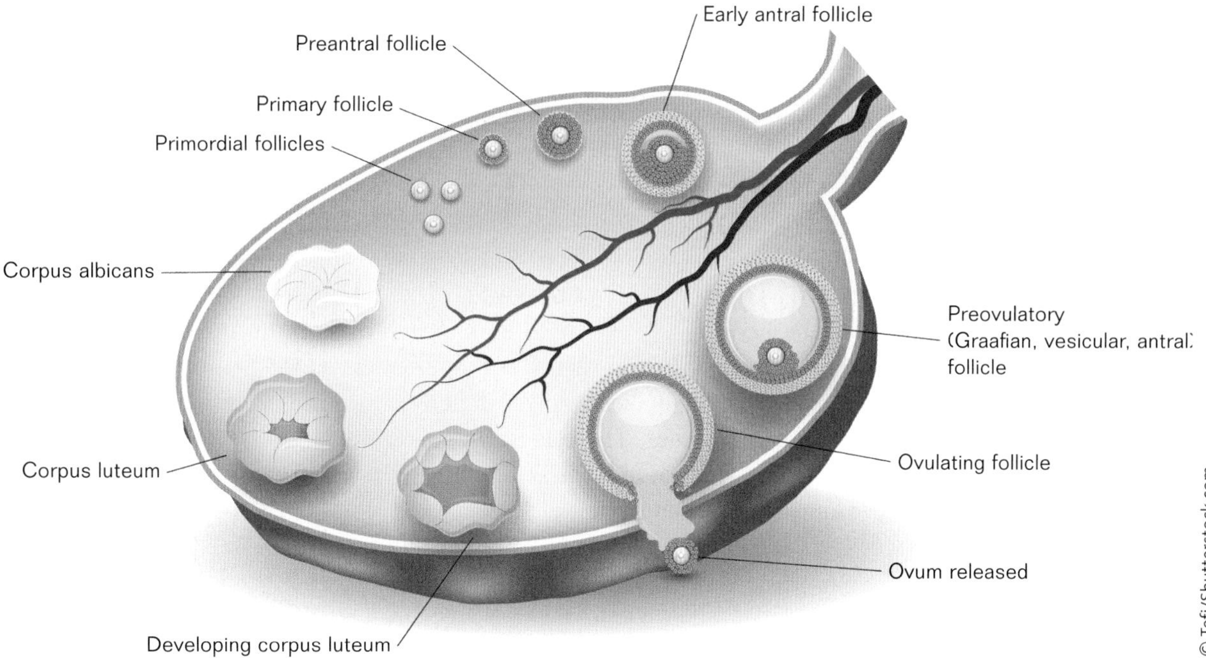

FIGURE 15-2 Ovulation in an ovary. When ovulation occurs, an egg is released and moves down the fallopian tube.

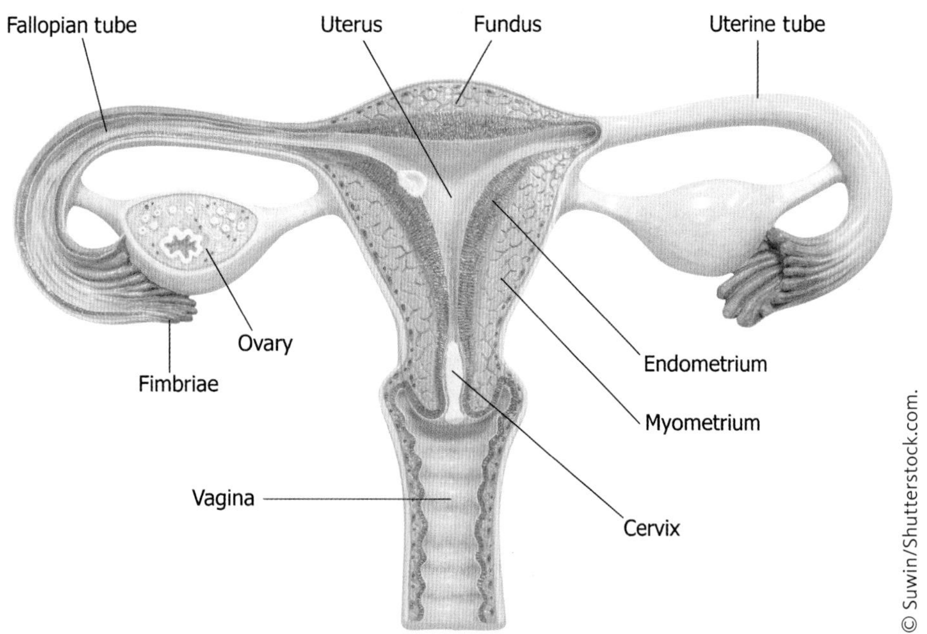

FIGURE 15-3 Female reproductive system.

the egg along the tubes. The infundibulum then leads to a widened region known as the ampulla, which narrows to a portion referred to as the isthmus, which leads into the uterus.

The uterus, located in the pelvis near the bladder, is a small (2–3-inch) pear-shaped organ with a thick muscular structure. The major portion of the uterus is called the body where a fetus develops. The area of the uterus near the fallopian tubes is called the fundus, and a narrow anterior region is known as the isthmus. The portion of the uterus that extends into the vagina is called the cervix, and the part that connects the uterus to the vagina is called the cervical canal.

The uterus wall is made up of three different layers. The perimetrium, also known as the visceral peritoneum, is the outermost layer. The middle layer is called the myometrium, which is made up of smooth muscle that provides contractions during the baby's birth. The endometrium, which lines the inside of the uterus, is highly vascular layer called the mucosa layer that can be further divided into two layers. The basal layer regenerates the uterine lining every month, and the functional layer is shed or sloughed about every 28 days during the woman's menstrual period.

15-3 VAGINA

The vagina (see Figure 15-3) is a tube about 10 centimeters long from the uterus to the outside of the body. It is lined with a mucous membrane and receives a man's penis during intercourse and is the birth canal through which the baby passes during delivery. It also allows for the passage of menstrual fluid from the uterus.

15-4 EXTERNAL ANATOMY

The external anatomy, shown in Figure 15-4, is collectively known as the vulva. A list of its structures and their definitions are given in Table 15-1.

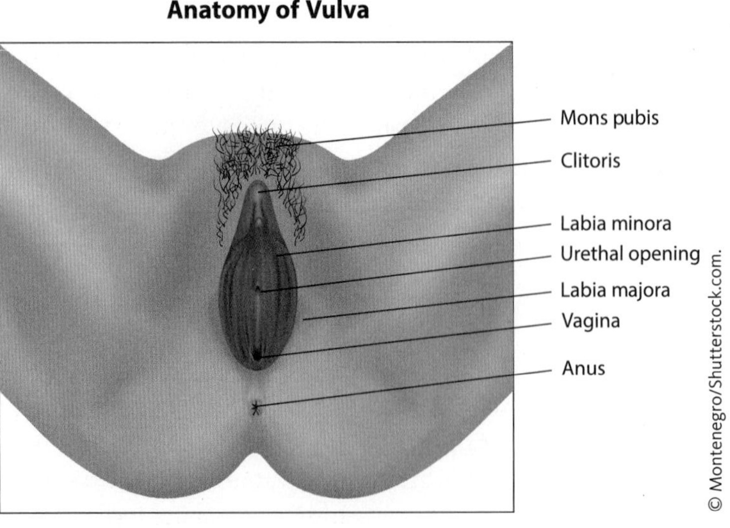

FIGURE 15-4 Anatomy of the vulva.

Table 15-1 The external structures

TERM	DEFINITION
Vulva	The external female genital structures
Labia majora	The outermost fold of the vulva
Labia minora	The smaller, inner folds of the vulva
Clitoris	A small, sensitive sexual organ located in front of the vagina
Vestibula	A space or entrance to a canal, in this case, the vaginal opening
Hymen	A membrane that partially covers the opening of the vagina
Vaginal orifice	Opening of the vagina
Vestibular glands	Two small, pea-like glands found near and on either side of the vaginal opening. The glands secrete mucus to lubricate the vagina.

15-5 BREASTS

The female breasts, external accessory sex organs, are located over the pectoralis major muscle between the second and seventh ribs of the chest. They contain the **mammary glands** for milk production. The tissue types that compose the breast are glandular, fibrous, and adipose. Usually, the breasts are almost symmetrical and the same size. However, breast size varies considerably from person to person as it depends on weight and body structure, along with other variables such as menstruation and pregnancy. The hormones secreted during those times can affect the composition and size of the breasts.

Before puberty, breast size in girls and boys is the same. After a girl reaches puberty, her breasts begin to develop and development occurs during the next 2 to 3 years. An adult woman's breast has 15 to 20 glandular lobes composed of smaller lobes called alveoli, which secrete milk. Breast milk is produced by a hormone called prolactin. The milk travels from the alveoli through a series of ducts to reach the nipple, from which it can be secreted. When a woman reaches menopause, breast tissue begins to decrease in size with atrophy. See Figure 15-5.

15-6 MENSTRUAL CYCLE

The **menstrual cycle** begins when a girl has her first period called menarche. The menstrual cycle involves the ovaries, uterus, pituitary gland, and hypothalamus and can range from 25 to 35 days. The menstrual cycle includes the **ovarian cycle**, which involves a monthly maturation and release of an egg from one ovary. The **uterine cycle** is made up of a monthly sloughing of the uterine lining. Fertilization and pregnancy stops the uterine cycle and allows the endometrial lining to build up and nourish the developing fetus. When a woman reaches her 50s, her menstrual cycles likely will end, representing the onset of menopause. See Figure 15-6.

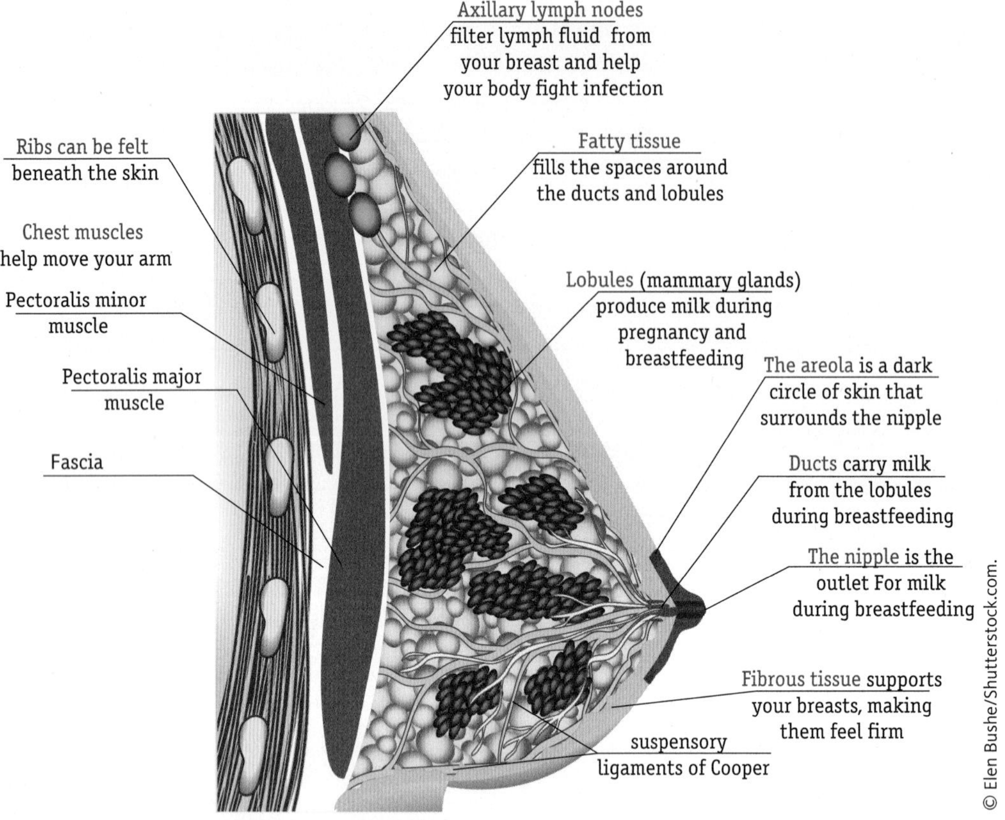
Medical Structure of the Female Breast
Axillary lymph nodes filter lymph fluid from your breast and help your body fight infection
Fatty tissue fills the spaces around the ducts and lobules
Ribs can be felt beneath the skin
Chest muscles help move your arm
Pectoralis minor muscle
Pectoralis major muscle
Fascia
Lobules (mammary glands) produce milk during pregnancy and breastfeeding
The areola is a dark circle of skin that surrounds the nipple
Ducts carry milk from the lobules during breastfeeding
The nipple is the outlet For milk during breastfeeding
Fibrous tissue supports your breasts, making them feel firm
suspensory ligaments of Cooper
© Elen Bushe/Shutterstock.com.

FIGURE 15-5 Anatomy of the female breast.

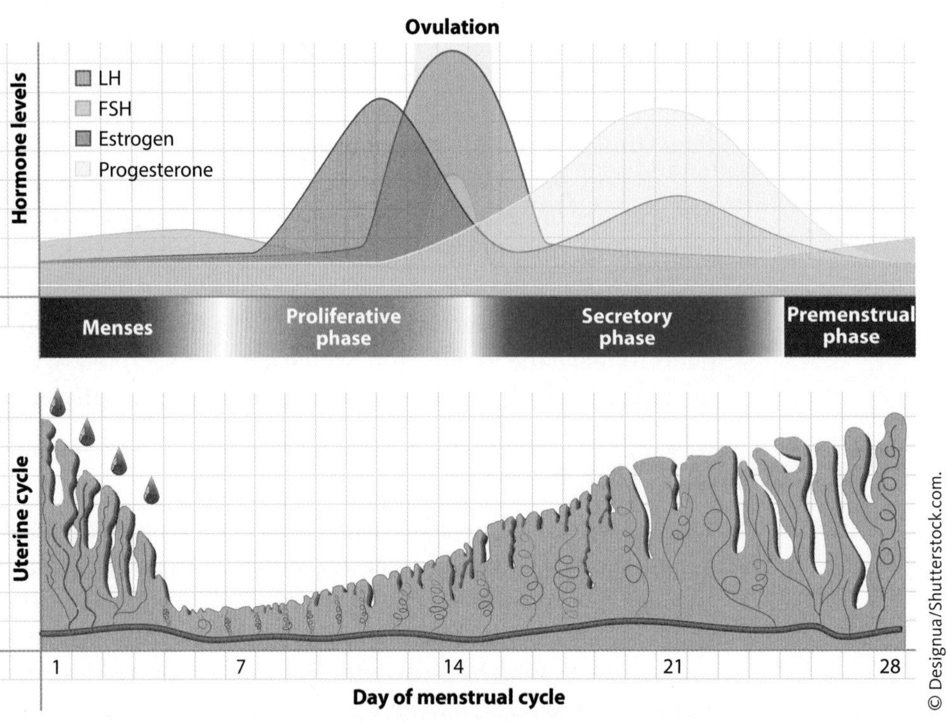
Menstrual Cycle
Ovulation
Hormone levels
LH
FSH
Estrogen
Progesterone
Menses
Proliferative phase
Secretory phase
Premenstrual phase
Uterine cycle
1
7
14
21
28
Day of menstrual cycle
© Designua/Shutterstock.com.

FIGURE 15-6 This chart contrasts the uterine cycle with the hormone levels of the menstrual cycle. Menses are the discharge from the uterus. The proliferation phase causes follicle-stimulating hormone (FSH) to increase circulation in the bloodstream, which increases the maturity levels of the follicles (small sac) that have developed inside the ovary for ovulation. The secretory phase is also known as the luteal phase; it is when a woman is most fertile.

LEARNING OBJECTIVE 15.2 Explain pathopharmacology of the female reproductive system.

KEY TERMS

Acid balance test (gynecologic) Used to test the pH of a vagina.

Amenorrhea Absence of menses.

Atrophic vaginitis Vaginal inflammation from decreased estrogen production.

Breast cancer Cancer of the breast tissue.

Cervical cancer Cancer of the cervix.

Cystocele Weakening of the anterior wall of the vagina that allows the bladder to bulge into the vagina.

Dysmenorrhea Painful menstruation.

Endometriosis A condition in which endometrial tissue that normally lines the uterus implants in other regions of the reproductive system and intestines.

Fibrocystic breasts Benign changes of the breasts that give a lumpy or rope-like texture.

Fibroid tumors Benign tumors found in the uterus.

Gynecologic speculum A medical device used to hold open the vaginal walls for inspection.

Gynecologist One who treats diseases of the reproductive system.

Kegel exercises Exercises used to strengthen the pelvic floor muscles to prevent prolapse and urinary incontinence.

Mammogram A radiologic image taken of the breast to check for cancer.

Mastitis Inflammation of the breast caused by a bacterial infection or breastfeeding.

Menopause The stage of a women's life when regular menses cease.

Menorrhagia Abnormal bleeding during menses.

Metrorrhagia Uterine bleeding between regular menses.

Obstetrician One who specializes in childbirth.

Ovarian cancer Cancer of the ovaries.

Ovarian cyst A fluid-filled sac in the ovary.

Pelvic inflammatory disease (PID) Inflammation of a woman's pelvic organs.

Pessary A device inserted into the vagina to support its walls and prevent prolapse.

Premenstrual syndrome A group of symptoms that occurs just days before menstruation.

Rectocele Weakening of the posterior wall of the vagina allowing the rectum to bulge into the vagina.

Toxic shock syndrome (TSS) A life-threatening, acute bacterial infection caused by an intrauterine device or tampon.

Uterine cancer Cancer of the uterus.

Uterine prolapse A condition in which the uterus falls into the vagina.

Vaginitis Inflammation of the vagina.

15-7 FEMALE REPRODUCTIVE SPECIALISTS

Numerous conditions affect the female reproductive system. Whether caused by hormone imbalances, cysts, tumors, inflammations, or infection, their effects range in severity. The physician who specializes in treatment of the female reproductive system with either surgery or medication is called a **gynecologist**. An **obstetrician** is a physician who deals with the branch of medicine that encompasses childbirth. See Figure 15-7.

Many of the conditions we will discuss pertain to disturbances of the normal menstrual cycle, which is illustrated in Figure 15-8.

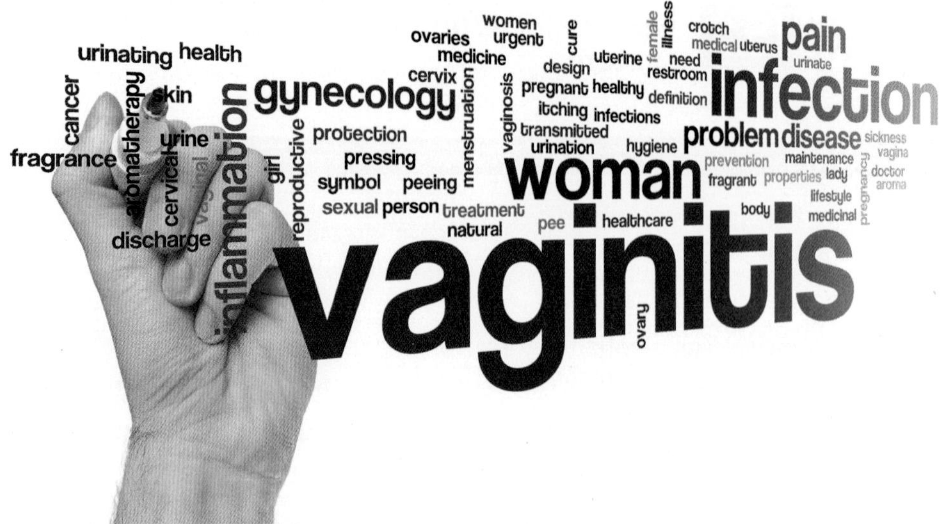

FIGURE 15-7 Gynecologic word cloud.

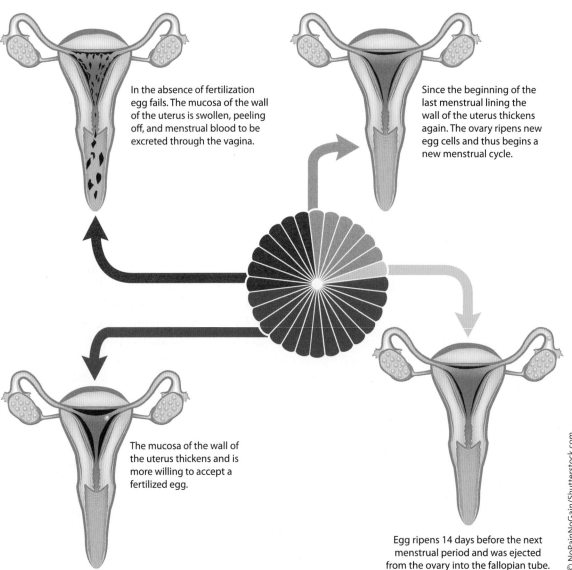

In the absence of fertilization egg fails. The mucosa of the wall of the uterus is swollen, peeling off, and menstrual blood to be excreted through the vagina.

Since the beginning of the last menstrual lining the wall of the uterus thickens again. The ovary ripens new egg cells and thus begins a new menstrual cycle.

The mucosa of the wall of the uterus thickens and is more willing to accept a fertilized egg.

Egg ripens 14 days before the next menstrual period and was ejected from the ovary into the fallopian tube.

FIGURE 15-8 Simplified illustration of the menstrual cycle.

Many of the conditions of this system require a pelvic examination to gather more information. Therefore, you should get an idea of how a pelvic exam and other special procedures are conducted.

15-8 PREMENSTRUAL SYNDROME

Most women have symptoms before their period (menses), but when the symptoms are severe and affect their quality of life, it is diagnosed as **premenstrual syndrome (PMS)**. While the cause is not known, potential causes include rapidly changing estrogen levels, vitamin deficiencies, and possible psychological disturbances.

15-8a PMS Signs and Symptoms

Signs and symptoms of PMS begin during the middle of the menstrual cycle with ovulation and become worse until a couple of hours after the onset of menses. Symptoms include mood swings, irritability, and depression. Other possible clinical presentations are:

- Edema (fluid retention)
- Weight gain
- Nausea
- Headache
- Joint pain
- Back pain
- Tender breasts
- Sleep difficulty.

15-8b PMS Diagnosis and Treatment

Diagnosing begins with ruling out other possible conditions because PMS is not completely understood and therefore the condition is difficult to pinpoint. Not everyone experiences the same signs and symptoms or responds favorably to certain treatments, so treatment must be tailored to each patient. Besides eating a healthy diet, avoiding caffeinated beverages, alcohol, and sugar, some medications can help. Drugs include diuretics to remove excess fluid, analgesics for body pain, and progesterone to facilitate menses and ease symptoms.

15-9 AMENORRHEA

Amenorrhea means without or no menses. There are two types of amenorrhea: primary and secondary. Primary amenorrhea is when a girl does not experience a period by 18 years of age. The condition might be caused by underdeveloped or missing female reproductive organs, anorexia, and hormone disturbances. Women who have had regular menses but then do not have a menstrual period in at least the last 6 months are diagnosed with secondary amenorrhea.

The causes of secondary amenorrhea can include depression, emotional stress, malnourishment, excessive exercise, pregnancy, hormone imbalances, and an ovarian tumor.

A physical examination will be performed, and hormone levels will be analyzed via blood and urine samples. Depending on the cause, treatment might include hormone administration to help initiate a menstrual cycle.

15-10 DYSMENORRHEA

Dysmenorrhea means difficult menses, with abdominal cramping that ranges from mild to severe discomfort. The causes of this painful condition include pelvic infections, endometriosis, cervical stenosis, and other unknown causes. Signs and symptoms also include pain in the lower back that can radiate upward to the upper back and down into the legs.

The causes of dysmenorrhea must be identified to have a favorable prognosis. Treatment can include applying a heating pad to the pelvic region to help ease pain, oral contraceptives to help regulate and decrease menstrual flow, and non-steroidal and inflammatory drugs to help reduce pain and inflammation.

15-11 MENORRHAGIA

Menorrhagia is a condition of excessive or prolonged menstrual flow that can be caused by hormone imbalances, pelvic inflammatory disease (PID), and uterine tumors. Treatment depends on the cause. A uterine tumor needs to be surgically removed; hormonal imbalances are treated with hormone therapy and antibiotics are given to treat pelvic inflammatory disease (PID).

15-12 METRORRHAGIA

Metrorrhagia is excessive bleeding or abnormal bleeding between periods. The primary cause is a hormone imbalance that causes the uterine lining to become abnormally thickened and shed. To treat the condition, however, the underlying cause of the imbalance must be determined. One potential treatment includes a procedure known as dilation and curettage (D&C), which entails dilating the cervix to remove a layer of tissue from the uterus.

15-13 MENOPAUSE

Menopause, or the cessation of menstruation, usually occurs in women in their 50s. As a woman ages, her ovaries produce less estrogen, eventually leading to a cessation of ovulation and, therefore, the menstrual cycle. During this time, a woman can experience common physical symptoms such as vaginal dryness, night sweats, and hot flashes, as shown in Figure 15-9. Other symptoms are psychological and can include a diminished sex drive, depression, and sleep disorders. The hormonal changes also put women at a greater risk of developing weakened bones (osteoporosis) and heart disease.

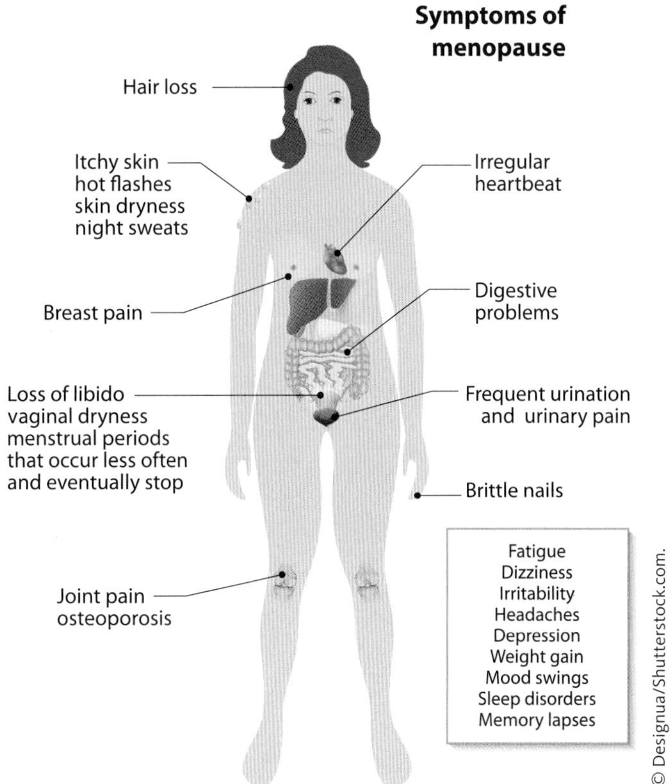

FIGURE 15-9 Symptoms of menopause.

15-13a Diagnosing and Treatment of Menopause

Diagnosis of menopause is typically made with a history of the woman's signs and symptoms. However, a blood sample can be ordered to analyze hormone levels to determine whether other factors might be causing the symptoms. For example, if estrogen and FSH are low, it is indicative of menopause. However, if the patient's thyroid-stimulating hormone (TSH) is low, it indicates hypothyroidism, which can present similar signs and symptoms.

Treatment for menopausal symptom relief includes hormone therapy, which may also benefit other conditions such as osteoporosis. Estrogen replacement, however, also can increase the patient's risk of heart attack, stroke, blood clots, and even breast cancer.

Low-dose estrogen therapy can be given to help relieve hot flashes. Estrogen can also be given through vaginal gels, creams, and rings to help relieve vaginal dryness symptoms. If a woman cannot take estrogen because of certain health risks, such as breast cancer, a low-dose antidepressant can be used instead. Antidepressant agents have shown to reduce vasomotor symptoms (hot flashes, night sweats, and flushes). Examples of antidepressant agents known as selective serotonin reuptake inhibitors (SSRIs) can be found in Table 15-2.

Table 15-2 Types of SSRIs

TRADE NAME	GENERIC NAME
Celexa	citalopram
Paxil	paroxetine
Prozac	fluoxetine
Lexapro	escitalopram

Also, if a woman cannot take estrogen and also suffers from migraines, an anticonvulsant drug called Neurontin (gabapentin), which is used to treat seizures, has been shown to be helpful in reducing menopause symptoms such as hot flashes and insomnia.

15-14 VAGINITIS

Many microorganisms can cause inflammation of the vagina, also known as **vaginitis**. Besides causing inflammation, they can ascend the urethra to the bladder and cause an infection. Symptoms can include:

- Swelling
- Painful intercourse and urination
- Change in odor of vagina
- Change in discharge of vagina
- Spotting of blood.

Types of infectious vaginitis include bacterial vaginosis, trichomoniasis, and candida vaginitis. Candida vaginitis is the most common and is caused by an opportunistic yeast that over-colonizes the normal lactobacillus bacteria in the vagina. The normal flora exists in the typically acidic vaginal environment of approximately 4–4.5 pH. This acidity prevents the growth of other microorganisms. Proper levels of estrogen also foster an environment for lactobacilli to grow. When the pH is disrupted, or estrogen levels are inadequate, opportunistic candida microorganisms can grow and cause a yeast infection as shown in Figure 15-10.

If a woman has multiple yeast infections, she should consult her physician. She also should abstain from having sexual intercourse to prevent the likelihood of a reinfection.

15-14a Vaginitis Treatment

Treatment depends on what caused the vaginitis. If it is infectious, the proper antimicrobial agent is indicated. If the inflammation is non-infectious, the cause of the inflammation must be removed. See Table 15-3.

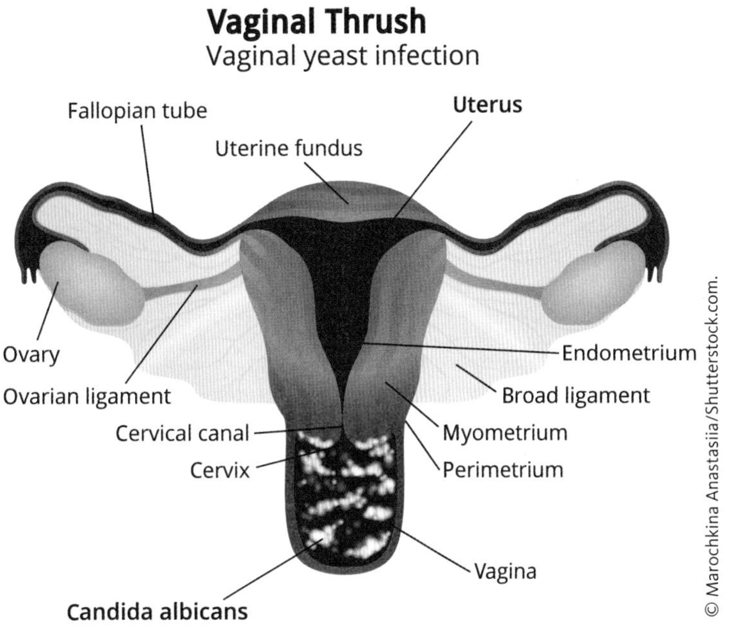

FIGURE 15-10 Vaginal yeast infection.

Table 15-3 Vaginitis treatment

CONDITIONS	TREATMENT
Bacterial vaginosis	• Flagyl (metronidazole) tablets by mouth • metronidazole (MetroGel) gel applied to the vagina • clindamycin (Cleocin) cream applied to the vagina
Yeast infections	Over-the-counter medications such as antifungal cream or suppository agents including Monistat 1 (miconazole), Gyne-Lotrimin (clotrimazole), Femstat 3 (butoconazole), and Vagistat-1 (tioconazole). Prescription oral antifungal medication includes Diflucan (fluconazole).
Trichomoniasis	metronidazole (Flagyl) and tinidazole (Tindamax) tablets
Genitourinary syndrome of menopause also known as vaginal atrophy	Estrogen in the form of vaginal creams, tablets, or rings
Non-infectious vaginitis	Avoid the source of irritation, such as a type of soap, detergent, or feminine hygiene product

15-15 ATROPHIC VAGINITIS

Another type of vaginitis is **atrophic vaginitis**, which is caused by a decreased release of estrogen that usually accompanies menopause, resulting in a poor vaginal lining. Associated symptoms are:

- Itchiness
- Burning sensation

- Frequent urination
- Incontinence
- Vaginal dryness
- Vaginal discharge
- Discomfort during intercourse
- Decreased vaginal lubrication during intercourse
- Increased risk of UTIs.

Diagnosis can be confirmed by a microscopic examination of vaginal secretions and finding pathogenic microorganisms. An **acid balance test** can be performed by placing vaginal secretions on an indicator paper to check the acidity level of the vagina. A pelvic examination, conducted with the help of an instrument called a **gynecologic speculum** (Figure 15-11), would indicate prolapse if there is a bulging in the pelvic walls.

Treatment can begin with over-the-counter moisturizers, such as Vagisil and Replens, which can be applied every three days. Over-the-counter lubricants can help relieve discomfort during intercourse. Water-based jelly is preferred because petroleum-based products can break down latex condoms. If these products do not relieve the symptoms, prescription medications with estrogen can be used. See Table 15-4.

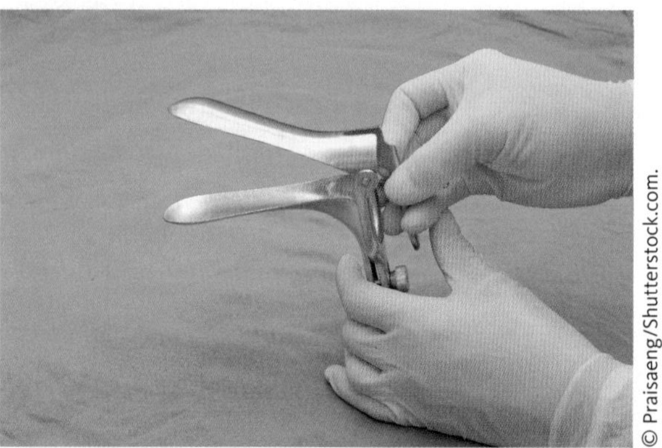

FIGURE 15-11 Gynecologic speculum used to inspect the female pelvic cavity.

Table 15-4 Medications used to treat Atrophic Vaginitis

PRODUCT TYPE	BRAND NAME/GENERIC NAME
Vaginal estrogen cream	estrace (estradiol)
Vaginal estrogen gel	estroGel 0.06% (estradiol) gel
Vaginal ring	estring (estradiol vaginal ring)
Estrogen inserts	vagifem (estradiol vaginal insert)

15-16 ENDOMETRIOSIS

Endometriosis is when there is an abnormal growth of endometrial tissue outside of the uterus. Complications arise because the tissue that is normally discharged out of the body can actually slough upward into the abdominal cavity, fallopian tubes, or bloodstream (see Figure 15-12). It is common for endometrial tissue to implant in the following areas:

- Ovaries
- Fallopian tubes
- Intestines
- Abdominal wall
- Diaphragm
- Bladder
- Vulva.

Although the cause of endometriosis is unknown, the abnormal tissue responds to menstrual cycles by increasing tissue thickness and bleeding. This results in further irritation and swelling of normal uterine tissue near the abnormal tissue and causes scar tissue to develop.

Signs and symptoms include:

- Pain and cramping in the vagina, pelvis, and lower back
- Dysmenorrhea (painful periods)
- Dyspareunia (painful intercourse)
- Thick discharge.

Other complications that result are:

- Infertility
- Miscarriages (spontaneous abortions)
- Ectopic pregnancy.

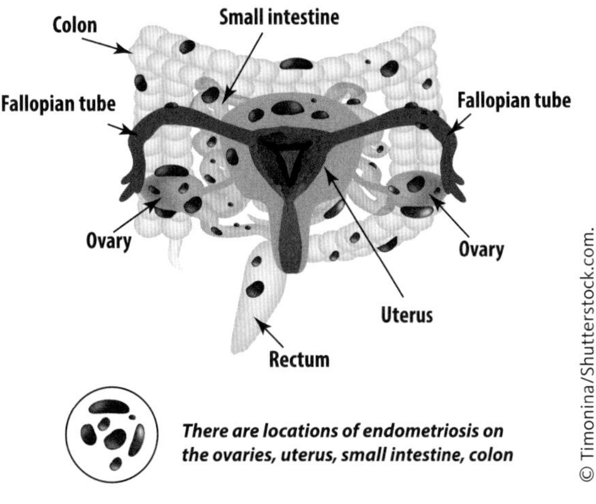

FIGURE 15-12 Areas endometriosis can be found.

Table 15-5 Hormone medications used to treat Endometriosis

TYPES OF THERAPY	MECHANISM OF ACTION	EXAMPLE MEDICATIONS
Hormonal contraceptives	Causes decreased menstrual flows	Apri (desogestrel and ethinyl estradiol tablets) Azurette (ethinyl estradiol and desogestrel) Caziant (ethinyl estradiol and desogestrel)
Progestin therapy	Decreases menstrual flow	Examples are Depo-Provera injection and Mirena intrauterine implant (IUD)
Gonadotropin-releasing hormone (GnRH) agonists and antagonists	Inhibits ovarian stimulating hormones, which decrease estrogen levels, and prevents menstrual cycles so endometrial tissue cannot thicken and be shed	An example of a GnRH agonist: Lupron (leuprolide) injection An example of a GnRH antagonist: Firmagon (degarelix)

15-16a Diagnosing and Treating Endometriosis

A diagnosis can be made by performing a pelvic examination. A laparoscopic examination can be made with an incision into the abdominal wall, and the scope inserted to examine the peritoneal cavity. An ultrasound can be used to view the reproductive organs, but it cannot definitely show if endometriosis is present. However, it can show any cysts that have developed as a result of endometriosis.

Treatment depends on the woman's age and desire to become pregnant. The abnormal tissue shrinks when a woman becomes pregnant, breastfeeds, or enters menopause. Hormone medication can be used to help treat as shown in Table 15-5.

15-17 PELVIC INFLAMMATORY DISEASE

Pelvic Inflammatory Disease (PID) is an inflammation of pelvic reproductive organs and is often caused by a bacterial infection, usually from a sexually transmitted disease. Childbirth and other events, however, can expose the vagina to bacteria which can ascend upward into the pelvic cavity. Signs and symptoms include:

- Pelvic pain
- Fever
- Chills
- White, foul-smelling vaginal discharge.

A pelvic exam can be done, and the discharge can be cultured. After confirmation, treatment involves antibiotics and analgesics to fight bacteria and pain. If not addressed, the infection can cause difficulty with pregnancy and even become deadly because it can cause sepsis.

Examples of antibiotics used are found in Table 15-6.

Table 15-6 Antibiotics used to treat Pelvic Inflammatory Disease (PID)

TRADE NAME	GENERIC NAME
Mefoxin	cefoxitin
Flagyl	metronidazole
Vibramycin	doxycycline
Rocephin	ceftriaxone

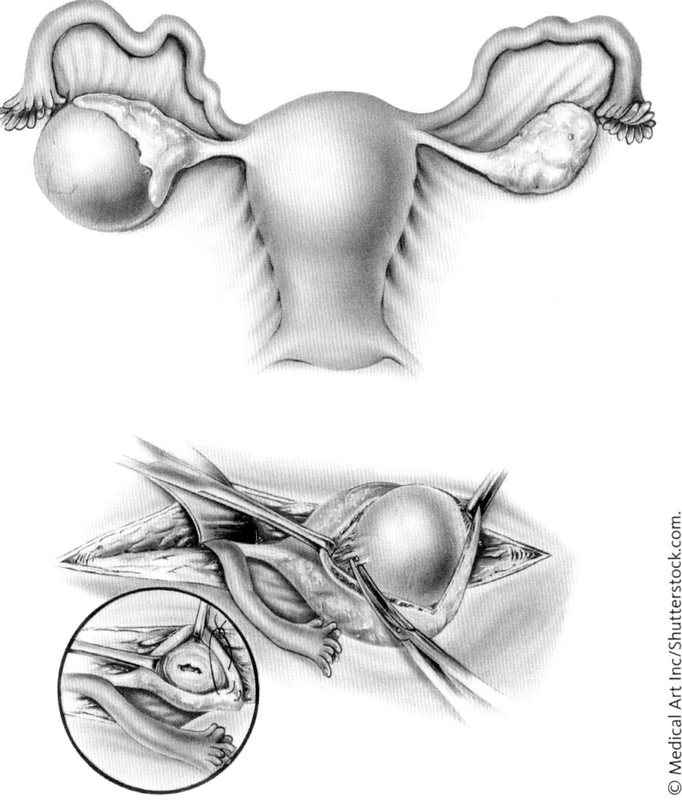

FIGURE 15-13 Cyst in the right ovary (top), surgical intervention to remove the cyst via cystectomy (middle), and surgical repair (bottom).

15-18 OVARIAN CYSTS

Ovarian cysts, as shown in Figure 15-13, are fluid-filled sacs found on or near an ovary. They are typically benign (non-cancerous), but they can cause many symptoms, including:

- Pain in the lower back and pelvic region
- Painful sexual intercourse
- Nausea and vomiting (the weight of the cyst can cause the ovary to become twisted).

To diagnose, a patient history, ultrasound, and pelvic examination are performed. It is important to find out what type of cyst is present and to determine whether it is cancerous. Treatment depends on how large the cyst is and what kind of cyst is present. Small cysts usually disappear on their own without treatment. Oral contraceptives can also help resolve small cysts. Large cysts can be either surgically removed or drained via a laparoscopy.

15-19 FIBROID TUMORS

Fibroid tumors, also known as leiomyomas, are the most commonly seen tumors of the female reproductive system. Fibroids are non-cancerous (benign) tumors of the smooth muscle of the uterine wall. Although the cause of these tumors is unknown, they are stimulated by estrogen. When small they are usually asymptomatic, but can increase in size when a woman is pregnant. See Figure 15-14.

Small fibroids are typically asymptomatic, but larger tumors can cause pain, excessive menstrual bleeding, and unusual uterine bleeding. Fibroid tumors can be diagnosed via a pelvic examination and ultrasound; treatment is surgical removal, if needed.

15-20 TOXIC SHOCK SYNDROME

Toxic shock syndrome (TSS) is typically seen in women who use tampons during menstruation. It is caused by *Staphylococcus aureus*, which is a normal bacterium found on the skin. When the bacterium comes into contact with the tampon material, however, it increases its production of toxins. TSS occurrence has declined over the years because there have been changes in the way tampons

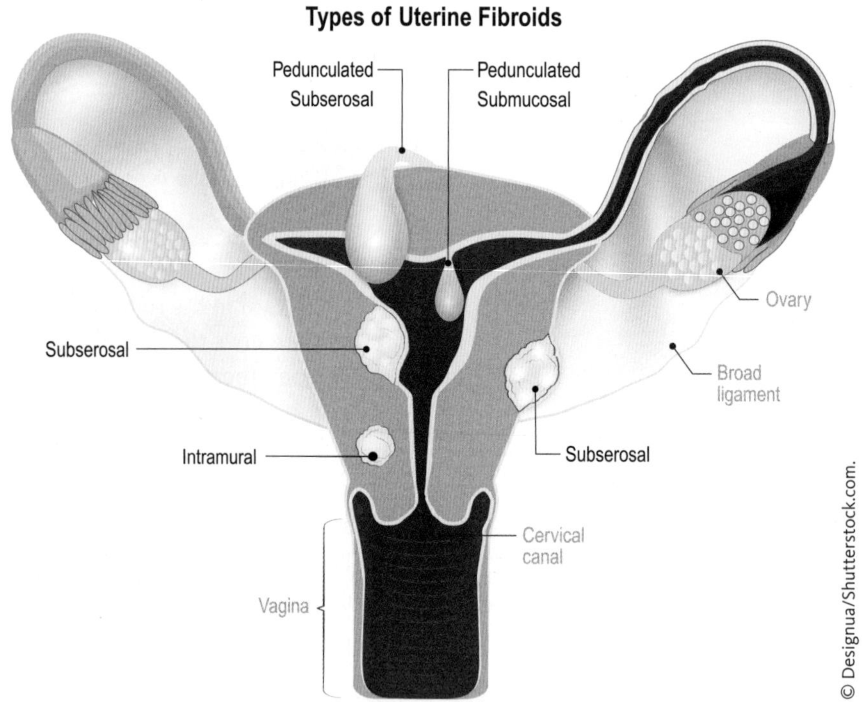

FIGURE 15-14 Types and locations of fibroids.

are made, Figure 15-15. This condition can be life-threatening because it causes a high fever and decrease in blood pressure. Other signs and symptoms include:

- Diarrhea
- Vomiting
- Chills
- Headache
- Pain
- Decreased urine output
- Rash all over the body.

A complete blood count (CBC), urinalysis, electrocardiogram (EKG), and chest X-ray (CXR) are helpful in making a diagnosis, as well as a patient history and physical examination to ensure the symptoms are not being caused by something else.

Intravenous antibiotic medications are given to combat the bacterial infection. IV fluids also can be given to treat dehydration and stabilize the blood pressure.

15-21 UTERINE PROLAPSE

Uterine prolapse, when the uterus falls downward into the vagina, is caused by a weakened pelvic floor muscle that can occur after childbirth and with increased age. Signs and symptoms include:

- Difficult urination
- Lower back pain
- Pressure in pelvic region
- Heaviness in pelvic region
- Incontinence
- Visualization of uterus bulging out of vagina.

Diagnosis is made with a pelvic exam; a hysterectomy, shown in Figure 15-16, is often the best choice of treatment.

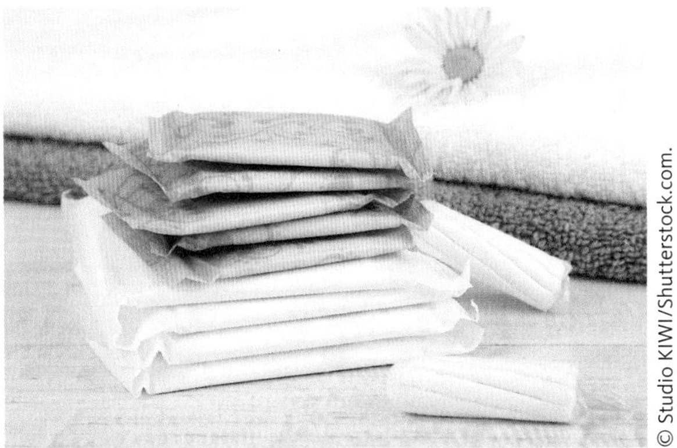

FIGURE 15-15 Before better materials were used to make tampons, there was an increased risk of TSS.

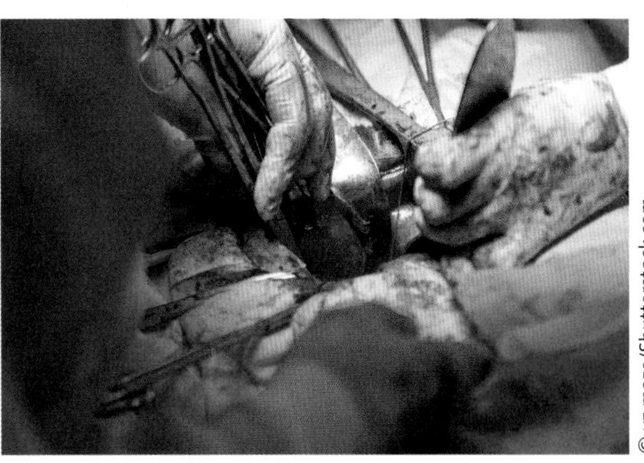

FIGURE 15-16 Uterus extraction during a hysterectomy.

15-22 CYSTOCELE

A **cystocele** is a herniation of the urinary bladder through the anterior wall of the vagina as shown in Figure 15-17. The causes include childbirth, old age, or an injury that results from actions such as heavy lifting and constipation, causing a weakened area of the vaginal wall. Cystoceles are categorized by degree: mild, severe, and advanced. Signs and symptoms include:

- Pain in the lower back
- Bulge in the vagina
- Heaviness or pressure in pelvic region
- Incontinence
- Frequent UTIs
- Urge to urinate often
- Painful intercourse.

Diagnosis is made with a pelvic examination. Treatment depends on the degree of the cystocele. **Kegel exercises** are used to help strengthen the pelvic floor muscles if the condition is not advanced. In moderate cases, a **pessary**, a device (rubber or plastic ring) inserted into the vagina to prevent the bladder from protruding into the vagina, is used. If the cystocele is large, surgery might be needed to put the bladder back to where it belongs.

15-23 RECTOCELE

A **rectocele** is when the rectum herniates into the posterior wall of the vagina as shown in Figure 15-18. The causes are the same as the cystocele. Signs and symptoms include:

- Constipation
- Feeling of not entirely emptying bowels after a bowel movement
- Pressure on rectum
- A bulge of tissue partially or totally occluding the vagina.

A pelvic examination and patient history are needed for diagnosis. Treatment can include Kegel exercises to strengthen the pelvic floor muscles, pessary procedure, or surgery to repair the posterior wall of the vagina.

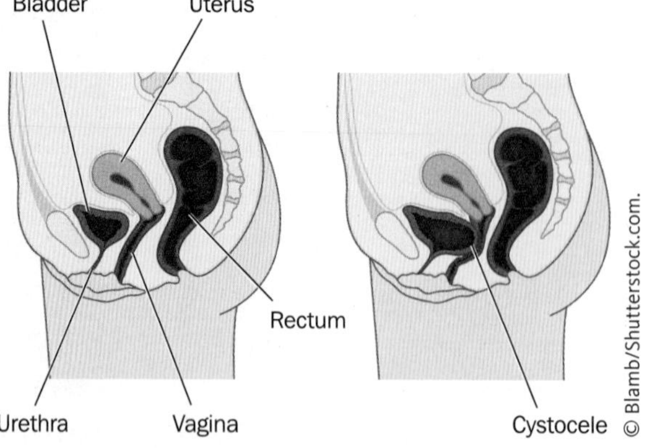

FIGURE 15-17 Urinary bladder herniating into the anterior wall of the vagina.

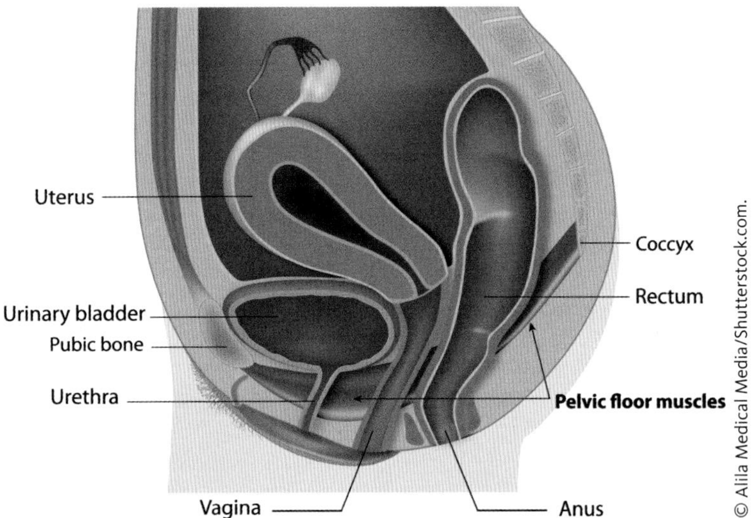

FIGURE 15-18 This image shows the normal female anatomy. However, if a rectocele were present, the rectum that is near the posterior wall of the vagina would herniate or bulge into the vagina.

15-24 CERVICAL CANCER

Cervical cancer begins growing in the lining of the cervix. As the cancer cells progress, deeper tissue is invaded, causing bleeding and ulcerations to develop. The cause of cervical cancer has been linked to human papillomavirus (HPV), which has more than 60 varieties. Some cases of HPV can cause warts on a patient's hands or feet, while in other cases the virus changes the cells in the uterus and cause cervical cancer. HPV can be acquired and remain dormant for up to 20 years before disturbing the cervical cells. An HPV vaccine is available to help lessen this threat. See Figure 15-19.

15-24a Cervical Risk Factors and Detection

The following risk factors increase the odds of developing cervical cancer:

- Family history of cervical cancer
- HPV infection
- Smoking, which disturbs cells in the uterus as nicotine levels concentrate in the cervix
- Drinking alcohol in excess
- Having intercourse with a male smoker
- Women with compromised immune systems
- Obesity
- Prolonged usage of birth control pills.

Although at one time cervical cancer was one of the most common causes of death in women, its rates have decreased with proper screening through a Pap smear exam. Signs and symptoms of cervical cancer occur slowly. Cervical bleeding is the most easily recognized sign leading to early detection, which significantly increases the curability rate.

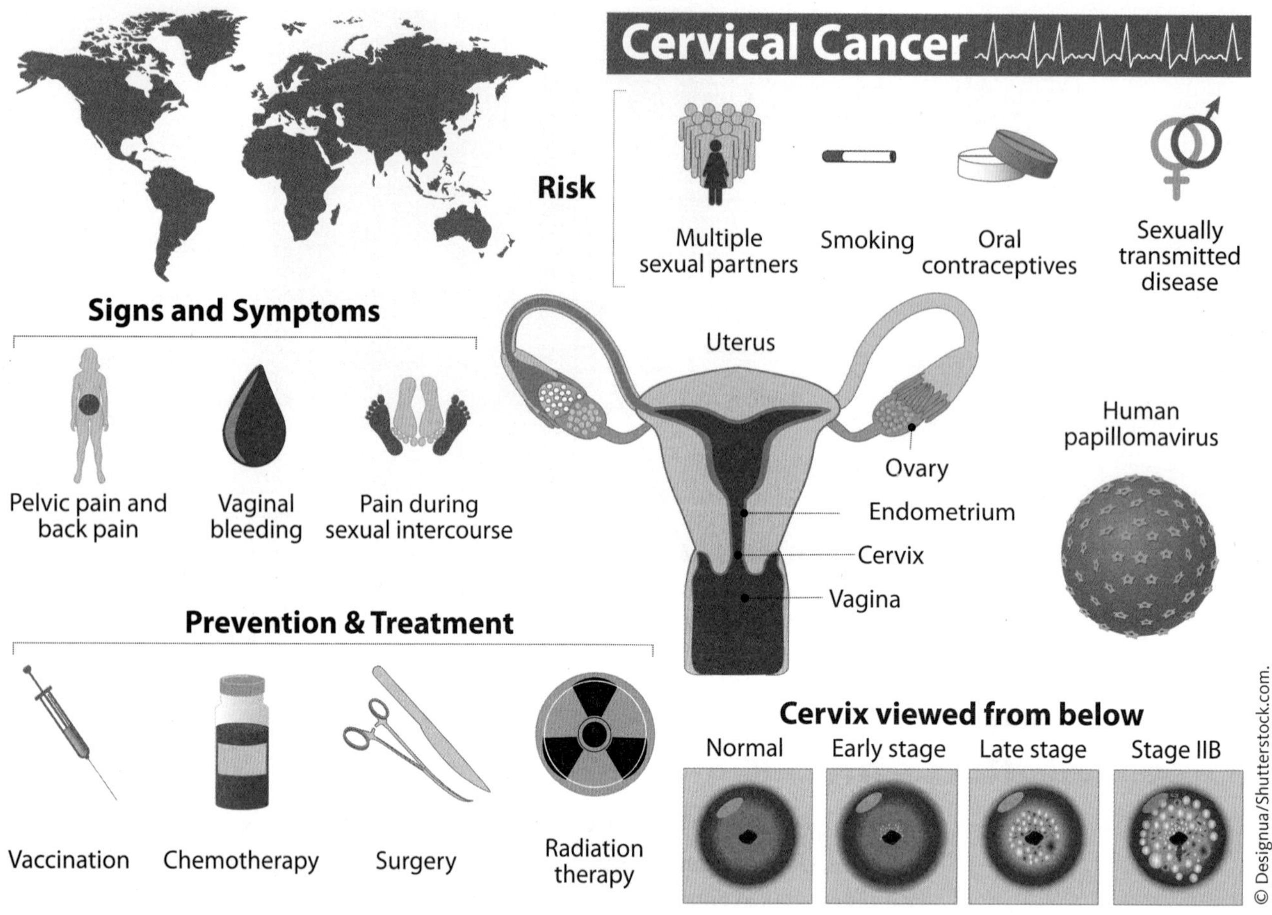

FIGURE 15-19 Cervical cancer infographic.

15-24b Cervical Cancer Treatment

Treatment depends on the stage of cancer. For early stages, surgical removal of the tumor and chemotherapy and radiation might be used, while in the later stages, radiation and chemotherapy are used. See Table 15-7 for chemotherapy drugs used to destroy cancer cells and prevent malignant cell replication.

CLINICAL CONNECTION 15-1

CERVICAL DYSPLASIA VS. CERVICAL CANCER

An irregular Pap smear test result can indicate the presence of cervical dysplasia even though the patient might not be experiencing symptoms. Cervical dysplasia causes cells in the lining of the cervix to become abnormal. This is not cancer, but it is a precancerous condition typically caused by HPV. Treatment depends on the severity of the condition, but the abnormal cells can be removed. Cervical cancer affects the same region as cervical dysplasia and can also be caused by HPV. However, cervical cancer is the rapid and unorganized growth of abnormal cells in the lining of the lower region of the cervix.

Table 15-7 Examples of chemotherapy drugs

TRADE NAME	GENERIC NAME
Platinol, Platinol-AQ	cisplatin
Paraplatin	carboplatin
Taxol	paclitaxel
Hycamtin	topotecan
Gemzar	gemcitabine

15-25 UTERINE CANCER

Uterine cancer, also known as endometrial cancer, develops in the lining of the inner uterus, endometrium, and walls of the uterus. This type of cancer is commonly seen in postmenopausal women who have never given birth. Other risk factors include obesity, extended use of hormone replacement therapy, and being infertile.

Uterine bleeding in a postmenopausal woman is a common sign of uterine cancer. The bleeding leads the woman to seek treatment in the early stages when treatment is most successful.

This condition can be diagnosed by a visual examination of the pelvic cavity and a biopsy of the endometrium tissue. After cancer is confirmed, treatment might include surgical removal of the uterus via a hysterectomy, radiation therapy, and chemotherapy.

15-26 OVARIAN CANCER

Ovarian cancer is the fifth-largest cause of cancer deaths in women and the No. 1 cause of death in cancer of the reproductive system. The number of diagnoses, however, has declined during the last two decades. Ovarian cancer is more common in Caucasian women than African Americans, and half of the women diagnosed are 63 years of age or older. There are many theories about what causes ovarian cancer, but the cause is not yet fully known. Women who have a family history of ovarian cancer should undergo preventative screening because inherited mutated genes are known to increase the risk of developing this cancer. Signs and symptoms include:

- Pressure sensation on bladder
- Frequent urgency to urinate
- Abdominal and pelvic pain
- Difficulty eating
- Quickly occurring sensation of fullness when eating.

Diagnosis includes a physical examination and imaging to determine if a tumor is present. A laparoscopic exam and blood tests can help assist in a diagnosis.

15-26a Treatment for Cervical Cancer

Treatment is based on the stage of cancer. Usually, more than two forms of treatment are used at once. The treatment options are surgery to remove reproductive organs, radiation, and chemotherapy.

A luteinizing hormone-releasing hormone (LHRH) medication can also be administered. These drugs lower the woman's estrogen levels by stopping the production of estrogen by the ovaries. Examples of these agents are listed in Table 15-8.

Other forms of hormone therapy can also be used to decrease the production of estrogen. Aromatase inhibitors, while more commonly used to treat breast cancer, block an enzyme called aromatase. Aromatase makes other hormones that turn into estrogen in postmenopausal women. Therefore, this inhibitor lowers the patient's overall estrogen level. These drugs are listed in Table 15-9.

Another drug class that can be used to treat ovarian cancer is a selective estrogen receptor modulator (SERM), meaning that these agents block receptors for estrogen in the breast tissue while allowing estrogen to reach other regions of the body such as the uterus and bones, which also have receptor sites. This prevents estrogen levels from stimulating cancer cell growth in breast tissue. Tamoxifen (Nolvadex or Soltamox), for example, is primarily used to treat breast cancer, but it can also be used to treat certain tumors such as ovarian stromal tumors.

Table 15-8 LHRH injections

TRADE NAME	GENERIC NAME
Lupron	leuprolide
Zoladex	goserelin

Table 15-9 Aromatase inhibitors

TRADE NAME	GENERIC NAME
Aromasin	exemestane
Arimidex	anastrozole
Femara	letrozole

15-27 FIBROCYSTIC BREASTS

Fibrocystic breasts, shown in Figure 15-20, are a common disorder in premenopausal women. This non-cancerous disorder causes breast tissue to become rope-like or lumpy. The term disease is not used to describe this condition because changes to breast tissue normally occur as a woman ages.

Many of the women affected tend not to have any symptoms. However, reported symptoms include:

- Lumpy breasts (commonly on the upper outer region)
- Breast pain during menstruation
- Breast tenderness
- Nipple discharge (brown or green)
- Heavy or fullness feeling in breast
- Change often felt in both breasts.

15-27a Fibrotic Breast Diagnosis and Treatment

The physician visually and manually inspects the breast and lymph nodes in the neck and armpit. If breast changes are normal, further testing might not be needed. However, if the changes are suspicious, more testing can be done.

If the patient is younger than 30 years, an ultrasound of the breast tissue is better than a mammogram because the breast tissue is denser in young women. A **mammogram** is a radiologic examination that uses an X-ray to target a specific area of the breast.

If the lump seems to be a cyst, as shown in Figure 15-20, the physician might use a fine-needle aspiration technique to withdraw fluid from it to relieve discomfort. If the physician is uncertain about a lump, a breast biopsy can be performed. This entails removing a very small tissue sample from the lump to be studied in a lab.

In addition to the needle aspiration to relieve discomfort, treatment includes NSAIDs such as Advil (ibuprofen) and Tylenol (acetaminophen) to help relieve pain. Oral contraceptives can help relieve discomfort by decreasing hormone levels responsible for causing breast changes.

Fibrocystic Breast Changes

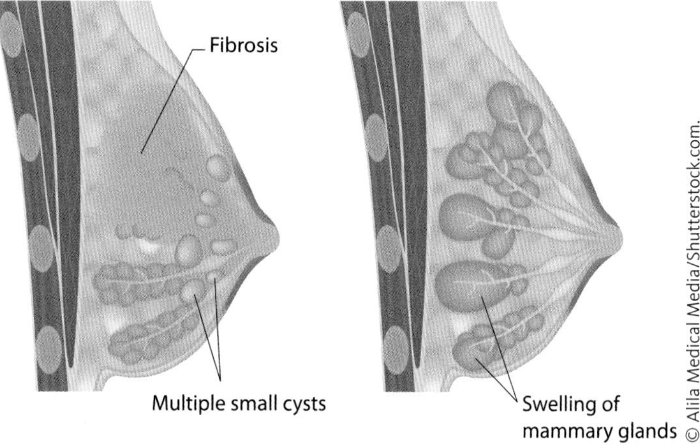

FIGURE 15-20 Fibrocystic breasts.

15-28 MASTITIS

Mastitis is a general term for inflammation of the breast tissue. It can be the result of an infection or from breastfeeding known as lactation mastitis. It might be caused by a blocked milk duct or bacteria entering the nipple from a breastfeeding baby's mouth.

Diagnosis is determined by a physical exam and the patient's signs and symptoms. Treatment involves antibiotics for infectious inflammation and over-the-counter pain relievers such as acetaminophen and NSAIDs.

15-29 BREAST CANCER

Breast cancer is an adenocarcinoma or cancer of the breast ducts. In the United States, breast cancer is the second most-common cancer affecting women, although it can also affect men. Although the exact cause is not known, many factors can contribute, including:

- Menstruation before 13 years of age
- Menstruation after 50 years of age
- Never giving birth
- Obesity
- Those 40 years and older
- Having the first child after 30 years of age
- Family history.

15-29a Signs and Symptoms of Breast Cancer

Signs and symptoms include: (See Figure 15-21.)

- Breast/nipple redness
- Thickening of nipple
- Breast scaliness
- Non-tender lump in breast (usually near upper outer area of breast)

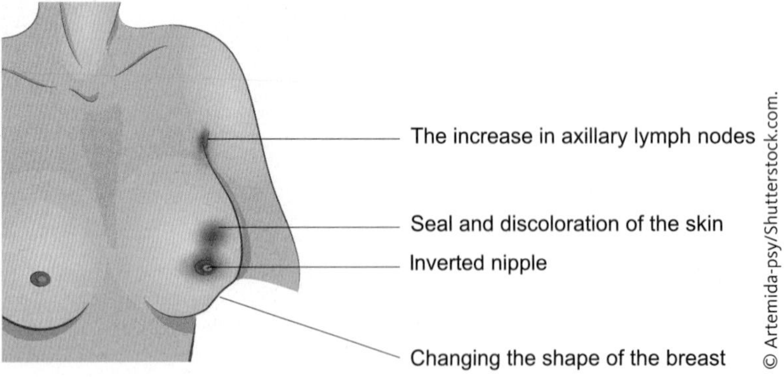

FIGURE 15-21 Signs of breast cancer.

- Nipple discharge
- Breast/nipple pain
- Nipple retraction
- Dimpling of breast.

15-29b Diagnosis of Breast Cancer

Many procedures and tests can be done to verify the presence of cancer, the type, and stage. The primary diagnostic tests for breast cancer are:

- A history and physical examination
- Clinical breast examination
- Ultrasound
- Mammogram, shown in Figure 15-22
- MRI
- Biopsy of tissue lump
- Fine-needle aspiration.

If a tissue sample is positive for cancer, more tests are done to learn more about the type and stage. For example, an estrogen and progesterone receptor test can test levels of these hormones. If the cancer tissue has more than normal levels, the patient's treatment should be tailored to block these hormones from being produced.

15-29c Treatment of Breast Cancer

Treatment of breast cancer is usually done by removing the lump (lumpectomy) or even the entire breast (mastectomy). The patient then might receive radiation

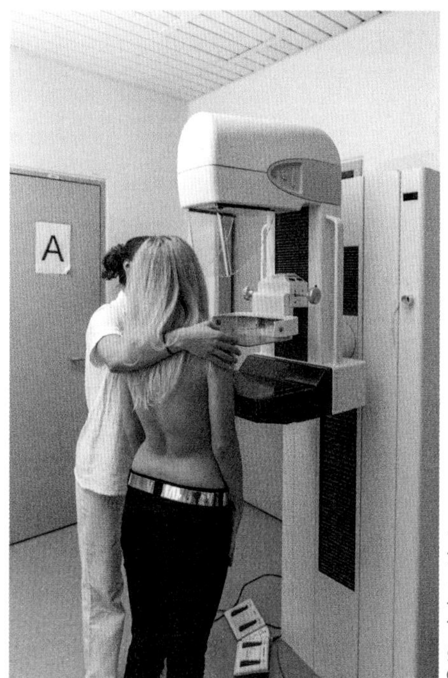

FIGURE 15-22 Mammogram.

Table 15-10 Chemotherapy agents used to treat breast cancer by destroying and stopping cancer growth

TRADE NAME	GENERIC NAME
Perjeta	pertuzumab
Herceptin	trastuzumab
Faslodex	fulvestrant
Adrucil	efudex, others (fluorouracil)

Table 15-11 Chemotherapy agents used to treat cancers that are hormone sensitive

TRADE NAME	GENERIC NAME
Arimidex	anastrozole
Zoladex	goserelin
Femara	letrozole
Nolvadex or Soltamax	tamoxifen

and chemotherapy. Also, since it is common for breast cancer to spread to lymph nodes and vessels, they also might be removed as well. The types of surgery are:

- Lumpectomy. Removal of lump only.
- Simple or total mastectomy. Removal of breast.
- Modified radical mastectomy. Removal of breast and lymph nodes.
- Radical mastectomy. Removal of breast, lymph nodes, and pectoral muscle.

For pharmaceuticals to treat breast cancer, see Table 15-10 and Table 15-11.

LEARNING OBJECTIVE 15.3 Identify male anatomy and physiology.

KEY TERMS

Bulbourethral glands Two pea-sized glands that participate in the production of a component of seminal fluid; also known as Cowper glands.

Ejaculatory duct A canal located between the vas deferens and the seminal vesicle duct that goes through the prostate and connects to the urethra.

Epididymis Duct located behind the testicle where sperm is stored.

Erectile bodies Allow for penis erection.

Foreskin Skin that surrounds distal tip of penis.

Glans penis Bulbous structure at the tip of the penis.

Penis Male genital organ that transports both sperm and urine.

Prostate gland Located below the bladder and in front of the rectum and provides fluid for the nourishment and transportation of semen.

Root (of penis) The part of the penis that attaches to the body.

Seminal vesicles Hold fluid that mixes with semen.

Shaft Body of the penis.

Spermatic cord A cord-like structure made of nerves, vessels, and ducts that go to and from the testicles.

Testicles Male gonad.

Testosterone Male sex hormone.

Vas deferens A duct that transports semen to the urethra.

15-30 OVERVIEW OF MALE ANATOMY

The male reproductive system, like the female system, has both internal and external organs. Figure 15-23 provides an overview of the various components of the male reproductive system.

15-31 TESTICLES (TESTES)

Testicles (testes), the external primary genitalia of the male reproductive system, secrete the male sex hormone called **testosterone**. The testes are a man's gonads and produce sperm, the male's germ cells. Men have two testicles that, when mature, descend from the abdomen and into the scrotum, and for a good reason. Sperm cells cannot be kept at body temperature or else they will die. The temperature in the scrotum is low enough for viable sperm.

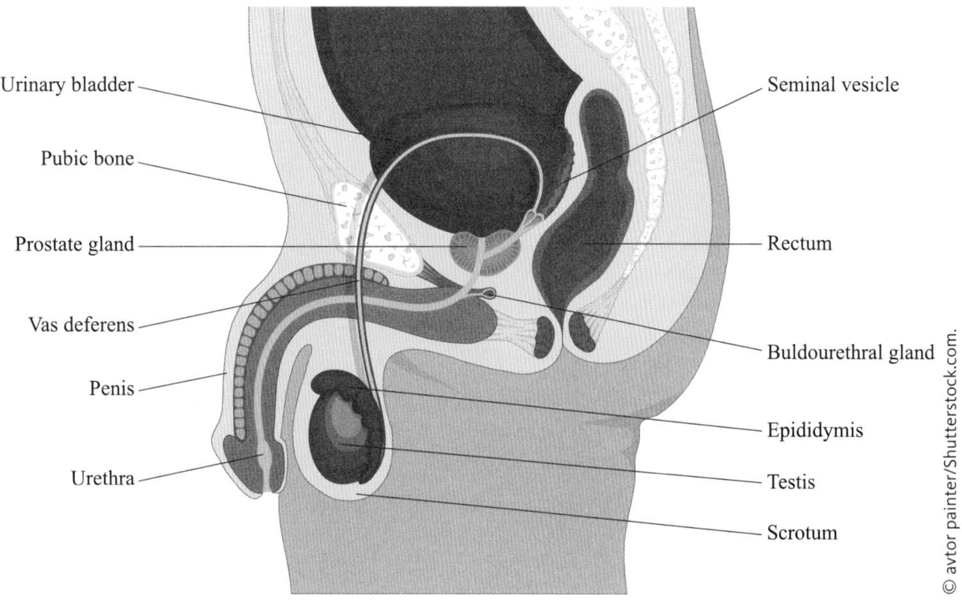

FIGURE 15-23 Male reproductive system.

Sperm is produced in coiled structures inside the testes called seminiferous tubules. Connected to each testis is an epididymis where sperm is matured and stored. The sperm are directed in the correct direction with the help of smooth muscle contraction. The sperm reach the ampulla, which is a dilation at the end of the duct (vas deferens), located near the prostate gland and next to the seminal vessel. Fluids from the seminal vessel are added to the sperm. The semen continuously moves forward through another duct called the ejaculatory duct. As semen passes through the prostate via this tube, the prostate also secretes fluid into the semen, giving it its milky appearance. As the semen continues to move forward, the bulbourethral gland releases fluid that thickens the semen. The semen, carrying sperm, is ejaculated out of the penis via the urethra.

15-32 PENIS

The **penis**, shown in Figure 15-24, is another external part of the male reproductive system. The term penis is derived from the Latin word for tail. Urine is

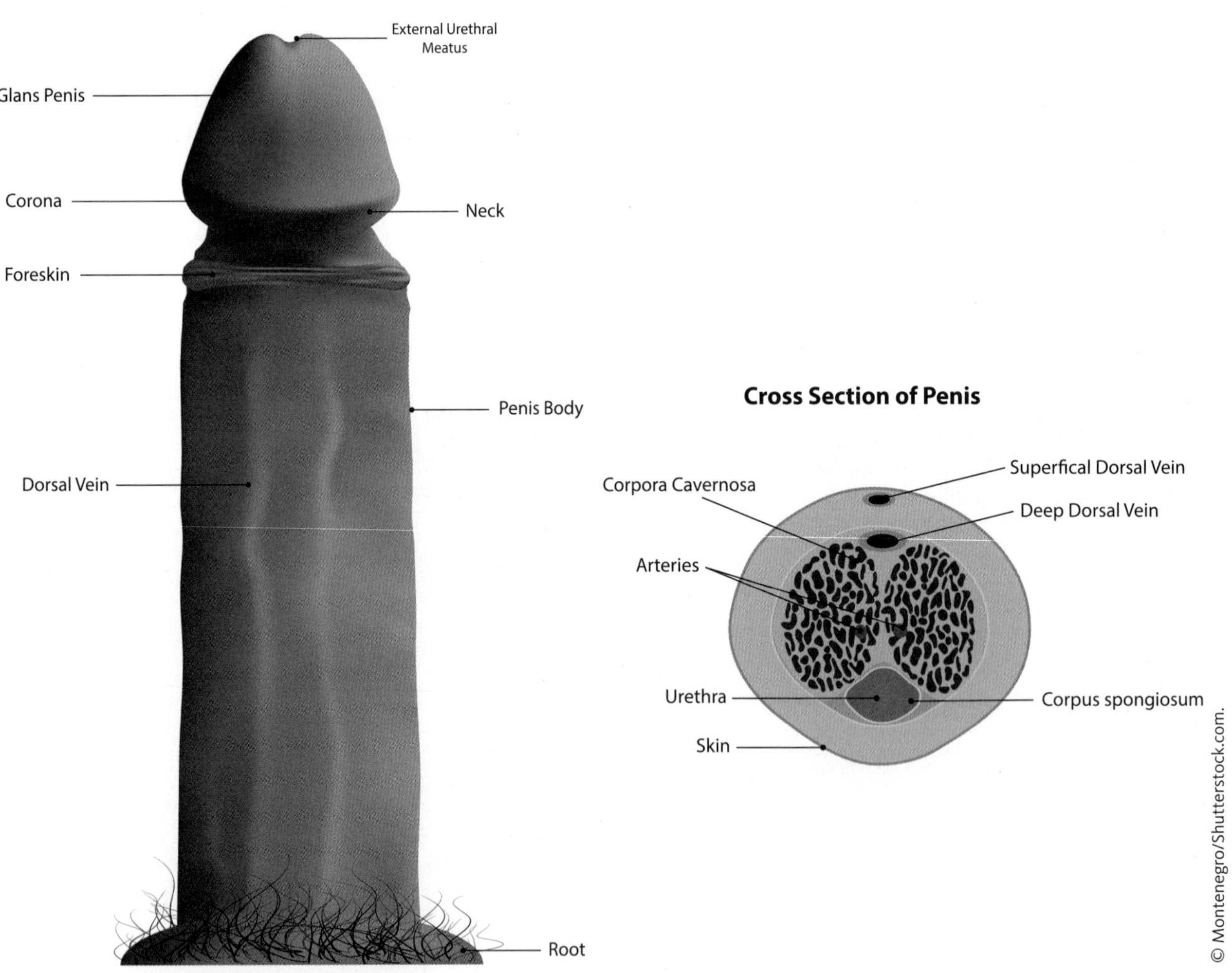

FIGURE 15-24 Anatomy of the penis.

transported outside the body from the bladder through the urethra, which runs through the penis. Sperm is transported via this same passageway. The end of the penis that is attached to the body is referred to as the **root**. The middle section is known as the body or **shaft**, while the tip of the penis is called the **glans penis**. The glans penis is covered by a loose skin called **foreskin** unless the male has undergone a circumcision to have the skin removed. Finally, to become erect, the penis has three **erectile bodies** that are similar to a spongy network of blood sinuses.

15-33 EPIDIDYMIS

The male reproductive system consists of many ducts. The **epididymis**, shown in Figure 15-25, is a duct located in the posterior and lateral part of the testes. The epididymis consists of coiled tubes that are connected between the testes and vas deferens. The epididymis, where sperm mature and are stored, is made of smooth muscle and pseudostratified ciliated epithelium.

15-34 VAS DEFERENS

The **vas deferens** are two long tubes that extend from each testicle to the penis. The tubes are made of pseudostratified ciliated epithelial tissue and a layer of smooth muscle called the adventitia. The vas deferens connects to the seminal vesicles, which form the ejaculatory duct. The **ejaculatory duct** moves through the prostate gland and finally empties into the urethra. The vas deferens can be found through a tube with nerves and blood vessels called the **spermatic cord**. See Figure 15-25.

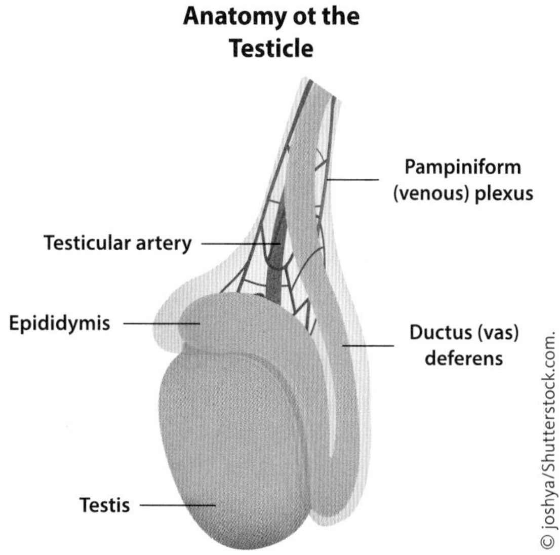

FIGURE 15-25 Anatomy of the testicle. The pampiniform is a network of blood vessels in the male's spermatic cord.

CLINICAL CONNECTION 15-2

VASECTOMY

While considered an invasive form of birth control, a vasectomy is much less invasive than a woman having her tubes tied. A vasectomy entails either cutting or clamping off the vas deferens so sperm cannot mix with seminal fluids, Figure 15-26. So instead of sperm exiting the body, they are reabsorbed. The amount of fluid ejaculated from the penis is still the same after a vasectomy, because the other fluids still operate as they did before the procedure. To be fully effective and to be sure that no sperm can still make their way out of the body, a semen sample is tested to ensure a semen count of zero. Otherwise, the man could still impregnate a woman.

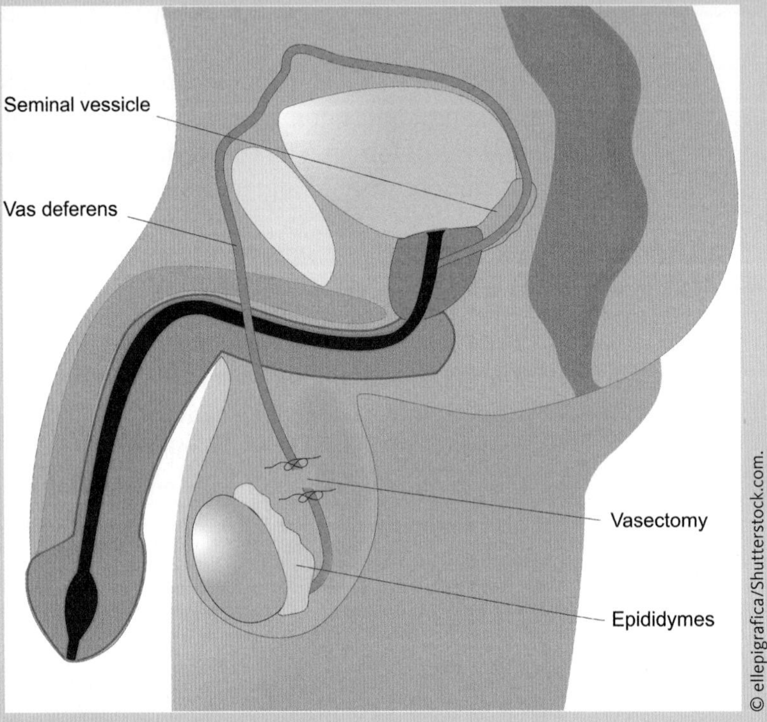

FIGURE 15-26 Location of a vasectomy.

15-35 ACCESSORY GLANDS

The male reproductive system has three accessory glands. The **seminal vesicles** are located posterior to the bladder and are coiled. The glands are constructed of pseudostratified epithelium, connective tissue, and smooth muscle. These vesicles are one of sites that produce fluid that mixes with semen.

The **prostate gland** is located just below the bladder, surrounds the urethra, is about the size of a walnut, and weighs about one ounce. The prostate also produces fluid that is used to carry sperm. The prostate has muscles that contract during ejaculation to push semen through the urethra.

The **bulbourethral glands** are pea-sized glands below the prostate that produce fluid that is added to semen during ejaculation via small ducts that connect to the urethra. This fluid thickens the semen to prevent it from being too watery. See Figure 15-27.

Human Anatomy: Male Reproductive System

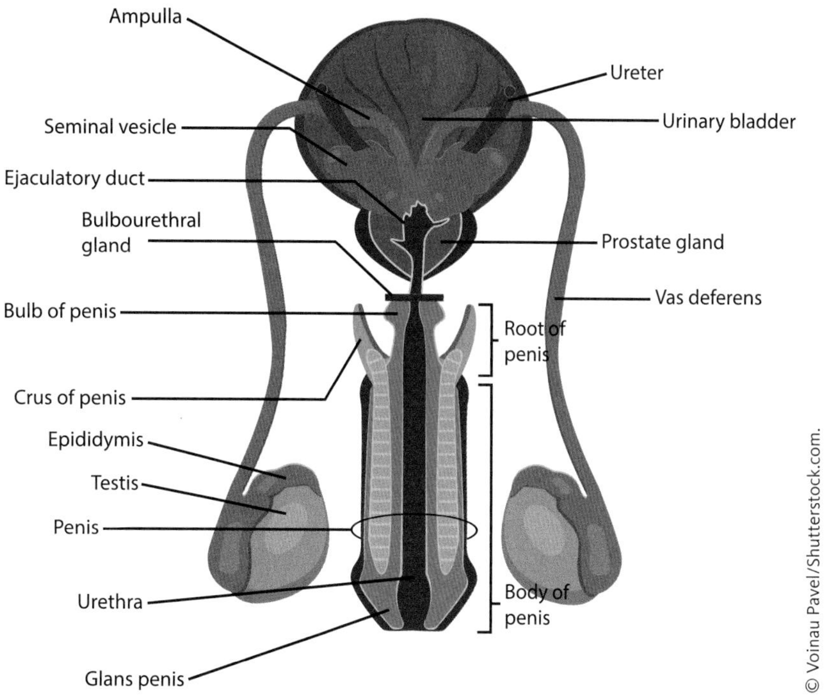

FIGURE 15-27 Note the location of the seminal vesicles, prostate gland, and the bulbourethral glands.

LEARNING OBJECTIVE 15.4 Discuss the pathopharmacology of the male reproductive system.

KEY TERMS

Acquired immunodeficiency syndrome (AIDS) An incurable syndrome caused by HIV, which severely compromises the immune system.

Benign prostatic hyperplasia Enlargement of the prostate gland as a result of increased age; causes difficult urination.

Chlamydia A curable sexually transmitted disease caused by the bacterium *Chlamydia.*

Epididymitis Inflammation of the epididymis.

Genital herpes A sexually transmitted disease causing genital sores from the herpes simplex virus.

Genital warts A sexually transmitted disease from the human papillomavirus (HPV).

Gonorrhea A curable sexually transmitted disease caused by bacteria *(Neisseria gonorrhoeae).*

Hepatitis B A contagious viral disease caused by the hepatitis B virus that attacks the liver; can be spread via contact with bodily fluids.

Hepatitis C A contagious viral disease caused by the hepatitis C virus that attacks the liver; can be spread via contact with bodily fluids.

Human immunodeficiency virus (HIV) An incurable acquired virus that attacks the body's immune system by hijacking healthy cells to reproduce.

Orchitis Inflammation of the testicle.

Prostate cancer Cancer of the prostate gland, which secretes seminal fluids.

Prostate-specific antigen (PSA) Special proteins released into the bloodstream from prostate cells; elevated in the presence of prostate cancer.

Prostatitis Inflammation of the prostate gland.

Syphilis A curable, but potentially serious sexually transmitted disease; if untreated, painful sores develop.

Testicular cancer Cancer of the testicle; usually affects only one testis.

Trichomoniasis A curable sexually transmitted disease caused by a parasite.

15-36 PROSTATITIS

Many of the complications that affect the male reproductive system arise from urinary tract infections, sexually transmitted diseases, and old age. We begin with one that often occurs with aging. **Prostatitis**, shown in Figure 15-28, is inflammation of the prostate gland. This condition is most prevalent in men older than 50. There are many different reasons for this condition to occur, but the causes are not always known. Prostatitis can occur suddenly or slowly over time. Common signs and symptoms of prostatitis include:

- Abdominal pain
- Groin pain
- Testicle pain
- Lower back pain
- Painful or burning urination
- Painful ejaculation
- Urge to urinate
- Frequent urination
- Blood in urine
- Cloudy urine.

15-36a Diagnose and Treatment of Prostatitis

To ascertain if an infection is the cause, a urinalysis and a urine culture to check for the presence of bacteria are usually ordered. To physically assess the size or

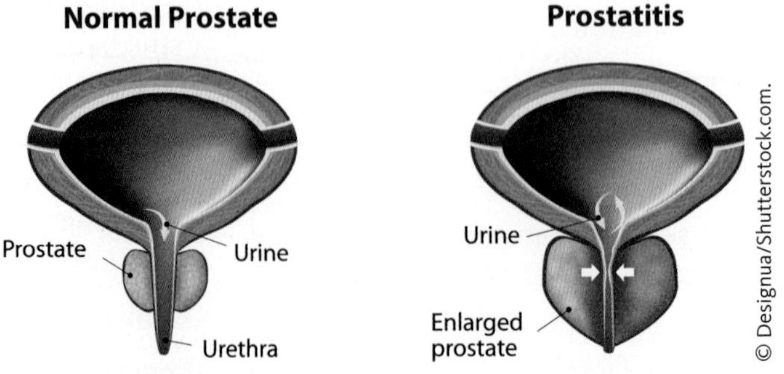

FIGURE 15-28 Comparison between a normal prostate and inflamed prostate.

Table 15-12 Antibiotics used for bacterial prostatitis

CLASSES	MECHANISM OF ACTION	EXAMPLES OF DRUGS
Fluoroquinolones	A type of antibiotics that inhibit the ability for bacteria to grow and replicate by changing certain DNA enzymes	Levaquin (levofloxacin), Floxin (ofloxacin), and Cipro (ciprofloxacin)
Sulfonamides	Inhibit the growth of bacteria by interfering with their folic acid	Bactrim (trimethoprim/ sulfamethoxazole)
Tetracycline	Inhibits bacterial growth by interfering with certain proteins they need to grow	Vibramycin (doxycycline)

Table 15-13 Alpha-Adrenergic Antagonists

EXAMPLES OF DRUGS	MECHANISM OF ACTION
Hytrin (terazosin)	Causes relaxation of the smooth muscle in the neck of the bladder and the prostate gland by blocking certain alpha-1 receptors
Flomax (tamsulosin)	Targets A1 receptors causing relaxation

any swelling in the prostate, a digital rectal exam (DRE) is performed. Also, to get an image of the prostate, a CT or ultrasound can be used.

To treat prostatitis, anti-inflammatory agents such as non-steroidal drugs can help reduce the swelling. If the prostatitis is of infectious origin, an antibiotic, such as those as shown in Table 15-12, can be used. Alpha-blockers are used to relax the neck and muscle of the bladder to facilitate urination and reduce urges to urinate. Sample alpha blocking drugs are shown in Table 15-13.

15-37 BENIGN PROSTATIC HYPERPLASIA

Benign prostatic hyperplasia (BPH) or benign prostatic hypertrophy is an enlargement of the prostate gland as a result of the overgrowth of its normal cells, as shown in Figure 15-29. Those most commonly affected by BPH are men older than 60. In fact, more than half of the men older than 65 have an enlarged prostate. While the cause of BPH is unknown, it is thought to be linked to the changes in hormones as a man ages.

The enlargement of the prostate puts pressure on the bladder and urethra, causing the following signs and symptoms:

- Weak flow of urine
- Difficulty starting urination
- Difficulty voiding all the urine in the bladder
- Frequent urination at night (nocturia)
- Infection from not voiding all of the urine from the bladder.

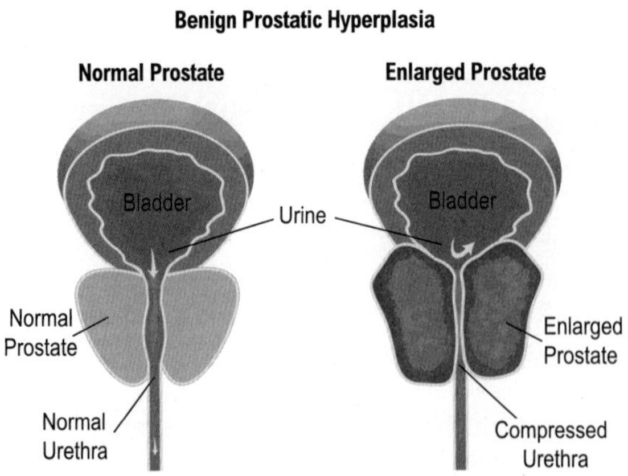

FIGURE 15-29 The comparison between a normal prostate and an enlarged prostate.

Table 15-14 Drugs used to treat BPH

TRADE NAME	GENERIC NAME	MECHANISM OF ACTION
Proscar	finasteride	Steroid reductase inhibitor used to decrease a hormone called dihydrotestosterone (DHT). This causes a reduction in the size of the prostate gland.
Rapaflo Cardura Avodart	silodosin doxazosin dutasteride	Alpha-1 blockers that block the alpha—adrenergic receptors in the smooth muscle of the prostate and bladder neck.

Diagnosis includes a digital rectal examination (DRE) along with a patient history. Drugs used to treat BPH include those shown in Table 15-14.

15-38 PROSTATIC CARCINOMA

Usually occurring in men older than 50, prostatic carcinoma is new growth or neoplasm of the prostate gland. **Prostate cancer** is the most common type of cancer in men, and the second-leading cause of death, second only to lung cancer.

While the exact cause is unclear, it might be linked to changes in hormone levels. This cancer begins in the outer layer of the prostate and usually does not have any signs or symptoms until it metastasizes or spreads elsewhere. Any signs and symptoms are similar to those of BPH. See Figure 15-30.

To diagnose prostate cancer, the physician will do a digital rectal exam (DRE) to determine whether the prostate feels harder than normal or has a mass growing on it. A blood test called a **prostate-specific antigen (PSA)** would have higher-than-normal levels if cancer is present. PSA levels, however, also can be increased by other factors, such as inflammation, so a tissue biopsy should be performed to confirm a diagnosis.

Treatment depends on the extent of the cancer and patient's condition. If the cancer has not spread, the prostate will be removed via a prostatectomy.

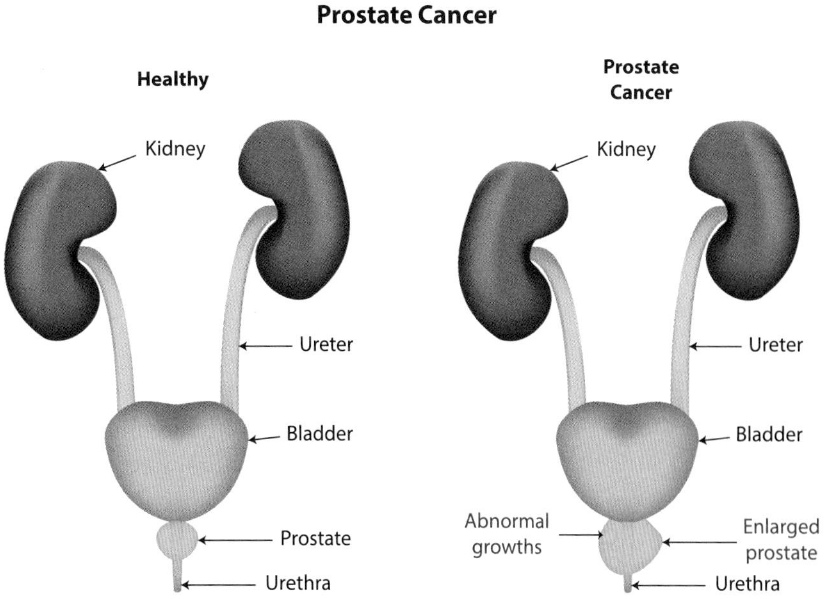

Prostate Cancer

FIGURE 15-30 Prostate cancer.

If it has metastasized, however, hormone therapy will be used to slow the growth.

15-38a Hormone Suppression Therapy for Prostate Cancer

Reducing testosterone levels can help treat prostate cancer. Drugs that reduce the amount of testosterone produced in the body include Eligard (leuprolide), which is given subcutaneously for monthly regimens, which vary depending on the dosage. Lupron Depot (leuprolide) is usually given intramuscularly. Another drug given in conjunction with leuprolide is Casodex (bicalutamide), an oral nonsteroidal antiandrogen that prevents testosterone from binding to androgen receptor sites in the prostate. It is used to treat prostate cancer that has metastasized.

Another hormone drug that can be used is Eulexin (flutamide), a luteinizing hormone-releasing hormone agonist or gonadotropin-releasing hormone (GnRH) agonist. It is used in cases where the cancer has spread to surrounding tissues and where cancer cells have spread throughout the body. Zoladex (goserelin), also a GnRH agonist, is given to patients along with radiation therapy.

Another way to treat prostate cancer is to use antiandrogen agents that block testosterone from getting to the actual cancer cells. An example of this type of agent is Nilandron (nilutamide).

15-38b Chemotherapy

Chemotherapy is used to prevent the growth of cancer cells by interfering with cellular division. One injectable chemotherapeutic agent is Taxotere (docetaxel anhydrous), which can be given with a steroid (dexamethasone) to prevent side effects. Another chemotherapy drug is Jevtana (cabazitaxel), which is used in conjunction with prednisone to reduce side effects. These drugs are used to treat prostate cancer that has not responded to hormone therapy agents.

15-39 EPIDIDYMITIS

Epididymitis is inflammation of the epididymis, which can be caused by many different conditions. Some of the most common are:

- Infection
- Urinary tract infection
- Prostatitis
- Gonorrhea
- Chlamydia
- Syphilis.

Signs and symptoms of epididymitis include swelling and discomfort in the scrotum. The epididymis will be hard and inflamed as shown in Figure 15-31. The patient may find walking difficult.

Diagnosis is made via a history of the patient's symptoms. The physician can feel for a hard and swollen epididymis. Also, a urine culture and urinalysis can be done.

Common antibiotics used to treat epididymitis include:

- Moxatag (amoxicillin)
- Vibramycin (doxycycline)
- Levaquin (levofloxacin)
- Cipro (ciprofloxacin)
- Floxin (ofloxacin)
- Rocephin (ceftriaxone).

To help relieve any pain and discomfort, the patient can take OTC NSAIDs such as Motrin IB, Advil (ibuprofen), or Aleve (naproxen).

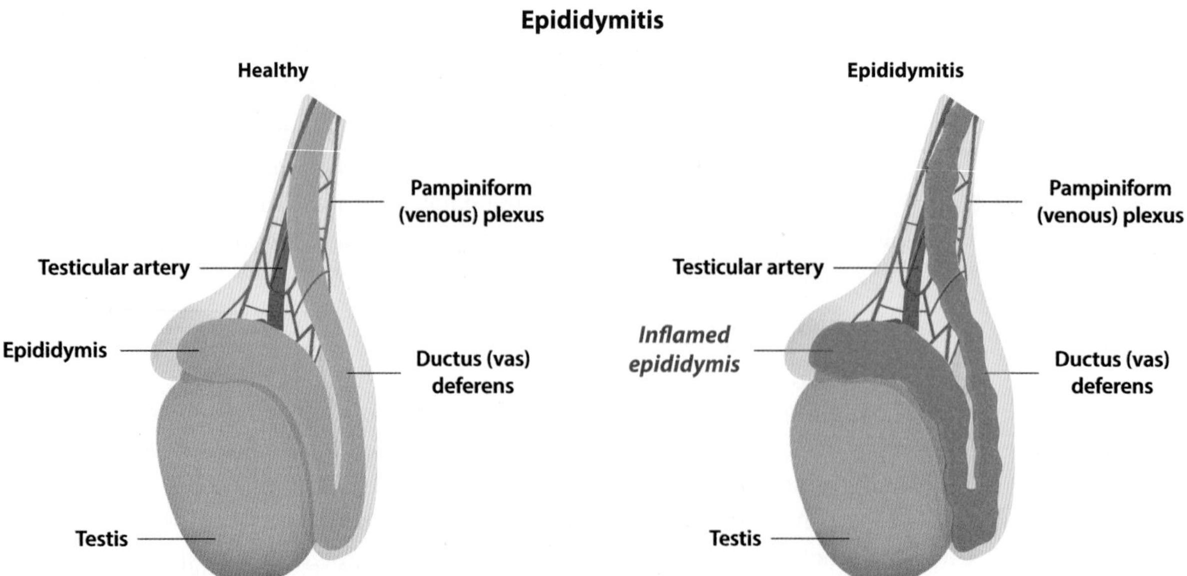

FIGURE 15-31 Comparison between a healthy epididymis and an inflamed epididymis.

15-40 ORCHITIS

Orchitis is inflammation of the testicle. This condition is caused by an infection, either the mumps virus or a bacterial infection such as chlamydia or gonorrhea. When it occurs, it can affect both testicles at once, or only one. Orchitis often occurs with epididymitis.

Signs and symptoms include:

- Pain/tenderness in one or both testicles
- Swelling in one or both testicles
- Nausea
- Fever
- Vomiting
- Discomfort.

Diagnostic testing can include a patient history and physical and other tests such as urinalysis, screening for sexually transmitted infections, and ultrasound imaging.

Typical antibiotic medications used to treat bacterial orchitis include:

- Vibramycin (doxycycline)
- Cipro (ciprofloxacin)
- Floxin (ofloxacin)
- Rocephin (ceftriaxone)
- Zithromax (azithromycin).

To treat pain and reduce inflammation of viral orchitis, the patient can take OTC NSAIDs such as ibuprofen and naproxen.

15-41 TESTICULAR CANCER

Testicular cancer typically affects young men between the ages of 15 and 35 and is less common in males older than 40. The cause of testicular cancer is unknown. It only affects one testicle and is known to start its growth in the structures of the testis that produce sperm. Men should perform routine self-examinations to check for lumps. See Figure 15-32.

15-41a Diagnosis and Treatment of Testicular Cancer

Signs and symptoms of testicular cancer are:

- Mass on the testicle
- Testicle, scrotal, or back pain
- Build-up of fluid in the scrotum
- Dull ache
- Enlarged breast tissue
- Scrotum feels heavy.

The two basic types of testicular cancer are seminoma and non-seminoma. See Table 15-15 for the differences between them and Table 15-16 for the stages of testicular cancer.

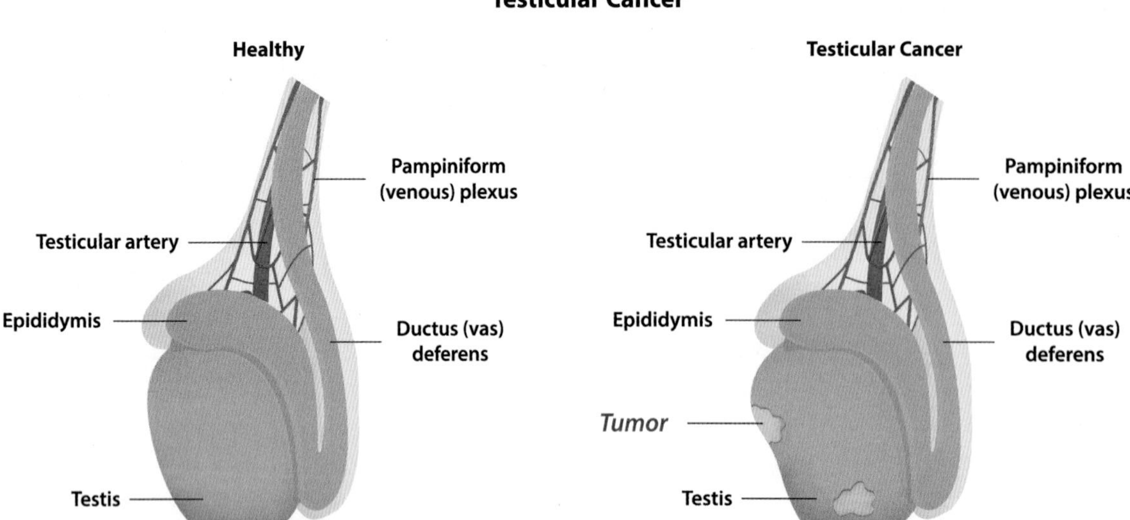

FIGURE 15-32 Testicular cancer.

Table 15-15 Differences between Seminoma and Non-seminoma

SEMINOMA	NON-SEMINOMA
Less aggressive More common in older men	More aggressive More common in young men More likely to metastasize

Table 15-16 Stages of testicular cancer

Stage 1	The carcinoma is contained to the testicle.
Stage 2	Metastasized to lymph nodes in the abdominal cavity.
Stage 3	Cancer has metastasized to other regions of the body, most commonly liver and lung tissues.

The first treatment for testicular cancer is surgical removal, regardless of the type or stage of the carcinoma. If only the testicle is removed, it is a radical inguinal orchiectomy; if the lymph nodes are also removed, it is a retroperitoneal lymph node dissection. Other therapeutic methods used are radiation therapy and chemotherapy. Chemotherapy agents used to treat testicular cancer are:

- Platinol and Platinol-AQ (cisplatin), which interfere with the cancer cells' ability to divide and slow their growth.
- Paraplatin (carboplatin), which stops the growth of cancer cells and kills them.

15-42 SEXUALLY TRANSMITTED DISEASES VS. SEXUALLY TRANSMITTED INFECTIONS

Sexually transmitted diseases are diseases that are transmitted to others through sexual contact. Because not every disease has signs and symptoms or develops into a disease, the term sexually transmitted infection is used. Sexually transmitted infections (STIs) also are spread through sexual contact, including contact with an infected person's blood, semen, or vaginal secretion during vaginal, anal, and oral sex. To prevent exposure to these diseases, condoms should always be used, and people should avoid sexual intimacy with anyone who is infected or those with an unknown sexual history. Although some STDs and STIs are non-life-threatening, some can be deadly. This is especially true for HIV and hepatitis that are untreated.

15-42a HIV/AIDS

Human immunodeficiency virus (HIV) is a blood-borne pathogen that can be transmitted through sexual intercourse and transfusions of blood from an infected person. The virus can lead to **acquired immunodeficiency syndrome (AIDS)**, which often caused death in the first decades of the epidemic in the United States and still does in third-world countries.

Six different classes of drugs can be used to treat HIV/AIDS.

- Nucleoside/nucleotide reverse transcriptase inhibitors (NRTIs) prevent the virus from replicating. Examples include Ziagen (abacavir) and Videx (didanosine).
- Non-nucleoside reverse transcriptase inhibitors (NNRTIs) adhere to certain cellular proteins to prevent the virus from replicating. Examples include Rescriptor (delavirdine), Intelence (etravirine), and Sustiva (efavirenz).
- Protease inhibitors (PIs) inhibit certain proteins from being used by the virus to prevent it from reproducing. Examples are Reyataz (atazanavir), Prezista (darunavir), and Lexiva (fosamprenavir).
- Fusion inhibitors prevent the virus from entering healthy cells in order to replicate. An example is Fuzeon (enfuvirtide).
- CCR5 antagonists work like fusion inhibitors by preventing the infection of healthy cells by preventing the virus from entering them. An example is Selzentry (maraviroc).
- Integrase inhibitors prevent the virus from using a certain protein, stopping the virus from transferring its DNA into the healthy cell. An example is Vitekta (elvitegravir).

Some pharmaceutical companies provide combination dosages, in which more than one of the previous mechanisms are included in one pill.

15-42b Hepatitis B and Hepatitis C

Both **Hepatitis B** and **Hepatitis C** are viral infections that attack the patient's liver. One of the ways the viruses can be spread is via sexual intercourse.

Treatment involves antiviral medications, including Epivir (lamivudine), Hepsera (adefovir), Baraclude (entecavir), and Tyzeka (valacyclovir).

15-42c Other STDs/STIs

In addition to HIV/AIDS and hepatitis, many other different types of STDs and STIs can be contracted.

Genital Herpes

Genital herpes is a viral infection that causes painful blisters to appear on an infected person's genitals. This recurring and highly contagious disease is caused by the herpes simplex virus (HSV), type II, and usually is spread by sexual contact with an infected person. Treatment involves antiviral medications such as Zovirax (acyclovir), Famvir (famciclovir), and Valtrex (valacyclovir).

Gonorrhea

Commonly referred to as the clap, **gonorrhea** is a highly contagious bacterial infection and the most common sexually transmitted disease. If untreated, it can be deadly, because it is known to cause endocarditis and meningitis. Treatment involves antibiotics. Penicillin can be used, in combination with newer antibiotics because of an increase in the number of penicillin-resistant strains. Ala-Tet, Brodspec, Panmycin, tetracyclines, Oracea (doxycycline), and Rocephin (ceftriaxone) have been used to treat the condition.

Syphilis

Syphilis is caused by the bacterium *Treponema pallidum*. This disease is transmitted sexually or by contact with a lesion. After the bacteria are on the surface of the skin or mucous membrane, they penetrate the tissue and enter the bloodstream, resulting in a systemic infection. Syphilis has three different stages: primary, secondary, and tertiary. Treatment is by antibiotics such as doxycycline, erythromycin, and tetracycline.

Chlamydia

Chlamydia is a very common STD that is usually asymptomatic, which is why it is called the silent STD. Lack of symptoms makes chlamydia especially dangerous because it is not recognized by the patient until serious complications arise. Treatment is by doxycycline, azithromycin, and amoxicillin.

Trichomoniasis

Trichomoniasis is an STD that is caused by a protozoan called *Trichomonas vaginalis*. While this disease can be asymptomatic, it also can cause inflammation of the prostate, urethra, and epididymis in men, and itching and burning of a woman's genitals, along with a frothy green discharge. This condition is treated with Flagyl (metronidazole), a commonly used antibiotic and antiprotozoal medication.

Genital Warts

Genital warts are caused by the human papilloma virus (HPV). This common STD usually makes an appearance within six months after exposure. Genital warts are mostly seen around the tip of a man's penis and at the vaginal opening in women. Treatment involves a topical antitumor medication, Condylox (podofilox), which inhibits structures called microtubules to prevent cellular division.

Glossary

1906 Pure Food and Drug Act. Forces manufacturers that produce drugs for sale in the United States to begin following minimum standards for drug purity, strength, and quality.

1938 Federal Food, Drug, and Cosmetic Act. Requires that all new prescription drugs and over-the-counter (OTC) drugs be deemed safe by the FDA before marketing drugs, cosmetics, and therapeutic devices to the public.

1970 Controlled Substances Act (CSA). Categorizes drugs by the acceptable medical uses, the potential for drug abuse, and/or potential for dependency; requires those with prescribing or distributing privileges to have a DEA registration number to prevent fraudulent dispensing of medication.

1983 Orphan Drug Act. Gives financial incentives to manufacturers that develop drugs to treat rare diseases.

24-Hour urine-free cortisol test. A diagnostic procedure used to measure the cortisol levels in urine over a 24-hour period.

A

Abscess. Localized collection of infected material or pus.

Absolute contraindication. Medication or procedure is life-threatening and the benefits do not outweigh the risks; should not be administered.

Absorption. Drug dissolution into the patient's bloodstream.

Acetylcholine (ACh). A chemical neurotransmitter found in both parasympathetic and sympathetic nervous system at the preganglionic sites and only the postganglionic sites of the parasympathetic nervous system.

Acetylcholinesterase (AChe). Deactivates acetylcholine.

Achlorhydria. Absence of hydrochloric acid in stomach acid.

Acid balance test (gynecologic). Used to test the pH of a vagina.

Acne. Skin condition characterized by hyperactivity of oil glands and red pimples on the face, back, and chest.

Acquired immunity. Immunity developed over time through pathogenic exposure.

Acquired immunodeficiency syndrome (AIDS). An incurable syndrome caused by HIV, which severely compromises the immune system.

Acrocyanosis. Bluish hue in the outer skin because of lack of oxygen, combined with hemoglobin in the peripheral area or extremities.

Actin. Thin myofilaments mainly constructed of a protein.

Active acquired immunity. Immunity occurring when the body is exposed to a pathogen and produces antibodies to defend itself against re-exposure.

Acute disease. Disease that has a rapid onset.

Acute glomerulonephritis. Sudden infection of the glomerulus.

Acute pain. A sudden onset of pain.

Acute respiratory distress syndrome (ARDS). Sudden life-threatening lung failure that develops within 24–48 hours of a major illness or injury.

Acute rhinitis. Symptoms of congestion and runny nose usually viral etiology, aka "a cold."

Addison's disease. A condition caused by the lack of cortisol produced by the adrenal glands.

Addisonian crisis. A severe complication of Addison's disease.

Additive. Effect that occurs when two drugs are taken separately, but at the same time together, summative affect when two drugs are taken together.

Adenomatous polyps. Gland-like growths that develop in the large intestines on the mucous membrane.

Adhesion. A normal scar that develops internally and that can cause structural problems.

Adhesive capsulitis. Also known as a frozen shoulder, the shoulder becomes stiff and painful to move due to the lack of movement over time.

Adoptive cell transfer. Cancer treatment using patient's own selectively grown T-cells.

Adrenal glands. Glands located on top of each kidney.

Adrenal medulla gland. Inner section of the adrenal gland.

Adverse reactions. Can occur suddenly or over time and range from patient discomfort to possible death; also known as side effects.

Agonist muscle. Muscle that causes other muscle to move.

Agonist. Substance that binds to a receptor site and causes a response.

AHFS Drug Information (American Health-System Formulary Service). A book primarily for pharmacists that covers such topics as drug stability and chemical information.

Airborne transmission. Pathogenic transmission by way of coughing, sneezing, talking, and laughing.

Albinism. Condition of lacking melanin that leads to loss of skin color resulting in very white skin and hair.

Allergens. Foreign substances to which the body is hypersensitive.

Allergic rhinitis. Inflammation of the mucous membranes from an *allergic reaction*, such as ragweed or grass allergies.

Allergies. Bodily reaction to an allergen exposure.

Alopecia. Condition of balding.

Alpha blockers. Group of drugs used to relax the muscles of the bladder neck and prostate to allow for improved urine flow.

Alpha-agonists (ophthalmic). Decrease the production of aqueous humor while increasing the outflow of aqueous humor from the anterior chamber to lower intraocular pressure.

Alveoli. Lung structure where gas exchange takes place.

Amenorrhea. Absence of menses.

Ampules. A glass bottle that is fused closed and must be broken to open.

Ampulla. Wide section of the fallopian tube.

Analgesics. Medications to reduce pain.

Anaphylactic reaction. A severe and potentially life-threatening allergic reaction to a drug.

Anaphylaxis reaction. A serious, sometimes life-threatening, allergic reaction.

Anastomoses. New connections developed between vessels that serve as a backup or alternative pathways to allow blood flow if a blockage occurs.

Anemia. Low hemoglobin commonly seen as a result of hemorrhage or a decrease in red blood cells.

Aneurysm. Weak spot in a vessel.

Angina pectoris. Chest pain caused by decreased oxygenation to the heart muscle.

Angiocardiography. Examination of the vessels and chambers of the heart performed with a special dye and an X-ray.

Angiogenesis inhibitors (AIs). Biological response modifier therapy that targets and destroys cancer-feeding blood vessels. Drug example: bevacizumab (Avastin).

Angiogenesis. Formation of new blood vessels.

Anhidrosis. Condition of decreased or lack of ability to sweat.

Ankle-brachial index (ABI). Non-invasive method used to check for the presence of peripheral artery disease.

Anoscope. Tube-like instrument that is inserted into the anus to examine the walls of the lower rectum and anal region.

Antacids. Medications taken to neutralize stomach acid.

Antagonist muscles. Muscles that inhibit certain movement and return a muscle contraction back to its original resting position by opposing the muscle contraction.

Antagonist. Blocks a desired effect; when two drugs are given and they cancel out the desired effect.

Anterior pituitary gland. Frontal portion of the pituitary gland.

Anthelmintics. A class of drugs used to treat worm infections.

Anthracosis. Lung disease as result of inhaling anthracite (hard coal) dust.

Antifungal. Agents used to treat fungal infections.

Antiandrogens. Medications that suppress the production and effects of testosterone and can be used to treat prostate cancer. Drug examples are Eligard and bicalutamide (Casodex).

Antiarrhythmics. Drugs used to treat an abnormal heartbeat.

Antibiotics. A class of drugs used to treat bacterial infections.

Anticholinergics. Group of drugs used to prevent bladder constrictions to prevent the frequent urge to urinate.

Anticoagulants. Drugs that prevent the blood from clotting.

Antidiabetic drugs. Drugs used to control Type 2 diabetes.

Antiemetics. Classification of drugs to treat nausea often given in conjunction with cancer treatment.

Antiestrogens. Drugs that modify or block the cancer-causing effects of the hormone estrogen on breast tissue. Tamoxifen is an example of a selective estrogen receptor modifier.

Antifungal agents. Medications used to treat fungal infections.

Antihistamines. Medications to prevent the release of histamine during an allergic response.

Antilipemic agents. Drugs that help decrease the amount of lipids in the blood.

Antimetabolites. Cancer medications that interfere with cellular metabolism and thus interfere with cellular repair and reproduction. Drug examples are methotrexate and fluorouracil.

Antineoplastic agents. Medications that counteract the growth and spread of malignant cells.

Antiplatelet drugs. Drug class that prevents platelets from sticking together to cause a clot.

Antipruritics. Medications used to relieve itching.

Antipyretics. Medications to reduce fever.

Antiseptics. Chemicals that inhibit the growth of bacteria.

Antithyroid. Drug that stops the thyroid from producing T3 and T4 hormones.

Antitussive agents. Reduces cough.

Antivirals. A class of drugs used to treat viral infections.

Anxiety disorder. Mental health condition in which anxiety becomes chronic and exaggerated or inappropriate for the given situation.

Apnea. The cessation of breathing.

Apocrine sweat glands. Glands found in the groin and anal regions that become active around puberty.

Apoptosis. Cellular death.

Appendicitis. Inflammation of the appendix.

Appendix. A long, thin pouch on the outside wall of the cecum.

Aqueous humor. Gelatinous fluid found in both anterior and posterior chambers between the lens and cornea of the eye.

Arrector pili muscles. Muscles that allow the hair to stand erect for thermoregulation of our body and in times of fright.

Arrhythmia. Abnormal heartbeat.

Arterial blood gases (ABGs). Sample of *arterial* blood to see if there are adequate oxygen and carbon dioxide levels.

Arteriography. Test that uses a special dye and an X-ray to check the inside of the arteries.

Arteriosclerosis. Develops when the vessels are no longer elastic and have become stiff, can cause an increase in blood pressure, can be caused by old age.

Arthritis. Inflammation of a joint.

Asbestosis. Lung disease as a result of the asbestos particles.

Ascending colon. The first of four segments of the colon that extends in an upright direction.

Asexual reproduction. Cellular division producing identical copies without the involvement of another cell.

Asphyxia. Extreme decrease in the amount of oxygen in the body to the point of unconsciousness and death.

Aspiration. Food or liquid entering the airway, which can cause serious obstruction and damage.

Asthma. Respiratory condition where the airways go into bronchospasm and narrow due to some stimulus; patient experiences dyspnea and wheezing.

Astigmatism. A refractive error condition that causes light to be unevenly scattered over the retina.

Astrocytes. Cells that keep blood vessels and neurons close together.

Asystole. Condition with no electrical heart activity and therefore no heartbeat.

Atelectasis. Lung collapse.

Atherosclerosis. A condition caused by plaque that builds up on the walls of the arteries causing the walls to become thicker.

Atherosclerosis. Hardening of blood vessels.

Atrophic vaginitis. Vaginal inflammation from decreased estrogen production.

Attention deficit hyperactivity disorder (ADHD). Mental health disorder that has hyperactivity along with the inability to concentrate and impulsive behaviors.

Audiogram. A graph that gives a detailed description of how well a patient can hear.

Audiologist. One who specializes in hearing impairments and disorders.

Auricle. Part of the external ear, the portion you can see. Also known as the pinna.

Auscultation. Listening with a stethoscope to examine breath, and heart and bowel sounds to determine if any abnormalities are present.

Autoimmunity. A situation in which the immune system fights against its own tissues and cells.

Autonomic nervous system. Involuntary portion of peripheral nervous system whose output controls cardiac muscle, smooth muscle, and glands.

Autonomic system. Controls functions automatically.

Autoregulation. Protection mechanism in our body used to protect fragile filters in the kidneys from pressure fluctuations that occur throughout the day.

Avulsion fracture. Fracture causing a small bone fragment to separate from the bone where the tendon or ligament is attached.

Axon terminal. The end of an axon.

Axon. Long portion of the neuron that transmits the received signal.

B

Bacteria. Single-celled microorganisms.

Barrett's esophagus. Damage caused by chronic acid reflux causing the cells to change from its normal squamous cells to a specialized intestinal metaplasia cell found in the small intestine.

Basal cell carcinoma. Most common form of skin cancer that does often not metastasize; appears as a raised nodule with depressed center or a smooth shiny tumorpinkish to whitish in color.

Bell. Side of the stethoscope used to listen to the patient's heart.

Bell's palsy. Disease affecting the facial nerve causing (one-sided) facial paralysis leading to face drooping.

Benign prostatic hyperplasia. Enlargement of the prostate gland as a result of increased age; causes difficult urination.

Benign. Non-cancerous.

Beta blockers. Drugs causing decreased heart rate.

Beta-adrenergic blockers (ophthalmic). Used to relieve the pressure of glaucoma by decreasing the fluid in the eye.

Bicuspid. A tooth with two cuspids, also referred to as a premolar tooth.

Bile acid sequestrants. Medications used to help lower cholesterol by binding to certain resins in the bile.

Binary fission. Asexual cellular reproduction forming two identical cells.

Binge eating disorder (BED). Eating disorder characterized by eating large quantities of food often very quickly to the point of discomfort on average at least once a week for three months.

Bioavailability. The measurement of how much of a drug is found in our bloodstream.

Biological response modifier therapy. This "targets" the cancer by manipulating the immune system to hunt down and specifically kill the cancer cells.

Biological vector. Animal or insect that spreads pathogen to other hosts by a bite or injection.

Biopsy. Procedure during which a tissue sample is obtained for testing.

Biotransforms. The chemical changes of a drug in the body as a result of metabolism.

Bipolar disorder. Mental health condition with extreme mood changes that include emotional highs (mania) and emotional lows or depressive states.

Black lung. General term for the inhalation of all the different types of coal dust.

Bladder. Expandable sac acting as a holding chamber for urine that has drained from the kidneys.

Blepharitis. Inflammation of the eyelid that results in redness, crusty dandruff-like skin flakes on the eyelashes, and itchiness.

Blood glucose. Sugar found in the bloodstream used for energy.

Blood thinners. Drugs used to prevent clotting and to increase the time it takes for blood to clot.

Blood urea nitrogen (BUN) test. Blood test used to check the function of the kidney.

Body. Largest portion of the stomach.

Bone Mass Density (BMD). Diagnostic test using X-rays to measure the amount of minerals (especially calcium) in a bone.

Booster dose. Given to maintain the desired immune response of a primary immunization.

Bradycardia. Heartbeat that is slower than normal.

Bradypnea. Slower than normal breathing.

Brain stem. Stalk-like structure inferior to the cerebrum that contains the medulla oblongata, midbrain, and pons.

Brand name. Proprietary drug name owned by a company.

Breast cancer. Cancer of the breast tissue.

Breath-actuated nebulizer (BAN). A type of nebulizer able to deliver an aerosol continuously or on inspiration only.

Bronchi. Large airways.

Bronchiectasis. Area of irreversible, abnormal, and irregular enlargement of the inner diameter of an airway, usually caused by repeated infections.

Bronchioles. Small airways (iole = small).

Bronchogenic carcinoma. Cancerous tumor, originating in an airway.

Bronchospasm. Narrowing of the airways due to smooth muscle contraction.

Buccal tablet. A tablet that is kept between the cheek and gum.

Bulbourethral glands. Two pea-sized glands that participate in the production of a component of seminal fluid; also known as Cowper's glands.

Bulimia. Eating disorder of binge eating followed by vomiting or purging the body of food.

Bundle of His. Collection of cardiac muscle nerve fibers for electric conduction.

Bursitis. Inflammation of the fluid-filled sac found in joints.

C

Cachexia. Describes thin and wasting away appearance.

Cachexia. Weakened and frail state because of nutrient deprivation, often seen in cancer patients.

Calyces (singular: calyx). Funnel- or cup-like structures that collect urine from the renal pyramids.

Cancer staging. Objective measurement system to determine the severity of the cancer based on the size and spread of the original or primary tumor.

Cancer. Malignant cell growth.

Candidiasis. Caused by the candida yeast, it is an opportunistic infection that surfaces if normal flora is wiped out by antibiotic use or an immunosuppressant condition. Infections can occur in the mouth (thrush), vagina (vaginitis), intestines, and fingernails (onychomycosis).

Canines. Long, pointed teeth used to hold onto food.

Capillaries. Very tiny blood vessels that connect to form a network.

Capsid. A virus's outer coating.

Capsule (cap). A pill with a gelatin coating, making it easier to swallow.

Carbonic anhydrase inhibitors. Agent used to decrease intraocular fluid production to decrease the pressure in the eye.

Carbuncle. Large grouping of furuncles.

Carcinogenic. Potential to cause cancer.

Carcinoma in situ. A cancer that is "just sitting there" in the particular tissue and hasn't broken through the basement membrane and invaded other tissues or sites.

Carcinoma. General term for cancerous tumor.

Cardiac (stomach). Portion of the stomach located around the lower esophageal sphincter.

Cardiac catheterization. Invasive procedure used to treat and diagnose cardiovascular conditions.

Cardiac cycle. Series of heart movements that repeat for every heartbeat.

Cardiac muscle. Involuntary muscle found only in the heart.

Cardiac output. Amount of blood pumped by the heart in 1 minute.

Cardiac sphincter. A circular or ring-shaped muscle leading to the stomach.

Cardiomyopathy. Disease of the heart muscle.

Carditis. Inflammation of the heart.

Carotene. Skin pigment that gives a normal yellowish hue to the skin.

Carotid endarterectomy. Surgical removal of the plaque within the arteries supplying the brain.

Carpal tunnel syndrome. Inflammation pressing on the median nerve in the wrists from strenuous or repeated movement.

Cataract. An opaque clouding of the lens of the eye resulting in vision impairment.

Cauterization. Electrical burning of tissue to prevent or stop bleeding.

Cautions. A list of certain patients for whom or conditions under which a drug should be used with close supervision.

Cavities. Small holes that can develop in teeth.

Cecum. A short pouch-like structure that connects the small intestine to the large intestine.

Cell cycle. Is the total life span of eukaryotic cells; two major phases are known as interphase and the mitotic phase.

Cell-mediated immunity. Consisting of specialized white blood cells (WBCs), it is the body's main defender from foreign substances.

Cellular reproduction. Is the process of one cell dividing into two cells, also known as cellular division.

Cellulitis. A potentially serious bacterial skin infection.

Cellulitis. Bacterial infection of the skin caused by *streptococcus* and/or *staphylococcus* bacteria.

Cementum. Surface of the tooth root that is a bone-like connective tissue adhering teeth to the jaw bone.

Centers for Disease Control and Prevention (CDC). Agency responsible for recording and tracking diseases not only domestically but also abroad.

Central diabetes insipidus. Caused by the lack of antidiuretic hormone.

Central nervous system (CNS). The portion of nervous system composed of the brain and spinal cord.

Cerebellum. Located posterior to the brain stem; plays an important role in sensory and motor coordination and balance.

Cerebral spinal fluid (CSF). Specialized fluid that bathes and protects the brain and spinal cord.

Cerebrovascular accident (CVA). Neurological condition caused by disruption of adequate blood flow to the brain, affecting its ability to function.

Cerumen. Earwax.

Cervical cancer. Cancer of the cervix.

Cervix. Lower portion of the uterus.

Chemical name. The drug name used to describe the anatomical or molecular structure of a substance.

Chemical neurotransmitter. Chemical substance such as acetylcholine that can carry the signal on to the next nerve, gland, skeletal, smooth, or cardiac muscle.

Chemoinformatics. The usage of analytical data about the properties, structure, and molecular activities of chemical compounds used to design a drug.

Chemotaxis. The ability of cells to move to a location.

Chemotherapy. Use of chemical substances or drugs to treat a disease, usually in reference to cancer.

Chest tube. Tube inserted into the pleural space to remove the air and allow re-expansion of the lung.

Chest X-ray (CXR). Imaging used to examine the thoracic cavity.

Chief complaint (CC). Main reason the individual sought medical attention.

Chlamydia. A curable sexually transmitted disease caused by the bacterium *Chlamydia*.

Cholecystectomy. Surgical removal of the gallbladder.

Cholecystokinin (CCK). Hormone that is released to assist in the digestion of protein and fat.

Choroid. The vascular layer of the eye found between the retina and the sclera.

Chromosomal disorders. Abnormality of a whole or partial chromosome.

Chronic bronchitis. Progressive and non-reversible obstructive respiratory disease characterized by swollen airways, bronchospasm, and excessive mucus production that affects the flow of air in and out of the lungs.

Chronic disease. A long-term disease.

Chronic glomerulonephritis. Ongoing or recurring infection of the glomerulus.

Chronic inflammation. Ongoing inflammation of 7 to 10 days.

Chronic Obstructive Pulmonary Disease (COPD). Category of non-reversible obstructive lung disease with distinct diseases, chronic bronchitis, and emphysema, that can occur singularly or in combination.

Chronic pain. Prolonged pain.

Chyme. Puree of acidic fluid containing partially digested food moving from the stomach to the small intestine.

Cilia. Microscopic hair-like structures that act like oars moving mucus up and out of the airways in a coordinated fashion.

Ciliary muscles. Muscles that flatten the lens to assist focusing.

Circulation. Movement of blood throughout the body.

Clean catch method. Method used to collect urine to prevent contamination of the sample.

Closed reduction. Required when fracture does not require a surgery and needs only a cast to fixate the fracture.

Cluster headache. Headache type occurring upon awakening with throbbing pain behind the nose and eyes.

CNS stimulant. Medication that stimulates the central nervous system, usually causing tachycardia, increased respirations, and high levels of energy and alertness.

Cochlea. Spiral cavity found in the inner ear that plays a major role in hearing.

Collagen. Fibrous protein in the connective tissue.

Colles' and Pott's Fracture. A fracture at the end of the radius of a bone, typically seen in wrist and ankle injuries.

Colon polyps. Growths developed from a cluster of cells on the intestinal wall that may become cancerous.

Colon. The large intestine.

Colonoscopy. A procedure that uses a scope to visually inspect the colon.

Colony-stimulating factors (CSFs). Biological response modifiers that stimulate the bone marrow to develop red and white blood cells and platelets, which are often deficient in many cancers. Example drug is Erythropoietin (Epogen and Procrit).

Colorectal cancer. Cancer of the colon or rectum.

Comminuted fracture. Fracture in which the bone breaks into two halves with many bone fragments at the site of the break.

Common vehicle. Any medium such as food or blood that acts as a vehicle to transport pathogens.

Communicable. Contagious and spread from one source to another whether it is person–person, animal–person, or even an object–person via bacterial or viral microorganisms.

Compact bone. Hard, very dense, and tightly compact bone tissue that covers the outer layer of bones.

Complete Blood Count (CBC). Blood sample analyzing types and numbers of cells within the bloodstream.

Complete fracture. Fracture that goes completely through the bone.

Compression fracture. Collapsing of the vertebrae in the spinal column.

Computerized tomography (CT or CAT) scan. Imaging utilizing X-rays and a computer to produce cross-sectional slices of the body.

Concussion. Traumatic head injury usually accompanied by temporary loss of consciousness.

Cones. Provide central vision and the ability to see color.

Congenital disease. An inherited disease at birth that may not be experienced until later in life or fetal damage due to maternal trauma.

Congestive heart failure (CHF). Fluid builds up in tissues around the heart because of heart failure.

Conjunctivitis. Inflammation of the lining of the eye known as the conjunctiva, commonly known as pink eye.

Contact dermatitis. Inflammation of the skin because of contact with an irritating substance.

Contagious. Potential to cause infection and spread rapidly.

Contractility. Ability of the muscle to shorten or contract.

Contraindications. A list of reasons why a certain drug should not be given.

Contusion. Physical bruising of brain tissue.

Cor pulmonale. Lung disease that leads to right-sided heart failure.

Coronary artery disease (CAD). Disease caused by the buildup of plaque in the arteries of the heart.

Corpus luteum. What remains of the follicle after ovulation.

Corticosteroids. (for integumentary use) Agents used to treat skin disorders from allergic reactions.

Corticosteroids. Medications that suppress both the inflammatory and allergic response.

Crackles. Popping sound upon inspiration, representing fluid in the alveoli.

Cranial nerves. Twelve pairs of nerves associated with the brain that conduct information to (sensory) and from (motor) the brain.

Creams. Thin semisolid topical drug form applied to the skin.

Creatinine clearance test. Blood test used to see how well the kidneys are functioning.

Crohn's disease. Common, chronic inflammatory bowel disease causing inflammation in the lining of the digestive system.

Croup. Inflammatory pediatric condition of viral or bacterial origin that is characterized by a barking cough.

Crown. Upper visible portion of a tooth usually consisting of enamel.

Cruciate Ligament Tear. Tear in the ACL (anterior cruciate ligament) or PCL (posterior cruciate ligament).

Culture and sensitivity (C&S). Laboratory sample from a patient that grows and identifies the pathogen and tests what drug will kill it.

Culture and sensitivity test (sputum C&S test). A lab test that grows (cultures) the bacteria found in a sample in order to identify the type of bacteria, then tests against (sensitivity) a variety of antibiotic medications to see which are effective.

Cumulative effect. Occurs when a drug is not eliminated from the body and the drug level accumulates.

Cushing's syndrome. A condition caused by too much cortisol in the body.

Cyanosis. Bluish hue in the outer skin because of lack of oxygen combined with hemoglobin.

Cystic fibrosis. Is an inherited disease causing exocrine glands to malfunction; as a result, the airways produce a thick mucus that is hard to eliminate, thus, leading to repeated lung infections or pneumonias.

Cystitis. Inflammation of the bladder.

Cystocele. Weakening of the anterior wall of the vagina that allows the bladder to bulge into the vagina.

Cystogram. Picture of the bladder.

Cystoscopy. Procedure done to inspect the inside of the bladder.

Cytokinesis. The division of the cellular cytoplasm.

D

D-dimer test. Test used to measure a specific substance that would be present if a clot has been broken up.

Death rate. A statistical measurement of deaths caused by a disease of a certain population over a specific time period.

Debridement. The process of removing foreign material and necrotic tissue from a wound.

Decongestants. Medications that constrict blood flow and inflammation, thereby, reducing passageway congestion.

Deep vein thrombosis (DVT). Clot that has formed within the deep veins.

Degenerative disc disease. Skeletal disease usually caused by aging that wears away the intervertebral disc, resulting in compression and damage to spinal nerves.

Dehiscence. The reopening of a wound because of weak scar tissue.

Dementia. Progressive deterioration of mental abilities because of changes in the brain.

Dendrites. Branch-like structures that receive information from other nerve cells or environments and transmits the signals to the body.

Dentin. Hard layer of the tooth found directly under the enamel.

Dependency. Psychological need for the drug that might or might not be accompanied by a physical need.

Dermal patches (transdermal patches). Deliver medication externally through the skin.

Dermatologist. Medical doctor who specializes in the treatment of skin conditions and diseases.

Dermatology. Study of skin and its related structures.

Dermatoplasty. Surgical repair of the skin such as skin grafting needed to replace damaged skin with healthy grafted skin.

Dermis. Considered the true skin containing nerve, blood vessels, elastic fibers, hair follicles, and glands; lies below the epidermis.

Descending colon. A section of the colon that moves in a downward direction and meets the sigmoid colon.

Diabetes insipidus. A condition caused by a lack of antidiuretic hormone, causing frequent urination and thirst.

Diabetes mellitus. A group of diseases caused by too much sugar in the blood.

Diabetic coma. Unconscious state caused by high blood sugar.

Diabetic gangrene. Dead tissue resulting from a loss of blood flow, peripheral artery disease caused by diabetes mellitus.

Diabetic retinopathy. Blindness caused by high blood sugar.

Diabetic retinopathy. Vascular changes on the retina; a complication from either Type I or Type II diabetes.

Diabetic shock. Life-threatening condition caused by too much insulin in the body.

Diagnosis. Identifying the disease.

Diapedesis. Movement of cells out of blood vessels during the inflammatory process to assist in the healing process.

Diaphragm. Main breathing muscle.

Diastole. Part of the cardiac cycle in which the heart relaxes and fills with blood.

Dilated cardiomyopathy. The left ventricle becomes stretched and enlarged, causing the heart not to beat properly.

Direct contact. Making physical contact with another person or body fluids that spreads infection.

Direct or closed questioning. Asking questions that require a yes or no answer.

Disinfectants. Chemicals that kill bacteria on surfaces.

Dislocation. Total or complete separation of a bone from a joint.

Disorder. Describes disruption from the normal functioning of the mind or body. Typically used when a disease is not an appropriate term to describe condition.

Displaced fracture. Bone fragments are not in the original correct position.

Diuretics. Class of medication used to eliminate excess water from the body to help control hypertension and edema.

Diverticula. Outward sac that develops in the wall of the large intestine.

Diverticulitis. Condition developing from the inflammation of diverticula.

Doppler echocardiogram. Test used to study the flow of blood through the heart.

Douche solution. A solution used to irrigate the vaginal canal.

Drops (gtt). Liquid drops of medication that can be instilled in eyes, ears, and nose.

Drug actions. The interactions between a drug and body at the cellular level.

Drug classification. A method used to group drugs in a meaningful way.

Drug Enforcement Agency (DEA). Established to enforce provisions of the 1970 Controlled Substances Act.

Drug legend. Statement warning that any distribution without a prescription is prohibited by federal law.

Dry powder inhaler (DPI). Portable inhalation device that delivers aerosolized powdered medication to the airway. Since the patient must generate high inspiratory flows for the delivery, this is only used prophylactically with maintenance medications.

Dual energy X-ray absorptiometry (DXA). Testing that uses X-rays to measure the amount of minerals (especially calcium) in a bone.

Duodenal ulcer. Peptic ulcer located in the duodenum.

Duodenum. First part of the small intestine between the stomach and the jejunum.

Dysentery. Bacterial infection of the intestines causing severe, infectious diarrhea.

Dysmenorrhea. Painful menstruation.

Dysphagia. Difficulty swallowing.

Dysphonia. Difficulty speaking.

Dysplasia. Abnormal tissue development.

Dyspnea. Difficulty breathing.

E

Eccrine glands. Sweat glands located over the body to allow perspiration and cool the body by evaporation to aid in temperature regulation.

Eczema. Genetic hypersensitivity skin reaction often found in infants.

Ejaculatory duct. A canal located between the vas deferens and the seminal vesicle duct that goes through the prostate and connects to the urethra.

Elasticity. Muscle's ability to return back to its original length after contracting.

Electrocardiogram (ECG or EKG). Recorded display of electrical impulses produced by the heart.

Electrocardiograph. Instrument used to record heart rhythms.

Electroencephalography (EEG). Measures the electrical activity of the brain; used to locate an abnormal area.

Electrolytes. Minerals dissolved in blood needed by the body to function properly, (calcium, potassium, sodium, phosphate, magnesium, and chloride).

Electromyography (EMG). Testing used to examine muscle disorders by inserting a small needle into the patient's muscle tissue and recording its electrical activity.

Elixir (elix). Liquid drug mixed with an alcohol base.

Emollients. Agents used to soothe irritation and protect skin damage.

Emphysema. Progressive and non-reversible obstructive respiratory disease characterized by the destruction of alveolar walls and the surrounding capillaries, and affects the exchange of gas between the alveoli and blood.

Empyema. Formation of pus in the pleural space, usually due to a bacterial infection.

Emulsion. Liquid drug preparation containing fats and oils in water.

Enamel. Hard, white outer layer of a tooth providing durability and protection against everyday wear and tear.

Encephalitis. Inflammation of the brain tissue caused by a variety of microorganisms.

Endemic. Disease found in a certain region or specific population.

Endocardium. The inner layer of the heart.

Endocrine system. System that produces and secretes hormones to control everyday bodily functions.

Endolymph fluid. Fluid found in the labyrinth.

Endometriosis. A condition in which endometrial tissue that normally lines the uterus implants in other regions of the reproductive system and intestines.

Endometrium. Innermost layer of the uterine wall.

Endomysium. Sheath of connective tissue around myofibrils.

Endoscopic mucosal resection. Removal of abnormal lesions with a scope instrument.

Endoscopy. Viewing of internal portions of body and/or body passageways through use of flexible fiber optic scopes through which tissue biopsies also can be taken.

Endotracheal intubation. Inserting a tube *within* the trachea, often connected to a machine called a ventilator to help the patient breathe.

Enema. Liquid solution instilled into the rectum with an applicator bottle.

Enteral route. Administering substances through the GI tract, including oral, feeding tubes, and rectal routes.

Enteral route. Giving drugs by way of the GI tract.

Enteric-coated tablet. Coated pill that prevents disintegration by gastric juices.

Environment. Surrounding in which one lives.

Enzymatic agents. Promote removal of necrotic and fibrotic tissues (aids in debridement).

Ependymal cells. Nerve support cells that act as epithelial cells by covering the surfaces of cavities.

Epicardium. The outer of three layers of the heart.

Epidemic. Sudden spread of illness to large amount of people.

Epidemiology. Study of disease transmission, occurrence, distribution, and control for a population.

Epidermis. Outermost, visible layer of skin.

Epididymis. Duct located behind the testicle where sperm is stored.

Epididymitis. Inflammation of the epididymis.

Epidural hematoma. Collection or pooling of blood between the skull and dura membrane that covers the brain, often resulting in increase in intracranial pressure.

Epidural. Injection into the epidural space of the spinal cord.

Epiglottis. Leaf-like fibrocartilage that, when you swallow, closes over the opening to the trachea, thus, directing food or liquid down the esophagus to prevent aspiration.

Epiglottitis. Potentially life-threatening illness, mainly affecting children, of epiglottic swelling, which can obstruct the airway leading to asphyxia; caused by the bacterium *Haemophilus influenzae* type b; the Hib vaccine can help protect children from developing epiglottitis.

Epilepsy. Chronic disease characterized by periodic episodes of abnormal electrical conduction resulting in seizures.

Erectile bodies. Allow for penis erection.

Erysipelas. Acute skin infection that extends into the underlying fat layer; more commonly found in children caused by group A *streptococcus* bacteria.

Esophageal varices. Dilated (varicose) veins in the lower portion of the esophagus.

Esophagogastroduodenoscopy (EGD). Upper GI endoscopy used to diagnose and treat.

Esophagus. Flexible, yet muscular tube that connects the pharynx with the stomach allowing food to pass through.

Etiology. Cause or origin of the disease.

Eukaryotic cells. Cells having a true nucleus bounded by a nuclear membrane and containing cellular organelles.

Eustachian tube. A tube that acts as a passageway in between the middle ear and nasopharynx.

Eversion. Ankle has moved or rolled outward.

Exacerbation. Acute disease flare up or attack from a chronic condition.

Excitability. Ability to respond to certain stimuli such as electric signals.

Excretion. Stage at which the drug has been broken down to be eliminated from the body.

Exophthalmos. Abnormal protrusion of the eyes.

Expectorants. Agents to help increase secretions that can then be expelled.

Extensibility. Ability for a muscle to be stretched.

Extracapsular fracture. Break that occurs in the outside of a joint capsule.

Exudates. Leakage of cellular debris from the bloodstream to the tissues of the body from an injury or irritation.

Eye ointment. Semi-solid substance used for ophthalmic purposes.

Eyelids. Skin folds located on the top and bottom of the eye that cover the eye when closed.

F

Facultative mitotic cells. Cell division process used to replace cells.

Fallopian tubes. Two tubular structures that transport the egg to the uterus.

Family history. Interview to identify diseases the patient is susceptible to according to heredity.

Fecal impaction. Hardened stool causing a blockage.

Femoral neck fracture. Crack in the neck of the femur near the hip joint.

Fibrinous exudate. Fluid containing fibrinogen that indicates a large injury and inflammation are present.

Fibroblasts. Cells found in connective tissue that fill the deep area of a wound and forms collagen.

Fibrocystic breasts. Benign changes of the breasts that give a lumpy or rope-like texture.

Fibroid tumors. Benign tumors found in the uterus.

Fimbria. Finger-like projections that direct an egg from the ovary to the fallopian tube.

Flat bones. Bones that have a plate-like structure.

Folliculitis. Infection of the hair follicle on the skin from *staphylococcus* bacteria.

Food and Drug Administration (FDA). Federal agency that ensures drugs and devices are safe to use.

Forceps. Set of surgical pinchers that can be advanced through an endoscope to sample a portion of a tumor for testing.

Foreskin. Skin that surrounds distal tip of penis.

Formulary. A list of medications offered in a particular hospital or healthcare system.

Freckles. Concentrated patches of melanin on the skin.

Frontal lobes. Section of the brain responsible for motor activities, conscious thought, and speech.

Fundus. Midportion and most superior part of the stomach.

Fungus. A plant-like organism spread by spores.

Furuncle. Small abscess developed around a hair follicle.

G

Gag reflex. Protective airway reflex to prevent aspiration.

Gallbladder. Sac-like organ which stores bile from the liver before releasing the bile to the small intestine.

Gallstones. Hardened deposits of bile that form in the gallbladder.

Gametes. Germ cells (sperm from the male; ovum from the female) that unite to form a fetus during reproduction.

Gastric cancer. Cancer of the stomach.

Gastritis. Inflammation of the lining of the stomach.

Gastroenteritis. Inflammation of the gastrointestinal tract.

Gastroesophageal reflux disease (GERD). Flow of gastric juices from the stomach into the esophagus.

Gastrointestinal stromal tumors (GIST). Tumors that develop from the walls of the GI tract from cells in the autonomic system responsible for regulating the body's digestion.

Gauge. The diameter or width of a needle.

Generalized anxiety disorder (GAD). Anxiety disorder characterized by excessive worrying.

Generic name. A name not owned by any particular pharmaceutical company.

Genetic immunity. General ability of our body to respond to an invader based on genetic traits we are born with.

Genital herpes. A sexually transmitted disease causing genital sores from the herpes simplex virus.

Genital warts. A sexually transmitted disease from the human papillomavirus (HPV).

Genitals. External parts of the reproductive system.

Gestational diabetes. Diabetes that develops because of pregnancy.

Glans penis. Bulbous structure at the tip of the penis.

Glasgow coma scale (GCS). Objective standardized scale used to measure the extent of a brain injury.

Glaucoma. An eye condition that affects the optic nerve and overtime may result in blindness.

Glial cells. Support tissue for the nervous system that lines cavities and provides functions such as producing myelin.

Glomerular capsule or Bowman's capsule. Double-layered membrane that encompasses the glomerulus, which is found inside the nephron of the kidney.

Glomerular filtrate. Material filtered by the glomerulus.

Glomerulonephritis. Group of diseases that results from an injury to the glomerulus.

Glomerulus. Network of capillaries surrounded by the glomerular capsule.

Gloves. Latex, vinyl, or nitrile; worn to protect hands from coming into contact with any type of patient fluid or mucous membrane secretions.

Gonads. Organs (testicles in males and ovaries in females) that produce germ cells or gametes for reproduction.

Gonorrhea. A curable sexually transmitted disease caused by bacteria (*Neisseria gonorrhoeae*).

Gout. Condition of build-up of uric acid in the blood causing pin like crystals to develop.

Gowns. Protective garment used to protect clothing and skin from infectious exposures.

Graafian follicle. The name of the mature follicle that ruptures and releases an egg.

Granuloma. Hardened tissue formed by the calcification of macrophages and fibrous tissues formed by collagen.

Greenstick fracture. Classification of bone fracture in which one side of the bone breaks while the other side is bent, just as if it were a green tree limb.

Guillain-Barre syndrome. A disease of an unknown etiology causing paralysis which progresses from the outer most extremities to the face.

Gynecologic speculum. A medical device used to hold open the vaginal walls for inspection.

Gynecologist. One who treats diseases of the reproductive system.

H

H-2 blockers. Medications used to block the production of stomach acid.

Hair shaft. Visible portion of hair on the epidermal layer.

Hairline fracture. Very thin fracture line that resembles a strand of hair on an X-ray.

Half-life (T 1/2). The time for a drug dose to decrease by half after it is administered.

Healthcare-associated infection (HAI). Infection caused by medical intervention.

***Helicobacter pylori*.** Gram-negative bacterium that can cause stomach ulcers.

Helminths. Parasitic worms.

Hemangiomas. Common benign, often cherry red, childhood tumor made up of blood vessels; usually appears on the face and neck.

Hematocrit (HCT). Ratio of total cellular volume to total volume of blood.

Hemodialysis. Method used to cleanse the blood of waste when the kidneys are unable to do so by placing a direct catheter line into the bloodstream.

Hemoglobin (Hgb). Protein in the red blood cell that carries oxygen.

Hemoptysis. Coughing up bloody sputum.

Hemorrhoids. Inflamed veins of the anus and rectum.

Hemothorax. Collection of blood in the pleural space.

Hepatitis A (HAV). Infectious liver disease caused by contaminated food or water.

Hepatitis B (HBV). A contagious viral disease caused by the hepatitis B virus that attacks the liver; can be spread via contact with bodily fluids.

Hepatitis C (HCV). A contagious viral disease caused by the hepatitis C virus that attacks the liver; can be spread via contact with bodily fluids.

Hepatitis. Inflammation of the liver.

Hereditary. Diseases are passed down from parents to their offspring.

Herniated nucleus pulposus (HNP). Herniated vertebral disc.

Herpes simplex. Viral infection causing clusters of fluid-filled vesicles called cold sores or fever blisters and genital herpes.

Herpes varicella. Viral infection causing chickenpox.

Herpes zoster. Viral infection causing shingles.

Hiatal hernia. Portion of the stomach pushes through the diaphragm.

Histamines. Chemical substances released to cause dilation of vessels in response to injury or irritation.

History of present illness (HPI). History of the current condition or disease.

Holistic medicine. A care plan that not only focuses on the disease, but the patient as a whole, including body, mind, spirit, and emotions, in a quest for optimal health and wellness.

Hookworms. Type of parasitic worms, found in tropical regions of the world, that enter the body through the bare feet of those walking on contaminated soil.

Hormones. Chemical signals that are secreted into the bloodstream to control bodily functions.

Host. The susceptible individual who can harbor pathogen.

Human immunodeficiency virus (HIV). A virus that progressively attacks the body's immune system by destroying specialized cells called helper T-cells.

Human papilloma virus (HPV). Viral infection causing warts. Genital warts, the most commonly sexually transmitted disease, has been shown to increase risk for cervical cancer.

Humoral immunity. A type of acquired immunity from circulating antibodies.

Hydronephrosis. Condition in which fluid (urine) is obstructed from leaving the kidney causing renal distention.

Hyperemia. Increases blood flow to a certain area causing redness and warm sensation.

Hyperglycemia. High blood sugar.

Hyperopia . A refractive error condition known as farsightedness, meaning objects at a distance can be seen clearly while objects nearby are blurry.

Hyperplasia. Excessive growth of normal cells.

Hypersensitivity. When a patient has an allergic reaction to a substance.

Hypertension. High blood pressure.

Hypertensive heart disease. Group of conditions that cause high blood pressure, which in turn affect the function of the heart.

Hyperthyroidism. Overproduction of thyroid hormones.

Hypertrophic cardiomyopathy. Condition in which a chamber of the heart becomes enlarged without a specific cause.

Hypodermal layer. Also known as the subcutaneous layer; innermost layer of skin that is composed of elastic and fibrous connective tissue and fatty tissue.

Hypodermic syringes. Commonly used to inject medication.

Hypoglycemia. Condition of low blood sugar.

Hypothyroidism. Underproduction of thyroid hormones.

Hypoxemia. Low levels of oxygen within the blood.

I

Iatrogenic. Disease caused by medical intervention.

Idiopathic. Disease occurring spontaneously with an unknown cause.

Idiosyncratic reaction. Type of adverse drug reaction that is uncommon in response to a drug.

Ileocecal valve. Valve attaching the ileum to the large intestine.

Ileum. Last portion of the small intestine after the jejunum that is connected to the large intestine.

Ileus. Inability of the intestines to move contents by way of peristalsis.

Immune system. Specialized cells, tissues, and organs that fight against and protect our bodies from disease.

Immunity. Ability to protect from illness.

Immunodeficiency. The inability of the body to defend and protect itself from pathogenic organisms.

Immunotherapy. Use of natural or synthetic substances to stimulate or suppress immune system.

Impacted cerumen. A blockage of earwax.

Impacted fracture. Bone fracture that is forced into the end of another bone.

Impetigo. Highly contagious pustule forming skin disease usually found in children and affecting the hands and face.

In and out catheterization. Temporary catheter used to drain urine and then be removed.

Incisors. Teeth located in the front of the mouth, used for cutting.

Incomplete fracture. Break that does not completely separate the bone.

Incubation period. Period of pathogen reproduction causing symptoms to occur within the host.

Incus. Anvil-shaped bone in the middle ear; located between the malleus and stapes.

Indirect contact. Host coming into contact with a contaminated surface.

Indwelling catheter. Catheter that remains in the patient over a period of time.

Infection. Invasion of pathogenic microorganisms.

Infectious. The ability to cause disease.

Inferior vena cava. Large vein that brings deoxygenated blood to the heart from the lower body.

Inflammation. A bodily process used to kill invaders to allow healing.

Inflammatory bowel disease. Conditions causing inflammation to the intestinal tract.

Inflammatory exudate. Cellular debris resulting from inflammation.

Inflammatory polyps. Type of polyp that usually occur in individuals who suffer from an inflammatory condition of the bowel.

Influenza. More commonly known as the flu; a highly contagious respiratory viral infection spread by coughing and secretions.

Infundibulum. Funnel-shaped end of the fallopian tube is proximal to the ovary.

Inguinal hernia. Intestinal tissue pushes through a weakened area of the abdomen wall.

Injectable routes. The ways in which a substance can be injected directly into the body.

Inner ear. Innermost section of the ear.

Inoculation period. Period of pathogen introduction without symptoms.

Inotropic agents. Drugs that change the heart's contraction. Positive inotropic agents increase the heart's contractility, while negative inotropic agents cause the heart to have a weaker contraction.

Inspection. Visually looking for anything out of the norm.

Insula. Section of the brain located deep inside the temporal lobe that coordinates information from the autonomic nervous system.

Insulin syringes. Special syringes used only to give insulin preparations to diabetics.

Insulin. Hormone required to control blood sugar.

Integumentary system. Composed of skin and other accessory organs that make up our outer covering. Other main parts of the integumentary system are hair, nails, sweat glands, and sebaceous glands.

Interaction. List of items that can interact and change a drug's effect.

Interatrial septum. Septum separating the right and left atria.

Interferons. Biological response modifier therapy that actively stimulates the body's immune response to fight cancer.

Interphase. Where the majority of the cell cycle is spent on normal functioning and stockpiling needed materials for cellular division.

Intertrochanteric fracture. Describes fractures in the trochanter of the femur.

Interventricular septum. Septum that separates the right and left ventricles.

Intestinal obstruction. Blockage of the intestines.

Intracapsular (intra-articular). Injection into the joint.

Intracapsular fracture. Fracture occurring inside a joint capsule.

Intracranial pressure (ICP). Measure of pressure within the cranial cavity.

Intradermal (ID). Injection right below the skin.

Intramuscular (IM). Administering a drug directly into a muscle.

Intraosseous. Injecting medication into the patient's marrow of the long bones for immediate systemic effect.

Intraspinal. Injection into the spinal cord.

Intravenous (IV). Directly injecting into a blood vessel.

Intravenous pyelogram (IVP). Radiological technique that uses dye to obtain a better visualization of the urinary system.

Intraventricular route. Medications are given through a catheter into the ventricle of the brain.

Intussusception. Condition occurring when part of the intestine folds into itself.

Inversion. Ankle turns inward.

Investigational new drugs (IND). Three-step process for a drug to be approved by the FDA for clinical use.

Involuntary muscles. Muscles that move without conscious effort.

Ionized. A charged state in which drugs will not be absorbed until they reach a certain environment that allows them to become non-ionized; then they can be absorbed.

Iris. Controls size and diameter of the pupil and therefore controls the amount of light allowed into the eye.

Irregular bones. Bones that are in many different shapes and sizes.

Irritability. (see excitability).

Irritable bowel syndrome. Chronic condition affecting the large intestine causing pain, cramping constipation, or diarrhea.

Isthmus. Narrow section of the fallopian tube.

J

Jaundice. Skin that has a deeper yellow or orangish coloration because of the build-up of bilirubin; often found with liver disease.

Jejunum. Second part of the small intestine located between the duodenum and ileum.

K

Kegel exercises. Exercises used to strengthen the pelvic floor muscles to prevent prolapse and urinary incontinence.

Keloid. Excessive scar tissue growth.

Keloids. Raised mass of scar tissue that usually develops after trauma or surgery.

Keratin. Protein that hardens cells and forms hair and nails.

Keratitis. Inflammation of the cornea.

Keratolytic agent. Loosens and breaks down epithelial skin scaling.

Ketoacidosis. Buildup of ketones (acid) in the blood when the body breaks down fat for energy.

Kidney-Ureter-Bladder (KUB). X-ray used to visualize the kidney, ureter, and bladder.

Kyphosis. Humpback curvature of the spine.

L

Labeled indications. Uses for what the drug is intended to treat.

Labyrinth. Bony outer wall of the inner ear.

Lacrimal apparatus. Consists of lacrimal glands and ducts, which secrete and drain lacrimal fluid.

Lacrimal glands. Glands that produce lacrimal fluid.

Large intestine. Located between the small intestine and the anal opening that plays a major role in absorption.

Laryngitis. Acute or chronic inflammation of the larynx and vocal cords leading to difficulty speaking.

Larynx. Voice box.

Late-night salivary cortisol level test. Salivary test done at night to measure cortisol levels.

Lesion. Damaged or defective area on the inside or outside of the body, such as scabs, ulcers, and tumors.

Lethal dose. A drug dose causing death.

Leukemia. Malignant neoplasms of the blood and blood-forming organs.

Leukocytes. A type of white blood cell.

Lifestyle. The way in which an individual lives his or her life.

Limbic system. Series of nuclei in the cerebrum and superior brain stem involved in mood, emotion, and memory.

Liniment. Medicated preparation used to soothe aches and muscle pains.

Lipid (fat) solubility. Ability to dissolve in lipids (fats); substances with low-fat solubility are absorbed at a slower rate, while those with a high-fat solubility are absorbed faster.

Lipocytes. Cells that produce fat needed to provide padding to protect the deeper tissues of the body and act as energy storage.

Liver. Large organ located below the right side of the abdomen with important digestive and metabolic roles.

Loading dose. Larger initial dose given to quickly establish the desired therapeutic effect.

Lobectomy. Surgical removal of a lobe of the lung.

Local effect. Stimulation of a certain part or region of the body.

Long bones. Bones that are longer than they are wide.

Long-term control or maintenance agents. Agents used in chronic respiratory disease to lessen or prevent exacerbations; not to be used in acute situations, examples include inhaled steroids, such as beclomethasone (Qvar) and budesonide (Pulmicort), and long-term bronchodilators, such as Serevent.

Longitudinal fracture. Vertical crack that goes the length of a bone.

Loop diuretics. Group of drugs used to block the reabsorption of water in the loop of Henle and the proximal and distal tubules.

Loop of Henle. U-shaped loop that develops a concentration gradient in the kidney's medulla, used in the reabsorption process of sodium and water.

Lordosis. Anteroposterior curvature of the lumbar of the spine.

Lotion. Topical cream that comes in both medicated and non-medicated forms.

Lower airways. Extend from the vocal cords down to the alveoli, where inspired air is transported to the alveolar region for gas exchange.

Lower esophageal sphincter (LES). A ring-like muscle that leads to the stomach.

Lozenge (troche). Flavored tablet held in the mouth, where it slowly dissolves.

Lumbar puncture. Procedure performed to obtain CSF fluid for analysis.

Lunula. White, half-moon shaped area at the base of the nail.

Lyme Disease. Transmitted by the bite of an infected deer or blacklegged tick that harbors the bacterium *Borrelia burgdorferi*; often forms a bull's eye rash.

Lymphomas. Malignant neoplasms of the lymphatic system.

M

Macular degeneration . A condition in which the macular region of the retina degrades, causing central vision impairment or loss.

Magnetic resonance elastography (MRE). An MRI with the ability to show the stiffness of body tissue.

Magnetic resonance imaging (MRI). Imaging uses magnets and radio waves to produce high resolution images of organs and soft tissue with no radiation exposure to patient.

Maintenance dose. Drug dose given to maintain a desired dose of drug in the blood.

Major depressive disorder (MDD). Clinical term for depression that affects quality of life.

Malabsorption syndrome. Condition preventing the absorption of nutrients in the small intestine.

Malignant growths. Neoplasms whose cells are uncontrolled and have no function and an irregular structure.

Malignant melanoma. Most deadly form of skin cancer often resulting from overexposure to the sun or harmful radiation.

Malignant. Cancerous cell growth.

Malleus. The outermost small hammer-shaped bone in the middle ear.

Malnutrition. Poor nutrition.

Mammary glands. Glands that produce milk in the female breast.

Mammogram. A radiologic image taken of the breast to check for cancer.

Masks. Facial covering to protect a clinicians face, nose, and mouth from body fluids and secretions.

Mastitis. Inflammation of the breast caused by a bacterial infection or breastfeeding.

Mastoiditis. Inflammation of the mastoid bone located behind the ear.

Maternal immunity. Strengthening of a baby's immune system by receiving antibodies from the mother's breast milk.

Maximum dose. The largest dose without causing a toxic effect.

Mechanical vector. Pathogen transmitted by an animal or insect simply by coming into contact with a microorganism and then physically transporting it to the host.

Medication error. A preventable mishandling of medication.

Medication history. Listing of all current prescriptions, over-the-counter (OTC) drugs, and herbal supplements and any adverse drug reactions.

Medication reconciliation. Comparing the patient's medications to the drugs currently ordered by the physician when a change of care occurs.

Medulla oblongata. Section of the brainstem continuous with the spinal cord that controls heartbeat, breathing, and blood pressure.

Melanin. Dark pigment produced by melanocytes that provides for skin color.

Melanocytes. Specialized cells located deep in the epidermal layers responsible for our skin color.

Meninges. Protective membranes of the brain and spinal cord.

Meningitis. Viral or bacterial inflammation of the protective coverings of the brain and spinal cord.

Meniscal tear. Tear in the semilunar pads in the knees that are a cushion between the femur and the tibia.

Menopause. The stage of a women's life when regular menses cease.

Menorrhagia. Abnormal bleeding during menses.

Menstrual cycle. A series of changes a woman's body undergoes in preparation for pregnancy.

Metabolized. When a drug is broken down or biotransformed, primarily done in the liver.

Metastasize. To spread from original site.

Metered Dose Inhaler (MDI). Pressurized inhalation device to deliver aerosolized medication to the airways.

Metered dose inhaler (MDI). Uses a propellant to propel the aerosolized drug from a canister into the airways; this form can be used to give both maintenance and rescue doses.

Methicillin-resistant staphylococcus aureus (MRSA). *Staphylococcus aureus* bacteria that has become pathogenic and resistant to antibiotic.

Metrorrhagia. Uterine bleeding between regular menses.

Microglia. Neural support cells that attack microbes and remove any debris.

Midbrain. Superior section of brain stem that acts as a two-way conduction pathway to relay visual and auditory impulses to the cerebrum.

Migraine headache. Most severe form of headache with incapacitating pain, visual disturbances, nausea, and vomiting.

Minimum dose. The smallest dose of a drug required to obtain the desired therapeutic effect.

Miotics. Agents used to constrict the pupil of the eye.

Mitosis. Cellular division used for tissue growth where daughter cells have same number of chromosomes as original mother cell.

Mitotic cells. A type of cell that always divides and continues to do so throughout our lifetime.

Mitotic inhibitors. Chemotherapeutic agents derived from natural substances used to inhibit cellular reproduction of cancer cells. The drug paclitaxel derived from the bark of the Pacific yew tree is an example.

Mitotic phase. Phase of actual cell division.

Mode of transmission. The way a pathogen is transported from the source of infection to the host.

Molars. Last teeth in the back of the mouth used to grind and crush food.

Monoclonal antibodies (MABs). Biological response modifier therapy that uses genetically engineered antibodies that are too large to enter the targeted cell but can attach to the outside surface of the cancer cell thus tagging it for destruction by immune system.

Morbidity rate. Statistical measurement of how often a disease occurs in a certain time-frame within a population.

Mortality rate. Statistical measurement of deaths caused by a disease of a certain population over a specific time period; also known as death rate.

Mortar and pestle. Used to crush pills into a powder.

Motor system. Portion of the nervous system that sends orders to skeletal, smooth, and cardiac muscles and to the body's glands.

Mucociliary escalator. The tissue layer mechanism that performs pulmonary hygiene.

Multifactorial disorders. Caused by the abnormality of many genes.

Multiple sclerosis. Neural disease that causes destruction of myelin sheath of neurons.

Muscle strain. A pulled muscle.

Muscular Dystrophy (MD). Disease caused by a defective gene resulting in the degeneration of the affected tissue.

Myasthenia gravis. Autoimmune disorder causing muscle weakness, beginning at the patient's face to the outermost extremities.

Mycosis. A disease caused by a fungus.

Myelin sheath. Soft, fatty, white covering for certain nerve fibers or axons.

Myelin. Lipid insulation produced by Schwann cells that line the neurons.

Myocardial infarction (heart attack). Also known as a heart attack; can be caused by a blockage of blood flow to the heart muscle.

Myocardium. Heart muscle.

Myofibrils. Tiny strands of muscle fiber that make up muscles.

Myometrium. Middle layer of the uterine wall.

Myopathy. General term for muscle disease (*myo* = muscle).

Myopia. A refractive condition known as near-sightedness, meaning objects that are close by are seen clearly, while objects at a distance are blurry.

Myosin. Thick myofilaments of protein.

Myxedema. Condition associated with hypothyroidism.

N

Nail root. Part of epidermis where specialized cells that form the nail are located.

Narcotics. CNS depressants such as morphine that are used primarily as prescribed painkillers (analgesics).

Nasal cavity. Beginning of the upper airway within the nose.

Nasogastric tube (NG). A tube that is passed through the nasal passage and into the stomach for a short-term feeding solution.

National Formulary (NF). Book of preparations and standards for pharmaceuticals.

Negative feedback loop. Physiological process used to bring the body back to its normal point.

Neoplasia. New growth formation.

Neoplasm. A new growth that results from overproduction of cells forming a lump or tumor.

Nephrogenic diabetes insipidus. Form of diabetes insipidus caused by kidney disease.

Nephrologist. Physician who specializes in the conditions and treatment of the kidneys.

Nephrons. Microscopic tubules that make up the actual functioning unit of the kidney.

Neuroglia. Cells that support and protect structures in the nervous system.

Neurons. Nerve cells that transmit signals in the nervous system.

Neutrophils. A specialized WBC that is part of the innate immune response.

Nicotinic acid (niacin). Class of drugs used to decrease the amount of triglycerides present in the blood.

Nitroglycerin. Drug that causes vasodilation; used to treat angina (chest pain).

NKA. Abbreviation for no known allergies.

Non-dividing cells. Cells that do not divide when damaged, resulting in loss of function.

Non-ionized. Non-charged state during which drugs can be absorbed through the membranes of the body and into the blood.

Non-labeled indication. When a drug or medication is used to treat a condition for which it is not approved; may be used if enough research proves it beneficial.

Non-specific inflammation. A quick response that locates the foreign invader, kills it, and cleans up the remaining debris to allow healing.

Normal flora. Native bacteria needed for normal body function.

Nothing by mouth (NPO). No food, beverage, or medication to be given orally.

Nystagmus. A condition of involuntary eye movements.

O

Oblique fracture. A transverse pattern of bone fracture.

Obsessive compulsive disorder (OCD). Anxiety disorder with both obsession or the repetition of a thought or emotion along with compulsion to do a repetitive act.

Obstetrician. One who specializes in childbirth.

Obstructive Sleep Apnea (OSA). Periods of cessation of breathing during sleep due to airway obstruction.

Occipital lobes. Sections of the brain responsible for vision.

Occult stool. Fecal test for blood in stool.

Occupational history. Listing of what the patient does or did for a living.

Official name. Name given by the USP/NF, after the drug has been approved for use.

Ointments. Thick semi-solid drug forms applied on skin or mucosal membranes.

Olfactory. Area in nasal cavity for your sense of smell.

Oligodendrocytes. Cells that hold nerve fibers together and also make up the fatty or lipid covering known as myelin.

Omnibus Budget Reconciliation Act (OBRA) of 1990. Legislation that mandates pharmacies to ask customers if they would like to be educated about their medication at time of purchase.

Oncologist. Specialist who treats cancer.

Open comedo. Blockage and stagnation of the sebaceous gland; a blackhead.

Open fracture. Classification of broken bones that protrude through the skin at the site of injury.

Open reduction. Fracture requiring surgical correction such as the insertion of pins, screws, plates, and rods.

Open-ended questioning. Asking the patient simple, broad questions that require more than a yes or no to answer.

Ophthalmologist. One who specializes in treating disease of the eye.

Opportunistic organisms. Invade regions of the body causing illness when given the opportunity.

Optometrist. One who practices optometry.

Oral cancer. Mouth cancer.

Oral cavity. Beginning of the GI tract where food and drink are mechanically broken down by chewing.

Oral route (PO). Taken by mouth.

Oral syringes. Needleless syringe used to deliver medication orally.

Orbital cavity. Two sockets located in the anterior portion of the skull that house the eyes.

Orchitis. Inflammation of the testicle.

Organ of Corti. A structure located in the cochlea that produces nerve impulses in response to sound.

Orthopnea. Difficulty breathing while lying down, and the patient needs to "straighten up" in order to breathe easier.

Osteoarthritis (OA). Degenerative joint disease.

Osteocytes. Mature bone cells found in the area surrounding the blood vessels in the bone.

Osteomalacia. Softening of the bones.

Osteomyelitis. Inflammation of bone tissue caused from a bacterial infection.

Osteons. Holes found in compact bone tissue.

Osteoporosis. Condition causing gradual decrease in bone density, causing the bones to become porous.

Otitis externa. Inflammation of the external ear canal.

Otitis media. Inflammation of the middle ear.

Otolaryngologist. One who treats conditions of the ears, nose, and throat.

Otosclerosis. A condition of abnormal hardening of the bones in the ear that reduces vibrations producing sound.

Otoscope. A device used to look into the ear.

Ova. Eggs released from the ovaries; singular: ovum.

Oval window. An opening covered by a membrane that leads from the middle ear to the inner ear.

Ovarian cancer. Cancer of the ovaries.

Ovarian cycle. Monthly release of eggs from the ovary.

Ovarian cyst. A fluid-filled sac in the ovary.

Ovary. Female reproductive organ.

Over-the-counter (OTC). Drugs or medications that do not require a prescription.

Oxygen therapy. Used in many of the diseases of the lower airway to provide adequate oxygen levels for gas exchange; therapy can include a nasal cannula or various types of oxygen masks.

P

Palate. The roof of your mouth.

Palliative therapy. Therapy aimed at alleviating symptoms such as pain or obstructions to improve the quality of life.

Palpation. Process of touching a patient in an effort to evaluate abnormalities.

Pancreas. Located behind the liver, this gland secretes digestive enzymes into the duodenum. Produces and secretes insulin.

Pancreatitis. Inflammation of the pancreas.

Pandemic. Disease affecting the population of a vast geographic area such as a country or possibly worldwide.

Pap tests. Named after the founder Dr. George Papanikolaou; stain the cells from the body sample (usually cervical smear) and look for abnormal cells.

Paper medicine cups. Disposable containers used to hold pills, tablets, and capsules.

Paradoxical reaction. Drug reaction that does the opposite of what was intended.

Paranasal sinuses. Air-filled chambers located *around* the nasal cavity.

Paraplegia. Paralysis of the lower body.

Parasympathetic branch. Division of the autonomic nervous system dedicated to maintenance activities of normal body functions.

Parathyroid glands. Four pea-sized regions in the posterior side of the thyroid.

Parenteral route. Any route that does not go through the GI tract, but term is commonly used for an injectable route.

Parenteral route. Substance given by an injection.

Parietal lobes. Sections of the brain involved with body senses and speech.

Parietal pericardium. The outer layer of the pericardium.

Parkinson's disease. Slow progressive degeneration of the brain because of deficiency of the brain neurochemical transmitter dopamine.

Parotid salivary glands. Glands that assist with chewing and swallowing of food by lubricating with saliva.

Passive acquired immunity. The body acquires antibodies for a specific disease from a vaccine.

Past medical history (PMH). Listing of previous medical illnesses and procedures.

Pathogen. Any organism causing disease to its host.

Pathogenesis. Creation or progression of disease development.

Pathogenic. Used to describe organisms that produce disease.

Pathologist. Individual who studies disease.

Patient care plan. Set of steps used to explain patient's care regarding possible treatments and expected outcomes.

Patient education. Instructing patients in various aspects of their care such as how to properly perform treatments.

Patient interview. Process where clinician gathers patient information.

Peak flow meter. Asthma monitoring device to measure exhaled flow rates.

Pediculicides. Agents used to treat lice infestation.

Pelvic inflammatory disease (PID). Inflammation of a woman's pelvic organs.

Penis. Male genital organ that transports both sperm and urine.

Peptic ulcers. Crater-like lesions that may occur in the esophagus, stomach, or duodenum.

Percussion. Tapping with fingers in areas on the body such as the chest, to check body cavities for excess fluid or air.

Percutaneous endoscopic gastrostomy (PEG) tube. The actual tube used to administer fluids, medications, and nutrition.

Percutaneous endoscopic gastrostomy procedure. The procedure for inserting a feeding tube through the abdomen and into the stomach.

Pericardial sac. Double-walled sac that surrounds the great vessels and heart.

Perimetrium. Outer layer of the uterus.

Periodontal disease. Destructive gum disease.

Peripheral artery disease (PAD). Narrowing of the arteries in the body other than the heart and brain.

Peripheral nervous system (PNS). The portion of the nervous system composed of all the nerves outside of the brain and spinal cord.

Peripheral perfusion. Amount of blood reaching the furthest extremities.

Peripheral resistance. The resistance to blood flow from the arteries.

Peripheral Vascular Disease (PVD). Disease of the blood vessels outside of the heart often resulting in partial or complete blockages of blood flow.

Peristalsis. Unconscious, wave-like motion or contraction of the smooth muscle in the intestinal walls necessary to move contents through the GI tract.

Peritoneal dialysis. Method used to remove wastes from the blood by using the patient's peritoneal membrane as a filter.

Personal Protective Equipment (PPE). Clothing and equipment used to prevent bodily fluid contact.

Pertussis. Preventable vaccinated pediatric disease that is also known as *whooping cough* based on the sound the patient produces when he or she coughs.

Pessary. A device inserted into the vagina to support its walls and prevent prolapse.

pH. In regards to drugs, it is the range from acidity to alkalinity in the GI tract.

Phagocytosis. The process of neutrophils escaping blood vessels and entering tissue to surround and attack the foreign invader to destroy it.

Pharmacist. Individual licensed to prepare and distribute medications.

Pharmacodynamics. Actions from a drug in the body.

Pharmacogenetics. Pertains to genetic differences that can cause a drug to affect us in different ways, whether therapeutically or adversely.

Pharmacogenomics. Analyzes human genes to better understand how an individual's genetics affects the way drugs affect his or her body.

Pharmacognosy. Studies the natural sources of pharmaceuticals.

Pharmacokinetics. The movement of a drug through the body from absorption to elimination.

Pharmacology. The study of the origin, uses, effects, and actions of chemicals in living organisms.

Pharmacotherapy. The act of giving drugs targeted to treat disease.

Pharmacy technicians. Individuals who assist and work under the direct supervision of pharmacists.

Pharmacy. Dispenses medications to the public.

Pharyngitis. Inflammation of the pharynx.

Pharyngoesophageal sphincter. Muscular ring located at the beginning of the esophagus.

Pharynx. Passageway more commonly referred to as the throat allowing for food and air to pass.

Phlebitis. Inflammation of a vein.

Phobia disorder. Most common anxiety disorder that exhibits an intense and irrational fear of an object, event, situation, or thing.

Phonation. The process of speech.

Photophobia. Light sensitivity.

Phrenic nerve. A nerve that innervates the diaphragm causing it to contract and flatten out creating more room in the thoracic space (chest cavity) and less pressure, allowing air to rush into the lungs for inspiration.

Physical examination. Process of physically examining a patient in a systematic manner.

Physicians' Desk Reference (PDR). Collection of specific drug information required by the FDA from drug manufacturers that includes photos of medications.

Pill crushers. Used to crush tablets into powder.

Pill splitter. Used to split a pill in half.

Pineal gland. A small gland located in the brain responsible for maintaining our circadian rhythm.

Pinworms. The most common parasitic intestinal worm infection in the United States.

Placebo effect. Fake pill or sugar pill that the patient believes is medicine to treat his or her condition.

Plantar fasciitis. Condition of pain and inflammation occurring from small tears in the plantar fascia ligament from activities causing repeated pressure on the bottom of the foot such as running or walking long distances.

Plasmapheresis. Procedure used to remove antibodies from the patient's bloodstream.

Plastic medicine cups. Disposable containers used to give liquid medications orally.

Platelets (PLT). Cellular fragments that clots blood.

Pleural cavity. Cavity where lungs are housed; contains a double-layered serous membrane, which creates the visceral pleura, which surrounds each lung; and the parietal pleura, which covers the inner wall of the thoracic cage.

Pleural effusion. Fluid entering the pleural space.

Pleural fluid. Fluid within the pleural space needed to make the movement of the pleural layers friction free as you breathe in and out.

Pleuritis. Also called *pleurisy*, is an inflammation of the pleura, which is characterized by a sharp pain when breathing.

Pneumoconiosis. General term for *conditions* caused by the inhalation of inorganic dust particles that can produce toxic effects.

Pneumonectomy. Surgical removal of entire lung.

Pneumonia. Inflammation of both the airways and alveoli due to infection by bacteria, viruses, fungi, and even chemicals that create an inflammatory response.

Pneumothorax. Condition that allows air into the pleural space and can collapse the lung or lungs.

Poliomyelitis. Major crippling viral disease affecting children prior to development of a polio vaccine in the 1960s.

Polycystic kidney disease (PKD). Inherited disease that slowly destroys the kidneys.

Polycythemia. Increased number of red blood cells in the blood.

Pons. Section of brainstem that plays a role in regulating breathing.

Portal of entry. Pathogen point of entry to host such as by way of mouth, eyes, and nose or other mucous membrane.

Portal of exit. A point where pathogen leaves the body.

Positive feedback loop. Physiological process that takes the body farther way from its normal point and will continue to do so until the cycle is broken.

Post-lumbar puncture headache. Headache that results after lumbar puncture procedure because of leakage of CSF from the puncture site.

Post-polio syndrome (PPS). Syndrome developed by polio survivors 10–40 years after the initial disease.

Post-traumatic stress disorder (PTSD). Mental health condition that develops after an intense psychological event that is outside the range of normal human experience, such as combat, rape, child abuse or incest, acts of violence/terrorism, or natural disasters.

Posterior pituitary. Rear portion of the pituitary gland.

Potassium-sparing diuretics. Group of drugs that work in the distal tubule to eliminate water and salt while saving potassium.

Potentiation. When two or more drugs have an increased response or a prolonged effect when given together.

Powder drug form. Drug in powdered form that must be mixed with fluid for oral or injection. In addition, fine powdered drugs can be administered via the inhalation route.

PPD test. Skin test to diagnose tuberculosis.

Prediabetes. Condition of slightly higher than normal blood sugar that is not high enough to be considered diabetes.

Prefilled syringes. Used to deliver a premeasured amount of a substance.

Pregnancy category A. Category of drug that has been studied and shown to have no adverse fetal effects.

Pregnancy category B. Category of drug tested on animals with no adverse effects but not tested on pregnant women.

Pregnancy category C. Category of drug with no convincing studies done on animals or pregnant women to determine adverse effects.

Pregnancy category D. Category of drugs showing adverse effects to fetus and given only when benefits to mother outweigh fetal risk.

Pregnancy category X. Category of drugs showing adverse fetal effects and not to be used under any circumstances.

Premenstrual syndrome. A group of symptoms that occurs just days before menstruation.

Premolars. Flat teeth located behind the canine teeth used to crush food.

Presbycusis. Hearing loss because of old age.

Presbyopia. Hyperopia caused by old age.

Prescription. Written orders for a certain therapy or medication; also called scripts.

Primary infection. Infection resulting from first exposure to pathogen.

Primary mover muscle. Main muscle causing movement.

Primary union (first intention). Small wounds with no debris or bacteria present, allowing a quick healing time.

Proctoscope. Slightly larger instrument than the anoscope used to examine the anus and rectum.

Prodrugs. Drugs that only become active as they are broken down into metabolites.

Prognosis. Expected outcome or the prediction of an ailment.

Prokaryotic cells. Cells that lack a nucleus such as bacteria.

Prophylactic treatment. Treatment to prevent the exacerbation or occurrence of a disease.

Prostaglandin analogs (ophthalmic) . A group of agents used to lower intraocular pressure by increasing the outflow of aqueous humor from the anterior chamber.

Prostate cancer. Cancer of the prostate gland, which secretes seminal fluids.

Prostate gland. Located below the bladder and in front of the rectum and provides fluid for the nourishment and transportation of semen.

Prostate-specific antigen (PSA). Special proteins released into the bloodstream from prostate cells; elevated in the presence of prostate cancer.

Prostatitis. Inflammation of the prostate gland.

Proton pump inhibitors. Medication used to reduce the amount of acid produced.

Prototype. A drug that typifies a certain drug classification.

Protozoa. One-cell members of the animal kingdom found in soil and water.

Psoriasis. Non-contagious, chronic, idiopathic skin disease that presents as a series of red raised lesions with silvery scaling generally on the elbows, knees, and scalp.

Pulmonary abscess. General term for a collection of infectious material in encapsulated regions of the lungs.

Pulmonary artery. Artery that carries deoxygenated blood from the heart to the lungs.

Pulmonary circulation. Part of the circulatory system that carries deoxygenated blood from the heart to the lungs.

Pulmonary function tests (PFTs). Volume and flow tests to measure airway function.

Pulmonary valve. Valve located between the right ventricle and pulmonary artery.

Pulmonary veins. Veins that carry oxygenated blood from the lungs to the left atrium.

Pulp. Connective tissue inside the tooth beneath the dentin layer supplying it with nerves and blood.

Pulse oximeter. Non-invasive device used to measure oxygen saturation in the blood.

Pupil. The opening in the center of the iris.

Purkinje fibers. Collection of special fibers that sends electrical impulses to the ventricles.

Purulent exudate. Pus containing cellular and tissue debris.

Pus. Viscous fluid containing primarily white blood cellular debris resulting from the inflammatory process.

Pustule. Small bump in skin filled with pus; a pimple.

Pyelitis. Inflammation of the lining of the renal pelvis.

Pyelonephritis. Inflammation of the structures inside the kidney.

Pyloric sphincter. Muscular ring that prevents stomach contents from prematurely moving into the duodenum.

Pylorus. Funnel-shaped, terminal end of the stomach.

Pyothorax. Formation of pus in the pleural space, usually due to a bacterial infection.

Q

Quadriplegia. Paralysis of all four limbs and resulting in loss of bladder and bowel control.

R

Rabies. Often fatal viral encephalomyelitis caused by an infected animal bite.

Rales. Older term for crackles (see crackles).

Reconstituted. Act of mixing fluid with a powdered drug form to create a solution.

Rectally (PR) or (R). Administering a drug by inserting into the rectum.

Rectocele. Weakening of the posterior wall of the vagina allowing the rectum to bulge into the vagina.

Rectum. A short, tube-like structure located between the sigmoid colon and outside of the body.

Red blood cells (RBCs). Cells within blood that transport oxygen.

Refractive errors. Symptoms of a group of conditions that prevent light rays from properly reaching the retina at a correct focal point.

Relapse. Reappearance of the disease or condition.

Relative contraindication. A drug or procedure that is only done if the benefits outweigh the risks.

Remission. Period where disease is treated successfully and the patient is free of symptoms.

Renal biopsy. Performed to remove tissue for study.

Renal calculi. Formation of hardened crystals in the kidney.

Renal capsule. Outer covering of the kidney made of fibrous connective tissue.

Renal cell carcinoma. Most common type of kidney cancer.

Renal columns. Columns of cortical tissue extensions that separate renal pyramids.

Renal cortex. Outer portion of the kidney.

Renal failure. Inability of the renal system to function and cleanse the blood of toxins.

Renal hilum. Indented area of the kidney where the renal artery, vein, and ureter connect, giving the kidney a bean-shaped appearance.

Renal medulla. Middle portion of the kidney.

Renal pelvis. Innermost region of the kidney that is shaped like a funnel and collects urine.

Renal pyramids. Triangle-shaped structures in the medulla that are made up of tubules that collect urine.

Rescue or quick-relief inhaled bronchodilators. Aerosolized medications used in acute bronchospasm, such as albuterol (Proventil, Ventolin), levalbuterol (Xopenex), and ipratropium bromide (Atrovent) to give relief of bronchospasm within minutes.

Respirator. Specialized mask used for droplet airway infections.

Restrictive cardiomyopathy. Disease in which the ventricle walls are too stiff, not allowing the heart walls to expand as it should.

Reticular system. Diffuse network of nuclei in the brain stem responsible for bringing the cerebral cortex to conscious awareness of the surroundings.

Retina. The light-sensitive portion of the eye that sends signals to the brain via the optic nerve.

Rh factor. Type of antigen found on the surface of red blood cells in some humans.

Rheumatic heart disease. Heart disease caused by rheumatic fever that damages the heart valves.

Rheumatoid Arthritis (RA). Common autoimmune condition that is known to attack the lining of joints.

Rhinorrhea. Runny nose.

Rhonchi. Low-pitched abnormal breath sounds, usually indicating airway secretions.

Rickettsiae. Non-motile bacteria.

Rods. Provide side vision and the ability to see at night or in a dimly lit room.

Root (of penis). The part of the penis that attaches to the body.

Rosacea. Chronic, non-contagious, idiopathic skin condition that presents as redness and inflammation of the face, especially around the nose and cheeks.

S

Sarcoma. Cancerous tumor found in the connective tissue of bone, fat, or muscle.

Sarcomeres. Protein threads of small contractile units of striated muscle.

Satellite fracture. Cracks in bone that appear to be in a star-like pattern.

Scabicides. Agents used to treat mite infestations (scabies).

Schedule I. Listing of drugs not currently used in medical treatment that have a high potential for abuse.

Schedule II. Listing of drugs that have usage in medical treatment but with severe restrictions because of a high potential for abuse.

Schedule III. Listing of drugs currently used in medical treatment that have less of a potential for abuse than drugs in schedules I and II.

Schedule IV. Listing of drugs currently used in the medical treatment but have a slight potential for abuse; less than schedules II and III.

Schedule V. Currently used for medical treatment with less potential for abuse than drugs in schedule IV; have a slight possibility for abuse and might cause limited physical or psychological dependence.

Schizophrenia. Type of psychosis with drastic personality changes and loss of reality.

Sclera. Outer layer of the eye made of connective and fibrous tissues; the white of the eye.

Sclerosing. Irritates tissue causing an inflammatory response to initiate fibrosis or scarring.

Sclerotherapy. Procedure usually involving the direct injection of a salt solution into a vessel causing inflammation and the vessel to stick together.

Scoliosis. Condition where spine appears to be in an S-shape from the lateral or sideways curvature of the spine.

Seasonal affective disorder (SAD). Type of depression associated with winter months because of lack of natural sunlight.

Sebaceous glands. Glands located around the eyes that secrete an oily substance to lubricate the eyes; known as meibomian glands.

Seborrheic keratosis. Non-cancerous overgrowth of skin cells that appears as a wart-like growth; tan or black.

Sebum. Oily secretion of the sebaceous glands that keeps the skin lubricated; also acts as an anti-infective agent because of its acidic nature.

Secondary infection. An infection developing as a result of another illness or injury.

Secondary union (secondary intention). A large wound loaded with debris and/or bacteria making it difficult to heal.

Sedatives. Medications that have a calming affect, such as the benzodiazepines (BDZs) and valium.

Selective distribution. Occurs when drugs have a greater affinity to reach a certain area than others, such as a cell or organ in the body.

Selective serotonin reuptake inhibitors (SSRIs). Drugs that increase the utilization of serotonin; used to treat depression.

Semicircular canals. Passageways in the bony labyrinth that help to control equilibrium.

Seminal vesicles. Hold fluid that mixes with semen.

Semisynthetic. Drug having a natural origin with a chemically altered variation.

Sensorineural deafness. Permanent loss of hearing caused by damaged nerves or cochlea in the inner ear.

Sensory system. Input portion of nervous system that receives information about the immediate environment.

Serotonin and norepinephrine reuptake inhibitors (SNRIs). Medications to increase serotonin production to treat depression.

Serous exudate. Thin watery fluid that exudes or escapes from blood vessels into the surrounding tissue.

Serous fluid. Clear fluid in the ear caused by pressure or allergy.

Serrated polyps. Flattened saw-toothed appearing growths.

Shaft. Body of the penis.

Shingles. Herpes zoster viral disease causing itchy, painful rash with blisters along the pathway of the affected nerve.

Shingles. Viral disease caused by herpes zoster that causes painful skin lesions that follow the course of a spinal nerve.

Short bones. Bones that are cube-like in appearance since they are similar in width and length.

Side effects. Undesirable experiences of medication that can occur quickly or over time; also known as adverse reactions.

Sigmoid colon. The portion of the large intestine that is in an "S" shape leading to the rectum.

Sigmoidoscopy. Procedure utilizing a scope to examine the sigmoid colon.

Signal transduction inhibitors (STIs). Targeted cancer therapy agents that block specific enzymes and growth factors in cancer cells. Imatinib (Gleevec) is an oral STI that is approved for chronic myelogenous leukemia and some rarer types of cancers.

Signs. Objective measurements of body functions.

Silicosis. Lung disease resulting from the inhalation of silicates, such as those found in sand, glass, ceramics, and rocks.

Simple fracture. Classification of bone fracture that does not break the skin surface.

Single gene. Likely to be a recessive or an inherited disorder.

Sinusitis. Inflammation of the mucous membranes lining the sinus cavities.

Skeletal muscle. Voluntary muscle fiber looks like striated, long cylinder-like strands and is found attached to bones.

Sleep apnea. Periods of cessation of breathing during sleep.

Small intestine. Nearly 20-foot-long, hollow organ consisting of three parts, the duodenum, jejunum and ileum that is located between the stomach and large intestine.

Small Volume Nebulizer (SVN). Special inhaled aerosol delivery device that is powered by compressed gas to deliver aerosolized medications to the airway over a several minute treatment.

Smooth muscle (visceral muscle). Involuntary muscle found within the lining of hollow organs such as the intestines and blood vessels and airways.

Social history. Information obtained on the type of lifestyle the patient lives such as marital status, social or frequent drinking history, smoking history, or illicit drug use.

Solution form. Solution that does not need shaken and the drug is uniformly distributed within the mixture.

Solution. Usually clear in appearance, the drug is in liquid form that is completely dissolved within the fluid.

Somatic nervous system. Voluntary portion of peripheral nervous system that controls movements of skeletal muscle.

Somatic system. Controls voluntary muscles.

Spacer. Reservoir that can be added to an MDI to assist in treatment administration.

Specific immune response. An immune action that kills the foreign organisms in a selective process by marking the foreign invader.

Spermatic cord. A cord-like structure made of nerves, vessels, and ducts that go to and from the testicles.

Sphygmomanometer. Blood pressure cuff.

Spinal cord. Structure in the CNS that represents the neural highway upon which nerve signals are transmitted to and from the brain and all parts of the body.

Spinal nerves. Thirty-one pairs of nerves named for their corresponding vertebrae that travel to various parts of the body.

Spinal stenosis. Narrowing of the spinal nerve root pathways.

Spiral fracture. Crack that twists around a bone.

Spongy bone. Porous, sponge-like appearing bone.

Sprain. Complete or partial damage done to the ligaments such as tearing or stretching.

Squamous cell carcinoma. Cancer developing from an abnormal growth of squamous cells.

Squamous cell skin cancer. Form of skin cancer with high cure rate that usually appears as a firm, red nodular lesion with a crusty-looking appearance; usually found on face, arms, or neck.

Stable angina. Stable and predictable chest pain caused by exertion and relieved with medication or rest.

Standard precautions. Set of steps and procedures that protects not only the clinician, but the patient from exposure to infectious microorganisms.

Stapes. A bone in the middle ear between the incus and oval window; also called the stirrup bone.

Statins. Class of drugs used to lower cholesterol.

Steady state. Method of drug administration where the same amount of drug is eliminated as administered therefore giving a predicable effect.

Sterile technique. Catheterizing an individual for a sample of urine.

Stomach. Pear-shaped organ located between the esophagus and small intestine.

Strabismus. A condition of abnormal eye alignments; also known as a lazy eye.

Stratum basale. Deepest layer of the epidermis where new cells are formed.

Stratum corneum. Outermost layer of the epidermis made up of flat, hardened dead epithelial cells.

Strep throat. Sore, swollen, red throat caused by the bacteria *streptococcus*.

Stroke volume. Amount of blood pumped from the left ventricle per heartbeat.

Sty. Inflammation of the top or bottom eyelid from a blocked gland resembling a pimple or boil. Also called stye.

Subcapital fracture. Describes a break in the femur at the proximal end.

Subcutaneous (subcu). Injection of a drug into the fatty tissue layer located just below the skin.

Subcutaneous layer. Also known as hypodermal layer; innermost layer of skin composed of elastic and fibrous connective tissue and fatty tissue.

Sublingual salivary glands. Salivary glands located between the tongue and mandible on each side of the mouth, which also happen to be the smallest of the three salivary glands.

Sublingual tablet. Placed under the tongue to slowly disintegrate and absorb into the mucosa under the tongue.

Subluxation. A partially separated bone from a joint injury.

Submandibular salivary glands. Salivary glands located under the jaw.

Subtotal gastrectomy. Removal of part of the stomach, usually the lower portion.

Sudoriferous glands. Sweat glands located in the skin for cooling and release of toxins.

Sun protection factor (SPF). Value of protectiveness of sunscreen.

Superior vena cava. Large vein that brings deoxygenated blood to the heart from the upper body.

Suppository (supp). Drug is suspended in a solid substance and inserted into the rectum.

Suppurative fluid. Pus accumulation in the ear from an infection.

Suprapubic catheter. Type of catheter that is placed through the pelvic wall to avoid the urethra.

Surfactant. Fluid produced within lungs that helps hold the alveoli open between breaths.

Survival rate. Length of time a patient's lives after being diagnosed with a disease.

Suspension (susp). A liquid drug form that must be shaken before using to mix the drug in the fluid.

Suspension form. Occurs when a drug is suspended in a solution mixture and must be shaken up to mix the particles sitting on the bottom of the bottle.

Sustained-release capsule or tablet. Medication with a coating to deliver a dose over an extended period time.

Sympathetic branch. Division of autonomic nervous system known as the fight-or-flight response system; prepares the body for high stress and emergency situations.

Symptoms. Observable subjective states or behaviors that rely on the patient to state how they feel.

Synapse. Gap at the end of an axon, also known as the synaptic gap, where the nerve signal can continue on via a chemical neurotransmitter.

Syndrome. A particular set of signs and symptoms that when grouped together is indicative or characteristic of a certain disease or disorder.

Synergism. Effect when two drugs work together to reach an increased effect much greater than if either drug was given alone.

Synergistic muscles. Move to help assist the primary muscle's movement.

Synthetic. Chemically manufactured drug.

Syphilis. A curable, but potentially serious sexually transmitted disease; if untreated, painful sores develop.

Syringes. Devices used to inject substances into or withdraw substances from the body.

Syrup. Sweetened, colorful liquid drug often masked with palatable flavors.

Systemic circulatory system. The part of the circulatory system that carries oxygenated blood from the heart to the tissues of the body and returns deoxygenated blood to the heart.

Systemic effect. Effect of a drug on the entire body.

Systemic Lupus Erythematosus (SLE). Chronic autoimmune disease where the body mistakes tissue such as joints, kidneys, skin, and other organs as a foreign invader.

Systole. The part of the heartbeat when contraction occurs.

T

Tablet (tab). Form of compressed drug that comes in a variety of colors and shapes.

Tachycardia. Faster than normal heart rate.

Tachypnea. Rapid breathing.

Tapeworms. Intestinal parasites found in both humans and animals.

Targeted therapy. Precision medicine that targets the desired abnormal cell (usually cancerous) for treatment and does not affect normal cells.

Telephone order (TO). Used to receive physician orders via telephone when the physician is not present.

Telephone order repeated back (TO/RB). Verbally repeating the physician's order over the phone; used to increase accuracy and reduce error.

Temporal lobes. Sections of brain involved in hearing, taste, and integration of emotions.

Temporomandibular Joint Dysfunction (TMJ or TMD). Inflamed disk-like joints in the jaw.

Tendonitis. Inflammation of the tendon.

Tension headache. Type of headache caused by high levels of stress and tension.

Teratogenic effect. Drugs that can cause physical malformations in a fetus.

Terminal. Condition or disease resulting in imminent death.

Testicles. Male gonads.

Testicular cancer. Cancer of the testicle; usually affects only one testis.

Testosterone. Male sex hormone.

Tetanus. Life-threatening bacterial condition, also known as lockjaw, that can cause respiratory failure by paralyzing muscles needed to breathe.

The chain of infection. Chain-like illustration made up of a series of steps or links that demonstrates how pathogens infect others.

Therapeutic dose. Is the dose needed to obtain the desired effect.

Therapeutic level. Preferred level of a drug required to treat disease.

Therapeutic range. Amount of a drug present in the blood that gives the desired effect without causing any toxicity or side effects.

Thiazide diuretics. Group of drugs that work in the distal tubule to prevent the reabsorption of water and salt.

Thoracentesis. Procedure using a large needle and syringe to remove fluid from the pleural space.

Thrombolytic agents. Clot-busting agents dissolve an existing clot.

Thrombophlebitis. Inflammation of a vein caused by a thrombus (clot).

Thymus gland. A gland found in the chest behind the breastbone that plays a role in our immune system.

Thyroid gland. Important structure located in the middle section of the neck that secretes thyroid hormones.

Thyroid storm. Life-threatening complication of hyperthyroidism.

Tinea barbae. Fungal infection affecting bearded area of neck and face; barber's itch.

Tinea capitis. Fungal infection of the skull or cap of head.

Tinea corporis. Fungal infection found on smooth skin of arms, legs, and body; called ringworm because of its appearance, but no worm is involved.

Tinea cruris. Fungal infection of the scrotal and groin area; jock itch.

Tinea pedis. Fungal infection of the feet; athlete's foot.

Tinea unguium. Fungal infection of the fingernails or toenails causing white patches on the nail; difficult to treat, can destroy the entire nail.

Tissue biopsy. Removal of small portion of a suspicious tissue for microscopic examination by a pathologist.

Tissue degeneration. Tissues cannot replace the cells as efficiently with old age.

Tissue infarction. Tissue death due to lack of oxygen.

Tissue necrosis. The death of healthy tissue.

Tolerance. Need for increasing levels of drugs to get the same effect.

Tolerance. Process that occurs when a dose of a drug is taken repeatedly and has less effect on the person, so a larger dose is required to reach the desired effect.

Tonsils. Masses of lymphoid tissue that fight infection.

Topical route. Drug administration applied to local area.

Torn rotator cuff. Stress injury in which a tear occurs in a tendon within a collection of muscles that hold the head of the humerus into the shoulder socket.

Total gastrectomy. Removal of the stomach in its entirety.

Total parenteral nutrition (TPN). All nutrition is received through a vein.

Toxic dose. Side effects that can result in poisoning the patient.

Toxic shock syndrome (TSS). A life-threatening, acute bacterial infection caused by an intrauterine device or tampon.

Toxicology. The study of a chemicals and pharmacologic actions on the body with poisons and antidotes.

Trabeculae. Irregular holes or pores come from the bars and plates that make up the bones' spongy structure.

Trachea. Also called the windpipe, it is the main airway of the tracheal bronchial tree.

Trade name. Proprietary name owned by a pharmaceutical company to market its creation to the public; also known as a brand name.

Transdermal route. Use of a skin patch to deliver various medications.

Transient ischemic attacks (TIAs). Mild mini-strokes.

Transitional cell carcinoma of the bladder. Cancer that develops in the lining of the bladder.

Transudate. Occurs when too much pressure is present, causing fluid to cross the semipermeable membrane of a blood vessel.

Transverse colon. The section of the large intestine that goes across the abdomen below the stomach and liver.

Transverse fracture. Horizontal lines spanning across a bone at a 90-degree angle.

Trauma. Physical injury or a disturbing experience.

Trichomoniasis. A curable sexually transmitted disease caused by a parasite.

Tricuspid valve. Heart valve located between the right atrium and right ventricle.

Tuberculin (TB) syringes. Used to deliver a small quantity of a substance intradermally.

Tuberculosis (TB). Contagious bacterial infection that affects the lungs, but can also impair other organs and affect the bones; the causative agent is *Mycobacterium tuberculosis*.

Turbinates. Shelf-like structures called *conchae* within the nasal cavity that heat and humidify inspired air.

Tympanic membrane. Eardrum.

Type 1 diabetes. Also called juvenile diabetes, caused by the pancreas's inability to produce insulin.

Type 2 diabetes. A chronic, lifelong condition of high blood sugar.

Type A blood. Blood that contains only A antigens on the red blood cell and B antibodies in the plasma.

Type AB blood. Blood that contains both A and B antigens on the red blood cells and no antibodies for A or B in the plasma.

Type B blood. Blood that contains only B antigens on the red blood cells and A antibodies in the plasma.

Type O blood. Blood that does not have any A or B antigens on the red blood cells, but both A and B antibodies in the plasma.

U

Ulcerative colitis. Inflammatory bowel disease causing ulcer-like lesions in the large intestine.

Ulcers. Cavitous or crater-like sores occurring either internally or externally, causing tissue to slough off.

Ultraviolet (UV) radiation. High-energy radiation from the sun or from tanning beds that can be carcinogenic with excessive exposure.

United States Adopted Names (USAN) Council. Group that gives names to generic medications.

United States Pharmacopeia (USP). Collection of drug standards and testing that determines the strength, purity, and quality of a drug.

United States Pharmacopeia and the National Formulary (USP–NF). A reference compiled by combining the USP and NF to form one source.

Unstable angina. Chest pain that has a longer duration than a stable angina and is not caused by exertion. It is not likely to be relieved by medicine.

Upper airway. Anatomically extends from the nose to the vocal cords, where inspired air is conditioned through heating or cooling and humidification.

Upper Respiratory Infections (URIs). General term for infections of the upper airway such as the common cold.

Uremia. Urine in the blood.

Ureters. Two hollow tubes, one from each kidney that drains urine from the kidney to the bladder.

Urethra. Hollow tube used to drain urine from the bladder to the outside of the body.

Urethritis. Inflammation of the urethra.

Urinalysis. Analysis of urine.

Urinary incontinence. Inability to control the bladder.

Urinary tract infection (UTI). Term used to describe an infection in any region of the urinary system.

Urine analysis (UA). Testing a urine sample for abnormalities.

Urine color. Observing urine color to help identify a disease or dehydration.

Urine concentration. Measurement to determine if kidney failure is present.

Urine culture and sensitivity test (C&S). Study performed on urine to identify the pathogen responsible for the infection and so determine what drug can be used to treat it.

Urine odor. Determining the smell of the urine to help determine presence of illness.

Urodynamic testing. Testing used to study the anatomic structure and function of the bladder and urethra.

Urologist. Physician who specializes in the conditions and treatment of the urinary system.

Urticarial. Raised reddened area of skin because of allergic reaction.

Uterine cancer. Cancer of the uterus.

Uterine cycle. Monthly sloughing of the uterus lining.

Uterine prolapse. A condition in which the uterus falls into the vagina.

Uterus. Muscular, hollow organ that carries a fetus; also known as the womb.

V

Vagina. Hollow canal that receives the penis during intercourse and acts as the birth canal during childbirth.

Vaginal creams. Medicated creams inserted into the vagina.

Vaginal suppositories. Drugs suspended in a substance that melts at body temperature after being inserted into the vagina.

Vaginitis. Inflammation of the vagina.

Vagus nerve. Tenth cranial nerve, responsible for motor and sensory input in the digestive tract organs.

Valvular heart disease. Any condition or disease that affects the heart valves.

Variant angina (Prinzmetal's angina). A severe pain brought on by the temporary spasm of a coronary artery; treated with medicine.

Varicose veins. Veins that are characterized by being twisted, bulging, and distorted.

Vas deferens. A duct that transports semen to the urethra.

Venography. Procedure that uses special dye and an X-ray to examine veins.

Vermiform. A slender, hollow, blind-ended tube connected to the cecum.

Verrucae. Medical term for warts caused by a virus (papilloma virus).

Vestibule chamber. An oval-shaped cavity in bony labyrinth.

Vestibulocochlear nerve. The nerve in the ear is responsible for transmitting information from the inner ear to the brain; responsible for balance and hearing.

Vial. Glass container with a lid and rubber stopper to hold one dose or many doses depending on bottle size.

Viruses. Microorganisms smaller than bacteria and that require a host cell to reproduce.

Visceral pericardium. The inner layer of the pericardium.

Vital signs. Measured signs that are vital for life; heart rate, respiration rate, blood pressure, and body temperature.

Vitreous humor. A clear jelly-like substance that fills the area between the lens and the retina.

Vocal cords. V-like structures found in the larynx that vibrate to give sound (phonation).

Volume of distribution (VD). Areas where a drug can be distributed in the body.

Voluntary. Muscle that requires conscious effort to move.

Volvulus. Condition where the intestine becomes twisted.

W

Wheal. Raised, reddened, swollen, and itchy area of the skin; hives

Wheals. Also known as hives or urticaria, are itchy, raised, red-colored circles resembling welts.

Wheezes. High-pitched abnormal breath sounds, indicating airway narrowing due to bronchospasm.

White blood cells (WBCs). Cells within bloodstream that fight infection.

Withdrawal. Unpleasant side effects and symptoms associated with abruptly stopping a substance to which one is addicted.

Wound debridement. Process of removing of foreign material, dead and damaged tissue from a wound to stimulate healing.

X

X-ray. Imaging technique utilized to determine any bone breaks and defects in the body.

Z

Z lines. Myofilaments striations (dark bands) repeated throughout the muscle.

Index

Note: Italicised page numbers indicate illustrations.

A

D

E

F

G

H

I

J

K

L

M

N

O

P

Q

R

S

T

U